Handbook of Adolescent
Behavioral Problems

Handbook of Adolescent Behavioral Problems

Evidence-Based Approaches to Prevention and Treatment

Edited by

Thomas P. Gullotta

Child and Family Agency of Southeastern Connecticut,
New London, CT

and

Eastern Connecticut State University, Windham, CT

Gerald R. Adams

University of Guelph
Ontario, Canada

Research Assistant

Jessica M. Ramos
Child and Family Agency of Southeastern Connecticut,
New London, CT

A Sponsored Publication of the Child and Family Agency of Southeastern Connecticut

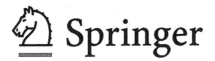 Springer

Thomas P. Gullotta
Child and Family Agency of Southeastern Connecticut
New London, CT 06320

Gerald R. Adams
Department of Family Relations and Applied Nutrition
University of Guleph
Ontario, Canada N1G 2W1

Library of Congress Cataloging-in-Publication Data

Handbook of adolescent behavioral problems : evidence-based approaches to
    prevention and treatment / edited by Thomas P. Gullotta, Gerald R. Adams ;
    research assistant, Jessica M. Ramos.
        p. cm.
    Includes bibliographical references and index.
    ISBN 0-387-23845-X (acid-free paper) — ISBN 0-387-23846-8 (eBook)
    1. Adolescent psychopathology.   2. Adolescent psychiatry.   3. Behavior
disorders in adolescence.   I. Gullotta, Thomas, 1948-   II. Adams, Gerald R.,
1946-   III. Ramos, Jessica M.

RJ503.H266 2005
616.89'00835—dc22   2004062642

ISBN-10:0-387-23845-X   e-ISBN 0-387-23846-8   Printed on acid-free paper.
ISBN-13:978-0387-23845-X

Printed in the United States of America.   (TBI/SBA)

9 8 7 6 5 4 3 2 1

springeronline.com

Contributors

Gerald R. Adams is Professor of Family Relations and Human Development at the University of Guelph. He has been awarded recognition as a Distinguished Professor of Teaching at the University of Guelph, received honors from the American Psychological Association and American Psychological Society, served as the editor of the *Journal of Adolescent Research*, and was one of three editors for a 10 volume series of Advances in Adolescent Development. He has recently coedited the Blackwell Handbook of Adolescence.

Jill Antonishak is a doctoral student in the Department of Psychology at the University of Virginia. She received her undergraduate degree from Goucher College and her master's degree from UVA. Her research focuses on adolescent risk-taking and problem behavior, with an emphasis on peer relations.

Andre P. Bessette received his B.A. in Psychology from Connecticut College in New London, CT. He and his family moved out to California where he completed his M.S. and Ph.D. in clinical psychology at Pacific Graduate School of Psychology in Palo Alto. He completed his predoctoral internship in Pediatric Psychology at Children's Hospital Oakland and his postdoctoral residency at The Learning Clinic in Brooklyn, CT, where he is currently a clinician. Dr. Bessette resides in northeast city with his wife, Donna, and their two daughters, Nathalie and Yvonne.

Brian Bishop is an Associate Professor at Curtin University or Technology. He is a community psychologist, and his areas of research interest include community theory and development, indigenous issues and social justice. Recent research he has been involved in includes developing strategies for prevention of depression and anxiety in Aboriginal children, and in community participation in large-scale regional natural resource management.

Mark B. Borg, Jr. is a community/clinical psychologist and interpersonal psychoanalyst who is affiliated with the William Alanson White Institute. He is co-founder and principal partner of the Community Consulting Group, which is a community revitalization organization. He lives and practices in New York City.

Jeanne Brooks-Gunn is the Virginia and Leonard Marx Professor at Teachers College and the College of Physicians and Surgeons of Columbia University. She is also co-Director of the National Center for Children and Families and the Institute for Child and Family Policy at Columbia University. A developmental psychologist, she does policy-relevant research on prevention and intervention programs, long-term longitudinal studies of the life course, work on neighborhood and family SES disparities in outcomes, and investigation of effects of biological and environmental interactions on behavior and achievement in children, youth, and families. She has written over a dozen books and 400 articles and chapters on these topics.

Joseph L. Calles earned a B.S. in zoology from U.C. Davis. His M.D. is from Michigan State University (M.S.U.), where he also completed his residency in general psychiatry. His child and adolescent psychiatry fellowship was at U.S.C. He is the Director of Child and Adolescent Psychiatry for the Psychiatry Residency program at Michigan State University/Kalamazoo Center for Medical Studies, and is a Clinical Associate Professor of Psychiatry at M.S.U.

Christina M. Camp holds a dual appointment as a faculty member with the Program on Recovery and Community Health (PRCH), Department of Psychiatry at Yale University, and as an Associate Director of Research Projects at Emory University, Rollins School of Public Health. Dr. Camp's research interests lie in the areas of biobehavioral processes, ethno-cultural issues in health and mental health and the interpersonal dynamics of male-female relationships.

Deborah M. Capaldi is a Senior Scientist at the Oregon Social Learning Center in Eugene, Oregon. She is currently conducting three linked studies to examine the causes and consequences of antisocial and co-occurring behaviors across the life span within a dynamic developmental-contextual framework.

Sucheta D. Connolly is Director of the Pediatric Stress and Anxiety Disorders Clinic and Assistant Professor of Clinical Psychiatry at the University of Illinois at Chicago (UIC). She graduated from Washington University Medical School in St. Louis, completed her residency in general psychiatry at UIC and her fellowship in child and adolescent psychiatry at University of Chicago. She provides consultation and professional development programming to schools and mental health agencies in the community.

Feyza Corapci is a clinical psychology graduate student in the Department of Psychological Sciences at Purdue University. She is completing her predoctoral clinical internship in the Child Track at the University of Illinois at Chicago (UIC), Department of Psychiatry. Her research interests include the operation of environmental risk and protective factors on low-income preschoolers' social competence and behavioral adjustment and the role of home context and child temperament on parent-child transactions.

Melinda Corwin is an assistant professor in the Department of Speech, Language, and Hearing Sciences at Texas Tech University Health Sciences Center. She is a clinical instructor and provides speech-language therapy to young children and adolescents with diagnoses including ADHD and language learning disability. Ms. Corwin is working toward her Ph.D. in Human Development and Family Studies at Texas Tech University. Her research involves family stress related to attention deficit hyperactivity disorder in adolescents.

Natalie Crespo is a graduate student in the Community and Culture Psychology program at the University of Hawaii at Manoa. She graduated with a B.A. from the

Ohio State University. Her employment and research experiences have revolved around issues pertaining to at-risk youth and families, including working with homeless teenagers, disadvantaged families in need of child care, and literacy aid for children.

Michael R. Dalla is Managing Director of UrbanSensor a market research and promotions company partnering with Fortune 1000 companies to provide Real Time Consumer Insights. He is co-founder and partner of the Community Consulting Group. He resides in San Francisco and conducts research abroad.

Ralph J. DiClemente is the Charles Howard Candler Professor of Public Health in the Rollins School of Public Health and Professor of Psychiatry and Pediatrics at the Emory University School of Medicine. His research focuses on adolescent health risk and protective behaviors and the socio-ecological influences that affect these behaviors.

Peter W. Dowrick is Professor of Disability Studies and Psychology at University of Hawaii. He has wide experience working with people marginalized by culture, disability, mental health, and other considerations. His consultation on prevention and intervention extends to New Zealand, Great Britain, Alaska, Kansas, Baltimore, Canada, Chicago, Philadelphia, New Jersey, Kentucky, Hawaii, Micronesia, and American Samoa, with consultation-from-a-distance to another 26 states and 16 countries. His principal contribution has been in the concepts of *feedforward* and *creating futures*, applied in situations of personal safety, serious mental illness, social behavior, sports and recreation, daily living, literacy, academic skills, health, housing, management, and jobs, among others.

Raymond W. DuCharme is the founder and director of The Learning Clinic, Inc. (TLC), a private nonprofit education and treatment program for children and adolescents. TLC has provided day education and residential services since 1980. Dr. DuCharme has been a researcher and teacher, and Adjunct Professor at The University of Connecticut and Assistant Professor at Brown University, a national consultant and author of numerous papers and articles on the subjects of treating and educating students with Autistic spectrum disorders and associated co-morbid conditions.

J. Mark Eddy is an Associate Director and a Research Scientist at the Oregon Social Learning Center. He has conducted several long-term, follow-up studies of preventive and clinical interventions conducted within the juvenile justice and the school systems. For the past four years, he has been working with the Oregon Department of Corrections on the development of a research-based parenting program for incarcerated mothers and fathers, and currently is studying the outcomes of the program.

Cassandra Fink received her bachelor's degree in psychology from the University of California, Los Angeles, and then went on to complete her master's degree in Public Health at Columbia University. She is currently working with the National Institute on Drug Abuse (NIDA) Clinical Trials Network (CTN). Her research in drug abuse has included contingency management in a methadone-maintained population, the efficacy of smoking cessation treatment in substance abuse rehabilitation programs, and tobacco use counseling among homeless, recovering drug abusers. She has also been involved with smoking cessation among other populations, including a United Nations Business Council project with employees of Fortune 500 companies in the Northeast. Ms. Fink is also interested in nutrition and physical activity. Her master's thesis was on the demographic, behavioral, and genetic familial influences on childhood obesity.

Daniel J. Flannery is Professor of Justice Studies and Director of the Institute for the Study and Prevention of Violence at Kent State University. Prior appointments include Associate Professor of Psychiatry and Pediatrics at Case Western Reserve University and Assistant Professor of Family Studies at the University of Arizona. Research interests are in aggression, delinquency, and youth violence with a focus on etiology and on the relationship between violence and mental health. He received his Ph.D. in clinical child psychology from The Ohio State University.

Michael J. Furlong is a professor and program leader of the Counseling/Clinical/School Psychology Program and Special Education, Disability and Risk Studies at the Gevirtz Graduate School of Education, University of California, Santa Barbara.

Lynn Gilman is a doctoral student in Counseling Psychology at Indiana University and Assistant Director of the training clinic in the Department of Counseling and Educational Psychology. The department training clinic provides individual, couples, and family counseling services to the local community. Her research interests include training and supervision, particularly the supervision of evidenced-based practice and the link between supervision and client outcome.

Patricia A. Graczyk is an Assistant Professor of Clinical Psychology at the Institute for Juvenile Research in the Department of Psychiatry at the University of Illinois at Chicago. She received her PhD in Clinical Psychology and School Psychology from Northern Illinois University in 1998 and completed an NIMH prevention research postdoctoral fellowship in 2001. Her primary research interests are childhood anxiety and mood disorders, school-based mental health, and children's social competence.

Mark Griffiths studied psychology at the University of Bradford, received his Ph.D. in 1991 from the University of Exeter, was a lecturer of psychology at University of Plymouth (1990–1995), and has been at Nottingham Trent University ever since. He is now Europe's only professor of gambling studies and has an interest in technological addictions. Mark has published over 120 refereed papers, two books, numerous book chapters, and over 350 other articles.

Thomas P. Gullotta is C.E.O. of Child and Family Agency and is a member of the psychology and education departments at Eastern Connecticut State University. He is the senior author of the 4th edition of *The Adolescent Experience*, co-editor of *The Encyclopedia of Primary Prevention and Health Promotion*, and is editor emeritus of the *Journal of Primary Prevention*. He is the senior book series editor for *Issues in Children's and Families' Lives*. Tom holds editorial appointments on the *Journal of Early Adolescence*, *The Journal of Adolescent Research*, and the *Journal of Educational and Psychological Consultation*. He has published extensively on adolescents and primary prevention. Tom was honored in 1999 by the Society for Community Research and Action, Division 27 of the American Psychological Association with their Distinguished Contributions to Practice in Community Psychology Award.

Tobias Hayer studied psychology at the University of Bremen and received his diploma in 2001. Since 2001 he has been a research assistant at the Institute for Psychology and Cognition Research (University of Bremen). He conducts research on issues related to problem gambling. Tobias is currently completing his doctoral dissertation on the prevention of problem gambling.

David Hussey is a Faculty Associate at the ISPV and Assistant Professor of Justice Studies at KSU. He is Director of Research at Beech Brook, a private center offering comprehensive mental health services for youth and families. Research interests are in systems of care and adoption studies. Dr. Hussey received his Ph.D. in social welfare from the Mandel School of Applied Social Sciences at Case Western Reserve University.

Eric Jefferis is a Research Associate at Kent State University's Institute for the Study and Prevention of Violence. He serves as project director for the Northern District of Ohio's Project Safe Neighborhoods initiative and as Co-Principal Investigator for the Internet Mapping and Analysis for Police Problems Solving (iMAPPS) project. Prior to joining the ISPV, Eric was a Social Science Analyst at the National Institute of Justice. He is completing his Ph.D. in Criminal Justice at the University of Cincinnati.

Christine Johnson-Erickson is a doctoral student in the Counseling Psychology program at Indiana University. She is a project leader at the Center for Adolescent and Family Studies, a research center dedicated to disseminating and studying effective treatments for at-risk adolescents and their families. She is trained in functional family therapy, an evidence-based family-focused intervention. Her research interests include marital distress and conflict, as well as process and outcome in marriage and family therapy.

John Kalafat is a faculty member of Rutgers Graduate School of Applied and Professional Psychology. He has published widely on suicide prevention and program evaluation and is co-author of Lifelines School Based Youth Suicide Response Program. He is also a consultant on the Maine Youth Suicide Prevention CDC-funded Targeted Injury Prevention Project, Past President and member of the Board of Directors of the American Association of Suicidology, and Member of the Scientific Advisory Council of the American Foundation for Suicide Prevention.

Kirti N. Kanitkar has a bachelor's in Psychology and an M.S. in Human Development and Family Relations from the University of Mumbai, India. After working for a year at the Tata Institute of Social Sciences in Mumbai, she entered the doctoral program at Texas Tech University in fall 2001. Her area of interest is adolescent risk-taking behaviors, the processes through which adolescents engage in them, and factors associated with increased risk, vulnerability, and resilient outcomes.

Tatyana Kharit is from Russia, and earned her M.D. from the Moscow Institute of Health Ministry. She practiced general medicine for several years before immigrating to the United States. She is a second-year resident in psychiatry at MSU/KCMS. She is a Clinical Instructor in the Department of Psychiatry, Michigan State University. She is involved in research that is looking at the use of antidepressant and mood-stabilizing medications in the treatment of fibromyalgia.

Theresa Kruczek is an Assistant Professor and Licensed Psychologist in Indiana. She is the Director of the Counseling Practicum Clinic at Ball State University. Her research focuses on identifying and promoting adaptive functioning in child survivors of sexual abuse. Previously, Dr. Kruczek was on faculty at the Medical College of Virginia Hospital's Virginia Treatment Center for Children, where she coordinated the child trauma services and conducted outcome research with adolescent survivors of sexual abuse.

Maritza Lagos is from Peru, but earned her M.D. from Volgograd State Medical Institute in Russia. She completed her general psychiatry residency at Michigan State University/Kalamazoo Center for Medical Studies (MSU/KCMS), where she served as Chief Resident. She is currently on the faculty at MSU/KCMS, practicing adult inpatient psychiatry, and is a Clinical Assistant Professor of Psychiatry at M.S.U. Dr. Lagos is fluent in the reading, writing, and speaking of Spanish, Russian, and English.

Carl G. Leukefeld is Chair of the Department of Behavioral Science and Director of the Center on Drug and Alcohol Research at the University of Kentucky. He was a commissioned officer and Chief Health Services Officer in the U.S. Public Health Service, and for much of that time he was assigned to the National Institute on Drug Abuse in various management and scientific capacities. He has given presentations and has written over 120 articles as well as 15 books and monographs on treatment, criminal justice, prevention, and AIDS. His research interests include judicial sanctions, drug abuse treatment, rural services, and HIV.

Michael P. Levine is Samuel J. Cummings Professor of Psychology at Kenyon College in Gambier, Ohio. Dr. Levine is a co-editor of *The Developmental Psychopathology of Eating Disorders* (Mahwah, NJ: Erlbaum, 1996) and of *Preventing Eating Disorders: A Handbook of Interventions and Special Challenges* (Philadelphia: Brunner/Mazel, 1999). He is a Fellow of the Academy for Eating Disorders and a member of the American Psychological Association.

Catherine Martin is an academic child psychiatrist and clinical researcher. The focus of her research, clinical care, and teaching involves tobacco, alcohol, and other drug-abuse risk in teenagers. Understanding the contribution of personality differences and differences in drug effects to drug-abuse risk is of particular interest. Dr. Martin's administrative is Vice Chair for Research in the Department of Psychiatry, a member of the University of Kentucky's Presidents Commission for Women, and a member of the University Faculty Senate.

Judy A. McCown is an Associate Professor of Psychology and Director of the Doctoral Program in Clinical Psychology at the University of Detroit Mercy in Detroit, Michigan. She received her Ph.D. in Clinical Psychology from Wayne State University and maintains a private practice in psychology in St. Clair Shores, Michigan.

Hope M. Smiley McDonald is a doctoral candidate in sociology at the University of Kentucky. Her work focuses on studies related to drug courts, prisoner health service utilization, substance abuse, and substance abuse treatment. Her interests include treatment for drug-involved offenders, juvenile delinquency, substance abuse policy, and prisoner re-entry.

Kathleen A. McGrady has been the Clinical Director of The Learning Clinic, Inc. (TLC) since 1994. TLC is a private nonprofit education and treatment program for children and adolescents. Dr. McGrady is a neuropsychologist and has been a researcher and author of numerous papers and presentations on assessment, diagnosis, and treatment of children and adolescents with autistic spectrum disorders, and the associated comorbid conditions.

Gerhard Meyer studied psychology at the University of Göttingen; received his PhD in 1982; and is an Associate Professor at the Institute of Psychology and Cognition Research (University of Bremen). He has conducted several research projects on problem gambling. Gerhard works as forensic expert witness and trainer for casino employees; gambling specialist on international level.

Brent C. Miller is Vice President for Research and Professor of Family, Consumer, and Human Development at Utah State University. His research has focused on adolescent sexual behavior and pregnancy, but recently he has been studying adjustment of adopted children and adoptive families. He is the author of several books and over 100 articles and chapters, mostly authored with graduate student collaborators.

Kathleen M. Morrissey is a Ph.D. student in Marriage and Family Therapy at Iowa State University. She is a research assistant under Dr. Werner-Wilson in the area of positive youth development and is a student member of the American Association for Marriage and Family Therapy. She has a social work background and has worked with adolescents in group home settings, community corrections, and as a substance abuse prevention specialist.

Miriam Mulsow is an Associate Professor and the Director of Graduate Programs in the Department of Human Development and Family Studies at Texas Tech University. She holds a Ph.D. in Child and Family Development from The University of Georgia. Her research involves family stress and resiliency, with particular emphasis on parenting stress, attention deficit hyperactivity disorder, and addictions. In addition, she performs and teaches program evaluation.

Michael W. Naylor is an Associate Professor of Child and Adolescent Psychiatry. He is the Division Chief of the Institute for Juvenile Research at the University of Illinois at Chicago and Medical Director of the Comprehensive Assessment Response Training System. Dr. Naylor has had numerous publications and has received many honors, including being listed in *America's Top Doctors, 1999*. Among many projects, he is currently working on a research project, Pharmacoepidemiology of DCFS Wards.

Ahsan Nazeer is from Pakistan, and graduated from Rawalpindi Medical College. He is currently a third-year resident in psychiatry at MSU/KCMS, and serves as Vice-Chief Resident. He is a Clinical Instructor in the Department of Psychiatry, Michigan State University. He has co-authored peer-reviewed articles on the use of neuroimaging in depression and in post-traumatic stress disorder. He plans on pursuing training in child and adolescent psychiatry and a career in academic psychiatry.

Vanessa M. Nyborg is an assistant researcher and adjunct professor at the Gevirtz Graduate School of Education, University of California, Santa Barbara.

Mani N. Pavuluri is the Director of the Pediatric Mood Disorders Clinic and Bipolar Research Program at the Institute for Juvenile Research (IJR) and Center for Cognitive Medicine (CCM).

Christina Paxson is Professor of Economics and Public Affairs at Princeton University, and the founding director of the Center for Health and Wellbeing, an interdisciplinary health research center in the Woodrow Wilson School of Public and International Affairs. She is a Research Associate of the National Bureau of Economic Research and a member of the MacArthur Foundation Research Network on Socioeconomic Status and Health. Her current research focuses on economic status and children's health outcomes.

Gary W. Peterson is Professor and Chair of the Department of Family Studies and Social Work at the University of Miami in Oxford, Ohio. His areas of research are parent-child/adolescent relations, cross-cultural influences on adolescent development, and family theory. He is Co-Editor of the *Handbook of Marriage and the Family (2nd Ed.)*, Editor of *Marriage and Family Review*, and Senior Editor of a book series entitled the *Haworth Series on Marriage and Family Studies*.

Niva Piran is a Professor at the Ontario Institute for Studies in Education of the University of Toronto. Dr. Piran is co-editor of *Preventing Eating Disorders: A Handbook of Interventions and Special Challenges* and of *A Day Hospital Group Treatment Program for Anorexia Nervosa and Bulimia Nervosa*. She is a Fellow of the Academy for Eating Disorders and the Prevention Editor of the *Eating Disorder Journal*.

Jessica M. Ramos received her B.A. in psychology from Eastern Connecticut State University. She is a Research Assistant at Child and Family Agency of Southeastern Connecticut. She has served as a research assistant editing, undertaking library research, and supporting the work of the editors, Thomas Gullotta and Martin Bloom, on the *Encyclopedia of Primary Prevention and Health Promotion*. She has also assisted in the editorial process in the *Asperger Syndrome: A Handbook for Professionals and Families; Handbook of Evidence-Based Approaches for the Treatment and Prevention of Challenging Behaviors in Adolescence*, as well as *Promoting Racial, Ethnic, and Religious Understanding and Reconciliation* and is involved in child observations and research for the Bingham *Early Childhood Prosocial Behavior Curriculum*.

Jody Reed is from Chicago, IL. He earned his M.D. from Meharry Medical College. He is a fourth-year resident in psychiatry at MSU/KCMS, and serves as Chief Resident. He is a Clinical Instructor in the Department of Psychiatry, Michigan State University. He has been involved in a project that screens high school freshmen for depression. His interests are in forensic and cross-cultural psychiatry. He will attend law school after completion of his residency.

LaDonya Reed is in the Child & Adolescent Psychiatry training program at the University of Kentucky. She attended Duke University for her undergraduate education and the University of Kentucky College of Medicine. She completed an internship in Pediatrics at the University of South Carolina then transferred to the University of Kentucky to Psychiatry. Her special interests include psychopharmacology with children and special issues in adolescent psychiatry. She has received an award for medical student teaching.

N. Dickon Reppucci has been a Professor of Psychology at the University of Virginia since 1976. He received his Ph.D. from Harvard University in 1968 and was an assistant and Associate Professor at Yale University from 1968 to 1976. He is an author, co-author, or editor of more than 135 books, chapters, and articles. His major research interests include children, families, and the law, especially juvenile justice and adolescent development, and the prevention of child abuse and neglect.

Clare Roberts is a clinical psychologist with 20 years of experience working with children and adolescents with psychological problems. She is an Associate Professor at Curtin University of Technology. Her research interests include the prevention of internalizing disorders in children and adolescents, and early intervention in developmental disabilities. She heads a research team conducting a large dissemination trial of school-based mental health promotion programs. Clare lives in Perth with her 12-year-old twin boys.

Rayna Sage was a doctoral student at USU, working on a project evaluating an extension-based prevention/intervention mentoring program for youth. She is interested in comprehensive youth and family programming how it can enhance resiliency and reduce risk processes for long-term positive development.

Laura F. Salazar is a Director of Research in Emory University's Rollins School of Public Health, Department of Behavioral Science and Health Education in Atlanta, GA. Dr. Salazar received her Ph.D. in Community Psychology from Georgia State University. Her research interests are in examining the intersection of exposure to intimate partner violence and sexual risk behavior among adolescents, and in determining the role societal and systems-level factors have in contributing to violence against women.

Jill R. Salsman is working toward her doctoral degree in Counseling Psychology at Ball State University in Muncie, IN. Her research interests are in the areas of eating disorders and childhood sexual abuse. Her clinical focus is the adolescent population. She received her bachelor's degree in psychology from Augustana College in Rock Island, IL, and a master's degree in counseling from Ball State University.

Adam Schwebach received his masters degree in Clinical Psychology from Eastern Kentucky University. He is a doctoral canidate in school psychology at the University of Utah. Mr. Schwebach works as a neuropsychology intern for the Neurology Learning and Behavior Center in Salt Lake City, UT, where he provides diagnostic and clinical services to children and adolescents having attention deficit hyperactivity disorder. Mr. Schwebach's research interests include attention-deficit/hyperactivity disorder, learning disabilities, and traumatic brain injury in children and adolescents.

Thomas L. Sexton is a Professor in the Department of Counseling and Educational Psychology at Indiana University, where he is the Director of the Clinical Training Center, Director of the Center for Adolescent and Family Studies, and teaches in the APA-accredited Counseling Psychology Program. Dr. Sexton has written extensively in the areas of outcome research and its implications for clinical practice and training. He is a national expert on family-based treatment interventions for at-risk adolescents and regularly presents workshops nationally and internationally.

Jill D. Sharkey is a postdoctoral researcher at the Center for School-Based Youth Development in the Gevirtz Graduate School of Education, University of California, Santa Barbara.

Suhail Sheikh is from Pakistan and graduated from Liaquat Medical College. He had extensive medical practice experience prior to immigrating to the U.S. He is a third-year resident in psychiatry at MSU/KCMS. He is a Clinical Instructor in the Department of Psychiatry, Michigan State University. He has been involved in a project that screens high school freshmen for depression.

William W. Stoops is a native of Pittsburgh, PA. He received a Bachelor of Arts degree in psychology from Davidson College in Davidson, NC, and a Master of Arts degree in psychology from the University of Kentucky in Lexington, KY. He is a doctoral candidate in psychology at the University of Kentucky and is interested in human behavioral pharmacology.

Erin L. Sutfin is a doctoral student in the Department of Psychology at the University of Virginia. She received her B.A. from William Smith College in 1996 and her M.A. in psychology from UVA in 2001. Her research focuses on the influence of mass media on children and adolescents. She is interested in the use of mass media as a prevention tool for unhealthy behaviors.

John A. Sweeney is Professor, Departments of Psychiatry, Neurology, and Psychology, and the Director of the Center for Cognitive Medicine at the University of Illinois at Chicago. Dr. Sweeney is a clinical investigator with interest in autism and schizophrenia, and has directed clinical neuropsychology services at Cornell University Medical College and at the University of Pittsburgh. He is a recipient of a NIMH Research Scientist Development Award, and is a standing member of the NIH study section BDCN6.

Stephanie Vitanza is a Licensed Psychologist in Arizona. She is the Director of Mental Health Services for Childhelp USA, an international nonprofit agency that specializes in child abuse treatment. Her current clinical specialty is working with children and adolescents who have been sexually abused and their families. She also treats children and teens who have been physically abused and/or neglected or who may have been witnesses to homicide or violence.

Ronald Jay Werner-Wilson is Associate Professor and Director of the Marriage and Family Therapy Program and Clinic at Iowa State University, which is accredited by the Commission on Accreditation for Marriage and Family Therapy Education. He is a clinical member and Approved Supervisor of the American Association for Marriage and Family Therapy and a member of the American Family Therapy Academy. Dr. Werner-Wilson has been investigating adolescence (particularly adolescent sexuality and positive youth development) since 1990.

Gina M. Wingood is an Associate Professor in the Department of Behavioral Sciences and Health Education at Emory University's Rollins School of Public Health; Co-Director, Behavioral and Social Science Core, Emory Center for AIDS Research. Dr. Wingood received her ScD from the Harvard University School of Public Health in Health and Social Behavior. Dr. Wingood's research interest is in developing gender-tailored HIV prevention programs for women and in examining social structural factors that Increase women's vulnerability to HIV.

Bryan Winward was a doctoral student at USU. He has been employed teaching adolescents for ten years and has a great interest in helping teens achieve worthwhile life skills. At Utah State University his research interests have focused on adolescent pregnancy and long-term outcomes for teens who have been adopted.

Foreword

Thomas P. Gullotta and Gerald R. Adams

As we review the chapters that represent the work of the many talented scholars who contributed to this volume, we cannot help but reflect back on our own careers. We were educated at a time when the dominance of psychoanalytic theory was waning and the importance of the environment and learning was emerging. *Family* was the "buzz word." *Social justice* was the "buzz phrase."

During the late 1970s, we witnessed the re-emergence of genetics and neurobiology, which were grounded not in eugenics but a new science that used CAT, MRI, and PET imaging and DNA unraveling as its methodologies. This interest would grow in subsequent years such that the buzz word of the 1990s would be *genes*, and the *decade of the brain* was the buzz phrase. During this time, we saw pharmacological treatment options grow from a small handful to a multitude of psychotropic drugs.

As the general public became increasingly focused on mental health issues, it expected managed health care companies to include coverage for services such as counseling and medications. Against this backdrop, our understanding of helping underwent a transformation (thanks to managed care) that is still in progress—no longer are we interested in the mental health of our clients, but in their behavioral health. Apparently, actions speak louder than thoughts and feelings. Whether this is indeed true is debatable.

Finally, across these decades, a small but vocal group within the helping professions questioned the noble but futile efforts of their clinical colleagues and dared to ask if there might be ways to reduce the incidence of mental illness/dysfunctional behavior and promote mental health/functional behavior.

As the new century begins, these different tracks are converging as social science seeks to identify effective practices leading to successful treatment and prevention approaches. The new buzz words are *bio-psycho-social theory*. The new buzz phrase is *evidence-based practice*. This handbook reflects not only this movement toward identifying best practices, it acknowledges that no single causal agent causes the pain of mental illness or the behaviors considered dysfunctional. Rather, most experts in the field agree that biology creates a susceptibility that can be exploited under certain circumstances. The growing consensus is that personality characteristics can enable an individual to handle adversity more effectively or to have a less-than-desirable, riskier reaction. And clearly, the environment matters.

Environment matters as a trigger for illness and a protective factor for health. We use environment in the broadest sense. Environment is the air we breathe that encourages the development of asthma, and it is the Clean Air Act. Environment is the media that exposes youth to desensitizing video games and sexually demeaning images on film and the internet. Environment is also *Sesame Street*. Environment is the family, friends, teachers, and others that nurture positive and less positive personality characteristics. These multiple elements merge to create the uniqueness that is found in each of us.

We hope that practitioners regularly use this reference work in their practices and that policymakers and human services directors use this state-of-the-art guide to pursue promising paths of helpfulness. For graduate students in the helping professions, we have provided a set of blueprints for fashioning intervention plans for addressing the needs of young people. We urge you to look beyond the immediate need of the client and to imagine how that client's issues might be prevented in others. If we work at it together, we can create a healthier society.

Contents

Handbook of Adolescent
Behavioral Problems

Section I

Introduction and Overview

Chapter 1

Adolescent Development

Gerald R. Adams

This chapter offers a broad overview of adolescent development and in so doing prepares the canvas for the remaining chapters in this volume.

There are a multitude of excellent sources that pertain to this chapter. In particular, I used *Developing Adolescents*, a reference guide, for professionals prepared by the American Psychological Association (2002); *The Blackwell Handbook of Adolescence* (Adams & Berzonsky, 2003); *The Adolescent Experience*, 4th E. (Gullotta, Adams & Markstrom, 1999); and an edited volume, *Reducing Adolescent Risk* (Romer, 2003). For further reading on adolescent development I recommend a ten-year series by Sage Publication called *Advances in Adolescent Development*.

A Definition of Adolescence

There is no single definition of adolescence. Some have called it the teenage years, others the second decade of life, and in North America it is being referred to as either adolescence and youth or adolescence and emerging adulthood. Any attempt to construct a worldwide definition is even more difficult given the growing appreciation for the kaleidoscope that is the adolescent experience. The experience of adolescence in one region of the world is very different from that in another. Even within a geopolitical state subcategories of the population have historical, economic, political, and religious differences that influence the nature of adolescence. On a global level, perhaps the most striking differences exist between North American and Europe and much of the remaining world, especially with regard to the rights and opportunities of young men versus young women.

My objective is not to solve the problem of definition. Rather, it is to recognize the challenges associated with deriving a single definition. We consider adolescence to be a stage of life that begins sometime around the onset of puberty and ends sometime when the individual obtains adult rights, responsibilities, and recognition by family, law, society, and such. Given the diversity of the population, even in North America, we appreciate that the pathways and trajectories of adolescence into young adulthood vary according to the historical, cultural, ethnic, and religious systems in which a young person grows and matures.

Theoretical Perspectives on Adolescence

To help understand what is considered normal during this life stage, it is useful to explore several general theories of adolescence. Given that the study of adolescence is of interest to several social science disciplines, I will review major theoretical notions from those disciplines. In the end, I will extrapolate what these theories suggest is normal and where deviance, pathology, or dysfunctional behavior might begin. In later chapters the notion of dysfunction is examined for a wide variety of behaviors, emotions, and cognitions. Therefore, I will consider broad issues, rather than specific diagnostic categories of dysfunctions, deviance, or pathos.

Psychiatric Perspectives

Sigmund Freud gave the first psychiatric perspective on the study of adolescence in the early 1900s at Clark University. He was invited by G. Stanley Hall, the first prominent scholar in the United States to popularized the study of adolescence. Briefly Freud contrasted two powerful and opposing forces—inherent instincts (sexuality and aggression) with social needs to live together. Human beings are seen as individualistic and selfish but still in need of social living to survive. Of course, the now well-known concepts *id* (instincts), *ego* (executive functions), and *superego* (a form of conscience), were his major contributions.

Freud proposed that human beings come to balance instinctual demands with social sanctions through a series of three life stages. When an imbalance between individual demands and societal pressures occur, the individual becomes anxious and the ego must deal with this discomfort. To deal with this anxiety an individual uses *defense mechanisms*. A defense mechanism is the way an individual deals with painful experiences, internal conflicts, personal inadequacy, and the associated anxiety (Gullotta et al., 1999).

It was Freud's daughter Anna who promoted the idea of adolescence as a period of internal disharmony. Anna Freud maintained that with the onset of adolescence the intrapsychic equilibrium between instinctual demands and ego mechanisms is temporarily disrupted, resulting in a period of storm and stress. New, strong sexual urges emerge during adolescence. The personality consolidation of childhood is threatened by a new genital or sexual orientation that revives the pregenital urges that have been controlled during childhood through ego defenses. This is referred to as the Oedipal fantasy. Repression is a primitive defense mechanism that guards against instinctual forces through hiding certain unthinkable fantasies, such as incestuous urges, from an individual's consciousness. The anxiety accompanying pregenital urges and Oedipal striving renews the use of old defense mechanisms. According to the Freuds, the adolescent is in a psychological struggle, where the demanding id (instinctual needs) is constantly confronting the ego, thus creating a state in which the adolescent is continuously undergoing vacillations in ego functioning and emotional tone. In time, this disharmony is reduced through the development of several major defense mechanisms.

Anna Freud suggested several major and appropriate defense mechanisms for adolescents. To mitigate the anxiety associated with regressive urges to possess the love and attention of a parent, *displacement* is used to withdraw love from a parent and extend it to a parent substitute. Often a parent is treated with callous indifference, while a teacher, neighbor or youth leader might receive admiration, respect, and caring. This displacement eases the adolescent's anxiety and defends against urges or desires focused on a parent. Another technique might be a defensive reversal of affect. The adolescent might act just the opposite of the way he or she really feels toward a parent. This is called a *reaction formation*. This negative reaction toward the displacement of love from a parent to a significant other does not diminish the regressive urges characteristic of adolescence. Rather, it further heightens the anxiety accompanying these urges and often heightens denial, uncooperativeness, and hostility toward the parent. In contrast, some adolescents withdraw into themselves. Unfortunately, withdrawal leads to an inflation of one's sense of self-importance and increases fantasies of narcissism and omnipotence. Freud describes other defense mechanisms; however, the foregoing provides a general picture of the defensive world of adolescents (Gullotta et al., 1999).

Sociological Perspective

In sociological theory the influences of norms on behavior, mores, cultural expectations, social rituals, group pressures, or technological factors are the key to understanding adolescence. For example, Kingsley Davis argued that modern society changes very rapidly, and so each new generation is reared in a social milieu different from that of the prior generation. Since each generation's experiences of its own cultural and historical content guides its actions and provides the basis for understanding the world, parents find it difficult to provide direction to the new generation, and conflict is inevitable. Davis indicates that parents cannot modernize their view because they are a product of a past historical time; their personality is fixed. Further, it is not acceptable to change because that would mean that all of the parent's prior experiences are meaningless.

It is argued that intergenerational conflict is inevitable. Further, as the adolescent comes to reach his or her peak physical ability, filled with energy and enthusiasm, parents are beginning to lose energy and are trying to conserve it. To adjust for this distinction, society limits competition between adolescents and their parents to reduce or limit competitive feelings and jealousy. Unfortunately, this process diminishes a wide variety of opportunities for adolescents to interact or compete with parents and other adults. Davis believes the result is heightened frustration in many adolescents and increased conflict between adolescents and their parents.

Conflict can occur for another reason. Adolescents are filled with utopian ideals, e.g., that life should be fair and just for all people. They usually see their pragmatic parents as too conservative. This creates a dichotomy about social reality, and provides parents and adolescents with fertile ground for conflict.

Davis suggested a last source of conflict. In North America children are expected to emancipate themselves and to individuate into independent beings. However, there are no formal institutional steps to guide the adolescent and family through this process. Because of the ambiguity of this transition, conflicts often arises over the relinquishing of parental authority (see Noller, 1994).

Margaret Mead has offered further observations on culture and social change. Mead suggests there are three general cultural types. In a *postfigurative culture*, parents and grandparents provide the guidance for cultural stability and continuity by expressing that their way of life is unchanging. In this case, group membership and identity are generally predetermined or ascribed at birth. Essentially, adolescents are told what to do and they do it. Parental expectations and values determine how children grow up.

In a *cofigurative culture*, each generation acquires different values, norms, or mores. Instead of acquiring them from parents, each generation acquires them from their peers. In a cofigurative culture each new generation is expected to be different. Some conflict is expected between generations because each generation has its own standards that can conflict with those of parents or grandparents.

Things are very different in *prefigurative cultures* in that adults actually learn from the children. In this case, adults emulate the new authority of children. Parents learn how to parent through their children's instructions on what is right and expected. In this cultural configuration adolescents shape their parents' expectations through instruction and guidance that is youth-centered (Mead, 1970).

Anthropological Perspective

Sociologists mostly focus on how society affects the adolescent. In the anthropological perspective the focus is often on how adolescents affect society. What contributions do adolescents make as workers, athletes, innovators, or bargaining assets in the negotiation of marriage, business, or politics? According to Alice Schlegel and colleagues, adolescence is best seen as learning and unlearning of important social processes. Indeed, they refer to this life stage as *social adolescence*. During social adolescence the individual learns how to engage in new behaviors, such as sexuality, or new occupational roles and unlearn old behaviors like family subordination and dependency or asexuality. Schlegel refers to his process as a *reorganization of thought and action* (Schlegel, 1995).

As in many theories of adolescence, this reorganization is driven by underlying physical maturity. Unlike most other theories, the anthropological perspective focuses largely on incest taboos, sexual gratification, and preparation for intimacy and reproduction. The role of family is recognized through such things as arrangement for marriage, promotion of occupational roles, and maternal and paternal management of restricted (or permissive) sexual behavior prior to marriage. The peer group is recognized as helping the reorganization process and the structure and activity of peer socialization.

Notions of conflict within the family are not dismissed in the anthropological perspective. Changing roles and a changing body can lead to family conflict. Anthropologists recognize that hormonal and endocrine changes can contribute to emotionality, arousal, and mood fluctuations. But much of this is not thought to create major conflict, but rather simple perturbations over mundane things. From an anthropological viewpoint, conflict is more likely to occur around economic or property issues, where the control of marriage or economic opportunities for the adolescent might cause financial or work problems for the family.

Anthropologists often explore issues of gender and social status. They frequently observe that girls are primarily socialized by older women. However, boys are often sent off to be socialized by unsupervised peer groups. Less freedom for girls means stronger socialization, bonding, and supervision. Freedom for boys often means strong peer effects and greater opportunities for individuation.

Cultural anthropologists look for both commonalities (universals) and variations in adolescents behavior across cultures. They examine the sociocultural structure, social organizations, values, and expectations. They expect to find meaningful patterns of organization in adolescent behavior according to the kinship system, family structure and form of marriage, economy and technology, and religious or traditional values and practices. Within all of these broad societal areas they examine the power of the onset of pubescence and the role of gender in order to understand adolescent behavior.

Evolutionary Perspective

This perspective is generally embraced by ethologists, sociobiologists, and evolutionary psychologists. Each endorses Darwinian notions of evolution and natural selection. Further, the focus is on the human ethnogram or inventory of human behavior. This perspectives compares and contrasts sets of adaptive behaviors between humans and other primate relatives to determine if there is a phylogenetic continuity and thus a set of evolving behaviors.

Glenn Weisfeld (1999) has proposed that many behaviors during adolescence can be explained through an evolutionary perspective. He indicates that culture must adjust to the time of evolution and that aspects of sex differences and pubertal timing account for many adolescent behaviors. It is argued that culture has to adjust to biology. Indeed, evolving sex differences might be overridden by strong socialization, but thus far this has not occurred. In particular, sex differences in human reproductive behavior need to be recognized. Any notions of equal male and female potential for nuturing are put into doubt by all of the evidence on parental care. Indeed, it is argued that mammals have taken over 50 millions years to evolve maternal care giving. In the end, Weisfeld argues that traditional sex roles and behavior have been adaptive for years and that it is difficult, maybe even impossible, to change this biological destiny.

In evolutionary theory there is considerable attention given to pubescent *rites of passage*. It is argued that puberty rites are important because they facilitate separation from parents. In particular for boys, these rites lead to young males' being socialized by a broader social matrix than just the family. Puberty rites are often accompanied by sex segregation that leads to the mastery of sex-specific tasks and behaviors. Often a same-sex non-parent (like a coach, teacher, mentor) provides formal or informal instruction. Through this process the youth gets some level of training that ultimately incorporates the novice into adult society. If a formal ceremony is held, the event for boys often focuses on accomplishments and reentry back into society after a period of separation and trial. For girls, the events often focus on reproduction, fertility, beauty, or the responsibility of caring for others.

Psychological Perspective

There are many psychological perspectives that have been advanced to help understand adolescence. In our own conceptual work (Adams & Marshall, 1996) we have proposed a developmental social psychology of identity that broadly describes the nature of identity development and the importance of psychological context in the formation of identity. *Identity* is a psychological construct that refers to how individuals make meaning for themselves through discovery and psychological construction. In research literature on identity there is wide recognition of four types of identity. At the least mature level there is *diffusion*—a state of avoidance in identity formation and emptiness of the self. The next level is *foreclosure*—where an individual develops a sense of self based on identification with authority figures and imitation behavior. A great advance is made for moratorium youth. *Moratorium* youth begin searching and trying to discover and construct a self-defined sense of identity. Once this process has occurred the individual develops relatively enduring identity commitments. This state of mind is referred to as identity achieved.

The power of *identity achievement* is that it is accompanied by important self-regulation mechanisms. That is, as one moves from diffusion through foreclosure and moratorium into identity achievement several important psychological strengths emerge. These includes, among other things, a secure sense of self and self-confidence; the identification of goals, values, and directions one's life is taking; a sense of free will and self-efficacy; and the recognition of many types of futures and possibilities.

For youth to have a chance to become identity achieved they need to experience an environment that facilitates a balance between individuality as a sense of uniqueness and connectedness, where the youth feels like the individuality he or she has assumed matters to those who are important to him or her.

Theoretical Perspectives and the Identification of Dysfunctionality

In each of these perspectives there is an assumption that adolescence is a time of change and advancement. The focus may differ on what is changing and why, but the general assumption is that adolescence is a period of transformation. But if an individual is in a state of transformation, how can we know if the change is normal or dysfunctional? Anyone living or working with adolescents must ask this question from time to time. Yet the answer to this question might be difficult to obtain.

Each perspective suggests what is normal or typical. One might therefore assume that when a designated process or development does not occur there is some basic problem that might predict a dysfunction. The possible dysfunction could reside in the individual, relationships, environments, or social climate. Whether the problem is considered a problem is probably based on whether those in authority consider it to be. Sometimes things occur that are defined as norm breaking but not substantially dysfunctional. It should be clear that what is considered normal is actually a social construction based on parental viewpoints, institutional expectations, legal and governmental positions, cultural definitions, and even by the adolescents' own perceptions. For example, the act of stealing some small item from a local store is, according to the law, a theft. But a single act may or may not be a defining moment in the practicing definition of delinquency in any given community. Further, such a single act might result in one community's stigmatizing a youth; in another, it might be seen as a single instance of acting-out or struggling to grow up and learn right from wrong. However, any dramatic act that has immediate health consequences, such as a serious act of aggression or an attempted suicide, is readily defined as dysfunctional behavior.

A psychoanalytic perspective of adolescence suggests that when anxiety becomes unmanageable or results in extreme forms of acting out, self-destruction, or compromises the health of an adolescent, this is dysfunctional behavior. From a sociological perspective the connections of the individual with society focuses on norms and mores. It is often thought that intergenerational conflict is a normal part of growing up. But when this conflict damages bonding within the family and unconventional behavior occurs, the situation moves from normative to dysfunctional. Further, behaviors that do not fit the cultural or subcultural norms are often described as dysfunctional. To elaborate on this idea consider the following. Listening to, and being guided by parental directions would be very functional in a postfigurative culture, but dysfunctional in a prefigurative culture where parents must learn through the child. From an anthropological perspective, if a youth fails to unlearn early behaviors regarding social reliance and dependence on parents and acquire a greater sense of individuality, the youth might be seen as enmeshed in a family and unable to achieve reorganization of self and acquire independence and self-construction. The evolutionary perspective likewise suggests that a failure by society to allow socialization beyond the family to other adults and peers may create unintended dysfunctional behavior among adolescents. Furthermore, attempts to diminish or eliminate biological imperatives may create little change and unnecessary stress among adolescents. For example, an over-exaggerated attempt to reduce masculinity might result in unforeseen resistance and dysfunctional behaviors. From a psychological perspective, psychological maturity, such as identity formation progression toward more mature levels, is associated with greater ego strengths, stress management, and well-being. Dysfunctional behaviors may emerge from diffuse identity states, for example, when families, schools, or society fail to provide a balance between individuality and connections with others.

Individual Differences and Progressions in Adolescent Development

In a recent document prepared by the American Psychological Association (2002) a guide for professionals was created through the cooperation of many organizations and government funding agencies. This document, along with various other handbooks and textbooks, offer an excellent overview of the nature of healthy development during adolescence. Some of the main points will be reviewed below and serve as the basis for further consideration of the question of normative versus dysfunctional development during adolescence.

Adolescent Physical Development

There is great variation in the timing and onset of puberty. This is caused by variations in genetic, biological, socioeconomic, nutritional, and life event factors. The most often cited age for normal patterns of growth ranges from age 10 to 12 years for girls and 12 to 14 years for boys. However, the gradual hormonal process actually begins around age 7, with full onset occurring earlier for African American than Caucasian youth. Therefore, there is considerable variation by gender, age, cultural heritage, and socioeconomic status.

PREPARATION FOR PUBERTY AND SEXUAL DEVELOPMENT. Few girls or boys are well prepared for the onset of puberty and the accompanying physical and emotional development. When adults present information on puberty, a positive presentation of personal experiences enhances girls' and boys' comfort level and perceptions. Mothers are more involved with their daughters (and possibly sons) than fathers. Most evidence suggests sons receive little to no information about nocturnal emissions or arousal. Nonetheless, there are both psychological and social impacts of body development.

TIMING OF PUBERTAL ONSET. The timing of the onset of puberty accounts for substantial differences in the psychological and social impacts of puberty. Special attention is recommended for early and late physical development. In particular, early-maturing girls are at-risk for such behavior as substance abuse and oppositional defiant and eating disorders. Early-maturing boys are often involved in high-risk behaviors such as sexual activity, smoking, and delinquency, while late-maturing boys appear to have higher levels of conflict with parents, school problems, and depression. Further, late-maturing boys may be at higher risk for being bullied.

Adolescent Cognitive Development

Considerable changes in intellectual functioning can occur during adolescence. Adolescent boys and girls do differ in their cognitive abilities. Although widespread differences are not observed, adolescent girls are more confident about their reading and social skills. Adolescent boys are more confident about their athletic and mathematical abilities. These differences are primarily accounted for by gender role stereotypes than actual differences. Nonetheless, self-perceived confidence differences do matter. Greater confidence in a particular ability often means greater involvement.

Regarding general patterns of intellectual development during middle childhood and adolescence, one major longitudinal study reported by Robert McCall and colleagues (1973) suggests several normal pathways in intellectual development. Many adolescents show a stable pattern of IQ change with a slow but steady increase from age 2 to age 17. This accounts for the majority of youth. Other patterns include either decreases from middle childhood into adolescence, or a sharp increase in middle childhood followed by a rapid decline in adolescence. McCall and colleagues report that between the ages of 3 and 17 a child's IQ score can vary by 28.5 points. They also found that one in every three children's scores increased by more than 30 points. From such evidence we can conclude that IQ is a changing and transforming ability and not necessarily fixed by heredity. Children and adolescents are flexible and evolving, with patterns of stability and flux well within normative ranges.

Regarding qualitative changes in intellectual functioning, the most widely recognized change involves the transformation from concrete to more abstract thinking. The onset of what is called *formal operational* thought brings with it many intellectual changes that are more advanced compared to early- or middle-childhood thinking. Adolescents move from an emphasis on the more concrete and sensible here-and-now to thinking about the world of possibilities. Considering both the observable world and the possibilities of the abstract world allows for more complete thought. Hypothetical reasoning emerges in which hypotheses can be used to eliminate unsupportable thoughts. Adolescents can spend time identifying the impossible versus the possible. So with formal operational thinking the adolescent can think about the future by planning and exploring possible causation. Further, adolescents can think about their own thoughts. They can become aware of cognitive processes that are inefficient, biased, or not productive or useful (Gullotta et al., 1999).

With the gradual onset of formal operational thought, adolescents begin to separate their own thoughts from those of others. As they begin to conceptualize this distinction, they begin to account for other people's thinking. During this process a sense of *egocentrism* emerges where the adolescent recognizes the thoughts of others but fails to differentiate the objects toward which the thinking of others are directed. There is confusion between others' thinking and one's own. Thus, adolescents falsely believe that others are as engrossed with their own thinking and behavior as the adolescent is him or herself. David Elkind (1985) indicates this egocentrism is demonstrated in the preoccupation with and self-consciousness about physical attractiveness, appearance, and body image. Elkind thinks that young people are inclined to anticipate the reactions of others in social situations and to assume that others are as admiring or as critical of them as they are of themselves. He calls this the *imaginary audience*.

Because of the imaginary audience adolescents regard themselves and their feelings as being unique and special. They feel that no one can ever know how intensely they feel. This feeling of uniqueness and intensity, which Elkind labels the *personal fable*, can create thoughts such as a belief in one's own immortality, the ability to influence animals, or similar imaginary conceits.

With ample experience in social perspective-taking the adolescent comes to differentiate between self-preoccupations and the interests of others, and to realize that others are concerned about different things. Thus, normally developing adolescents gradually merge the feelings of others into their own thoughts and feelings, but recognize differences between their own and others' thoughts, and, in fact, come to recognize their own limitations.

Any failure in gaining formal operational thinking will leave a youth unable to develop a "critical habit of mind" (Keating & Sasse, 1996). This includes three broad categories of thought. *Conceptual flexibility*, which involves the creation of links between ideas and the application of a particular concept to novel content. Types of conceptual flexibility include divergent thinking, analogical thinking, or applying algorithms. *Reflective thinking* is the core of critical thought and involves making qualifying conclusions about the value of ideas. While conceptual flexibility is essential for generating new ideas, reflective thinking is necessary to determine right or wrong and the usefulness of ideas or information. The final aspect of an adequate critical habit of mind involves *cognitive self-regulation*. This involves the selection and organization of cognitive activities needed to problem-solve effectively and efficiently. Cognitive self-regulation encompasses inquiry, information gathering, questioning, and comprehension.

Any youth is disadvantaged if the emergence of formal operations and the development of a critical habit of mind does not appear. Failure to develop these cognitive abilities will leave a youth functioning at less adaptive levels of concrete thinking. Potentially, limited cognitive capacity can create poor interactions with others.

Adolescent Emotional Development

It is a widely held belief that a healthy sense of *self-esteem* makes for a positive and emotionally balanced adolescent. It is also argued that a healthy self-concept includes a positive sense of self-esteem. The late Morris Rosenberg argued that a good *self-concept* includes, among other things, high self-esteem, a sense of mattering to others, stability in self-concept, low vulnerability, a sense of personal control, low levels of public anxiety, and harmony of all aspects of the self.

Self-esteem is recognized as a powerful motivational force. It is thought to be based on a human need to be valued or to hold a positive self-evaluation. It does not mean exaggerated feelings of superiority, feelings of perfection, or feelings of competency or efficacy. Instead, it is an unexaggerated sense of self-acceptance, a personal liking for one's self, and respect for oneself. When a healthy sense of self-esteem does not exist, adolescents are often appear hostile, bitter, disenchanted, depressed, or alienated from others.

It is often assumed that low self-esteem develops with a disparity between one's self-concept and what one believes one should be. The most common indicators of low self-esteem include feeling depressed, lacking energy, disliking one's appearance, rejecting complements, feeling inadequate, holding unrealistic expectations of oneself, having serious self-doubts, and acting submissive to others' demands. It comes as no surprise that low self-esteem is correlated to a wide range of negative outcomes—e.g., depression, suicidal ideation, eating disorders, delinquency, and adjustment problems, among other things.

Reed Larson and colleagues (1996) completed a series of studies on emotional states among adolescents. Among the many findings his team reports, is that compared to parents, adolescents experience greater extremes of emotion, and wider ranges between the lows and highs of daily emotions. Anyone living with an adolescent knows first hand that adolescents also experience more frequent negative emotions. However, Larson and colleagues also found that adolescents report more frequent positive moods, too. Fortunately, negative moods in adolescents dissipate much faster than they do in adults. This fleeting quality of low to high and rapid diminution of negative emotions gives some credibility to adults' perceptions that adolescents are moody and changeable.

There are many emotional skills or competencies that adolescents must master. When compared with children, adolescents must acquire the ability to (a) regulate intense and vacillating emotions, (b) learn self-soothing techniques, (c) learn how to be aware of their own emotions while not being overwhelmed by them, (d) understand the consequences of emotions for others, (e) distinguish feelings from facts to avoid biased emotion-driven behavior, (f) manage emotional arousal regarding empathy and sympathy, and (g) learn how to manage feelings of love, hate, or indifference in relationships with the opposite sex.

Adolescent Social Development

Contrary to popular media reports, families maintain a strong influence on adolescents. Adolescents turn to their families in time of need and ask parents for advice. Family closeness and attachment remains a major factor in predicting adolescents' adjustment and serves as a buffer against engaging in unhealthy behaviors such as smoking, drinking, using drugs, and leaving school.

To gain greater autonomy and independence, adolescents begin to orient themselves toward their peers. Some believe this orientation is supported more strongly for boys than girls. Nonetheless, peers remain important for both genders, and peer groups serve many important functions for adolescents. Both family and peers serve as reference points for identity formation. Identification with peers promotes modeling for the development of moral reasoning, judgments, and values. This helps youth to differentiate between family and peer judgments on moral or social issues. While parents are major sources of information for decision-making, peer groups provide an important source of information about the world outside of the family. Further, peer groups can provide powerful reinforcement during adolescence through such things as degree of popularity, social status, prestige, and general acceptance. These factors can go a long way in determining and understanding why adolescents behave the way they do.

The nature of peer groups and friendship patterns change during adolescence. In middle childhood to early adolescence, children have friends who are often their own gender and are simply available playmates. Often these friends have similar interests, gender, and are proximally available. In early adolescence there is a strong conformity to peer pressure and expectations and considerable compliance. Indeed, young adolescents are generally preoccupied with peer pressure because of their desire to "belong" or to be a part of a fun group. Unfortunately, peer pressure and conformity can result in engaging in social deviance. At this age it is extremely hard to resist peer pressure. In middle adolescence (roughly 14 to 16 years of age) the peer group often gets larger and there is more gender mix; however, rarely does this group have mixed races or ethnic backgrounds. With age there is less conformity to peer pressure, more tolerance of individual differences, and less focus on appearance or beliefs. By late adolescence, peer groups typically become groups of couples and become the ground for intimacy, sexual experimentation, and dyadic relationships.

Each adolescent will have varying numbers of friends. They all differ in the amount of time they spend with their peer group and how they spend it. Shy or socially unskilled youth tend to have fewer friends. However, their friendships tend to be intense and intimate. As gender role theory suggests, boys tend to engage in more action-oriented activities with friends. Girls tend to spend more intimate time talking and gossiping. Both boys and girls value trustworthiness and loyalty among their friends. Although some research suggests girls value intimacy in a friend more than boys, the difference may actually be due to the definitions used in survey research. Both boys and girls need friends, sexual partners, and companions. Social isolation is associated with a variety of undesirable correlates for boys and girls—including among other things depression, loneliness, poor social skill development, maladjustment, and delinquency, to name a few.

Adolescent Behavioral Development

The majority of adolescents have life experiences that involve no major dysfunction. They go to school, earn decent grades, work part-time or engage in extracurricular activities, attend church or report a sense of spirituality, get along with parents and adults, and mature into productive young adults. Although estimates vary, the general notion is that in each generation about 20% of adolescents have issues serious enough to be classified as dysfunctional. This means, of course, that close to 80%

of teenagers behave in acceptable ways: i.e., parents, teachers, community members, and other teenagers judge these youths as good citizens.

This volume focuses primarily on those 20% or so who manifest serious problems. Elsewhere, I have referred to the concept of a *"window of vulnerability"* that emerges for adolescents when they turn approximately 12 years of age. This window grows larger as the adolescent grows older. Indeed, it gets increasingly wider for adolescents until they are 18 to 21 years of age. It appears that many youth fall out of the window into serious social, emotional, criminal, or physical problems.

There is one concept within normal adolescent development that might account for the emergence of this window of vulnerability. It has to do with the *risk-taking* that is a natural part of growing up. In that experimentation is a foundational process of contemporary adolescence, it is not surprising that it underlies many aspects of shaping identity and learning new decision-making skills. Unfortunately, when taken to extremes, risk-taking can have severe consequences, and is connected to approximately 70% of teenage deaths due to motor-vehicle crashes, homicides, suicide; countless unintentional injuries for boys, and nearly one-half million unplanned pregnancies for teenage girls.

There are a multitude of reasons for risk-taking behavior among adolescents. Many spend unsupervised time after school before parents return home. Some adolescents use this time to experiment with sex, delinquent acts, or using drugs. Most don't. Most adolescents use the time to study, work, do errands, play sports, talk to friends, or engage in other productive behaviors. The few that do engage in risky behavior are often seeking excitement, fun, or novelty. Others engage in risky behaviors to go along with the crowd in response to peer pressure. Still others are likely trying to emulate modeled behavior in movies, TV shows, or songs. It might also be that many fear being teased by their friends; so they are motivated to act out of fear of ridicule.

It can be difficult to determine when risk-taking behaviors move from normal experimentation to problem behavior. There is no absolute rule to determine the boundaries. However, when adolescents begin risk-taking at far too early an age we should be concerned. When the behavior is consistent and ongoing and across multiple contexts we should be alarmed. Further, when a youth engages in a cluster of multiple risk-taking behaviors the window of vulnerability is widened, and interventions should be considered.

As the various chapters in this handbook demonstrate, there are many factors that serve as protective mechanisms that reduce risk-taking behavior. In *Developing Adolescents* (American Psychological Association, 2002) there is an excellent list of protective factors. Among others, a stable positive relationship with at least one adult caregiver, religious or spiritual values, realistic academic expectations, a positive family environment, and an adequate level of emotional intelligence are excellent protective factors that reduce adolescent risk-taking behaviors.

Adolescent Development and Dysfunctional Behavior

The various theoretical perspectives provide some general notions on what aspects of the adolescent experience would suggest dysfunctional features of adolescence. Extrapolations from theoretical perspectives on adolescence suggest that the following factors are indicative of immediate or impending problems for the adolescent:

- excessive anxiety associated with ineffective or extreme defense mechanisms
- extreme intergenerational or familial conflict that weakens emotional bonds or support by the family in general and parents in particular
- failures within the family to recognize the increasing need for autonomy through an absence of psychological or ceremonial events that recognize the maturation of the adolescent
- unsupervised or oversupervised socialization experiences for adolescents
- patterns of early or late onset of puberty
- delayed identity formation, particular in the form of identity diffusion, that results in poor self-regulation functions

Again, extrapolations from the general patterns of adolescent development suggest the following risk factors regarding dysfunctionality for adolescents:

- early pubertal development for girls may introduce them to heterosexual or social experiences they aren't prepared to manage
- late pubertal development for boys may diminish opportunities for experimentation and social activities due to slow physical development
- early-maturing boys may engage in risk-taking behaviors before they are psychological prepared for the consequences
- slow development of formal operational thought can leave a youth with limited cognitive skills and an inability to understand complex social interactions or events
- failure to establish abstract formal operational thinking reduces an adolescent's ability to create the factors associated with a critical habit of mind
- low self-esteem is associated with restrictions in social interactions, need for approval, and susceptibility to negative peer influences
- exaggerated self-esteem may reflect problems in understanding the self and interactions with others
- failure to develop age-appropriate emotional skills is likely to be associated with poor self-regulation and internal problems
- poor social skills are likely to be accompanied by isolation or even rejection by peers
- risk-taking behavior that is unsupervised or extreme is associated with unhealthy outcomes for many youth

When theoretical extrapolations, which help us to understand the psychological and social processes of adolescence, are combined with evidence from research on individual differences and patterns of development for adolescence, a rather large list of features emerges that can be used to predict or understand aspects of dysfunctionality. In reading this handbook one might add to this list of extrapolations in order to expand a personal understanding of social problems during adolescence.

References

Adams, G.R., & Berzonsky, M.D. (Eds). (2003). *Blackwell Handbook of Adolescence*. Blackwell Publishing: Oxford.

Adams, G.R., & Marshall, S.K. (1996). A developmental social psychology of identity: understanding the person in context. *Journal of Adolescence*, 19, 429–422.

American Psychological Association (2002). *Developing Adolescents: A Reference for Professionals*. American Psychological Association: Washington, DC.

Elkind, D. (1985). Egocentrism redux. *Developmental Review, 5*, 218–226.

Gullotta, T.P., Adams, G.R., & Markstrom, C.A. (1999). *The Adolescent Experience* (4th edition). Academic Press: New York.

Keating, D., & Sasse, D.K. (1996). Cognitive socialization in adolescence: critical period for a critical habit of mind. In G.R. Adams, R. Montemayor & T.P. Gullotta (Eds.), *Psychosocial Development During Adolescence: Progress in Developmental Contextualism*. Sage: Thousand Oaks, CA.

Larson, R.W., Richards, M.H., Moneta, G., Holmbeck, G., & Ducket, E. (1996). Changes in adolescents' daily interactions with their families from ages 10 to 18: disengagement and transformation. *Developmental Psychology, 32*, 744–754.

McCall, R.B., Appelbaum, M.J., & Hogarty, P.S. (1973). Developmental changes in mental performance. *Monographs of the Society for Research in Child Development, 38*(3), Serial No. 150, 60–93.

Mead, M. (1970). *Culture and Commitment: A Study of the Generation Gap*. Garden City, NY: Morrow.

Noller, P. (1994). Relationships with parents in adolescence: Process and outcome. In R. Montemayor, G.R. Adams & T.P. Gullotta (Eds.), Personal relationships during adolescence. Advances in Adolescent Development, Vol. 6. Sage Publications: Thousand Oaks, CA.

Romer, D. (Ed.) (2003). *Reducing adolescent risk: toward an integrated approach*. Sage Publications: Thousand Oaks, CA.

Schlegel, A. (1995). *A Cross-Cultural Approach to Adolescence*. Ethos, 23(1), 15–32.

Weisfeld, G.E. (1999) *Evolutionary principles of human adolescence*. New York: 1 Books.

Chapter 2

Understanding Primary Prevention

Thomas P. Gullotta

Why Is Illness Prevention / Health Promotion Important?

Why must illness prevention and health promotion be a central part of any national plan to improve mental health services for its citizens? It is as simple as this: "Preventing an illness from occurring is inherently better than having to treat the illness after its onset" (Surgeon General, 1999, p. 62). The majority of emotional problems are not diseases that can be traced to some microorganism, chemical imbalance, or gene. As the former Surgeon General of the United States C. Evert Koop (1995, p. 760) observed, "diseases are of two types: those we develop inadvertently and those we bring upon ourselves by failure to practice preventive measures. Preventable illness makes up approximately 70% of the burden of illness and associated costs."

As the National Commission on Children (1991, p. 126–127) noted in the report *Beyond Rhetoric: A New American Agenda for Children and Families*,

> Malnourishment, obesity, and the incidence of many illnesses are related to nutritional intake. Sexually transmitted diseases, accidents and injuries, and physical and mental impairments are directly attributable to early, unprotected sexual activity, drug and alcohol use, and delinquent behavior. . . . In fact, better control of a limited number of risk factors . . . could prevent at least 40% of all premature deaths, one-third of all short-term disability cases, and two-thirds of all chronic disability cases. Changes in health behaviors can also reduce medical costs and limit losses in productivity. Illnesses attributable to smoking cost individuals and society more than $65 billion a year. The total cost of alcohol and drug abuse exceeds $110 billion each year.

While some human characteristics like height are highly inheritable, with 90% of a person's height can be attributable to the genetics, other characteristics or behaviors do not have this effect size. As one of the world's most respected geneticists has stated,

> [Genetic research] provides the strongest available evidence for the importance of environmental influence. That is, twin and adoption studies usually find more than half the variance in behavioral development cannot be accounted for by genetic factors. For example, if identical twins are 40% concordant for schizophrenia, as recent studies

suggest, no genetic explanation can account for the 60% discordance between these pairs of genetically identical individuals (Plomin, 1994, p. 28).

Prevention does not yield a utopia. Illness and suffering requiring expert treatment and a full range of interventions from quality accessible out-patient care and medication to in-patient and rehabilitation services must also be provided. But the United States is experiencing an epidemic of suffering that overwhelms and will continue to overwhelm the service capacity of the nation and in the absence of preventive and treatment options impair the life potential of millions of children, youths, and adults. How so?

The Surgeon General's report (1999) supports previously published epidemiological studies suggesting that in any given year one in five citizens will experience a mental disorder. Of this number roughly 15% will experience a co-occurring alcohol or other drug-use disorder. With an estimated United States population of 300,000,000 individuals, this means that roughly 60,000,000 individuals are in need of help each year. Yet, the treatment and rehabilitation capacity of the United States is but a small fraction of this number. Each year millions of seriously ill individuals struggle without the necessary help to address problems that interfere with their ability to lead productive lives. If prevention were to reduce this population by only 20%, or 12,000,000 cases a year, it would have exceeded the total treatment capacity of the United States for any given year. Given that not all clinical interventions are either successful or are directed at those defined as most seriously ill, the cost-benefit ratio of prevention becomes readily apparent (Durlak & Wells, 1997; Yodanis & Godenzi, 2003). But even more important than prevention's favorable cost-benefit ratio is that millions of children and adults would avoid unnecessary suffering.

What is Primary Prevention?

Briefly put, prevention involves universal, selective, and indicated actions ". . . that protect existing states of health . . . promote psychosocial wellness and prevent . . . problems" (Bloom & Gullotta, 2003, p. 13). What does promoting health and psychosocial wellness mean? It means taking actions that encourage resiliency, coping, adaptation, and developing human social capital. What does preventing illness mean? This refers to reducing, modifying, and avoiding the risks known to foster ill health.

The terms *universal, selective,* and *indicated* are borrowed from Gordon's (1983) work as adopted by the Institute of Medicine (Mrazek & Haggerty, 1994) to describe the domain for preventive interventions. *Universal* is synonymous with the word *all.* For example, to reduce the incidence of tooth decay many communities add fluoride to their public water supplies. Thus everyone who drinks from that water supply is a recipient of this intervention known to reduce tooth decay. Childhood immunizations for polio and other crippling illnesses and automatically deploying car airbags are other examples of universal preventive interventions.

A *selective* intervention focuses more narrowly on populations at risk. In this instance, epidemiological evidence exists to suggest that a group of people is at higher than average risk for developing a disorder. To prevent that disorder and to promote the health of that group, interventions are offered. To illustrate, school teachers, who as a population have high contact with young people with runny noses, might be encouraged to receive flu shots to avoid influenza, an illness that peaks during the school year.

An *indicated* intervention draws on epidemiological evidence, but in this instance the risk for the group in question is considered very high. To use the flu shot example again, a teacher who is elderly and has heart disease would move from the selected group into an indicated group. Notice that in each instance the intervention for health promotion and illness prevention is occurring before the onset of disease. Intervention is not focused on individuals, but on entire populations, and is information driven. That is, risk determines need for intervention exposure. The purpose of the intervention is to prevent the development of the illness or disorder by either strengthening the health of the individual (the flu shot) or by preventing its onset (the deployment of the airbag).

Stress Theory

Stress theory offers a useful theoretical framework for designing efforts to reduce risk and promote health in individuals, families, and larger groups. A simple definition of stress is any change in life. Thus, the life events that mark off the life cycle carry with them positive stress (eustress) and negative stress (distress). Life can be filled with boredom and a lack of challenge (hypostress), or it can be filled with excessive demands on time, labor, and energy. These stressful situations mark transition points that, if coped with successfully, facilitate a healthier individual, family, and group environment.

An initial understanding of how stress affects organisms was developed Cannon (1939) and Selye (1982). Selye's laboratory work with animals found that stress-producing agents (called stressors) create a reaction that Selye called the general adaptation syndrome. When stress exceeds some threshold, Seyle found, laboratory animals enter into a stage of alarm. During this stage the organism is on alert, calling on its defensive systems to combat the stressor. The period during which the body fights the noxious stressor is called the stage of resistance. If the body cannot defeat the noxious stressor, it enters the stage of exhaustion. Unable to overcome the damaging virus, bacterium, or other adverse stimulus, the body surrenders to the stressor and expires.

The ABCX Stress Model

Of the stress models, Hill's (1949, 1958) *ABCX* model is particularly useful for preventive action as it identifies three areas for intervention. While recent theoretical work has elaborated on Hill's writings (the double *ABCX* model; see McCubbin & Patterson, 1982), it remains a very viable explanation with practical application on its own. In this model the letter *A* represents some event that brings discomfort, such as death of a loved one, a divorce, or school failure. *B* stands for the internal and external resources the person can use to fight the discomfort—wealth, friends, level of self-esteem, internal locus of control, coping abilities, and so on. *C* is the meaning the individual, family, or group attaches to the event. *X* is the crisis. Together *A*, *B*, and *C* result in *X*. That is, the magnitude of the crisis, its duration, and the individual's or family's level of reorganization after the crisis are determined by the sum of *A* (the event) + *C* (its meaning) − *B* (the available resources).

The second part of Hill's model predicts how most individuals or groups will react in a crisis. The crisis (X) sends the individual into a period of disorganization in which the group marshals its resources to meet the crisis. The angle of recovery reflects the time necessary for the group to find a solution to its distress; the level of reorganization reflects the group's success in returning to a pre-crisis state.

Now let's take a closer look at the *ABCX* model by examining its components individually.

A, the stressor. *A*, the event that causes discomfort, can also be called the "stressor." Stressors are events "of sufficient magnitude to bring about change in the family system" (McCubbin et al., 1980, p. 857). In line with our earlier definition of stress as any change in life, a stressor may be either a good or a bad event.

Life is filled with stressors. Some of these are sudden changes, such as an unexpected relocation or death of a loved one. Others can be more insidious, slowly sapping an individual's energy over a period of years, such as poverty, alcoholism, or chronic physical or emotional illness. Still others mark the flow of life. These include the addition of family members, entry into school, adolescence, dissatisfaction over a marriage, possibly divorce and remarriage, and the loss of family members.

C, the meaning. *C* in Hill's model represents the meaning the person, family, or group attaches to the event. Events are not stressors unless they are perceived to be, and the degree of positive or negative disruption is again determined by the individual. Suppose a job promotion has been offered to a family member. At first glance this would seem to be a positive event for the family, but it may not be. It may require the promoted member's extended absence from the home to meet increased job responsibilities, or it may mean a move to a new community. A promotion may then become a negative event in this family's life and acquire the status of crisis.

B, resources. The *B* in Hill's *ABCX* equation stands for the strengths that the individual, family, or group calls on in time of need. These *B* factors include personal resources, a family system's internal resources, social support, and coping. Personal resources include humor, religious faith, financial resources, self-respect, and an internal locus of control.

An individual's, family's or group's internal resources are its integrative abilities. Integration refers to the degree of unity existing in the family or group. Where there are common interests, a common agenda for the future, and affection for one another, there is a high degree of integration. Social support involves people outside the family or group who, in time of need, lend their strength to the family or group. This is accomplished by helping the family or group to feel loved, cared for, valued, and worthy, and by communicating to the individual, family, or group that it belongs.

The last factor, coping, involves the adaptive ways families use their *B* resources to handle a crisis. A family's adaptive capability is judged by its ability to mobilize its resources to confront a challenge and adjust to overcome that challenge.

X, the crisis. The *X* in Hill's model represents the state of disorganization after a crisis-producing event. There are two types of crisis events. The first are called developmental or normative crises and are considered a normal part of living life. The birth of a child, a child's entry into school, entry into adolescence, and the death of an aged family member are illustrations of normative crises. These events confront the individual with developmental tasks that, if coped with successfully, move the person on to another life stage. The second type of crisis is called situational or catastrophic. These events affect only some individuals, groups, or families and are tragic events. They may be circumstances that occur over time like living in a violent household or may be sudden like a close sibling dying in an automobile accident.

Primary Prevention Has Technologies

To achieve illness prevention and health promotion, prevention uses four technologies. They are overlapping and in and of themselves rarely effective. However, when they are combined, they prevent illness and promote health.

The first technology is **education**. The most often used of all prevention's technologies, alone it rarely, if ever, is effective. The reason for this is that while education increases knowledge, only occasionally does it affect attitudes, and it almost never changes behavior. Thus, the tobacco user will acknowledge the hazards of tobacco use and might wish to give up the habit, but rarely acts on the motivation. This said, education nevertheless plays an important role in health promotion and illness prevention in concert with other technologies.

Education can take one of three forms. The first is **public information**. This can be found on the side of a cigarette package, an alcohol beverage bottle, or on the visor of an automobile. Information can be provided by means of print, radio, internet, television, or film. It can be read, spoken, sung, or acted. In all instances the intention is to increase knowledge about a given subject and offer ways to handle that subject that promotes health or prevents illness.

A more specific form of education is **anticipatory guidance**. In this case, information is used to educate a group prior to some expected event. Drawing on the folk wisdom that to be forewarned is to be forearmed, the group will be better prepared to cope with the circumstances and adapt to the demands the event may place on them. Adaptation may be as simple as decreasing speed and braking as a traffic signal turns from yellow to red to heeding a weather report and packing sun protectorant to the beach, to childbirth preparation classes, children's visits to hospitals prior to elective surgery, and preretirement planning.

Education's third form is found in the **personal self-management** of behavior. In this instance, the individual or group learns how to control emotional, neurological, and physical aspects of their behavior. The methods to achieve this outcome range from yoga, transcendental meditation, and biofeedback to cognitive behavioral approaches.

Prevention's second tool is the promotion of **social competency**. To be **socially competent requires that one belong to a group, that the group value the membership of the individual, and that the individual make a meaningful contribution to the group's existence**. Socially competent people tend to possess the following individual characteristics: a positive sense of self-esteem, an internal locus of control, a sense of mastery or self-concept of ability, and an interest beyond themselves that extends to a larger group. Thus, a feedback loop is established between belonging, valuing, contributing, and individual characteristics that is self-perpetuating.

Effect prevention programs contain exercises aimed at nurturing these individual characteristics, which are demonstrated in the ways in which groups embrace and value their members, and afford them opportunities to contribute to the welfare and well-being of the group. This meaningful contribution can entail being the elected spokesperson for a group, becoming a literacy tutor, or donating blood. This value to the group can be that of the philanthropist or of the soup kitchen volunteer. This belonging is reflected in hundreds of ways from flags hung from homes, draped on rear view car mirrors, and worn on clothing to songs and stories that celebrate the group's existence. To achieve the solidarity that is the essence of social competency requires not only education but also prevention's next technology.

Prevention's third technology is "**natural caregiving**," which is a term used to draw a distinction between the services offered by mental health professionals and those afforded by others. Natural caregiving takes three different forms. The first is the **mutual self-help group** in which individuals are drawn together by some common experience. This experience may be the expected death of a loved one (hospice), a personal problem behavior like alcoholism (Alcoholics Anonymous), or a challenging behavior of another (attention-deficit/hyperactivity disorder parent's group). In the self-help group members are both caregivers and care-receivers. Reliance is not on a professional but on each other. Pathology is not the governing dynamic but rather navigating through life's swamp with a companion who knows the stress the affected individual is experiencing. By acknowledging the failures celebrating the small successes, and relying on each other for support and advice, self-help group members discover competency—the competency that goes with belonging, with being valued, and with being a contributing member.

The phrase "**indigenous trained caregiver**" describes the second form of natural caregiving that individuals turn to in time of need. While not trained as mental health professionals, people such as ministers, teachers, and police officers provide advice, comfort, and support that enables many in society to lead healthy and productive lives.

In times of need, individuals turn first to friends and loved ones, then to trained indigenous caregivers. Why? Because the power of a single caring relationship over time is both nurturing and healing. As with other forms of caregiving, **indigenous caregiving** involves behaviors such as the sharing of knowledge, the sharing of experiences, compassionate understanding, companionship, and, when necessary, confrontation (Bloom, 1996; Cowen, 1982). The indigenous caregiver accepts responsibility for her or his life and ideally invests in the life (health) of at least one other person.

Prevention's fourth technology is its most powerful. **Community Organization and Systems Interventions** (COSI) are concerned with the promotion of a community's social capital. That is, how does a community motivate its members to participate actively in the process of governance and how are inequalities are addressed? COSI addresses these issues in three ways. The first is **community development** and takes a variety of forms: the neighborhood civic association formed to be a local voice on zoning issues; the local recreation league created to afford after-school opportunities; and the neighborhood watch started to deter crime are but three examples. In each example, a group of people with concerns about property, youth activities, or crime prevention draw together and act to express their concerns and develop solutions in response to those concerns.

The second form COSI takes is **systems intervention**. The assumption is that every institution has dysfunctional elements within it that contribute to the needless suffering of individuals in society. Identifying those dysfunctional elements and correcting them is the purpose of this form of COSI. To illustrate, Tadmor (2003) describes her efforts to reform the medical practices used for treating children in one hospital. Policies and procedures that harmed children like restraining them to force compliance with the treatment regimen and separating them from parents during the treatment process were identified as dysfunctional and subsequently changed. For the outsider, while the identification of these dysfunctional practices might appear obvious, they are not necessarily evident to individuals within the system. Institutions—whether schools, hospitals, social service agencies, child care centers, or larger entities like child protective services and other state agencies—develop unique internal cultures very removed from those of society at large. Often, elements of these internal cultures are dysfunctional and needing change. This change rarely occurs without external COSI pressure.

The final form that Community Organization and Systems Intervention takes is **legislative change and judicial action**. Drawing on the earlier illustration of the difficulty that accompanies institutional change, it should be remembered that no legislation or judicial action benefits all. In these legislative and judicial contests, there are winners and losers. For example, while a universal family leave policy may be good for employees needing to care for loved ones, for the employer preserving a job for someone who may not return to work, the policy can be detrimental to business. While advocating civil rights legislation in the 1960s, it was Lyndon Johnson who observed that this just action would break the hold of the Democratic Party on the South, and it did. While offering a limited prescription benefit to Social Security recipients enables them to stretch their retirement savings, without a corresponding tax increase it hastens the eventual bankruptcy of the Social Security program.

This last form of COSI is a battleground where special interests strive to dominate the field. Over time and with growing public impatience, seat belt laws do become enacted. Wetlands are protected from development. Clean air standards are enacted. Tobacco laws restricting youth's access to cigarettes and other tobacco products are passed. Interestingly, it is often through the efforts of organizations like MADD and the NAACP, whose origins reflect many of the characteristics of self-help groups, that these laws capable of correcting injustice and improving public health are passed.

Thus, we come to see that when prevention's technology is fully utilized, a circle is completed. Education informs. Natural caregiving unites. Social competency enables, and COSI serves as a means to achieve community change.

Implementing Preventive/Health Promotion Interventions

Healthy communities are achieved from within. That is, the members of a community as small as a person or as large as the world must want change. In that desire for change a search for new ideas leading to new practices eventually leading to new behavior is undertaken. At times that search can be conducted without assistance; one or more community leaders may offer ideas that catch the imagination of the larger group and with group support transform those ideas into reality.

At other times assistance is necessary. This assistance can take one of three forms. The least intrusive form is **consultation**. Here, the advisor studies a program, a situation, a condition, or a behavior and offers advice. In its most elemental form, this consultative advice may be taken in whole, in part, or not at all. An illustration of this form of involvement is the architect who is asked to draw preliminary plans for a structure. After interviewing the client, visiting the site, and speaking with local zoning officials, this person renders a plan which may be accepted, modified, or rejected. The architect's involvement with the client ceases with the completion of the assigned task.

A higher level of involvement is **collaboration**. Here, the advisor has a personal stake in bringing the given advice to fruition. A junior partner in the enterprise, the advisor now argues his case and actively works for change. Imagine a political consultant in this instance. A person working for the election of a candidate, this advisor develops a position for the candidate, obtains the candidate's approval and then champions that position with the candidate and others in the campaign. It is important to note again that the collaborator is not the leader of the group but a trusted actively involved participant.

The highest level of involvement is **coaching**. In this instance the advisor is empowered to work with the client to bring about the desired change. Consider the personal trainer. This is a person who instructs the client in how to exercise, how long the exercise period will last, and the type of exercise to be engaged in. In some settings, like a spa, this level of control extends to control over daily activities, the types of food consumed, even when one rises and when the day ends. With coaching, the client voluntarily surrenders a part of their control to achieve the desired end. Yet, even in this instance, the individual being coached retains the power to dismiss the coach. Thus, while the coach can use a wide range of motivational techniques to achieve change, the ultimate authority remains not with the coach but with the person, institution, or community.

Conditions for Successful Prevention Activities

The challenge facing preventionists is that their interventions are frequently afterthoughts. When the community's discomfort with an issue reaches widespread public expression, it reacts with a pledge and a program. Both tend to be short-lived. Rather than the layering approach of adding an additional curriculum, the successful preventive intervention teaches a set of skills that can be used in multiple settings for multiple purposes.

New behaviors develop over time and require practice to be learned. Even when individuals are immersed in information, and some knowledge is retained, retention is measured in days—perhaps weeks—rarely in months or years; and any unfamiliar skill requires repeated practice in a variety of settings and circumstances in order to improve overall performance.

New behaviors are best learned in small groups. Small groups afford the opportunity for natural caregiving to occur, for competencies to be nurtured, and change agendas to be developed.

New behaviors are best learned by experiences that are lived through. Experiential learning offers opportunities to manipulate the learning experience, to vary its content, and to alter its intensity and duration. It allows the learner to interpret the information across a variety of intelligences (Gardner, 1993) best suited to the learner.

Finally, new behaviors need nurturance. Unless supported by the environment, new skills will rapidly disappear. Simply put, BE WANTED!

References

Bloom, M. (1996). *Primary Prevention Practices*. Thousand Oaks, CA: Sage.

Bloom, M. & Gullotta, T.P. (2003). Evolving definitions of primary prevention. In T.P. Gullotta & M. Bloom (Eds.), *Encyclopedia of Primary Prevention and Health Promotion*. New York: Kluwer Academic Press.

Cannon, W.B. (1939). *The Wisdom of the Body*. New York: Norton.

Cowen, E.L. (1982). Help is where you find it: Four informal helping groups. *American Psychologist, 37*, 385–395.

Durlak, J.A., & Wells, A.M. (1997). Primary prevention mental health programs for children and adolescents: A meta-analytic review. *American Journal of Community Psychology, 25*, 115–152.

Gardner, H. (1993). *The Multiple Intelligences: The Theory in Practice*. New York: Basic Books.

Gordon, R. (1983). An operational classification of disease prevention. In J.A. Steinberg & M.M. Silverman (Eds.), *Preventing Mental Disorders*. Rockville, MD: Department of Health and Human Services.

Hill, R. (1949). *Families Under Stress*. New York: Harper and Row.

Hill, R. (1958). Social stresses on the family. *Social Casework, 34*, 139–150.

Koop, C.E. (1995). A personal role in health care reform. *American Journal of Public Health, 85* (6), 759–760.

McCubbin, H.I., Joy, C.B., Cauble, A.E., Comeau, J.K., Patterson, J.M., & Needle, R.H. (1980). Family stress and coping: a decade review. *Journal of Marriage and the Family, 42*, 855–871.

McCubbin, H.I., and Patterson, J.M. (1982). Family adaptation to crises. In H.I. McCubbin, A.E. Cauble and J.M. Patterson (Eds.), *Family Stress, Coping, and Social Support*. Springfield, IL: Thomas.

Mrazek, P.J. & Haggerty, R.J. (Eds.). (1994). *Reducing Risks for Mental Disorders: Frontiers for Preventive Interventions*. Washington, DC: National Academy Press.

National Commission on Children (1991). *Beyond Rhetoric: A New American Agenda for Children and Families*. Washington, DC: U.S. Government Printing Office.

Plomin, R. (1994). *Genetics and Experience*. Thousand Oaks, CA: Sage.

Selye, H.A. (1982). History and present status of the stress concept. In L. Goldberger & S. Breznitz (Eds.), *Handbook of Stress*. New York: Free Press.

Tadmor, C.S. (2003). Perceived personal control. In T.P. Gullotta & M. Bloom (Eds.), *Encyclopedia of Primary Prevention and Health Promotion*. New York: Kluwer Academic Press.

Surgeon General (1999). *Mental Health: A Report of the Surgeon General*. Washington, DC: National Institute of Mental Health.

Yodanis, C., & Godenzi, A. (2003). Cost benefit analysis. In T.P. Gullotta & M. Bloom (Eds.), *Encyclopedia of Primary Prevention and Health Promotion*. New York: Kluwer Academic Press.

Chapter 3

Family Influences on Adolescent Development

Gary W. Peterson

Introduction

The topic "family influences on adolescent development" often has conjured up popular images in western societies of emotional turmoil, conflict, and rebellion by the young in reference to their parents. Fueled by dated theories and media stereotypes, parent–adolescent turmoil was supposed to be a normal occurrence triggered, in part, by raging hormones, dramatic physiological changes, re-emerging sexual impulses, and rapidly changing social expectations for the young. Throughout much of the past century, adolescence was thought to be a developmental stage characterized by "storm and stress," declining family influences, and a growing separation from parents (Arnett, 1999; Blos, 1979; Davis, 1960; Freud, 1969; Hall, 1904). In marked contrast, much less attention was focused, until recent decades, on the development of adaptive qualities, such as how social competence is fostered in adolescents through their socialization experiences within families (Peterson & Leigh, 1990; Peterson & Bush, 2003).

Although such popular images of youthful turmoil persist today, much of the current research on adolescent development within families fails to support the view that parent–youth relationships chronically involve severe conflict and dramatic growth in emotional distance. For most youth, the family remains the primary arena of social influence and security, both for fostering positive and negative consequences. Although a significant minority of adolescents certainly do experience a persistent pattern of troubled family relationships (Arnett, 1999), for the majority, a more balanced and positive view prevails about the influence of home life in adolescent development. In fact, a significant majority of adolescents report feeling close to their parents, value their parents' opinions, believe that their parents love and care for them, respect their parents as authority figures, and wish to be like them (Allen & Land, 1999; Gecas & Seff, 1990; Moore, Chalk, Scarpa, & Vandivere, 2002). Adolescents tend to agree with their parents on attitudes toward work, occupational and educational goals, as well as values based in particular religious, moral, ideological, and political belief systems. Current research indicates that differences of opinion are greater *among adolescents* than *between teenagers* and their parents (Gecas & Seff, 1990; Offer & Schonert-Reichl, 1992; Wyatt & Carlo, 2002).

The purpose of this chapter, in turn, is to provide an overview of the most prominent aspects of diverse family forms that influence the development of both prosocial and problematic outcomes by adolescents. Based on current social science research and theory, a complex array of family structural variations (i.e., family socioeconomic standing, poverty, maternal employment, divorce, remarriage, and the presence of siblings), parental styles, dimensions of parental behavior, parent–adolescent conflict, and interparental (or marital) have been identified as some of the factors that influence adolescent development. Before we delineate these influences, the process of socialization within families, the concept of family system, and the nature of socialized outcomes in the young (i.e., adolescent social competence or problem behaviors) will be described.

Socialization in Families

From the perspective of the social sciences, families influence adolescents through the socialization process—or the social dynamics that make the young capable of participating in interpersonal relationships and through which a society reproduces itself (Elkin & Handel, 1988). Socialization is a complex, multidirectional process involving the family, as perhaps the most important source of influence, but also involving all the major institutions and social settings in which individuals (i.e., adolescents) have direct or indirect experiences (e.g., religious institutions, work settings, schools, the mass media, political and governmental institutions, as well as neighborhoods and communities). A pattern of dynamic interaction exists between developing adolescents and their social environments, which includes influential factors from different levels of ecological analysis at the biological, physical, psychological, and sociocultural levels (Bronfenbrenner, 1979, 1994; Lerner, 2002).

Traditional conceptions of socialization within the family relationship are dominated by the idea that the young must be *influenced* by parents and other family members to internalize and become responsive to societal expectations (Inkeles, 1968; Parsons & Bales, 1955). Central components of this process within families are the socialization strategies (e.g., parental styles and behaviors) used by parents to encourage (or discourage) the young to participate effectively (or ineffectively) in a society's major institutions and inhibit the development of undesirable behavior. Although this is certainly true in part, numerous observers have countered with the idea that too much emphasis has been placed on how adolescents are shaped and guided by parents (and other social agents) to become members of society. According to this *deterministic* or *social mold* conception of socialization (Kuczynski, 2003; Peterson & Hann, 1999), the young are conceptualized primarily as passive recipients of parental influence (or the influence of other social agents). For a variety of reasons, in turn, the social mold perspective continues to dominate research concerned with studying adolescents in the context of their family relationships. Continued dominance of deterministic models of parent–adolescent research is based, in part, on the pragmatic or heuristic needs of scientific methodologies to focus on limited aspects of the social context within any particular study. Consequently, the parent–adolescent literature should be read with the awareness that current conceptions of socialization are substantially more complex than what is captured in the methodologies of most research studies.

A more accurate view of socialization recognizes that adolescents, to some degree, are initiated into society by parents, but also that youth are active participants in this social discourse. Instead of being unidirectional in nature, parent–youth socialization is conceptualized as being at least a bidirectional, if not a more complex, process (Corsaro, 1997; Kuczynski, 2003; Peterson & Hann, 1999). Socialization is a complex reciprocal or even multidirectional process between active organisms and a variety of responsive, encompassing contexts. Adolescents both influence and are influenced by many social agents in their interpersonal (e.g., family) environment. Neither specific kinds of socialization experiences, such as those within the family, nor specific biological factors, such as genetic influences, can be isolated as sole factors that drive development. Instead, a combination of youthful socialization, genetic, and maturational factors form the overall structure of adolescent development (Lerner, 2002).

The socialized adolescent, therefore, emerges from social interaction within families, not simply by internalizing norms and conforming to society, but in terms of responses shaped by meanings, individual interpretations, negotiations with others, and shared experiences (Corsaro, 1997; Kuczynski, 2003; Peterson & Hann, 1999). Parent–youth socialization is a dialectical process in which continuity, creativity, and change are complementary components of a larger whole (Kuczynski, 2003; Peterson, 1995). Consequently, the parent–adolescent relationship is a process of continuity and change in which both partners increasingly share meanings, but are always changing in respect to each other.

Adolescent Social Competence and Problem Behavior: Outcomes of Socialization

Despite more complex conceptions of socialization, the oldest and still dominant tradition of parent–adolescent research is the *parental influence perspective*, which explores the extent to which parental styles, behaviors, and characteristics contribute to various social-psychological qualities in the young. From this perspective, parents are conveyors of social reality who "mold" or "shape" the young into functional or deviant participants in society (Maccoby & Martin, 1983; Peterson & Bush, 2003; Peterson & Hann, 1999; Peterson & Rollins, 1987; Rollins & Thomas, 1979). From this perspective, parents are social agents who are teachers of social norms, models of behavior, managers of conduct, and providers of emotional support. Despite the growth of more complex theories of socialization, parental influence perspectives persist, in part, due to scientific requirements for parsimony and methodological constraints.

Before describing some of the ways parents and families influence adolescents, it is important to consider the goals or social outcomes that parents either seek to foster or inhibit in the young. Along these lines, it is proposed that most parents desire to instill *social competence* in their young by expecting them to adopt normative social behaviors that are adaptive in relationships with parents, peers, and other interpersonal relationships (Bloom, 1990; Gillespie, 2003; Peterson & Leigh, 1990;

Peterson & Bush, 2003). A general definition of social competence is a set of attributes or psychological resources that help adolescents adapt to their social circumstances and cope successfully with everyday life sufficiently to ward off problematic behavior (i.e., externalizing and internalizing behavior) (Baumrind, 1991; Peterson & Bush, 2003). Recent conceptions of social competence (i.e., particularly in European American cultures) identify some of its subdimensions as (1) a balance between autonomy and connectedness in reference to parents (and others), (2) an achievement orientation, (3) psychological or cognitive resources (e.g., self-esteem, identity achievement, and problem-solving skills), and (4) social skills with peers and other interpersonal relationships.

These aspects of social competence and the family circumstances that foster such outcomes are sources of social-psychological *resilience* that assist adolescents in successfully adapting to and coping with challenges that can lead to risky behavior (Gillespie, 2003; Hauser, 1999; Hawkins, Catalano, & Miller, 1992). Consequently, the inverse of social competence is *risk* or *problem* behavior, conceptualized here as either *internalizing* or *externalizing* attributes. Internalizing attributes are those outcomes in which the difficulties of adolescents become evident due to psychological disturbances that focus on the self (e.g., depression, suicidal thoughts, and eating disorders). Externalizing attributes, on the other hand, are based on psychological difficulties that take the form of "acting out" against society (e.g., violent behavior, delinquent behavior, substance abuse, conduct disorders in school) (Meyer, 2003). Extensive involvement in externalizing and internalizing behavior, or the inverse of social competence, can be a major obstacle to developmental progress during adolescence and early adulthood.

Most if not all cultures probably emphasize the general dimensions of social competence (i.e., balancing autonomy and connectedness, achievement, psychological resources, and social skills) to some degree in the socialization process. However, the specific manner in which each dimension of social competence is emphasized and resolved in reference to specific content within each culture may vary substantially. This is particularly true in the manner that socialization values focus on fostering either individual interests (i.e., individualism) or those of the social group (i.e., collectivism) or some combination of two (Arnett, 1995; Kagitcibasi, 1996). European American families with adolescents, for example, may value individualism through the promotion of autonomy rather than by emphasizing family connections, achievement as an expression of self-interest, conceptions of the self (e.g., self-esteem) rooted in the ideals of privacy and personal uniqueness, as well as by encouraging the development of assertive social skills to foster personal advancement. In contrast, families from non-western societies and specific ethnic groups within the United States (e.g., Hispanic American and Asian American families) may emphasize family connections over individual autonomy, personal achievement that serves group interests, self-conceptions based on relationships with others, and social skills emphasizing cohesive relationships with others. Some have proposed, in turn, that these seemingly opposite value orientations (i.e., individualism and collectivism) can be complementary not contradictory outcomes. Most cultures and ethnic groups strike some form of unique balance between these general belief systems as part of defining social competence within particular constructions of cultural reality (Arnett, 1995; Kagitcibasi, 1996; Peterson, 1995).

The Family System and Adolescents

A general means of conceptualizing the role of adolescents within families is that most are members of family *systems*, though these environments are substantially varied in structure, process, and socioeconomic resources. An initial way of recognizing how adolescents engage in relationships with other family members is to understand that family systems differentially accommodate or inhibit the adaptive development of adolescents (P. Minuchin, 2002).

Highlighting the *systemic* qualities of domestic life entails that family systems are complex social entities whose members (e.g., adolescents, parents, and siblings) are tied together as part of a larger relationship whole (Bodman & Peterson, 1995; Broderick, 1993). Consequently, all elements of the family system are interrelated through dynamic, mutual, and circular processes that link together the constituent individuals and relationships within families. Although each family is characterized by relationship qualities that generalize throughout the system, *subsystems* also exist within the larger family (e.g., the parent–child relationship or the marital relationship).

Part of a family's systemic qualities results from patterns of communication that are unique to each family, define the nature of their relationships with each other, and provide structure to their associations through redundant patterns of information exchange (Bodman & Peterson, 1995). A systems view of family relationships involving adolescents is often concerned with the degree of openness in information exchange that occurs between parents and their young. Interest in such communication patterns is stimulated by the belief that open communication between parents and adolescents will foster closer ties, help to prevent or solve problems, assist parents and teenagers to manage conflict, and allow parents and adolescents to negotiate adaptive developmental change (Noller, 1994).

Much of the time, families seek to provide stable environments, common routines, a sense of order, and daily security for the young. Despite this emphasis on stability, however, established family communication patterns must become challenged from time to time so that the family system and its members can develop. An important period of family change and adjustment occurs when children enter the stage of adolescence and begin making progress toward adulthood. Parents and adolescents must undergo challenging shifts in the established ways of dealing with each other (Carter & McGoldrick, 1999) and allow adolescents more complex social relationships beyond the family (e.g., with peers), more personal decision-making and autonomy, as well as expanded freedom for identity exploration. At the same time, parents of adolescents must continue to supervise, protect, communicate with, and provide guidance to diminish the likelihood that teenagers will become involved in problem behaviors (Bodman & Peterson, 1995; Peterson & Bush, 2003).

Family systems must strike a balance between allowing change that encourages greater individual competence, while maintaining stable connections that prevent teenagers from drifting into deviant behavior (Peterson, Bush & Supple, 1999). As this period of development progresses, parents and adolescents must gradually renegotiate (or change) their relationships from one in which parents are clearly in charge toward new arrangements in which greater equality, more autonomy, and more self-responsibility are granted to adolescents. The most common approach in western cultures, therefore, is one that strikes a middle ground between excessively controlling teenagers and granting too much autonomy before adolescents are capable of handling this responsibility (Silverberg & Gondoli, 1996). A delicate balance between being flexible and being firmly in control is needed so that greater autonomy can be granted within an atmosphere of standards, limits, and guidance (Carter & McGoldrick, 1999; Peterson, Madden-Derdich & Leonard, 2000). From the standpoint of the larger family system, such complicated negotiation processes can be conceptualized as "differentiation," or the degree to which family systems tolerate individuality and difference along with accommodating intimacy and belongingness (Anderson & Sabatelli, 1990; Bartle-Haring, Kenny & Gavazzi, 1999).

Another notable aspect of the family system is the construct "boundary" or the conceptual mechanism used to demarcate the difference between subsystems within families. Boundaries are social mechanisms that define how relationships between mothers and fathers are expected to function in reference to their adolescent sons and daughters (Day, 1995; S. Minuchin, 1974). Boundaries vary widely as to how firmly they maintain parental authority, but many observers believe effective parent–adolescent boundaries in western culture are those that maintain the position of parents as the primary authority figures in their relationships with adolescents. However, such "executive" positions of parents should be tempered by being open to mutual influence, allow two-way expressions of affection, be reasonably tolerant of mutual efforts to exercise control, and be selectively open to change. Such a partially open boundary emphasizes the importance of both parents having shared policies, consistent rules, and similar parenting approaches in reference to the young (Bodman & Peterson, 1995, S. Minuchin, 1974).

Family Structural Variation

Despite extensive focus on the socialization process (i.e., internal family process, relationship, and social psychological dimensions) within families, continuing interest exists in examining how variations in family structure contribute to adolescent development. Attention to family structure, in turn, refers to the formal or external patterns of family life such as whether parents are married, whether a biological relationship exists between parents and children, the number of members in families (e.g., adults, children, and siblings) in families, and the location of families in the larger socioeconomic structure of society (Furstenberg, 2000). Structural variation in families implies that important role adjustments must occur within families to accommodate such things as maternal employment, divorce, step-parenting, and the presence of siblings.

Although debate continues, growing evidence indicates that only modest if any differences in youthful social and personality outcomes can be *directly* traced to structural variations per se. In fact, particular structural effects that do exist often have *indirect* influences on adolescent development that are conveyed through specific family process and social-psychological variables (e.g., parental behavior or patterns of communication) that are brought directly to bear on adolescents (Demo & Cox, 2000; Teachman, 2000; Wilson, Peterson, & Wilson, 1993). Another way of viewing this issue is that distinguishing between "structure" and "process" in families may be simply a somewhat artificial distinction. The logic here is that variations within family structure may, indeed, increase the probability that certain relationship environments will either exist or not exist within families. In fact, many relationship and social psychological issues may either be present, absent, or differ substantially, depending on the particular kind of family structure variation that exists (e.g, the presence and number of siblings, the presence or absence of fathers in families).

Family Socioeconomic Standing (SES)

An example of such *indirect* effects is the influence of a family's socioeconomic standing on parenting processes, which, in turn, may have influence on dimensions of adolescent social competence or problem behavior (Gecas, 1979; Kohn, 1977; Kohn & Schooler, 1983). The roots of socioeconomic variations in child-rearing are the different conditions of life (e.g., in the workplace, school, or neighborhood) experienced by parents of particular SES levels. Lower socioeconomic status is commonly associated with diminished resources for youthful achievement, less likelihood of adjusting to schools, unemployment for parents, less desirable work conditions, poor nutrition, deficient health care, higher rates of emotional distress, unsafe neighborhoods, and greater opportunities for involvement in risk behaviors (McLoyd, 1998). Moreover, despite a booming economy in the 1990s, the number of children and adolescents who live in severely distressed neighborhoods increased significantly between 1990 and 2000 (O'Hare & Mather, 2003). Consequently, parents of different socioeconomic status often have distinctive conditions of life as well as values and priorities that reflect these circumstances. These values and priorities, in turn, are used by parents to place demands on the young for forms of social competence that will be adaptive for the social world as they experience it. For example, blue-collar and lower SES parents seem more inclined than white-collar parents to emphasize obedience and conformity with the young and to use more direct, coercive forms of discipline. In contrast, white-collar parents tend to use more moderate, rational forms of control as a means of encouraging such attributes as autonomy, self-control, and individual achievement (Gecas, 1979; Peterson & Hann, 1999; Peterson & Rollins, 1987).

Family socioeconomic issues that may influence adolescent development (i.e., maternal employment, maintenance of family income, and economic distress) illustrate how family structural linkages to the larger economic system may have consequences for adolescent development through the mediating influences of parent-youth relationships. Poverty, economic distress, and the need to maintain family income persist as challenges that families must address to avoid adverse consequences for the well-being of parents, their relationships with youth, and the developmental health of the young. An important aspect of such socioeconomic challenges has been the increasing trend for mothers to enter the labor force in response to economic circumstances that require more than one family income to maintain family SES. This trend is particularly prominent in families with children in middle childhood and adolescence and has increased as the normative American family has changed from the "nuclear" or two-parent family (i.e., both parents are married and biologically related to the children/adolescents) to greater frequencies of mother-headed families (i.e., single-parent and divorced families) (Peterson & Rose, 2003).

Maternal Employment and Economic Distress

In terms of the first issue, maternal employment, most research indicates that the simple structural issue of mothers working outside the home may have few adverse effects on the young, both in terms of the quantity and quality of time that is spent with adolescents. Instead, any negative or positive consequences for teenagers may depend on a variety of circumstances at work and at home that affect mothers' psychological state and capacity to parent effectively (Hoffman, 1989; Williams & Radin, 1993). Employed mothers who do not wish to work outside the home, are highly stressed by their work, unsupported at home, and unhappy in their jobs may have difficulty providing support, being involved with, and monitoring adolescents. In contrast, mothers who are working voluntarily, satisfied with their work, and supported at home may actually be better parents than mothers who are not employed outside the home (Lichter & Jayakody, 2002). The work circumstances of both mothers and fathers can, of course, interfere with effective parenting, particularly when job pressures elevate parents' stress levels and when they work an excessive amount of time (Crouter & Bumpus, 2001; MacDermid, Lee, & Smith, 2001). A key variable seems to be whether mothers (or both parents) can avoid leaving adolescents unsupervised every day for several hours between the time school ends and the time that parents return home from work (Galambos & Ehrenberg, 1997).

Some evidence indicates that maternal employment may have positive effects on the cognitive development, emotional adjustment, and the career aspirations of girls (Hofferth, Smith, McLoyd & Kindelstein, 2000; Hoffman, 1989; Zaslow, McGroder, Cave & Mariner, 1999). Employed mothers may function as positive models of employment values and aspirations for attainment and provide effective everyday structure for the young. Other studies point to nonexistent, mixed, or modestly adverse consequences of maternal employment for middle-class or upper middle-class boys (Lichter & Jayakody, 2002). Of particular importance is the tendency for boys from middle- and upper-middle-class backgrounds to argue more frequently with employed mothers and to perform in school less effectively (Montemayor, 1984; Bogenschneider & Steinberg, 1994), perhaps because boys resist the greater amount of household responsibilities required and are monitored less effectively when their mothers are employed. The overall trend, however, has been for greater similarities than differences to be found between adolescents who are from homes with employed versus nonemployed mothers.

Poverty and economic distress are other aspects of family socioeconomic circumstances that place adolescents at risk for a variety of problems by creating stressful circumstances. Chronic economic disadvantage involves dealing on a daily basis with poor housing, lack of food, dangerous neighborhoods, and illnesses that go untreated, all of which are sources of chronic stress, demoralization, and depression for parents (McLoyd, 1998). A primary means through which poverty places adolescents at risk is through the stress and depression experienced by parents that leads, in turn, to higher levels of marital conflict and ineffective parenting. Economic distress undermines competent parenting as mothers and fathers who experience stress and suffer from depression become more punitive, monitor less effectively, and are less supportive of teenagers (Conger & Conger, 1999). Problematic child-rearing practices used by parents have been linked, in turn, to higher levels of adolescent alcohol use, anxiety, depression, hostility, and conduct problems, as well as decreases in school performance (Conger & Conger, 1999; Conger, Conger, Elder, Lorenz, Simons, & Whitbeck, 1992; Conger, Lorenz, Elder, Melby, Simons, & Conger, 1991; McLoyd, Jayaratne, Ceballo, & Borquez, 1994).

Divorce and Remarriage

For many adolescents, an important family structural transition in family life occurs when their parents divorce. A primary concern is that adolescents whose parents divorce may be at risk for a variety of problematic outcomes commonly blamed on the fact that both parents no longer share the same household.

Frequently reported consequences of divorce for adolescents include anxiety, depression, psychological withdrawal, lower self-esteem, behavior problems, alcohol and drug use, and difficulties in school (Amato & Keith, 1991; Buchanan, 2000; Cherlin, 1999; Hetherington & Stanley-Hagan, 2002; Jeynes, 2002; Wallerstein, Lewis & Blakeslee, 2000). Adolescents are at greatest risk for these divorce-related problems both during the divorce crisis and for a time after their parents separate, with significant recovery occurring for the majority of youth by 1 to 2 years after the separation and/or divorce (Hetherington & Stanley-Hagan, 2002).

Other researchers indicate, however, that substantial variability exists in how adolescents respond to their parents' divorce, either in terms of long- or short-term consequences. Some evidence indicates, for example, that long-term or "sleeper" effects may appear during adolescence that were either less obvious or completely hidden earlier in childhood. These problems may include adjustment difficulties, interpersonal problems, drug and alcohol use, conduct problems, and poorer school performance (Amato, 2000; Amato & Keith, 1991; Wallerstein, Lewis, & Blakeslee, 2000). As the young enter early adulthood, painful memories of their parents' marriage may linger, problems in forming romantic relationships may develop, and reluctance to pursue educational objectives (e.g., lower college attendance) may result (Herzog & Cooney, 2002; Wallerstein, Lewis & Blakeslee, 2000).

An alternative perspective on the consequences of divorce identifies many inconsistencies in the current research and points only to moderate, if any, differences in youthful outcomes resulting directly from the structural reality of a divorced home. These observers conclude that the structural transitions of divorce do not lead directly to serious problems for adolescents. Instead, the specific developmental outcomes and well-being of adolescents depend immediately on a variety of psychological and relationship dynamics within families that occur before, during, and after marital disruption (Emery, 1999). Consequently, instead of asking why divorce is detrimental to adolescents in a simplistic way, the more accurate question is how the structural transitions (e.g., broken homes and father's absence) commonly associated with divorce contribute to (1) changes in psychological experiences and relationships within families, which, in turn, (2) may have socio-emotional consequences for adolescents.

Several psychological and relationship circumstances within divorcing or divorced families have been identified which make adolescents either more or less vulnerable to negative consequences. The most frequently identified circumstances are (1) the personal adjustment of custodial parents, (2) the extent to which parents maintain effective child-rearing practices, (3) whether adolescents maintain ties with noncustodial parents, (4) the degree of conflict between parents, (5) the degree of economic hardship caused by divorce, (6) the accumulation of other stressful life circumstances (e.g., moving to a new home and economic losses) associated with divorce; and (7) the adolescent's age-specific abilities and social competence (Amato, 2000; Amato & Keith, 1991; Emery, 1999; Hetherington & Stanley-Hagan, 2002).

Research has indicated that custodial parents, who are most frequently mothers, are often greatly preoccupied with and distressed by the divorce process. This emotional "trauma of divorce" is further exacerbated by increased pressure to be gainfully employed, the experience of greater economic distress (i.e., with the loss of former spouse's income), more involvement in the parental role, and greater responsibility for managing the daily hassles of family life (Hetherington & Kelly, 2002; Wallerstein, Lewis & Blakeslee, 2000). These stressful circumstances can lead, at least temporarily, to continued conflicts between former adult partners and declines in their parental abilities to effectively support, guide, monitor, and discipline the young. As a result, many parents who have recently experienced divorce often use less reasoning, less nurturance, more punitiveness, and engage in more frequent coercive exchanges with the young. Of particular importance is the issue of exposure to conflict between parents (i.e., interparental conflict) that may contribute to the adjustment problems of adolescents (Amato, 2000; Emery, 1999; Kelly, 2000). Instead of "divorce effects" being based on structural changes, therefore, recent studies have indicated that the frequency and severity of conflict between parents, both before and after divorce, may be the primary factors that lead to adverse consequences for adolescents (Amato, 2000; Buchanan, 2000; Emery, 1999). The implication here is that many problematic consequences of divorce for adolescents can be ameliorated, especially if the distress of custodial parents can be reduced, their inclination to engage in marital and postmarital conflict minimized, and the quality of their parenting sustained (Buchanan, 2000; Hetherington & Kelly, 2002; Hetherington & Stanley-Hagan, 2002).

Other evidence indicates that adolescents benefit when both parents (custodial and noncustodial) remain involved with them in positive ways during and after the divorce. Both adolescents and younger children cope with divorce more effectively when parents can put their own relationship differences aside, keep conflicts to a minimum, and agree on policies and strategies for dealing with the young (Amato, 2000; Hetherington & Stanley-Hagan, 2002). After divorce occurs, continued relations with fathers are particularly difficult to maintain, with the common pattern being for contact between adolescents and fathers to decline steadily (Hetherington & Kelly, 2002). An associated result is that adolescents from divorced households tend to have less positive feelings toward their fathers compared to youth from families with intact marriages (Cooney, 1994). Other adverse consequences result when divorcing families, especially those headed by women, experience financial hardships resulting from divorce and its impact on family income (Hernandez, 1997; Jeynes, 2002). Adolescents experience the best of circumstances in those divorcing homes where both parents are employable, child support payments are maintained consistently, and public assistance is available.

Some evidence exists that adolescents may be more capable of dealing with the traumas of divorce than younger children (Hetherington & Kelly, 2002). The elaborate cognitive abilities of teenagers may make them more capable than younger children of understanding the reasons for their parents' divorce. Adolescents appear to protect themselves more effectively than younger children from self-blame and experience their parents' divorce more objectively than younger children. Compared to younger children, the expanding peer involvements of adolescents also may provide sources of support outside the family that allow youth to insulate themselves from the worst traumas of divorce. Examples of external support include extended family relatives or close family friends who function as role models and sources of guidance. Some ethnic-minority families (e.g., African American families), in particular, have long-standing traditions of providing external support for single-parent families. Extended family relatives (e.g., grandmothers) or individuals outside the family (e.g., close friends or neighbors) may become important sources of support and guidance for the young (Hetherington & Kelly, 2002).

Although teenagers may be more capable than younger children of coping with divorce, recent research indicates that adolescents may have more problems dealing with remarriage, another major structural transition, than their youthful counterparts. Such problematic outcomes include depression, anxiety, conduct disorders, deficient academic achievement, and delinquent activities (Ganong & Coleman, 1999; Hetherington & Stanley-Hagan, 2000, 2002; Jeynes, 2002). These difficulties often result despite seemingly positive family developments, such as greater contentment by custodial parents with their new relationship (i.e., most often the mothers), the return of psychological resources to function effectively as a parent, and the easing of economic stress by adding an employed adult to the family system (Ganong & Coleman, 1999). Remarriage is another stressful disruption of the family system involving the need for adaptation to the challenge of integrating a new person into the family system. Of particular concern is the circumstance of early adolescent girls who appear to resist and have negative relationships with newly introduced stepfathers. These difficulties often develop when stepfathers are viewed as lacking authority and as "dethroning" daughters from almost exclusive relationships with their divorced mothers (Ganong & Coleman, 1999). In contrast, adolescent boys seem to fare better than teenage girls in stepfamilies, perhaps because new stepfathers function as new sources of economic support and same-gender role models for them (Hetherington, 1993; Hetherington, Henderson & Reiss, 1999).

Stepfamilies are faced with many new adjustments that may add to existing problems resulting from the earlier divorce. Recent evidence indicates that the best strategy for stepparents (especially stepfathers) is to establish their authority and build emotional ties gradually with adolescents. This is further complicated by the fact that adolescents often remain loyal to their biological fathers, have difficulty forming attachments to stepfathers, and may be uneasy about their mother's sexual relationship with their new stepfather (Ganong & Coleman, 1999; Hetherington & Stanley-Hagan, 2000, 2002). The most effective course of action is for stepparents to ease themselves into family roles that support biological parents without trying to assert their authority too rapidly (Hetherington, 1993).

Siblings

Another aspect of structural variation that complicates family socialization processes is the presence and number of siblings in families. Sibling relationships often are emotionally charged, characterized by conflict and competitiveness, but they also serve as sources of support and closeness for adolescents (Lempers & Clark-Lempers, 1992). Recent studies indicate that siblings become less influential for adolescents as the young expand their associations beyond family boundaries. The sibling relationships of adolescents, particularly those with younger siblings, become more distant, egalitarian, and periodically emotionally charged across the teenage years (Hetherington, Henderson, & Reiss, 1999; Teti, 2002; Updegraff & Crouter, 2003). Generally, conflict with siblings is highest during early adolescence, but tends to subside during the middle and later years of this stage. Adolescents report more negativity and less intimacy with siblings than with friends (Buhrmester & Furman, 1990; Updegraff & Crouter, 2003), though the amount of companionship, intimacy, and emotional support provided by siblings to the young should not be minimized (Updegraff & Obeidallah, 1999).

Older siblings often function as teachers, managers, helpers, sources of advice, and role models when they interact with their younger brothers and sisters (Brody, 1998; Tucker, Barber & Eccles, 1997). Social experiences with older siblings contribute both to positive and negative outcomes for younger siblings. Similar to the impact of parent–adolescent relationships, for example, current research has indicated that sibling relationships affect the development of social competence in terms of successful adjustment in school, sociability, conflict-management skills, autonomy, and self-worth (Brody, 1998; Hetherington, Henderson & Reiss, 1999; Rowe, Rodgers, Meseck-Bushey & St. John, 1989; Seginer, 1998). Sibling relationships also may serve as training grounds for relationships with peers and close friends (Brody, Stoneman & McCoy, 1994; McCoy, Brody & Stoneman, 1994; Teti, 2002). Unfortunately, sibling relationships also serve as contexts in which problematic outcomes such as substance abuse, antisocial behavior, and early sexual behavior are learned (Conger, Conger & Scaramella, 1997; Teti, 2002). The presence of siblings is, indeed, a structural circumstance that has complex relationship effects for those adolescents who have brothers and sisters.

Overall, the influences of family structural variation on adolescent development are primarily indirect through the provision of particular organizational contexts that make different relationship (or process) circumstances more likely to occur within families. Subsequently, the resulting relationship dynamics have direct consequences for the development of either adolescent social competence or youthful problem behaviors.

Family Process and Relationship Variables

As indicated earlier, the aspects of family life that have the strongest *direct* influences on both adolescent social competence and problem behavior are not dimensions of family structure, but family process and relationship variables. What follows, therefore, is a review of the most prominent parental influence and process dimensions of the parent–adolescent relationship having consequences for either youthful prosocial or problematic outcomes. Specifically, two ways of conceptualizing how parents socialize adolescents from a social mold perspective (i.e., parental styles and parental behavior) as well as two bidirectional process dimensions (i.e., parent–adolescent and interparental or marital conflict) are examined.

Parenting Styles and Behaviors

Parents who are members of diverse family structures (e.g., nuclear, divorced, single-parent, and stepfamilies etc.) influence adolescent development through a variety of child-rearing approaches conceptualized either as parenting styles or parental behaviors. The first means of conceptualizing these socialization strategies, *parenting styles*, involves complicated configurations or collections of several parental practices and attributes. Each configuration or style is composed of a different pattern of child-rearing strategies, such as control, warmth (i.e., support), communication, rule enforcement, as well as the particular attitudes and values of parents (e.g., values emphasizing obedience to authority versus values emphasizing autonomy). In contrast, *parental behavior* refers to specific or discrete dimensions of child-rearing actions that are often thought to be independent. A continuing focus of research on parent–adolescent relations has been to identify how distinctive parental styles or behaviors contribute differentially to dimensions of either social competence or problem behavior in the young (Darling & Steinberg, 1993; Peterson & Hann, 1999; Steinberg, 2001).

Parental Styles

The most widely known set of parental styles or configurations are those developed by psychologist Diana Baumrind (1978, 1991) and referred to as authoritarian, authoritative, and permissive approaches. *Authoritarian parents,* for example, use very strict and quite harsh control to encourage unquestioning obedience in youth. Harsh or punitive behavior is used regularly to impose the parent's will, whereas open communication, reasoning, and affection are either not used or applied very sparingly. A second child-rearing style, *permissive parenting,* identifies parents who make few demands upon and rarely seek to control adolescents, either through punitive or more moderate forms of control. The general style of permissive parenting is composed, in turn, of two subtypes of parenting, referred to as *indulgent* and *indifferent* child-rearing. Indulgent parents are supportive, emphasize democracy, foster trust, but use little if any form of control with the young. Indifferent or neglectful parents are neither supportive or controlling and are best described as being disengaged from (or disinterested in) their young. Although both indulgent and neglectful parents share a reluctance to assert control over adolescents, they differ in their willingness to be affectionate. Indulgent parents are supportive and emotionally close to teenagers, whereas indifferent parents are emotionally distant from their young.

The third blend of attributes, the *authoritative style,* identifies parents who use firm control to implement a consistent set of rules. Authoritative parents value both autonomous self-will and disciplined conformity from their young. These parents use reason in an issue-oriented manner and apply rewards and punishments that are clearly related to the adolescent's behavior. Authoritative parents assert their positions as authority figures, but are responsive to efforts by the young to exercise influence and are open to relationship change over time. These parents tend to encourage two-way communication and to foster an atmosphere of warmth and acceptance (Baumrind, 1991; Maccoby & Martin, 1983; Peterson & Leigh, 1990; Peterson & Hann, 1999).

Recent research tends to support Baumrind's view that authoritative parenting fosters a collection of prosocial qualities in adolescents often referred to as social or instrumental competence (Baumrind, 1978, 1991; Peterson & Hann, 1999; Steinberg, 2001). Specific outcomes encouraged include independence, responsible compliance, self-assurance, creativity, and skill in social relationships (Baumrind, 1991; Fuligni & Eccles, 1993; Lamborn, Mounts, Steinberg, & Dornbusch, 1991; Steinberg, 2001). Compared to the general population of adolescents, youth who are raised in authoritative homes tend to perform more successfully in school and to relate more effectively to peers and adults (Steinberg, 2001; Steinberg, Lamborn, Dornbusch & Darling, 1992).

Research on the other styles of parenting indicates that negative outcomes are more frequent results, though the specific outcomes vary with the particular style used. Adolescents from authoritarian homes, for example, are more inclined to be dependent, passive, conforming, less self-assured, less creative, and less socially adept than other adolescents. Compared to their contemporaries, youth from homes with indulgent parents tend to be more immature, irresponsible, and to conform more readily to peers. Recent research also indicates that indifferent or neglectful parenting tends to foster higher rates of impulsivity and involvement in delinquency as well as early experimentation with sexual activity and substance use (Baumrind, 1991; Fuligni & Eccles, 1993; Kurdek & Fine, 1994; Lamborn, Mounts, Steinberg & Dornbusch, 1991; Steinberg, Lamborn, Darling, Mounts & Dornbusch, 1994; Steinberg, Mounts, Lamborn & Dornbusch, 1991; Steinberg, 2001).

A serious problem with parental styles is their complexity and the difficulty that researchers face in understanding how specific aspects of style contribute to adolescent development. Because parental styles provide a general context consisting of many parental qualities (Darling & Steinberg, 1993), it is difficult to identify precisely which aspect of a parent's child-rearing approach is the primary factor that truly influences a specific aspect of adolescent development. A related issue is that none of the parental styles incorporate either all the dimensions of parental practice currently identified in the research literature or the full range of variation in each of these dimensions. Consequently, the existing typologies fail adequately to represent the many parental styles that are conceptually possible in the overall population of parents (Peterson & Hann, 1999; Peterson & Rollins, 1987).

Parental Behaviors

As a result of such problems with parental styles, many researchers have preferred to study specific dimensions of parental behavior rather than deal with the many complexities of parental styles (Darling & Steinberg, 1993; Lim & Lim, in press; Maccoby & Martin, 1983; Peterson & Hann, 1999). The most frequently studied child-rearing behaviors are parental warmth or support, autonomy-granting behavior, intrusive control, reasoning, monitoring, and punitiveness.

Perhaps the closest thing to a general law of parenting is that warm, supportive, nurturant, and accepting behavior by mothers and fathers is associated with the development of social competence by adolescents (Barber & Thomas, 1986; Maccoby & Martin, 1983; Peterson, Bush & Supple, 1999; Peterson & Rollins, 1987). Parental *support* consists of behaviors like touching, hugging, kissing, praising, approving, encouraging, and spending positive time with adolescents (Barber & Thomas, 1986; Fuligni & Eccles,

1993, Rohner, 1986). This behavior communicates that adolescents are valued, fosters close ties, and communicates the parents' confidence in the adolescent's abilities. A large amount of research indicates that parental support is associated with several positive characteristics in adolescents like higher self-esteem, identity formation, conformity to parents, and autonomy. Adolescents who receive support or nurturance from parents often report lower amounts of anxiety, depression, and behavior problems (Maccoby & Martin, 1983; Peterson & Rollins, 1987; Peterson & Hann, 1999).

An important way that many parents seek to influence adolescents is through the use of *reasoning* or induction. Parents use induction or reasoning for appealing to the adolescent's concern for others, their desire to be mature, and their abilities to understand and voluntarily accept the parent's point of view (Baumrind, 1991; Hoffman, 1980, 1994; Maccoby & Martin, 1983; Peterson & Hann, 1999). The purpose of reasoning or induction is to help adolescents understand why rules are necessary, why their misbehavior is unacceptable, how their behavior affects others, and how their behavior might become more acceptable. Parents who use induction do not impose authority on adolescents, but communicate respect for adolescents and their abilities to make good decisions, and their capacities to voluntarily comply (Maccoby & Martin, 1983). Reasoning is a moderate form of control that legitimizes parental authority, communicates respect for adolescents' viewpoint, and is unlikely to produce hostile feelings in the young toward parents. The use of reason may be particularly important for appealing to the abstract thinking abilities that are developing during adolescence. Parental reasoning often has been found to foster adolescent outcomes like moral development, conformity to parents, and higher self-esteem (Hoffman, 1980, 1994; Maccoby & Martin, 1983).

Monitoring or supervision refers to efforts by parents to become aware of and manage their teenager's schedules, peer associations, activities, and physical whereabouts. Parents monitor adolescents by supervising their dating and sexual relationships, preventing antisocial behavior and deviant peer associations, checking to see that homework is completed, being vigilant for the symptoms of drug use, and overseeing the popular media accessed by the young (e.g., movies, television, books, the internet) (Barber, Olsen & Shagle, 1994; Fuligni & Eccles, 1993; Patterson, 1986; Patterson & Capaldi, 1991 Small, 1990). Monitoring designates the extent to which parents are knowledgeable of adolescents' behavior and activities (Kerr & Stattin, 2000; Stattin & Kerr, 2000). Successful monitoring implies that parents must maintain a clear set of rules about the time that adolescents should be home, when they should return from peer activities, with whom they may associate, and places where the young are forbidden to go. The primary role of parental monitoring is to prevent the drift of teenagers toward problematic peer relationships, risk behavior, and deviant activities.

Psychological autonomy granting designates the extent to which parents employ non-coercive behavior, democratic discipline, and encouragement for the young to express their individuality within families (Gray & Steinberg, 1999). Fostering autonomy in this manner often encourages self-worth, self-competence, and self-confidence (Barber, 1996). The inverse of autonomy granting, in turn, is *intrusive psychological control,* or efforts made by parents that intrude upon the psychological independence and emotional development of adolescents. Parents exercise intrusive control by invalidating adolescent's feelings, constraining verbal expression, withdrawing love, or attempting to induce guilt by reasoning. Frequent use of this behavior by parents has been linked primarily to internalized forms of youthful outcomes such as depression, withdrawal, loneliness, eating disorders, less adequate perception of self, lower self-efficacy, and less effective identity development. (Barber, 1996, 2002a,b).

Parental punitiveness refers to arbitrary verbal or physical attempts to influence the behavior and internal qualities of teenagers. These actions involve the use of excessive force to impose the will of parents without the tempering influence of reason (Maccoby & Martin, 1983; Peterson & Rollins, 1987; Straus, 1994; Turner & Finkelhor, 1996). Punitiveness varies from nagging, name-calling, or yelling to corporal punishment (i.e., spanking) or violence (Day, Peterson, McCracken, 1998; Straus, 1994). Some evidence does exist that cultural norms in our society are much less supportive of using physical punitiveness with teenagers compared to younger children. Although this appears to be true, over 40% of teenagers continue to receive physical punishment from parents on a frequent basis (Straus, 1994). Physical or verbal punitiveness often leads to hostile feelings, resistance, and tendencies by teenagers to reject parental authority over the long term (Rollins & Thomas, 1979; Turner & Finkelhor, 1996). Other research indicates that children and adolescents often respond to parents' punitive behavior by "counterattacking" with their own forms of punitive behavior (Patterson, 1986; Patterson & Capaldi, 1991).

The use of harsh, punitive behavior by parents is associated with youngsters who have lower self-esteem, depression, less advanced moral development, lower success in school, but higher rates of substance abuse and delinquent activities (Eckenrode, Laird, & Doris, 1993; Eisenberg, 1989; Straus, 1994). Although mild forms of punitiveness do not always lead to adolescent problems (Baumrind, Larzelere, & Cowan, 2002), this may occur because parents use other practices (e.g., support or reasoning) that offset or dilute the worst effects of being subjected to punitiveness. From the perspective of current research, mild physical punishment (e.g., spanking or slapping) does not inevitably result in serious negative outcomes for the young. The danger does exist, however, that some parents will not be able to control their anger, with the result being that the mild punitiveness of an angry parent may escalate into physical abuse (Baumrind et al., 2002; Day, Peterson & McCracken, 1998). Rather than risk the danger of such escalation, the most effective course of action for parents is to use alternative forms of discipline and control that are less arbitrary and coercive (e.g., monitoring, reasoning, or consistent rule enforcement).

Cultural Complications

An important precaution about current research on parent–child relationships is that scholars have recently begun to question the application of results from European American samples to non-western cultures and ethnic populations in the United States. Of particular concern are tendencies to overgeneralize about the specific effects of western parental styles without recognizing cultural and ethnic differences in the goals, conduct, and consequences of parenting (Chao, 2000, 2001; Kagitcibasi, 1996; Lim & Lim, 2003).

It should be pointed out, however, that most of this criticism has been directed at parental styles rather than the study of specific dimensions of parental behavior (Chao, 2000, 2001; Lim & Lim, in press). Researchers have found, for example, that authoritative parenting is less prevalent among Asian American, Hispanic American, and African American families. Despite this, however, current evidence also indicates that ethnic minority adolescents in the United States benefit from authoritative parenting about as much as European American adolescents in terms of adjustment and social competence (Dornbusch, Ritter, Liederman, Roberts & Fraleigh, 1987; Steinberg, 2001; Steinberg, Mounts, Lamborn & Dornbusch, 1991; Steinberg, Dornbusch & Brown, 1992). Recent studies also have indicated that authoritarian parenting (i.e., high punitive or arbitrary control and low support) is more commonly used by ethnic minority families than among European American families. In contrast to findings for authoritative parenting, however, results indicate that authoritarian styles or punitive behavior may have less problematic results for ethnic-minority adolescents (e.g., African American youth) than their European American peers (Chao, 1994; 2000, 2001; Deater-Deckard, Dodge, Bates, Pettit, 1996; Dornbusch et al., 1987; Steinberg et al., 1994).

A variety of explanations have been provided for these findings about authoritarian or punitive parenting. One proposal, for example, is that authoritarian parenting may be adaptive for risk-laden neighborhoods and communities in which many ethnic-minority families with adolescents tend to live (McLoyd, 1998). More rigid forms of control used by parents may help to shelter ethnic-minority adolescents from some of the worst influences in the neighborhood and community beyond family boundaries (e.g., gang activity, delinquency, and substance abuse) (Day, Peterson & McCracken, 1998).

Other observers propose that the cultural roots of parenting styles or behaviors are underestimated in the current research (Chao, 1994, 2000, 2001; Lim & Lim, 2003; Peterson, Steinmetz, & Wilson, 2003). An important point, for example, is that parental approaches, like the authoritative or authoritarian styles, are concepts based in European American cultural values and may not be consistent with the cultural values of Asian American, Hispanic American, or African American families. A possible consequence is that parenting practices used by ethnic-minority parents may be studied "out of context" and misunderstood.

Compared to European American cultures, several ethnic-minority and non-western cultures place greater emphasis on collectivistic values consisting of group connections, family harmony, community interests over individual priorities, respect for authority, and the importance of tradition. This contrasts with basic European American values that underscore the importance of individuality, autonomy, democracy, and self-interest over the welfare of the group. Collectivistic values, therefore, may encourage very different meanings, even for behaviors that seem harsh or excessively rigid by European American standards. In other words, behavior that is viewed as harsh or intrusive in one culture might be viewed as an expression of concern to maintain group togetherness in another. Moreover, non-western parents may express cultural values by using styles composed of disciplinary, controlling, nurturing, and rejecting behavior that differ either substantially or in nuance from western conceptions of parenting (i.e., authoritarian and authoritative styles as well as other identified or completely novel styles) (Chao, 1994, 2000, 2001; Kagitcibasi, 1996; Lim & Lim, 2003; Peterson et al., 2003). A reasonable amount of caution is required, therefore, when the substance, meaning, and consequences of parental styles and behavior are examined across cultures.

Parent–Adolescent and Interparental Conflict

A prominent bidirectional process within families is the study of conflict within families that occurs both between adolescents and parents as well as between one parent and the other (i.e., studied as marital or interparental conflict). The degree of conflict within families, rather than family structural transitions (e.g., divorce), is often assigned greater importance as a primary factor (or direct influence) leading to adverse consequences (i.e., maladjustment or youth problem behaviors) for adolescent development (Amato, 2000; Buchanan, 2000; Emery, 1999; Kelley, 2000). Recent studies indicate that conflict occurs with some regularity within most families, but tends to be moderate in character, and to involve mostly mundane, everyday phenomena, rather than issues of major substance (Arnett, 1999; Collins & Repinski, 1994).

Parent–Adolescent Conflict

The first form of family conflict, *parent–adolescent conflict*, has been subject to a long history of scholarship in the social sciences (Arnett, 1999; Hall, 1904). One way social scientists have studied parent-adolescent conflict is by comparing the attitudes, values, and personal tastes of the younger generation with those of their elders, or the search for the prevalence of a "generation gap" between parents and adolescents. This search for generational disparities concerns how parents and adolescents feel about each other as well as their similarities or differences relating to basic value domains such as political attitudes, religious beliefs, ethical principles, career ambitions, and educational goals. Instead of support for a generation gap, the weight of the evidence indicates that most parents and adolescents love and respect each other. Moreover, most parents and adolescents have not been found to have fundamental differences in values, beliefs, and attitudes (Steinberg, 2001; Moore, Chalk, Scarpa, & Vandivere, 2002). Instead, parents and adolescents differ most frequently in the area of personal life-style choices, including styles of dress, tastes in music, curfews, and selection of leisure-time activities (Gecas & Seff, 1990; Steinberg, 1990, 2001; Steinberg & Levine, 1997).

A similar view is reported by investigators who examine parent–adolescent conflict in terms of the frequency and severity of arguments, bickering, and verbal interruptions. These exchanges have been found to originate from daily issues involving household chores, clothing preferences, music tastes, choice of friends, and leisure activities, but not usually from concerns about basic values (Montemayor, 1983, 1986; Steinberg & Levine, 1997). From the perspective of parents, however, these seemingly "surface" differences of opinion may be symptomatic of parental concerns for the safety and well-being of adolescents within social contexts where growing autonomy may expose the young to involvement in risk behavior (e.g., autonomy in leisure activities and peer choices may provide opportunities for substance use). Although not typically severe, parent–adolescent conflict tends to occur somewhat frequently (about once every three days for an average duration of 11 minutes) and happens more often than conflicts occur between couples experiencing some marital distress (Buchanan, Maccoby & Dornbusch, 1996). Adolescents and parents have their most frequent conflicts during the early years of adolescence, which subsequently stays high for several years and then declines in later adolescence (Arnett, 1999; Dworkin

& Larson, 2001; Larson & Richards, 1994; Laursen, Coy & Collins, 1998). The higher levels of conflict during early adolescence may result as teenagers try to play a more significant role in family life, but also when parents may not be ready to accept this change. Some have proposed, for example, that puberty and associated hormonal changes play key roles in stimulating parent–youth conflict during early adolescence, a social mechanism for adolescents to distance themselves from parents, but especially from their mothers. Several studies have indicated that conflicts (or negative exchanges) intensify when hormonal activity is high as adolescents reach the midpoint of puberty and become more sexually mature (Arnett, 1999; Steinberg, 1990; Paikoff & Brooks-Gunn, 1991). Parent–adolescent conflicts tend to be the most frequent and intense between mothers and daughters (Steinberg, 1990).

Other observers disagree that increased parent–adolescent conflict is rooted primarily in the physiological changes of adolescence. Instead, moderate conflict is viewed as a process that fosters adaptive forms of change within parent–adolescent relationships. According to this view, conflict encourages parents and adolescents to revise their expectations and renegotiate autonomy or the degree of relationship flexibility, without fundamentally changing their feelings of being connected to each other (Collins, Laursen, Mortenson & Ferreira, 1997). This flexibility within the context of continued bonds allows adolescents to become more autonomous and competent in relationships beyond family boundaries. Moderate conflict plays an important, even necessary role, in changing family relationships so that autonomous development can occur.

The possibility that conflict may be a normal and necessary part of family relationships does not mean that the potential should be completely neglected for parent–adolescent conflict to become problematic (Arnett, 1999). Instead, conflict requires intuitive or intentional forms of management to keep the frequency and severity of this process at moderate levels. Escalating conflict in terms of frequency and severity often becomes a central feature of troubled parent–youth relationships that leads, in turn, to greater involvement in deviant and antisocial behavior by the young (Patterson & Capaldi, 1991). Conflicts can become a major source of dissatisfaction for parents and adolescents, especially if few efforts exist to resolve or manage these disagreements. Other difficulties may result when conflicts are routinely resolved either through the submission or withdrawal of the adolescent or parent. Conflicts commonly resolved through these less effective means often ignore the needs, interests, and welfare of either person involved. More constructive strategies involve reaching reasonable compromises or finding ways for parents and adolescents to agree to disagree (Patterson & Capaldi, 1991). Although parents and adolescents may experience distress, some conflict may be useful in contributing to a new equilibrium in the family system that allows the young to have greater autonomy (Collins, Laursen, Mortenson & Ferreira, 1997; Laursen & Collins, 1994).

A prominent explanation for parent–youth conflict is that adolescents and their elders may have differing perceptions or assign distinct meanings to issues that arise in their relationship (Larson & Richards, 1994). For parents, a meaningful objective is to function as authority figures and prepare youth for social competence and success in one's culture. In contrast, for adolescents, life-style issues are important for defining one's identity, becoming more autonomous, and affirming personal choices. Consequently, parents may expect adolescents to comply with their wishes because a particular issue (e.g., about styles of dress or curfews) is perceived as one of required compliance due to custom, convention, or continuity in parental authority. Another possibility is that parents may view a particular adolescent life-style issue (e.g., curfew time) as a surface level substitute for deeper level issues that may place adolescents at risk (e.g., the absence of a curfew may create more potential or unsupervised free time that, in turn, leads to early sexual activity). In contrast, adolescents may view the same issue as one of personal choice or as a means to assert their autonomy, perhaps the most highly valued developmental goal by adolescents in Western societies (Smetana, 1988, 1989; Smetana & Asquith, 1994). Thus, adolescents and parents may be in conflict based on the different meanings that each assign to life-style issues. These distinctive ways of seeing things are framed in terms of different developmental priorities that adolescents and parents must deal with during their respective phases of the life-course.

An important point about parent–adolescent conflict is the extent to which this process may vary across cultures and ethnic groups. Extensive theory and a growing body of empirical evidence offers the view that parent–adolescent conflict is likely to be less frequent in cultures and ethnic groups emphasizing extensive economic interdependence, social interdependence, collectivism, parental authority, and the priority of family bonds over the need for personal autonomy. Many non-western and traditional cultures as well as some ethnic groups (e.g., Asian and Asian American, Latino and Latino American) have cultural and economic pressures that diminish conflicts based on needs for autonomy and individualistic preferences in social relationships (Arnett, 1999; Phinney & Ong, 2002). Youth from these "collectivistic" cultures seem less inclined to seek autonomy and challenge authority figures due to social-cultural and economic forces that reinforce group solidarity. However, such cultural differences in parent–adolescent conflict may be diminishing as forces of globalization spread either the norms of western individualism or a form of social-emotional "interdependence" (a complex of values that is particularly prominent in non-Western cultures) in which both autonomy and continued connections with others are complementary aspects of youthful social competence (Kagitcibasi, 1996).

Interparental or Marital Conflict

A second form of family conflict, marital *or interparental conflict*, appears to have substantial consequences for adolescent development and has received growing attention in the research literature (Buehler, Anthony, Krishnakumar, Stone, Gerard & Pemberton, 1997). Although conflict between parents appears to have important implications for adolescent development, some evidence also suggests that adolescents may be more resilient and less vulnerable to the adverse consequences of interparental conflict than are younger children (Acock & Demo, 1999).

Some of the research distinguishes between two forms of interparental conflict, overt and covert conflict. The first of these, *overt conflict,* is defined as hostile behavior and affect that are indicative of negative relationships between parents (e.g., belligerence, contempt, derision, screaming, insulting, slapping, threatening, and hitting) (Buehler, Anthony, Krishnakumar, Stone, Gerard & Pemberton, 1997; McHale, 1997). *Covert conflict,* on the other hand, refers to hostile behaviors and affect that reflect indirect ways of manifesting conflict between parents (Buehler & Trotter, 1990) (e.g., trying to manipulate an adolescent to take a particular parents' side, denigrating the other parent in front of an adolescent, and scapegoating the adolescent).

Interparental conflict appears to contribute in complex ways to foster the development of problematic behavior or inhibit the development of social competence by the young. Because conflict is commonly present in families, and may have some benefits in moderate levels (e.g., for maintaining a sense one's individuality), we cannot assume that all conflict between parents is problematic. Many subtleties exist and it is important to recognize conceptual distinctions, such as the difference between the *frequency* and *severity* of conflict. There is some evidence, for example, that, compared to the frequency of interparental conflict, the severity of strife (or the degree of hostility conveyed) between parents seems to operate independently of and to be more strongly predictive of adolescent problem behaviors (Buehler et al., 1997).

Another complication is that the influence of interparental conflict has both a *direct* and *indirect* effect on youthful problem behaviors. The direct effects are the most obvious in the sense that simply exposing the young to frequent, severe parental fights places them in disturbing, threatening, and anxiety-provoking psychological circumstances. Consequently, in families where the frequency and severity of such parental disagreements are high, the likelihood is increased that internalizing and externalizing responses will be evoked from the young (e.g., learned aggressiveness, insecurity, or psychological withdrawal), simply by observing and assigning negative meanings to their parents' interactions (Cummings & Davies, 1994).

Indirect effects of marital or interparental conflict on adolescent development also occur through a phenomenon referred to as *spillover*. The explanation for spillover involves the idea that marital conflict is psychologically disturbing to the parent, which, in turn, "spills over" into the parent–adolescent relationship negatively affecting the quality of socialization behaviors that parents use with their young. That is, parents who experience psychological distress and disorganized thinking in response to marital conflict often experience diminished abilities to maintain their supportiveness of adolescents and high-quality involvement with them. Moreover, high interparental conflict and the resulting psychological distress may eventuate in parents' being more punitive and more psychologically intrusive into the lives of their young. The resulting declines in supportiveness, reduced quality of involvement, increased punitiveness, and enhanced parental intrusiveness are behaviors that commonly predict the development of externalizing and internalizing behavior in the young (Buehler & Gerard, 2002; Stone, Buehler & Barber, 2002).

An important overall idea, therefore, is that some conflict probably occurs in all families and, when maintained at moderate levels, may even have positive developmental consequences. Probably the best course is to foster relationship mechanisms that manage strife within both the parent–adolescent and interparental relationships in ways that prevent conflict from escalating to unusually frequent and severe levels.

Recommendations

A primary conclusion of this review is that families remain strong and perhaps predominant influences on adolescent development. An extensive array of family structure, process, and relationship variables continue to have both direct and indirect influences on the development of adolescent social competence and problem behaviors. Despite the growth of influences from social agents beyond families during adolescence, families of diverse structure are sources of complex, complementary, and contradictory influences on adolescents. A key challenge for future research is to demonstrate how family influences are distinctive from, contradictory to, or complementary with the influence of other social agents such as schools, peer groups, neighborhoods, churches, and government/political institutions. More research in this area is needed to examine the efficacy of human ecological models that convey more realistic conceptions of the complex social world that adolescents must face each day (Lerner, 1995; Bronfenbrenner, 1994).

Although some progress is being made in developing socialization models that are more complex than the social mold perspective (e.g., Bates, Pettit, Dodge & Ridge, 1998; Beyers, Bates, Pettit & Dodge, 2003; Kuczynski, 2003), greater emphasis is needed on research that tests these more elaborate conceptions about how adolescent development is influenced. Part of this complexity involves examining how multiple contexts of socialization operate either in cojunction or at odds with each other as influences on adolescent development. More research is needed on bidirectional and multidirectional influences that adolescents, their parents, and their siblings experience in families (Kuczynski, 2003; Peterson & Rollins, 1987; Peterson & Hann, 1999). An emphasis on more complex socialization models also will require greater efforts to disentangle genetic from family environmental influences. Greater emphasis on twin studies and other behavioral genetic designs is needed to more precisely identify aspects of adolescent development that are truly a product of nurture rather than nature (Cleveland, Jacobson, Lipinski & Rowe, 2000; Collins, Maccoby, Steinberg, Hetherington & Bornstein, 2000). More complex research strategies also should include the more frequent use of cross-lagged designs that first can address how changes in parental and sibling attributes within families predict (or influence) changes in youthful social competence and problem behavior over time. Subsequently, these designs also provide insight into how such changes in adolescent social competence and problem behavior predict changes in subsequent patterns of parental and sibling attributes.

Another conclusion is that, although a great deal has been learned by studying parental styles and behaviors as predictors of adolescent development, it may be time to expand beyond being so disproportionately preoccupied with these aspects of the parent–adolescent relationship (Steinberg, 2001). Preoccupation with parental styles and behaviors in parent–adolescent research may lead to underestimating how the sophisticated cognitive abilities of youth provide them with the capacity to be either responsive or nonresponsive to parents based on their interpretations or meaning of the long-term relationships they have with their elders. Both parental styles and behaviors seem best suited for examining parent–child relations with younger children and may have somewhat less utility with adolescents. Such is the case because, compared to younger children, adolescents have greater abstract thinking capacities, more extensive relationship memories, enhanced social perceptions, and greater experience with parents. These abilities allow adolescents, in turn, to construct increasingly complex images or assessments of their parent's competence, wisdom, and authority. As a result, more complicated interpretations of the meaning of parent–adolescent relationships may be structured in ways that may be equally as influential for youth as reports of child-rearing behaviors of the moment. For example, adolescents may be influenced extensively by whether they view their parents as being competent, as having wisdom, and as being recognized as authority figures (Peterson & Hann, 1999). Compared to momentary displays of child-rearing behavior, these social constructions of their parents are more abstract and summarized products of long-term relationships. Adolescents increasingly develop abilities to "size up" their parents' worthiness or unworthiness as social agents (i.e., their degree of parental competence) and choose in complex ways the extent to which they will be influenced.

A general implication of the current research on families and adolescents indicates that family-based prevention/intervention models should be focused primarily on the social, psychological, and process dynamics of families rather than the structural dimensions. Family-based prevention/intervention approaches should be applied as part of a larger strategy involving components implemented across social contexts such as the family, school, peer group, and community. Such a broad-based strategy recognizes that no single approach can promote social competence when social contexts contradict each other in addressing multiple influences. Instead, greater success will be attained through a major public health effort that provides a coordinated package of approaches designed to address both general issues across contexts but also having sufficient flexibility for varied community circumstances.

References

Acock, A.C. & Demo, D.H. (1999). Dimensions of family conflict and their influence on child and adolescent adjustment. *Sociological Inquiry, 69,* 641–658.

Allen, J., & Land, P. (1999). Attachment in adolescence. In J. Cassidy & P.R. Shaver (Eds), *Handbook of Attachment: Theory, Research, and Clinical applications.* New York: Guilford.

Amato, P.R. (2000). The consequences of divorce for children and adults. *Journal of Marriage and the Family, 62,* 1269–1287.

Amato, P.R., & Keith, B. (1991). Parental divorce and the well-being of children: meta-analysis. *Psychological Bulletin, 100,* 26–46.

Anderson, S.A., & Sabatelli, R.M. (1990). Differentiating differentiation and individuation: Conceptual and operational challenges. *American Journal of Family Therapy, 18,* 32–50.

Arnett, J.J. (1995). Broad and narrow socialization: The family in the context of cultural theory. *Journal of Marriage and the Family, 54,* 339–373.

Arnett, J.J. (1999). Adolescent storm and stress, reconsidered. *American Psychologist, 54,* 317–326.

Barber, B.K. (1996). Parental psychological control: Revisiting a neglected construct. *Child Development, 67,* 3296–3319.

Barber, B.K. (2002a). *Intrusive parenting: How psychological control affects children and adolescents.* Washington, DC: American Psychological Association Press.

Barber, B.K. (2002b). Re-introducing psychological control. In B.K. Barber (Ed.), *Intrusive Parenting: How Psychological Control Affects Children and Adolescents.* Washington, D.C.: American Psychological Association Press.

Barber, B.K., Olsen, J.E., & Shagle, S.C. (1994). Associations between parental psychological and behavioral control and youth internalized and externalized behaviors. *Child Development, 65,* 1120–1136.

Barber, B.K., & Thomas, D.L. (1986). Dimensions of fathers' and mothers' supportive behavior: The case for physical affection. *Journal of Marriage and the Family, 48,* 783–794.

Bartle-Haring, S., Kenny, D.A., & Gavazzi, S.M. (1999). Multiple perspectives on family differentiation: analyses by multitrait multimethod matrix and triadic social relations model. *Journal of Marriage and the Family, 61,* 491–503.

Bates, J.E., Pettit, G.S., Dodge, K.A., & Ridge, B. (1998). Interaction of temperamental resistance to control and restrictive parenting in the development of externalizing behavior. *Developmental Psychology, 34,* 982–995.

Baumrind, D. (1978). Parental disciplinary patterns and social competence in children. *Youth and Society, 9,* 239–276.

Baumrind, D. (1991). Effective parenting during the early adolescent transition. In P.A. Cowan & M. Hetherington (Eds.), *Family Transitions* (pp. 111–163). Hillsdale, NJ: Lawrence Erlbaum.

Baumrind, D., Larzelere, R.E., & Cowan, P.A. (2002). Ordinary physical punishment: Is it harmful? Comment on Gershoff (2002). *Psychological Bulletin, 128,* 580–589.

Beyers, J.M., Bates, J.E., Pettit, G.S., & Dodge, K.A. (2003). Neighborhood structure, parenting processes, and the development of youths' externalizing behaviors: A multilevel analysis. *American Journal of Community Psychology, 31,* 35–53.

Bloom, M. (1990). The psychsocial constructs of social competency. In T.P. Gullotta, G.R. Adams, & R. Montemayor (Eds.), *Developing social competency in adolescence.* Newbury Park, CA: Sage Publications.

Blos, P. (1979). *The Adolescent Passage.* New York: International Universities Press.

Bodman, D., & Peterson, G.W. (1995). Parenting processes. In R.D. Day, K. Gilbert, B. Settles, W.R. Burr (Eds.), *Research and Theory in Family Science* (pp. 205–225). Pacific Grove, CA: Brooks/Cole.

Bogenschneider, K., & Steinberg, L.D. (1994). Maternal employment and adolescent academic achievement: A developmental analysis. *Sociology of Education, 67,* 60–77.

Broderick, C.B. (1993). *Understanding Family Process: Basics of Family Systems Theory.* Newbury Park, CA: Sage Publications.

Brody, G.H. (1998). Sibling relationship quality: Its causes and consequences. *Annual Review of Psychology, 49,* 1–24.

Brody, G.H., Stoneman, Z., & McCoy, J. (1994). Forecasting sibling relationships in early adolescence from child temperaments and family processes in middle childhood. *Child Development, 65,* 771–784.

Bronfenbrenner, U. (1979). *The Ecology of Human Development: Experiments by Nature and Design.* Cambridge, MA: Harvard University Press.

Bronfenbrenner, U. (1994). Ecological models of human development. In T. Husen & T.N. Postlethwaite (Ed.), *The International Encyclopedia of Education* (2nd ed., pp. 1643–1647). New York: Elsevier Science.

Buchanan, C.M. (2000). The impact of divorce on adjustment during adolescence. In R.D. Taylor & M. Weng (Eds.), *Resilience Across Contexts: Family, Work, Culture, and Community.* Mahwah, NJ: Erlbaum.

Buchanan, C.M., Maccoby, E.F., & Dornbusch, S.M. (1996). *Adolescents After Divorce.* Cambridge, MA: Harvard University Press.

Buehler, C., Anthony C., Krishnakumar, A., Stone, G., Gerard, J., & Pemberton, S. (1997). Interparental conflict and youth problem behaviors: A meta-analysis. *Journal of Child and Family Studies, 6,* 233–247.

Buehler, C., & Gerard, J. (2002). Marital conflict, ineffective parenting, and children's and adolescents' maladjustment. *Journal of Marriage and Family, 64,* 78–92.

Buehler, C., & Trotter, B.B. (1990). Nonresidential and residential parents' perceptions of the former spouse relationship and children's social competence following marital separation: Theory and programmed intervention. *Family Relations, 39,* 395–404.

Buhrmester, D., & Furman, W. (1990). Perceptions of sibling relationships during middle childhood and adolescence. *Child Development, 61,* 1387–1396.

Carter, B., & McGoldrick, M. (1999). *The expanded family life cycle: Individual, family and social perspectives* (3rd ed.). Needham Heights, MA: Allyn and Bacon.

Chao, R. (1994). Beyond parental control and authoritarian parenting style: Understanding Chinese parenting through the cultural notion of training. *Child Development, 65,* 1111–1119.

Chao, R.K. (2000). Cultural explanations for the role of parenting in the school success of Asian-American Children. In R. Taylor & M.C. Wang (Eds.), *Resilience Across Contexts: Family, Work, Culture, and Community* (pp. 333–363). Temple University: Center for Research in Human Development.

Chao, R.K. (2001). Extending research on the consequences of parenting style for Chinese Americans and European Americans. *Child Development, 72,* 1832–1843.

Cherlin, A.J. (1999). Going to extremes: Family structure, children's well-being, and social science. *Demography, 36,* 421–428.

Cleveland, H.H., Jacobson, K.C., Lipinski, J.J., & Rowe, D.C. (2000). Genetic and shared environmental contributions to the relationship between the home environment and child and adolescent achievement. *Intelligence, 28,* 69–86.

Collins, W.A., Laursen, B., Mortenson, N., & Ferreira, M. (1997). Conflict processes and transitions in parent and peer relationships: Implications for autonomy and regulation. *Journal of Adolescent Research, 12,* 178–198.

Collins, W.A., Maccoby, E.E., Steinberg, L.D., Hetherington, E.M., & Bornstein, M.H. (2000). Contemporary research on parenting: The case for nature and nurture. *American Psychologist, 55,* 218–232.

Collins, W.A., & Repinski, D.J. (1994). Relationships during adolescence: Continuity and change in interpersonal perspective. In R. Montemayor, G.R. Adams & T.P. Gullotta (Eds.), *Personal Relationships*

During Adolescence: Advances in Adolescent Development (Vol. 6) (pp. 7–36). Thousand Oaks, CA: Sage Publication, Inc.

Cooney, T.M. (1994). Young adults' relations with parents: The influence of recent parental divorce. *Journal of Marriage and the Family, 56,* 45–56.

Conger, K.J., Conger, R.D., & Scaramella, V. (1997). Parents, siblings, psychological control, and adolescent adjustment. *Journal of Adolescent Research, 12,* 113–138.

Conger, R., & Conger, K.J. (1999). Pathways of economic influence on adolescent adjustment. *American Journal of Community Psychology, 27,* 519–541.

Conger, R., Conger, K.J., Elder, G.H., Jr.; Lorenz, F.O., Simons, R.L., & Whitbeck, L.B. (1992). A family process model of economic hardship and adjustment of early adolescent boys. *Child Development, 63,* 526–541.

Conger, R.D., Lorenz, F.O., Elder, G.H., Jr., Melby, J.N., Simons, R.L., & Conger, K.L. (1991). A process model of family economic pressure and early adolescent alcohol use. *Journal of Early Adolescence, 11,* 430–499.

Corsaro, W.A. (1997). *The Sociology of Childhood.* Thousand Oaks, CA: Pine Forge Press.

Crouter, A.C., & Bumpus, M.F. (2001). Linking parents' work stress to children's psychological adjustment. *Current Directions in Psychological Science, 10,* 156–159.

Cummings, E.M., & Davies, P. (1994). *Children and Marital Conflict: The Impact of Family Dispute and Resolution.* New York: Guilford Press.

Darling, N., & Steinberg, L.D. (1993). Parenting style as context: An integrative model. *Psychological Bulletin, 113,* 487–496.

Davis, K. (1960). Adolescence and the social structure. In J. Seidman (Ed.), *The adolescent* (pp. 5–25). New York: Holt, Rhinehart, & Winston.

Day, R.D. (1995). Family-systems theory. In R.D. Day, K.R. Gilbert, B.H. Settles & W.R. Burr (Eds.), *Research and Theory in Family Science* (pp. 91–101). Pacific Grove, CA: Brooks/Cole.

Day, R., Peterson, G.W., & McCracken, C. (1998). Predictors of frequent spanking of younger and older children. *Journal of Marriage and the Family, 60,* 79–94.

Deater-Deckard, K., Dodge, K., Bates, J., & Pettit, G. (1996). Physical discipline among African American and European American mother: Links to children's externalizing behaviors. *Developmental Psychology, 32,* 1065–1072.

Demo, D.H., & Cox, M.J. (2000). Families with young children: A review of research in the 1990s. *Journal of Marriage and the Family, 62,* 876–895.

Dornbusch, S.M., Ritter, P.L., Liederman, P.H., Roberts, D.F., & Fraleigh, M.J. (1987). The relation of parenting style to adolescent school performance. *Child Development, 56,* 326–341.

Dworkin, J.B., & Larson, R. (2001). Age trends in the experience of family discord in single mother families across adolescence. *Journal of Adolescence, 24,* 529–534.

Eckenrode, J., Laird, M., & Doris, J. (1993). School performance and disciplinary problems among abused and neglected children. *Developmental Psychology, 29,* 53–62.

Eisenberg, N. (1989). Prosocial development in early and mid-adolescence. In R. Montemayor, G.R. Adams, & T.P. Gullotta (Eds.), *Advances in Adolescent Development, From Childhood to Adolescence: A Transitional Period?* (pp. 240–268). Newbury Park, CA: Sage.

Elkin, F., & Handel, G. (1988). *The Child and Society: The Process of Socialization.* New York: McGraw Hill.

Emery, R.E. (1999). *Marriage, Divorce, and Children's Adjustment* (2nd ed.). Newbury Park, CA: Sage Publications.

Freud, A. (1969). Adolescence as a developmental disturbance. In G. Caplan & S. Lebovici (Eds.), *Adolescence: Psychosocial Perspectives.* (pp. 5–10). New York: Basic Books.

Fuligni, A., & Eccles, J. (1993). Perceived parent-child relationships and early adolescents' orientation toward peers. *Developmental Psychology, 29,* 622–632.

Furstenberg, F.F. (2000). The sociology of adolescence and youth in the 1990s: A critical commentary. *Journal of Marriage and the Family, 62,* 4, 896–910.

Galambos, N.L., & Ehrenberg, M.F. (1997). The family as health risk and opportunity: A focus on divorce and working families. In J. Schulenberg, J.L. Maggs, & Hurrelman (Eds.), *Health Risks and Developmental Transitions During Adolescence* (pp. 139–160). New York: Cambridge University Press.

Ganong, L.H., & Coleman, M. (1999). *Changing Families, Changing Responsibilities: Family Obligations Following Divorce and Remarriage.* Mahwah, NJ: Erlbaum.

Gecas, V. (1979). The influence of social class on socialization. In W.R. Burr, R. Hill, F.J. Nye, & I.L. Reiss (Eds.). *Contemporary Theories About the Family,* Vol. 1 (pp. 365–404). New York: Free Press.

Gecas, V., & Seff, M.A. (1990). Adolescents and families: A review of the 1980s. *Journal of Marriage and the Family, 52,* 941–958.

Gillespie, J.F. (2003). Social competency, adolescence. In T.P. Gullotta & M. Bloom (Eds.), *Encyclopedia of Primary Prevention and Health Promotion* (pp. 1004–1009). New York: Kluwer Academic/Plenum Publishers.

Gray, M., & Steinberg, L.D. (1999). Adolescent romance and the parent-child relationship: A contextual perspective. In W. Furman, B. Brown, & C. Feiring, (Eds.), *Contemporary Perspectives on Adolescent Romantic Relationships* (pp. 235–265). New York: Cambridge University Press.

Hall, G.S. (1904). *Adolescence: Its Psychology and its Relation to Physiology, Anthropology, Sociology, Sex, Crime, Religion, and Education (Vols. I & II).* Englewood Cliffs, NJ: Prentice-Hall.

Hauser, S.T. (1999). Understanding resilient outcomes: Adolescent lives across time and generations. *Journal of Research on Adolescence, 9,* 1–24.

Hawkins, J.D., Catalano, R.F., & Miller, J.Y. (1992). Risk and protective factors for alcohol and other drug problems in adolescence and early adulthood: Implications for substance abuse prevention. *Psychological Bulletin, 112,* 64–105.

Hernandez, D.J. (1997). Child development and the social demography of childhood. *Child Development, 68,* 149–169.

Herzog, M.J., & Cooney, T.M. (2002). Parental divorce and perceptions of interparental conflict: Influences on the communication of young adults. *Journal of Divorce and Remarriage, 36,* 89–109.

Hetherington, E.M. (1993). An overview of the Virginia longitudinal study of divorce and remarriage with a focus on early adolescence. *Journal of Family Psychology, 7,* 39–56.

Hetherington, E.M., Henderson, S., & Reiss, D. (1999). Adolescent siblings in stepfamilies. Family functioning and adolescent adjustment. *Monographs of the Society for Research on Child Development, 64.*

Hetherington, E.M., & Kelly, J. (2002). *For better or worse: Divorce reconsidered.* New York: Norton.

Hetherington, E.M., & Stanley-Hagan, M. (2000). Diversity among stepfamilies. In D.H. Demo & K.R. Allen (Eds.), *Handbook of Family Diversity* (pp. 173–196). New York: Oxford University Press.

Hetherington, E.M., & Stanley-Hagan, M. (2002). Parenting in divorced in remarried families. In M.H. Bornstein (Ed.), *Handbook of Parenting: Vol. 3: Being and Becoming a parent (2nd ed.)* (pp. 287–315). Mahwah, NJ: Erlbaum.

Hofferth, S.L., Smith, J., McLoyd, V.C., & Kindelstein, J. (2000). Achievement and behavior among children of welfare recipients, welfare leavers, and low-income single mothers? *Journal of Social Issues, 56,* 747–773.

Hoffman, L.W. (1989). Effects of maternal employment in the two-parent family. *American Psychologist, 44,* 283–292.

Hoffman, M.L. (1980). Moral development in adolescence. In J. Adelson (Ed.), *Handbook of Adolescent Psychology (pp. 20–41).* New York: Wiley.

Hoffman, M.L. (1994). Discipline and internalization. *Developmental Psychology, 30*(1), 26–28.

Inkeles, A. (1968). Society, social structure, and child socialization. In J.A. Clausen (Ed.), *Socialization and Society* (73–129). Boston, MA: Little Brown.

Jeynes, W. (2002). *Divorce, Family Structure, and the Academic Success of Children.* New York: Haworth Press.

Kagitcibasi, C. (1996). *Family and Human Development Across Cultures: A View from the Other Side.* Mahwah, NJ: Lawrence Erlbaum Associated.

Kelly, J.B. (2000). Children's adjustment in conflicted marriage and divorce: A decade review of research. *Journal of the American Academy of Child & Adolescent Psychiatry, 39,* 963–973.

Kerr, M., & Sattin, H. (2000). What parents know, how they know it, and several forms of adolescent adjustment: Further support for a reinterpretation of monitoring. *Developmental Psychology, 36,* 1–15.

Kohn, M.L. (1977). *Class and Conformity: A Study in Values (2nd ed.).* Chicago, IL: University of Chicago Press.

Kohn, M.L., & Schooler, C. (1983). *Work and Personality: An Inquiry into the Impact of Social Stratification.* Norwood, NJ: Ablex.

Kuczynski, L. (2003). Beyond bidirectionality: Bilateral conceptual frameworks for understanding dynamics in parent-child relations. In L. Kuczinsky (Ed.), *Handbook of Dynamics in Parent-Child Relations* (pp. 3–24). Thousand Oaks, CA: Sage Publications.

Kurdek, L., & Fine, M.A. (1994). Family acceptance and family control as predictors of adjustment in young adolescents : Linear, curvilinear, or interactive effects. *Child Development, 65,* 1137–1146.

Lamborn, S.D., Mounts, N.S., Steinberg, L.D., & Dornbusch, S.M. (1991). Patterns of competence and adjustment among adolescents from authoritative, authoritarian, indulgent, and neglectful families. *Child Development, 62,* 1049–1065.

Larson, R., & Richards, M.H. (1994). *Divergent Realities: The Emotional Lives of Mothers, Fathers, and Adolescents.* New York: Basic Books.

Laursen, B., & Collins, W.A. (1994). Interpersonal conflict during adolescence. *Psychological Bulletin, 115,* 197–209.

Laursen, B., Coy, K.C., & Collins, W.A. (1998). Reconsidering changes in parent-child conflict across adolescence: A meta-analysis. *Child Development, 69,* 817–832.

Lempers, J., & Clark-Lempers, D. (1992). Young, middle, and late adolescents' comparisons of the functional importance of five significant relationships. *Journal of Youth and Adolescents., 21,* 53–96.

Lerner, R.M. (1995). *America's Youth in Crisis: Challenges and Options for Programs and Policies.* Thousand Oaks, CA: Sage Publications.

Lerner, R.M. (2002). *Concepts and Theories of Human Development* (3rd ed.). Mahwah, NJ: Lawrence Erlbaum.

Lichter, D.T., & Jayakody, R. (2002). Welfare reform: How do we measure success? *Annual Review of Sociology, 28,* 117–141.

Lim, S., & Lim, B. (2003). Parenting style and child outcomes in Chinese and immigrant Chinese families: Current findings and cross-cultural considerations in conceptualization and research. *Marriage and Family Review, 35,* (3/4) 21–43.

Maccoby, E.E., & Martin, J.A. (1983). Socialization in the context of the family: Parent-child interaction. In P.H. Mussen (Series Ed.) and M.E. Hetherington (Ed.), *Handbook of Child Psychology: Vol. 4, Socialization, Personality, and Social Development* (pp. 1–101). New York: Wiley.

McCoy, J., Brody, G., & Stoneman, Z. (1994). A longitudinal analysis of sibling relationships as mediators of the link between family processes and youths' best friendships. *Family Relations, 43,* 400–408.

MacDermid, S.M., Lee, M.D., & Smith, S. (2001). Forward into yesterday: Families and work in the 21st century. In K.J. Daly (Ed.), *Minding the Time in Family Experience: Emerging Perspectives and Issues.* Amsterdam: Elsevier Science.

McHale, J. (1997). Overt and covert coparenting processes in the family. *Family Process, 36,* 183–201.

McLoyd, V.C. (1998). Socioeconomic disadvantage and child development. *American Psychologist, 53,* 185–204.

McLoyd, V.C., Jayaratne, T., Ceballo, R., & Borquez, J. (1994). Unemployment and work interruption among African American single mothers: Effects on parenting and adolescent socioemotional functioning. *Child Development, 65,* 562–589.

Meyer, A.L. (2003). Risk-taking, adolescence. In T.P. Gullotta & M. Bloom (Eds.), *Encyclopedia of Primary Prevention and Health Promotion* (pp. 895–900). New York: Kluwer Academic/Plenum Publishers.

Minuchin, S. (1974). *Families and Family Therapy.* Cambridge, MA: Harvard University Press.

Minuchin, P. (2002). Looking toward the horizon: Present and future in the study of family systems. In J.P. McHale & W.S. Grolnick (Eds.), *Retrospect and Prospect in the Study of Families.* Mahwah, NJ: Erlbaum.

Montemayor, R. (1983). Parents and adolescents in conflict: All families some of the time and some families most of the time. *Journal of Early Adolescence, 3,* 83–103.

Montemayor, R. (1984). Maternal employment and adolescents' relations with parents, siblings, and peers. *Journal of Youth and Adolescence, 13,* 543–557.

Montemayor, R. (1986). Family variation in parent-adolescent storm and stress. *Journal of Adolescent Research, 1,* 15–31.

Moore, K.A., Chalk, R., Scarpa, J., & Vandivere, S. (2002). Family strengths: Often overlooked, but real. *Child Trends Research Brief, August,* 1–8.

Noller, P. (1994). Relationships with parents in adolescence: Process and outcome. In R. Montemayor, G. R. Adams, & T.P. Gullotta (Eds.), *Personal Relationships During Adolescence: Advances in Adolescent Development* (Vol. 6) (pp. 37–77). Thousand Oaks, CA: Sage Publications, Inc.

Offer, D., & Schonert-Reichl, K.A. (1992). Debunking the myths of adolescence: Findings from recent research. *Journal of American Academy of Child & Adolescent Psychiatry, 31,* 1003–1014.

O'Hare, W. & Mather, M. (2003). The growing number of kids in severely distressed neighborhoods: Evidence from the 2000 Census. *The Annie E. Casey Foundation and the Population Reference Bureau, KIDS COUNT,* revised, October, 2003.

Paikoff, R.L., & Brooks-Gunn, J. (1991). Do parent-child relationships change during puberty? *Psychological Bulletin, 110,* 47–66.

Parsons, T., & Bales, R. (1955). *Family Socialization and Interaction Process.* New York: Free Press.

Patterson, G.R. (1986). *Performance Models for Antisocial Boys. American Psychologist, 41,* 432–444.

Patterson, G.R., & Capaldi, D.M. (1991). Antisocial parents: Unskilled & vulnerable. In P.A. Cowan & E.M. Hetherington (Eds.), *Family Transitions* (pp. 195–218). Hillsdale, NJ: Lawrence Erlbaum Associates.

Peterson, G.W. (1995). Autonomy and connectedness. In R.D. Day, K.R. Gilbert, B.H. Settles, W. R. Burr (Eds.) *Research and Theory in Family Science*. Pacific Grove, CA: Brooks/Cole.

Peterson, G.W., & Bush, K.R. (2003). Parenting, adolescence. In T.P. Gullotta & M. Bloom (Eds.), *Encyclopedia of Primary Prevention and Health Promotion* (pp. 780–788). New York: Kluwer Academic/Plenum Publishers.

Peterson, G.W., Bush, K.R., & Supple, A. (1999). Predicting adolescent autonomy from parents: Relationship connectedness and restrictiveness. *Sociological Inquiry, 69*, 431–457.

Peterson, G.W., & Hann, D. (1999). Socializing parents and children in families. In M.B. Sussman, S.K. Steinmetz, & G.W. Peterson (Eds.). *Handbook of Marriage and the Family*, (pp. 327–370). New York: Plenum Press.

Peterson, G.W., & Leigh, G.K. (1990). The family and social competence in adolescence. In T.P. Gullotta, G.R. Adams, & R. Montemayor (Eds.), *Developing Social Competency in Adolescence: Advances in Adolescent Development, Vol. 3*, (pp. 97–138). Newbury Park, CA: Sage.

Peterson, G.W., Madden-Derdich, D., & Leonard, S.A. (2000). Parent-child relations across the life-course: Autonomy within the context of connectedness. In S.J. Price, P.C. McKenry, & M.J. Murphy (Eds.), *Families Across Time: A Life Course Perspective*. Los Angeles, CA: Roxbury Publishing Co.

Peterson, G.W., & Rollins, B.C. (1987). Parent-child socialization. In M. Sussman and S. K. Steinmetz (Eds.), *Handbook of Marriage and the Family* (pp. 471–507), New York: Plenum Press.

Peterson, G.W., & Rose, H.A. (2003). Nuclear families, childhood. In T.P. Gullotta & M. Bloom (Eds.), *Encyclopedia of Primary Prevention and Health Promotion* (pp. 705–713). New York: Kluwer Academic/Plenum Publishers.

Peterson, G.W., Steinmetz, S.K., & Wilson, S.M. (2003). Parent-child relationships: Cultural and cross-cultural perspectives. *Marriage and Family Review, 35*, 5–17.

Phinney, J.S., & Ong, A.D. (2002). Adolescent-parent disagreement and life satisfaction in families from Vietnams and European American backgrounds. *International Journal of Behavioral Development, 26*, 556–562.

Rohner, R.P. (1986). *The warmth Dimension: Foundation of Parental Acceptance-Rejection Theory*. Beverly Hills, CA: Sage Publications.

Rollins, B.C., & Thomas, D.L. (1979). Parental support, power, and control techniques in the socialization of children. In W.R. Burr, R. Hill, F.I. Nye, & I.L. Reiss (Eds.), *Contemporary Theories About the Family, Vol. 1, Research Based Theories* (pp. 317–364). New York: Free Press.

Rowe, D.C., Rodgers, J., Meseck-Bushey, S., & St. John, C. (1989). Sexual behavior and nonsexual deviance: A sibling study of their relationship. *Developmental Psychology, 25*, 61–69.

Seginer, R. (1998). Adolescents' perceptions of relationships with older siblings in the context of other close relationships. *Journal of Research on Adolescence, 8*, 287–308.

Silverberg, S.B. & Gondoli, D.M. (1996). Autonomy in adolescence: A contextualized perspective. In G.R. Adams, R. Montemayor, & T.P. Gullotta (Eds.), *Psychosocial Development During Adolescence: Progress in Developmental Contextulism* (pp. 12–61). Thousand Oaks, CA: Sage Publications.

Small, S. (1990). Preventive programs that support families with adolescents. Working paper: Carnegie Council on Adolescent Development. Carnegie Corporation, Washington, DC.

Smetana, J.G. (1988). Concepts of self and social convention: Adolescents' and parents' reasoning about hypothetical and actual family conflicts. In M.Gunnar & W.A. Collins (Eds.), *Minnesota Symposium on Child Psychology, Vol. 21* (pp. 79–122). Hillsdale, NJ: Erlbaum.

Smetana, J.G. (1989). Adolescents' and parents' reasoning about actual family conflict. *Child Development, 59*, 1052–1067.

Smetana, J.G. & Asquith, P. (1994). Adolescents' and parents' conceptions of parental authority and personal autonomy. *Child Development, 65*, 1147–1162.

Stattin, H., & Kerr, M. (2000). Parental monitoring: A reinterpretation. *Child Development, 71*, 1072–1085.

Steinberg, L.D. (1990). Autonomy, conflict, and harmony in the family relationship. In S.S. Feldman & G.R. Elliot (Eds.), *At the Threshold: The Developing Adolescent* (pp. 255–276). Cambridge, MA: Harvard University Press.

Steinberg, L.D. (2001). We know some things: adolescent-parent relationships in retrospect and prospect. *Journal of Research on Adolescence, 11*, 1–20.

Steinberg, L.D., Dornbusch, S.M., & Brown, B.B. (1992). Ethnic differences in adolescent achievement: An ecological perspective. *American Psychologist, 47*, 723–729.

Steinberg, L.D., Lamborn, S.D., Darling, N., Mounts, N.S. & Dornbusch, S.M. (1994). Over-time changes in adjustment and competence among adolescents from authoritative, authoritarian, indulgent, and neglectful families. *Child Development, 65*, 754–770.

Steinberg, L.D., Lamborn, S.D., Dornbusch, S.M. & Darling, N. (1992). Impact of parenting practices on adolescent achievement: Authoritative parenting, school involvement, and encouragement to succeed. *Child Development, 63,* 1266–1281.

Steinberg, L.D., & Levine, A. (1997). *You and Your Adolescent: A Parents' Guide for Ages 10 to 20* (rev. ed.). New York: Harper Collins.

Steinberg, L.D., Mounts, N., Lamborn, S. & Dornbusch, S. (1991). Authoritative parenting and adolescent adjustment across various ecological niches. *Journal of Research on Adolescence, 1,* 19–36.

Stone, G., Buehler, C, & Barber, B.K. (2002). Interparental conflict, parental psychological control, and youth problem behavior. In B.K. (Ed.), *Intrusive Parenting: How Psychological Control Affects Children and Adolescents* (pp. 53–95). Washington, DC: American Psychological Association.

Straus, M.A. (1994). *Beating the Devil Out of Them: Corporal Punishment in American Families.* New York: Lexington Books.

Teachman, J.D. (2000). Diversity of family structure: Economic and social influences. In D.H. Demo, K.R. Allen, & M.A. Fine (Eds.), *Handbook of Family Diversity* (pp. 32–58). New York: Oxford University Press.

Teti, D.M. (2002). Retrospect and prospect in the psychological study of sibling relationships. In J.P. McHale & W.S. Grolnick (Eds.), *Retrospect and Prospect in the Psychological Study of Family* (pp. 193–224). Mahwah, NJ: Erlbaum.

Tucker, C., Barber, B., & Eccles, J. (1997). Advice about life plans and personal problems in late adolescent sibling relationships. *Journal of Youth and Adolescence, 26,* 63–76.

Turner, H.A. & Finkelhor, D. (1996). Corporal punishment as stressor among youth. *Journal of Marriage and the Family, 58,* 155–166.

Updegraff, K., & Crouter, A.C. (2003). Adolescents' sibling relationships and friendship experiences: Developmental patterns and relationship linkages. *Social Development, 11,* 182–204.

Updegraff, K., & Obeidallah, D.A. (1999). Young adolescent's patterns of involvement with siblings and friends. *Social Development, 8,* 53–69.

Wallerstein, J.S., Lewis, J.M., & Blakeslee, S. (2000). *The Unexpected Legacy of Divorce.* New York: Hyperion.

Williams, E., & Radin, N. (1993). Parental involvement, maternal employment, and adolescents' academic achievement: An 11-year follow-up. *American Journal of Orthopsychiatry, 63,* 306–312.

Wilson, S.W., Peterson, G.W., & Wilson, P. (1993). The process of educational and occupational attainment of adolescent females from low-income, rural families. *Journal of Marriage and the Family, 55,* 158–175.

Wyatt, J.M., & Carlo, G. (2002). What will my parents think? Relations among adolescents' expected parental reactions, prosocial moral reasoning, and prosocial and antisocial behaviors. *Journal of Adolescence, 17,* 646–666.

Zaslow, M.J., McGroder, S., Cave, G., & Mariner, C. (1999). Maternal employment and children's health and development among families with a history of welfare receipt. In T. Parcel (Ed.), *Research in the Sociology of Work, Vol. 7, Work and Family* (pp. 233–259). Stamford, CT: JAI Press.

Chapter 4

Community Influence on Adolescent Development

Jill Antonishak, Erin L. Sutfin, and N. Dickon Reppucci

Capturing what encompasses "community" in the lives of adolescents presents a continuing challenge for both researchers and interventionalists. Community often represents an amorphous influence on the lives of adolescence. Depending on the purpose, *community* has been defined as a geographic locality or as a group of individuals who share common goals. For the purposes of this chapter, we cast a wide net with our definition of community to capture the complex and intertwined ecological influences that create shared bonds and experiences among adolescents. Our definition of community encompasses multiple factors that shape the culture of adolescence. We draw on Bronfenbrenner's (1979, 1995) ecological theory, which emphasizes the importance of social contexts in the study of the influence of the community on the adolescent. Contexts such as schools, churches, the workplace, race/ethnicity, and the policy climate represent important influences, but reviewing all aspects of the community is beyond the scope of this chapter. As such, we have selected three components of the community to demonstrate various proximal and distal influences affecting adolescents: (1) peers, (2) neighborhoods, and (3) media. We present a selective review of the literature related to these topics in order to highlight the critical role that community contexts play in adolescent development. We begin by providing a brief overview of Bronfenbrenner's person-process-context model as a foundation for discussing community influence. Within our three selected community components, we examine the role of the context in the lives of adolescents and its potential to serve as both a risk and protective factor.

Ecological Theory

Ecological theory emphasizes the importance of the development of individuals within embedded, interconnected contexts. Bronfenbrenner's (1986, 1995) person-process-context-time model emphasizes the importance of a particular environment on process as a function of individual characteristics. We find this paradigm a helpful heuristic in understanding how the community influences the adolescent at multiple levels. The person component represents the psychological, biological, and behavioral characteristics of an individual adolescent, and although work is increasingly concerned with external factors, much of the body of research related to development focuses on person-level variables. The process component refers to the interactions the adolescent has with other individuals and systemic levels within his or her environment that occur on a regular basis. The context component includes four hierarchical contexts in which the development and interaction of persons and processes occur: the microsystem, mesosystem, exosystem, and the macrosystem.

The *microsystem* is the most proximal setting and represents patterns of relationships, social roles, and interactions that occur in a specific setting. This system includes settings in which the adolescent has direct contact with, as well as distinctive qualities within the setting (Bronfenbrenner, 1989). This system includes settings such as the family, peers, or school, and the majority of research related to development focuses on these settings. However, research on adolescents' development has been increasingly more inclusive of larger contextual factors (Steinberg & Morris, 2001) and the connections between systems. The *mesosystem* represents these linkages between microsystems. For example, Steinberg, Darling, and Fletcher (1995) investigated the interaction of peers and parents on academic achievement of adolescents. Their results demonstrated that although parents have the most influence on long-term educational goals, the peer group had the most influence on daily school activities.

A more distal influence on adolescents is the *exosystem*. The exosystem represents the settings in which a person does not actively participate, but is affected by nonetheless (Bronfenbrenner, 1986). Many exosystemic factors represent mediating or moderating influences. For example, the parents' workplace setting and social support networks influence the parents, which in turn, influence the adolescents. The final level, the macrosystem, represents the broadest social context, and includes cultural or subcultural features and the patterns of interactions that are embedded in these features. Media images, social policies, and ethnic/cultural influences all represent larger macrosystem factors.

The final component of Bronfenbrener's ecological paradigm is *time*. Bronfenbrenner added this component to the framework after original publication of the person-process-context model (Bronfenbrenner, 1995), but consistently has asserted that we need to study how individuals and environments change over time. Within these embedded and changing contexts, processes can promote or impede development, depending on the nature of the setting.

Bronfenbrenner's (1986) ecological framework encourages the investigation of the behavioral, psychological, and biological characteristics of the individual adolescent, but also the interactions between the adolescent and his or her environment, and the interactions between multiple contexts. Characteristics or features within contexts can serve as risk factors, which can increase the likelihood of problem outcomes, or as protective factors, which can decrease the likelihood of a problem outcome or buffer the effect of a risk factor. In addition to context, Bronfenbrenner emphasized the importance of examining multiple facets of interactions, especially, the process or mechanisms which influence adolescents. Understanding these mechanisms provides valuable information for designing interventions, yet there is little research that investigates functional dynamics and contextual specificities that may reduce adolescent problem behavior or promote positive developmental outcomes. Throughout this chapter, we examine contexts at various systemic levels with an understanding that contexts serve as both proximal and distal influences. We highlight the potential of contexts to serve as a risk or protective factor and as a setting for intervention.

Peers

Peers play an important role during the transition from childhood to adolescence (Newcomb & Bagwell, 1995), and adolescents increasingly spend more time with peers over the course of adolescence (Buhrmester & Furman, 1987). Adolescents may also have greater levels of intimacy with friends than younger children (Buhrmester, 1990). Peer group relations have been linked to such diverse developmental constructs as self-esteem (Brown & Lohr, 1987), gender identity (Maccoby, 1990), body image (Paxton, Schutz, Wertheim & Muir, 1999), and academic achievement (Ryan, 2001). They also play an important role in problem behaviors, such as delinquency (e.g., Thornberry & Krohn, 1997), cigarette smoking (e.g., Ennett & Bauman, 1994), drug use (e.g., Dishion & Skaggs, 2000), and risk-taking (e.g., Patterson, Dishion & Yoerger, 2000). In this section, we consider how peer influence may differentially affect adolescents based on the context of the relationship and characteristics of the individual. Specifically, we focus on dyadic (reciprocated) friendships, peer groups, and social networks, and examine outcomes for victimized and rejected youth, who may be particularly vulnerable to negative social adjustment outcomes. We conclude by discussing the potential of the peer group as a protective factor.

The Role of Peers in the Lives of Adolescents

Relationships between adolescents occur within several different contexts and the strength and type of peer influence is likely to differ based on this relational context. To examine this process, we examine dyadic friendships, cliques, and social groups, and then consider the role that status within the peer groups and the social network may play in the influence of peers. The larger social network represents an exosystemic context from which dyadic friendships emerge. These close, reciprocal relationships represent a microsystem context. Adolescents who report having such friendships utilize these relationships as a source of support and advice (Brown, Dolcini & Leventhal, 1997) and report a greater sense of well-being (Hartup & Stevens, 1997). Social groups represent more distal contexts for youth. Researchers typically delineate two types of peer groups: cliques and crowds. Cliques are groups of peers who choose to associate with each other, while crowds represent more reputation-based groups of peers (Brown, 1990), often labeled based on perceived characteristics, such as jocks, brains, or burnouts (e.g., La Greca, Prinstein & Fetter, 2001).

One of the strongest findings on friendships is the similarity of friends' attitudes and behaviors, commonly known as *homophily* (Kandel, 1978). However, the mechanism through which homophily occurs may result from dual processes: peer selection and peer conformity. Selection effects imply that adolescents select into friendships with adolescents who are similar to themselves. For example, Urberg, Degirmencioglu, and Tolson (1998) found that adolescents later became friends with individuals who had similar levels of substance use and delinquency. The idea of conformity suggests that adolescents become increasingly similar to their friends, because they model themselves after their friends, or their friends pressure them to conform. Although it is likely that adolescents select into peer groups that are similar to themselves, researchers have found that the effect of peers on problem behavior goes beyond simply selection into friendships (e.g., Keenan, Loeber, Zhang, Stouthamer-Loeber & van Kammen, 1995), and adolescents may provide positive reinforcement, or implicit threats of rejection to encourage conformity. A process of reciprocal socialization appears to increase similarities between peers (Cairns, Leung & Cairns, 1995).

Research increasingly suggests that both models may be useful in understanding the influence of peers (e.g., Urberg, Luo, Pilgrim & Degirmencioglu, 2003). Thornberry and Krohn (1997) postulate an interactional theory to explain peer effects on delinquency and drug use, in which peers reinforce problem behaviors while providing a supportive context for such behavior. So while peers can provide supportive contexts for the promotion of positive development, peers can also exacerbate problematic pathways to negative outcomes. The duration of the relationship likely plays an important role in the strength of peer influence. For example, Brendgen, Vitaro, and Bukowski (2000) have suggested that the effect of delinquent peers on subsequent delinquent behaviors depends both on duration the adolescent has been exposed to the influence of the delinquent peers and the recency of affiliation with such friends, relative to the period of assessment. Over a two-year period, Bredgen et al. found adolescents who had stably affiliated with delinquent peers, *and* those who changed affiliations from non-delinquent to delinquent peers, participated in the highest levels of delinquent activity.

Given these types of influence, adolescents are likely to be differentially affected by peers. Cairns and Cairns (1994) suggest that some groups may be more powerful in exerting influence over members, and some individuals within the group may possess characteristics that make them more powerful models of socialization. Similarly, Kindermann (1998) suggests that some adolescents may be differentially resistant to influences within the peer group. Those who are firmly embedded in a peer group and perceive high levels of social support may be less susceptible to peer influence than those who perceive little social support. For example, for adolescents in antisocial peer groups, Bender and Lösel (1997) found that a lack of embeddedness in the group served as a protective factor. Peripheral members may differentially participate in peer group activities in order to gain inclusion; alternatively, they may feel less compelled to participate in risk-taking with other group members if they feel less invested in the group, but the characteristics of the person and the context are likely to play an important role. This relationship will have implications for intervention efforts targeting peer influence on problem behaviors.

Status within the larger social network exosystem may also play an important role in the process of peer influence. Adler and Adler (1995) delineated a hierarchy within peer groups, in which some group members exhibit greater social dominance than other group members. Status within a peer group is likely to be based on members' ability to compete for and control resources (Hawley, 1999). Those with higher social status are likely to have access to and attention from peers, choose the group's activities, and control information within the network, while individuals with lower social status may have more problem social adjustment outcomes. Researchers primarily determine perceptions of social status based on a peer nomination process, where participants nominate peers they like and dislike. Youth are then classified as either popular (receiving many like nominations), rejected (receiving many dislike nominations), neglected (receiving few nominations for either category), or controversial (receiving nominations in both like and dislike nominations) (Coie, Dodge & Coppotelli, 1982).

The relative influence of these different relational contexts and roles within the social network is unclear, although these relationships may be more important than the presence of friends. Bagwell, Newcomb, and Bukowski (1998) found that sociometric status predicted academic performance, rather than presence of friends. Bearman and Brückner (1999) found that girls' sexual initiation was influenced more by the peer group than by individual risk factors or close friends. On the other hand, Urberg and colleagues (1997) found that close friendships were more important influences for substance use than crowd affiliation. Although promising research has emerged to study these contexts and suggests that these different peer relationships provide unique contexts for influence (e.g., Kiesner, Poulin & Nicotra, 2003), further research is needed to elucidate these processes and the types of influence that may serve as risk and protective factors.

Peers as a Risk or Protective Factor

In an effort to understand mechanisms by which peer selection and reciprocal socialization may serve to exacerbate or buffer possible negative outcomes, we first discuss the peer group as a context for the development of aggressive behaviors, and then examine two groups of adolescents who may be particularly vulnerable to problem outcomes: rejected and victimized youth.

Parker and Asher (1987) identified aggressive behaviors as one of the strongest predictors of problems in the peer group. Aggressive acts have traditionally been seen as physical behaviors, in which the target is harmed through damage to his/her physical well-being; however, non-physical forms of social and relational aggression may also cause harm. *Relational aggression* is defined by Crick and colleagues (1999) as "behaviors that harm others through damage (or the threat of damage) to relationships or feelings of acceptance, friendship, or group inclusion" (p. 77). While physically aggressive acts include hitting, punching, or threatening to beat someone up, relationally aggressive acts include giving someone the silent treatment, excluding a person from a social activity, threatening to end a friendship, or spreading rumors about a person. Such acts are typically used to hurt someone emotionally by damaging social relationships, but these tactics may also be used to establish dominance in a group, maintain the aggressor's sense of belonging, or protect the integrity of the group. Adolescents may refine their use of relational aggression compared to younger children with an increased capacity for planning and greater understanding of sarcasm and innuendo.

Friendships formed by aggressive youth are frequently marked by problems. Physically aggressive youth establish friendships with other physically aggressive youth, but these relationships are marked by low levels of intimacy and a high number of coalitional acts in which they join forces to gang up aggressively on other children (Cairns, Cairns, Neckerman, Ferguson & Gariépy, 1989; Dishion, Andrews & Crosby, 1995). Aggressive youths who coalesce into aggressive peer groups and become dominant in a social network are likely to be at risk for conduct problems (e.g., Underwood, Kupersmidt & Coie, 1996). For example, in the school setting, these youths may challenge school authority and social conventions (Cairns, Cadwallader, Estell & Neckerman, 1999). Henrich, Kuperminc, Sack, Blatt, and Leadbeater (2000) examined school cliques and found that one clique of four boys accounted for 7% of all discipline referrals recorded for the entire sample of 499 students.

With regard to relational aggression, Grotpeter and Crick (1996) found that relationally aggressive children identified mutual friendships; however, while relationally aggressive friends tend to have high levels of intimacy (such as self-disclosure and feelings of closeness), these dyads are also marked by high levels of betrayal and demands for exclusivity. Research is needed to examine the role of relational aggression within adolescent peer groups. Although individuals who are highly relationally aggressive may continue to be rejected by peers, those with sophisticated relationally aggressive skills may actually be successful in negotiating peer dynamics and making a relationship more cohesive.

Aggressive behaviors may also be related to status within the peer group. Xie, Swift, Cairns & Cairns (2002) found that boys who were more central to the peer group exhibited higher levels of physical aggression, while girls who were central to the peer group exhibited more social aggression. Social status is often associated with greater linkages to peers and control of peer resources in the network, which may provide a greater arsenal of relationally aggressive strategies for those central to the peer group. Similarly, physically aggressive adolescents firmly embedded in the peer group may receive greater support for the use of aggressive behaviors (such as back-up during a physical fight). Research related to aggressive peer groups and experiences of victimization can inform interventions for both aggressive and victimized youth by elucidating the process in which an aggressive peer group forms.

Adolescents can target physical and relational aggression towards individuals within their peer group and those outside of their circle of friends. Victimization by physically aggressive peers has been found to be related to multiple emotional, behavioral, and social problems (e.g., Graham & Juvonen, 1998). Similarly, victimization by relational aggression has been related to negative adjustment outcomes, such as depression, loneliness, social anxiety, and other emotional difficulties (Crick & Grotpeter, 1996; Prinstein, Boergers & Vernberg, 2001). Victims of physical and relational aggression were more likely to be rejected by peers and feel socially anxious than non-victimized children (Crick and Bigbee, 1998) and report using verbal or physical aggression to retaliate (Schwartz et al., 1998; Roecker-Phelps, 2001). Hodges and Perry (1999) suggest that children's ability to form and maintain friendships may be damaged by peer victimization because peers are unlikely to associate with youth who are perceived as targets and are unable to defend their social status. Furthermore, aggressive children are likely to target victims who lack friends who could provide support and protection. Traditional views of bullying assume that victimization occurs in non-equivalent power relationships; however, bullying can also occur within the context of a friendship dyad (Grotpeter & Crick, 1996). Crick and colleagues (1999) suggest that some low-status peers may form relationships with aggressive youth and tolerate relationally aggressive victimization because they have few friendship choices and are seeking protection from larger peer threats in the social network. This research suggests that some members of the peer network may be particularly vulnerable to victimization. Identification of these youth can assist in targeting intervention efforts to those who may be at greater risk for negative social and psychological outcomes.

Similarly, youth who are rejected within the social network may be vulnerable to negative adjustment outcomes. Bagwell, Coie, Terry, and Lochman (2000) found that rejected youth were likely to be peripheral members of a peer group and associate with other low-status peers. Thus, rejected group members may experience relatively few opportunities to associate with pro-social youth and almost no modeling of positive social competencies. Laird, Jordan, Dodge, Petit, and Bates (2001) found that peer rejection in childhood was related to externalizing behavior in adolescence, particularly for those youth who had been repeatedly rejected by others in the social network. Laird and colleagues found that affiliation with antisocial peers was related to externalizing behaviors, but that peer rejection accounted for the variance above and beyond affiliation with peers.

Although much of the focus has been on peers as negative influences on adolescents, they can also serve as a protective factor. Dyadic friendships provide support and feelings of connectedness and security (Bukowski, Hoza & Boivin, 1994; Furman & Buhrmester, 1985). High-quality friendships can also increase feelings of social competence and self-esteem (Buhrmester, 1990, 1996). By providing information and support, and modeling positive social behaviors, peers can serve as prosocial influences (Berndt & Keefe, 1995; Berndt, 1996). Elliott (1994) found that adolescents who associated with peers who disapproved of delinquency served as a protective factor. Even disagreement within a positive close friendship can serve a constructive purpose in the development of conflict management skills (Hartup, 1992). Reciprocated close friendship may also buffer peer rejection in the larger social group (Parker & Asher, 1993).

Peer relations may also buffer poor relationships within the family. For example, having a reciprocal best friend or high-quality friendships served as a buffer between child abuse and lower self-esteem for younger children (Bolger, Patterson & Kupersmidt, 1998). In adolescence, high-quality friendships serve as a protective factor for adolescent social competence and self-worth in families with poor cohesion and adaptability (Gauze, Bukowski Aquan-Assee & Sippola, 1996). Lansford and colleagues (2003) found that although externalizing behaviors were related to negative parenting and low supervision, particularly for adolescents with antisocial peers, positive peer relationships attenuated the relationship.

Peer Groups as a Context for Intervention

The protective nature of some friendships may serve as an important context for intervention, although there is considerable evidence that the peer group may not be an ideal mechanism for some types of problem behaviors. Peer-based interventions are relatively common for delinquent and problem behaviors among youth, but Dishion, McCord and Poulin (1999) found iatrogenic effects for adolescents who had participated in a peer-based intervention focusing on problem solving skills, peer support, and resisting negative influence. They found that the youth's rule-breaking talk, usually outside the actual treatment group, predicted an increase in problem behaviors. These findings suggest caution in the development of peer-based interventions, but does not rule out peers as an important prosocial influence. Interventions that give youth an opportunity to interact with positive peer models may have more positive effects than those that aggregate youth with problem behaviors. For example, Hudley and Graham (1993) found a reduction in aggressive boys' hostile attributions after an intervention program that targeted both aggressive and non-aggressive boys. Programs which partner rejected children with average or popular youth may increase the target child's likeability and protect against victimization within the social network.

In summary, although peers can provide supportive contexts for positive social skills and outcomes, they can also be a risk factor for some problem behaviors. The type and context of the relationship and status within any peer relational context contribute unique influences to adolescent development. The qualities of the individual person and the context can affect the process through which peers influence outcomes. Peer-based interventions have potential if they target prosocial behaviors, but the dynamics of negative peer influences can also endanger intervention efforts. Intervention would benefit from using positive peer influences.

Neighborhoods

There has been increasing interest related to the role that neighborhoods may play in adolescent development. Research on neighborhood effects have found links to outcomes such as academic achievement (e.g., Duncan, 1994), delinquent behavior (e.g., Peeples and Loeber, 1994), child-bearing (e.g., Brooks-Gunn, Guo & Furstenberg, 1993), and maltreatment (Lynch & Cicchetti, 1998). Despite their importance, neighborhoods often represent relatively amorphous influences on individual outcomes. Depending upon conceptualization, neighborhoods may represent a proximal influence on the adolescent through his or her involvement in and perception of the neighborhood and use of public spaces and the modification of those spaces. Neighborhoods also may represent an exosystemic and distal influence in the lives of adolescents in that many of their components cannot be influenced by the adolescents. These unidimensional influences include neighborhood financial resources, racial/ethnic diversity, and external social support. The context of neighborhoods differs based on whether it is being considered a direct mechanism of influence on adolescent development or an indirect influence. In many instances, neighborhoods function in both capacities.

In this section, we review some methodological challenges for studying neighborhoods and some mechanisms by which neighborhoods affect adolescents. While an exhaustive review is beyond of the scope of this chapter, we do highlight two critical features of neighborhoods that have been linked to adolescent outcomes: (1) neighborhood characteristics and (2) relationships and social support within the neighborhood. We also review ways that neighborhoods can serve as both risk and protective factors.

Neighborhoods in the Lives of Adolescents

Research on neighborhoods presents complex methodological and theoretical challenges. One basic issue is related to the way neighborhoods are defined. In most studies, neighborhoods are defined in terms of geographic boundaries, primarily census tracts (Gephart, 1997) (although some studies and ethnographic work allow residents to determine their neighborhoods based on perceptions of boundaries [Leventhal & Brooks-Gunn, 2000]). Parents and youth, however, rarely view the dividing lines of the neighborhoods in the same way as the Census Bureau. Even within a neighborhood, residents may have different views on the boundaries, possibly based on perceptions of their own social networks (Jarrett, 1997). Children's concepts of neighborhood and community usually change as they develop. As children, their perception of neighborhood may include only the block on which they play or explore. During adolescence, as their perception of space develops and their network of peers and schools expands past their apartment building or block, so does their concept of their neighborhood. Census tract definitions of neighborhoods may be inadequate because they omit residents' subjective feelings and perceptions and present only a limited description of factors such as living conditions, composition of families, and cultural practices that describe the neighborhood.

Gephart (1997) discusses the difficulty researchers face in categorizing neighborhoods as a single measure or constructing multivariate indices based on cumulative risk factors. Moreover, determining unbiased neighborhood effects and causal relationships between neighborhood characteristics and adolescent outcomes is complicated by potentially confounding variables (Duncan & Raudenbush, 1999) and multiple pathways of neighborhood influence. Neighborhoods can serve as direct influences on adolescent outcomes, or more often, as moderators or mediators of other functional characteristics in the neighborhood (Boyce et al., 1998). Neighborhoods can directly and independently affect outcomes for adolescents. For example, the availability of public spaces in a neighborhood can affect adolescents' patterns of social congregation. Neighborhoods can also indirectly influence adolescents through other contextual factors, such as schools and the family. For example, high crime rates and violence in the neighborhood could increase parenting stress, which leads to lower levels of parental monitoring of youth. The combination of these multiple contextual factors influence adolescent outcomes, such that in some contexts of parenting, neighborhoods serve as risk factor, while in others, they can serve as a protective factor (see Leventhal and Brooks-Gunn [2000] and Brooks-Gunn, Duncan, and Aber [1997a, b] for excellent reviews).

Neighborhoods as a Risk or Protective Factor

Although low-income urban neighborhoods have a high mobility rate for residents, it appears that the essential characteristics of neighborhood are greater than the individuals living there (Aber, Gephart, Brooks-Gunn & Connell, 1997). Usually, a set of values and beliefs exist in a neighborhood that remains stable, regardless of who is moving in or out. This is not to say that neighborhoods do not change, and over time housing policies or employment opportunities may alter the neighborhood and its values, but the effects of these shifts unfold slowly over time. We first examine environmental characteristics within a neighborhood as potential risk factors for adolescents, and then present information about how relationships and social support within a community can serve as protective factors.

Research has demonstrated that the environmental characteristics of a neighborhood can influence adolescents. Factors at the mesosystemic level, such as residential mobility, vacant housing, or neighborhood violence or crime can serve as a risk factor for youth outcomes. The majority of studies, however, examine demographic characteristics of residents, such as family-level socioeconomic status (SES) as aggregate variables to represent neighborhood risk factors, and focus on urban areas. We know very little about how neighborhoods may influence adolescent development in rural or suburban areas. Moreover, the focus on poor, urban areas presents a methodological challenge in untangling the effects of poverty and neighborhood and isolating causal variables from SES (Duncan & Raudenbush, 1999).

High-risk neighborhoods tend to have a constellation of problem outcomes for youth. Coulton, Korbin, Su & Chow (1995) found that family hardship, poverty rate, unemployment rate, frequency of vacant housing, population loss, percentage of black residents, and percentage of female-headed households were linked to high rates of violent crime and delinquency, child maltreatment, adolescent deviant behavior, and teenage pregnancy. These multiple factors highlight the challenge of untangling the effects of SES and neighborhoods in determining which construct serves as a stronger influence and which truly represents neighborhood. As the number of risk factors within the neighborhood increases, so does the likelihood of problem outcomes among residents. We now focus on neighborhood violence as an example of an environmental neighborhood-level variable that may affect adolescent outcomes.

Some neighborhoods have particularly high concentrations of neighborhood violence and crime. For example, Bell and Jenkins (1993) found that 75% of students, aged 10–19, living in a Chicago neighborhood had witnessed either a robbery, stabbing, shooting, or killing. In a follow-up study, Jenkins and Bell (1997) found that almost half of a sample of 200 high school students had been shot at. Such exposure may be one of the strongest predictors of adolescents' use of violence (DuRant, Cadenhead, Pendergrast, Slavens & Linder, 1994). Youth exposed to neighborhood violence are also likely to experience post-traumatic stress disorder-like symptoms and anxiety (Horn & Trickett, 1998).

Spencer, McDermott, Burton, and Kochman (1997) examined the qualities of neighborhoods and crime rates and found that crime statistics were more related to neighborhood characteristics, such as quality of housing or patterns of teenage meeting places, than they were to individual family economic characteristics, such as single-parent households or family income. The link between low-SES and communities with high violence rates is difficult to separate. Hill, Levermore, Twaite, and Jones (1996) found that communities with high violence rates were affected by poverty, inadequate health care, poor schools, and lower maternal education. Most studies examining community violence attempt to control for low SES, but the two are strongly linked.

The problem of neighborhood violence may be especially important for African American youth, particularly males because they are over-represented in low-income neighborhoods (Cooley-Quille, Turner & Beidel, 1995). When Peeples and Loeber (1994) compared delinquency rates of African American and Caucasian boys, they found significant differences in the frequency and seriousness of delinquent acts, with African American boys being higher on both indices. However, when comparing African American boys who did not live in underclass neighborhoods (characterized by high rates of family poverty, use of public assistance, single-parent families, families with no one employed, unmarried births, and male joblessness) to Caucasian boys, these differences disappeared. Hyperactivity and parental supervision were correlated with delinquency; however, the strongest predictor of violence was living in an underclass neighborhood. Ethnicity was not related to either seriousness or frequency of delinquent acts when the contextual setting was controlled. Hammond and Yung (1993) suggest that regardless of the findings related to SES, the practical implication for African American youth remains because they are overly represented in low-income families.

The environmental characteristics of the neighborhood and relationships between residents in the neighborhood are inextricably linked and reciprocally influence each other, and in turn, influence the development of adolescents. Wilson (1991) suggests that poor environmental conditions in the neighborhood lead to feelings of isolation for families, which can lead to strained parenting and negative outcomes for children and youth. However, in these neighborhoods, a network of social support for adolescents and their families can buffer negative environmental conditions. For example, Gorman-Smith, Tolan, and Henry (2000) found that supportive social processes protected adolescents from chronic delinquency compared to children from similar neighborhoods without social support. The protective nature of these relationships is likely to vary based on the presence and quality of social networks, and the degree of personal responsibility that residents assume within the neighborhood (Wilson, 1995).

Sampson, Raudenbush, and Earls (1997) suggest that an important source of protection for youth and families is a sense of collective efficacy within a neighborhood. Collective efficacy represents networks of mutual trust and shared norms, where residents are involved in community organizations and willing to intervene for the common good of the neighborhood. Chavis and Wandersman (1990) suggest that parents in cohesive neighborhoods may be less restrictive toward their children because of the availability of neighborhood resources and high levels of neighborhood monitoring. These neighborhoods are likely to have high levels of social monitoring, and Sampson, Raudenbush, and Earls (1997) found that such neighborhoods have lower levels of crime and community violence. Although most work on social support within neighborhoods has focused on low-SES areas, Luthar (2003) suggests that affluent neighborhoods may be at risk for problematic outcomes such as internalizing problems or substance use, due to residents' relative independence. A lack of issues within the community may fail to activate a sense of collective efficacy within such neighborhoods.

Neighborhoods as a Context for Intervention

Interventions at the neighborhood-level have primarily focused on building social resources within the neighborhood. Brown (1996) reviewed components of programs designed to support neighborhoods and found that the general goals are to increase opportunities for social interactions. These types of interventions have the potential to increase social capital and collective efficacy within a neighborhood, which we know provides a buffer for adolescents.

In summary, research related to neighborhood represents a challenge for researchers due the complexity of modeling its effects and isolating neighborhood level variables. However, environmental characteristics and relationships within the neighborhood represent unique influences on adolescent outcomes. Neighborhood characteristics may also serve as a protective factor, and therefore an important context for intervention.

Media

The images portrayed through media represent multiple contexts of interaction. They may represent macrosystemic influences, in that they portray the culture of adolescence and representations of social norms. At the same time they may serve as an exosystemic influence, and influence our culture's all too often negative perceptions about adolescents. For example, youth are often portrayed as engaged in delinquent or violent acts. Woodruff (1998) analyzed local news coverage throughout California and found that 53% of stories about youth involved violence. Such negative appraisals influence how youth are treated and opportunities they are afforded. Media may also represent a microsystemic influence, particularly through video games and internet use. Adolescents using the internet create on-line relationships and communities, and although limited research exists, these relationships are likely to represent important contexts of influence. Media use also represents a salient example of proximal processes because adolescents have greater freedom to select the form and content they consume, either through their purchase of music and movie tickets, or by changing television channels. In this section we focus mainly on the influence of television on adolescents, as the research on that medium is the most prolific.

Media in the Lives of Adolescents

In today's culture, media is omnipresent in the lives of teens. On average, children aged eight years and older spend $6\frac{3}{4}$ hours using media each day (Roberts, Foehr, Rideout, & Brodie, 1999). In fact, children are surrounded by media in their homes. According to a survey done by the Kaiser Family Foundation, the average American child lives in a home with two television sets, three tape players, three radios, two VCRs, two CD players, one video game console, and one computer (Roberts et al., 1999). However, children divide their time unequally between these different forms of media, sometimes even using more than one medium at the same time. For instance, teens with internet access at home report spending about 46 minutes on line each day (Woodard & Gridina, 2000), and adolescents report listening to music for an average of between three and four hours daily (Roberts & Christenson, 2001). In addition, adolescents typically watch between three and four hours of television per day (Comstock, 1991). Television use peaks in early adolescents and then declines a bit before leveling off. As it declines, listening to music typically increases (Brown, Childers, Bauman & Koch, 1990).

Just as teens use a variety of media sources, the reasons for their use of media are varied. According to Strasburger and Wilson (2002), teens use music for relaxation and mood regulation, socializing with peers, self-expression, and background noise. Likewise, they use the internet for various reasons, including social communication (sending e-mail, participating in chat rooms, instant messaging), information seeking (news, health information, research for schoolwork), game-playing, shopping, and downloading music (Kaiser Family Foundation, 2001). With regard to television, Dominick (1987) suggests four purposes: (a) cognition (to obtain information), (b) diversion (for stimulation, relaxation, or emotional release), (c) social integration (to overcome loneliness, to allow quasi-social relationships with TV characters, etc.), and (d) withdrawal (to avoid chores or escape reality). As discussed below, understanding why teens use a certain medium may be helpful in understanding how they will be influenced by that medium.

Over the past several decades, many theories have emerged to explain the effect of mass media on children and adolescents. Because television has been the most widely studied medium, theories used to explain mass media were mainly developed with television in mind. Although these theories may be successfully applied to other media, research examining the applicability to newer forms, such as video games and internet use, is in the early stages. Bandura's (1967) *social learning* theory provided an early explanation of television's influence on children. This theory posits that viewers learn new skills and behaviors by watching and imitating models on television. However, the extent to which a viewer imitates a given model depends on several factors, including similarities between the viewer and the model, the credibility of the model, similarities between the model and other models in the viewer's life, the perceived reality of the observed behavior, the motivation of the viewer, and whether or not the model is rewarded or punished for his/her behavior (Van Evra, 1998). These determinants of imitation of televised models are complex and involve many characteristics of the viewer and the model.

In the 1980s, Gerbner, Gross, Morgan, and Signorielli's (1986) *cultivation theory* proposed that media influences viewers through extensive exposure which shapes the viewers' perceptions of social reality. In essence, the more time spent watching television, the more likely the viewer is to accept television's portrayal of the world, however inconsistent it may be with reality (Van Evra, 1998). According to this theory, the amount of time spent watching television is more important than the particular content of the programming watched. As with social learning theory, perceived reality is the critical variable. For example, if content is seen as being realistic, then it is likely to have a larger effect on the viewer's attitudes and beliefs. Younger viewers are more vulnerable to cultivation effects than are adults because they have fewer competing sources of information in their lives and are more likely to perceive content as realistic, thus enhancing the cultivation effects.

Van Evra (1998) suggests that the integration of social learning theory and cultivation theory can contribute to our understanding of the ways in which media influences viewers. Van Evra (1998) suggests that we need to consider the use made of television, the perceived reality of the content, the amount of viewing, and other competing sources of information to understand television's influence. In addition, we must take into consideration viewer variables such as age, gender, socioeconomic level, cognitive ability, and general experience fully to understand the influence of media. Therefore, predicting how media will affect viewers is a complicated and challenging endeavor; however, we have a large body of literature which suggests that media have an important influence on problem behaviors.

Media as a Risk or Protective Factor

Media can be both a risk factor and a protective factor for problem behaviors depending on the particular content viewed. In this section, we focus on media portrayals of violence, sexual activity, and substance use as potential risk factors for adolescents, and also examine how prosocial and educational content on these three activities may act as a positive influence.

VIOLENCE.   American media have long been considered extremely violent and have prompted decades of research to determine what, if any, impact this content has on viewers. To understand this, we explore first how much violent content a teen sees on average. The amount of violence on television is far greater than the amount of violence in the real word. In fact, by the time a child reaches his 18th birthday, he will have witnessed 200,000 acts of violence on television, including 40,000 murders (Huston et al., 1992). Not only is the sheer amount of violence on television a major concern for parents and researchers alike, the way in which it is portrayed must be considered. Research from the National Television Violence Study found that violence on television is typically glamorized, sanitized, and trivialized (for an extensive review, see Strasburger & Wilson, 2002). Over a three-year period at least 40% of violence on television was perpetrated by attractive characters, 75% of violent scenes contained no punishment, 85% of violence showed no long-term consequences, and almost half of the violence showed no physical harm or pain to the victim. In addition, violence was often coupled with some type of humor. These positive portrayals of violence may be likely to encourage modeling by viewers.

Decades of research have confirmed that exposure to violent content on television has a real and serious impact on viewers. We highlight three primary ways violent content affects adolescents: (a) increasing aggressive behavior, (b) desensitization, (c) increased fear. The bulk of the research has focused on whether watching violent television increases aggressive behavior. After 30 years of correlational, experimental, and longitudinal research, the results demonstrate a clear, causal relationship between viewing violence and behaving aggressively (Paik & Comstock, 1994). This is not to say that violent media are the single cause of aggressive or violent behavior in youth. Rather violent media are one of many possible causes (Bushman & Huesmann, 2001). As suggested by social learning theory, when violence is portrayed by attractive characters who get rewarded and not punished for their behavior, viewers are likely to model violent behavior.

In addition to increasing aggressiveness among youth, research also found that viewing violent television may lead to desensitization among viewers. As predicted by cultivation theory, heavy television viewers have been found to be less disturbed by violence, more likely to believe violence is justified, and more tolerant of it (Van der Voort, 1986). Viewers appear to cultivate the attitudes similar to those shown on television, such that violence is seen as acceptable, rather than problematic.

Finally, research has shown that viewing violent content may lead to fear and mistrust of the real world, a phenomenon known as the "mean world syndrome" (Signorielli, 1990). According to cultivation theory, heavy viewers of television will come to see the world as a more violent and frightening place than it is in reality. In fact, heavy television viewers believe the world is more violent than light viewers and that they are more likely to be the victims of violence (see Signorielli & Morgan, 1990).

In sum, violent television does lead viewers to be more aggressive, desensitized to its consequences, and fearful of the world around them. The results are particularly troubling given that a majority of television programs contain some form of violence, most of which is portrayed in a way that would increase, rather than decrease, learning and modeling the violent behavior. Therefore, violent content is a potential risk factor for adolescent aggressive behaviors.

SEXUALITY. In the absence of a comprehensive school or home-based sex education program, media have become the leading source of sex education in the United States (Strasburger & Wilson, 2002). Teens may be particularly drawn to television as a sex educator for several reasons. First, it allows them to gather information in an anonymous, non-threatening, non-embarrassing way. Second, while school-based sex education programs typically focus on the more physical aspects of sex, media usually focuses on the social aspects, such as providing scripts for dating. Finally, adolescents are often dissatisfied with the information that they get from their parents and search for additional information (Selverstone, 1992). Unfortunately, teens use of television as a sex educator is particularly troublesome. On average, teens view 14,000 sexual references, innuendos, and behaviors each year on television, with less than 170 scenes incorporating some sort of responsible behavior (Harris & Associates, 1988).

Although there have only been a few studies that address the impact of sexual content on adolescents, theory suggests that such consistent messages are likely incorporated by adolescents (Huston & Wright, 1997). There have been two documented studies that found a positive correlation between viewing television and having intercourse (Brown & Newcomber, 1991; Peterson & Kahn, 1984, as cited in Strasburger & Wilson, 2002). Although the research is limited, it does suggest that watching television, which is composed of "a consistent set of messages portraying erotic sexuality as a casual, recreational activity with little emotional or personal commitment and few negative consequences" (Huston & Wright, 1997, p. 1033) can have an impact on adolescents' sexual attitudes and behaviors. Therefore, television content, which is saturated with careless sexual imagery, can be a risk factor for irresponsible, early sexual behavior.

Research has found that when television programs incorporate positive educational messages about sexuality into the plot of the show, teens learn the information. For example, the producers of *ER* and the Kaiser Family Foundation worked together to develop storylines with information about emergency contraception and human papilloma virus (HPV). After the episodes aired, people reported that they knew of HPV and emergency contraception at greater rates than before they watched the episodes (Brodie et al., 2001). Therefore, media can act as a positive influence in the lives of teens, helping them to learn useful and important information.

SUBSTANCE USE. Alcohol and tobacco use are quite regularly shown in American movies and television programs. In fact, Roberts, Henriksen, and Christenson (1999) found that of the 200 most popular movie rentals of 1996 and 1997, 93% portrayed alcohol use and 89% showed tobacco use. In one longitudinal study, Robinson and colleagues (1998) found that for ninth-graders, watching a heavy diet of television and music videos was one risk factor for alcohol use. Adolescents are also regularly exposed to extensive advertising for these products. Teens see between 1,000 and 2,000 advertisements for beer and alcohol each year (Strasburger, 1997). The old Joe the Camel advertising campaign was so successful that six-year-olds could identify Joe as readily as they recognized the Disney logo (Fischer, Schwartz, Richards, Goldstein & Rojas, 1991). It is not only to the sheer number of ads viewed, but also the way in which the ads portray alcohol and tobacco use that is troubling. The ads are crafted to appeal to teens, depicting attractive people in enjoyable activities (Strasburger & Wilson, 2002) to make the viewer believe that smoking and/or drinking alcohol is a positive normal activity that will make you attractive to others (Strasburger, 1997).

Research shows that alcohol and tobacco ads are particularly effective. Eighty-four percent of teens who smoke, smoke the three most heavily advertised brands of cigarettes (Marlboro™, Camel™, and Newport™) (Centers for Disease Control, 1992). A series of studies by Atkin and colleagues (Atkin & Block, 1983; Atkin, Neuendorf & McDermott, 1983; Atkin, Hocking & Block, 1984) found that adolescents who were exposed to larger amounts of alcohol advertising had more positive beliefs about drinking, viewed drinkers as very much like the people shown in the ads, and were more likely to drink themselves. Although this research suggests that alcohol and tobacco use in media has a negative impact on adolescents, more research needs to be done to help understand the direction of effect and the magnitude of the impact (Strasburger & Wilson, 2002). However, at this point, it is clear that exposure to alcohol and tobacco ads and portrayals on television are important risk factors for adolescents that need to be addressed.

Just as media can act as a risk factor for increasing adolescent substance use, it can also act as a prevention tool if the content is prosocial or educational. As such, mass media has long been used as a method for delivering important public health messages to teens. Adolescent tobacco prevention is one particular topic that has been targeted by both state and national counteradvertising media campaigns. For example, in early 1998, Florida began a comprehensive, state-wide anti-tobacco campaign targeting teens aged 12 to 17 (Sly, Hopkins, Trapido & Ray, 2001). The intervention featured a multi-pronged approach to tobacco prevention, including youth-directed community prevention programs, school-based educational programs, retailer education, and a youth-led mass media campaign (Bauer, Johnson, Hopkins, Brooks, 2000). One prominent component was a concentrated counteradvertising media campaign that focused on the fact that the tobacco industry had knowledge of and tried to conceal evidence of the harmful effects of tobacco use (Sly, Hopkins, Trapido & Ray, 2001). Research showed that after the first year of the mass media campaign, Florida youth had stronger anti-tobacco attitudes and also lower uses of tobacco as compared to national youth (Sly, Heald & Ray, 2001). In addition, researchers found a 40% decrease in smoking among Florida middle-school students and an 18% decline among high-school students two years after the prevention program began (Bauer, Johnson, Hopkins & Brooks, 2000). Although it is difficult to separate the effects of mass media from other aspects of the Florida Tobacco Control Program, this research suggests that the mass media anti-tobacco campaign was a significant and important part of their multi-pronged prevention program.

In summary, although the research is very limited, it suggests that media can provide supportive contexts for positive social skills and outcomes. At the same time, research has shown that media can serve as a risk factor for adolescents by increasing their aggressive and sexual behavior and their alcohol and tobacco use. Therefore, content plays an essential role in determining how media will affect adolescents. Media's potential as an intervention tool needs extensive investigation.

Conclusion

The intent of this chapter was to highlight the need to look beyond the microsystem context of adolescence. Adolescents are embedded within contexts that differentially affect development. Peers, neighborhoods, and the media represent but three levels of the widening ecology that affects adolescent development. Bronfenbrenner's model focuses on the process, or mechanisms of influence. These influences vary based on individual or context characteristics. Understanding these mechanisms and the interplay between context and the individual provides valuable information about the development of problem behaviors. Changes at one contextual level, such as modification of public space within a neighborhood, could change characteristics at another level, such as where youth hang out or how they structure their free time.

Ecological theory presents a useful framework for the development of interventions and prevention programs to ensure healthy outcomes for adolescents. Most successful interventions are those that operate on multiple ecological levels. Peer, neighborhood, and media-based interventions represent efforts to incorporate community influences, and programs targeting multiple contextual levels are strengthened by incorporating multiple process. Researchers have found that comprehensive community based programs are effective at alleviating multiple problem behaviors, such as delinquency (Tate, Reppucci & Mulvey, 1995), cigarette smoking (Jason, Pokorny, Curie & Townsend, 2002), conduct disorder (Henggeler, Schoenwald & Pickrel, 1995), and HIV/AIDS (Galbraith et al, 1996). Although a comprehensive review of community-based interventions was beyond the scope of this chapter (see Reppucci, Woolard & Fried, 1999; Wandersman and Florin, 2003), such programs offer a promising opportunity for intervention and prevention of adolescent problem behaviors.

Community contexts represent important influences in the lives of adolescents. The inclusion of both proximal and distal influences in research about adolescent problem behavior, in conjunction with individual level characteristics, enhances our ability to understand the mechanisms that affect the development of problem behaviors and how to utilize the potential within the community to promote healthy development.

References

Aber, J.L., Gephart, M., Brooks-Gunn, J., & Connell, J. (1997). Development in context: Implications for studying neighborhood effects. In J. Brooks-Gunn, G. Duncan, & J. L. Aber (Eds.), *Neighborhood Poverty: Vol. 1. Context and Consequences for Children.* (pp. 44–61). New York: Russell Sage Foundation.

Adler, P.A. & Adler, P. (1995). Dynamics of inclusion and exclusion in preadolesent cliques. *Social Psychology Quarterly, 58,* 145–162.

Atkin, C.K., & Block, M. (1983). Effectiveness of celebrity endorsers. *Journal of Advertising Research, 23,* 57–61.

Atkin, C.K., Hocking, J., & Block, M. (1984). Teenage drinking: Does advertising make a difference? *Journal of Communications, 28,* 71–80.

Atkin, C.K., Neuendorf, K., & McDermott, S. (1983). The role of alcohol advertising in excessive and hazardous drinking. *Journal of Drug Education, 13,* 313–325.

Bagwell, C.L., Coie, J.D., Terry, R.A., & Lochman, J.E. (2000). Peer clique participation and social status in preadolescence. *Merrill-Palmer Quarterly, 46,* 280–305.

Bagwell, C.L., Newcomb, A.F., & Bukowski, W.M. (1998). Preadolescent friendship and peer rejection as predictors of adult adjustment. *Child Development, 69,* 140–153.

Bandura, A. (1967). The role of modeling processes in personality development. In W.W. Hartup & N.L. Smothergill (Eds.), *The Young Child: Reviews of Research* (pp. 42–58). Washington, DC: National Association for the Education of Young Children.

Bauer, U.E., Johnson, T.M., Hopkins, R.S., & Brooks, R.G. (2000). Changes in youth cigarette use and intentions following implementation of a tobacco control program: Findings from the Florida Youth Tobacco Survey, 1998–2000. *Journal of the American Medical Association, 284,* 723–728.

Bearman, P., & Brückner, H. (1999). *Peer Effects on Adolescent Sexual Debut and Pregnancy: An Analysis of a National Survey of Adolescent Girls.* Washington, DC: National Campaign to Prevent Teenage Pregnancy.

Bell, C.C., & Jenkins, E. (1993). Community violence and children on Chicago's southside. *Psychiatry, 56,* 46–54.

Bender, D. & Lösel, F. (1997). Protective and risk effects of peer relations and social support on antisocial behaviour in adolescents from multi-problem milieus. *Journal of Adolescence, 20,* 661–678.

Berndt, T.J. (1996). Exploring the effects of friendship quality on social development. In W.M. Bukowski, A.F. Newcomb, & W.W. Hartup (Eds.), *The Company They Keep: Friendship in Childhood and Adolescence.* (pp. 346–365). New York: Cambridge University Press.

Berndt, T.J., & Keefe, K. (1995). Friends' influence on adolescents' adjustment to school. *Child Development, 66,* 1312–1329.

Bolger, K.E., Patterson, C.J., & Kupersmidt, J.B. (1998). Peer relationships and self-esteem among children who have been maltreated. *Child Development, 69,* 1171–1197.

Boyce, W.T., Frank, E., Jensen, P.S., Kessler, R.C., Nelson, C.A., & Steinberg, L. (1998). Social context in developmental psychopathology: Recommendations for future research from the MacArthur Network on Psychopathology and Development. *Development and Psychopathology, 10,* 143–164.

Brendgen, M., Vitaro, F., & Bukowski, W.M. (2000). Stability and variability of adolescents' affiliation with delinquent friends: Predictors and consequences. *Social Development, 9,* 205–225.

Brodie, M., Foehr, U., Rideout, V., Baer, N., Miller, C., Flournoy, R., & Altman, D. (2001). Communicating health information through entertainment media. *Health Affairs, 20,* 1–8.

Bronfenbrenner, U. (1979). *The Ecology of Human Development.* Cambridge, MA: Harvard University Press.

Bronfenbrenner, U. (1986). Ecology of the family as a context for human development. *Developmental Psychology, 22,* 723–742.

Bronfenbrenner, U. (1989). Ecological systems theory. *Annals of Child Development, 6,* 185–246.

Bronfenbrenner, U. (1995). Developmental ecology through space and time: A future perspective. In P. Moen, G.H. Elder, & K. Luscher (Eds.), *Examining Lives in Context: Perspectives on the Ecology of Human Development* (pp. 619–647). Washington, DC: American Psychological Association.

Brooks-Gunn, J., Duncan, G.J., & Aber, J.L. (Eds.) (1997a). *Neighborhood Poverty: Vol. 1. Context and Consequences for Children.* New York: Russell Sage Foundation.

Brooks-Gunn, J., Duncan, G.J., & Aber, J.L. (Eds.) (1997b). *Neighborhood Poverty: Vol. 2. Policy Implications in Studying Neighborhoods.* New York: Russell Sage Foundation.

Brooks-Gunn, J., Guo, F., & Furstenberg, F.F. (1993). Who drops out of and who continues beyond high school? A twenty-year follow-up of Black urban youth. *Journal of Research on Adolescence, 3,* 271–294.

Brown, B.B. (1990). Peer groups and peer cultures. In S. Feldman & G. Elliott (Eds.), *At the Threshold: The Developing Adolescent* (pp. 171–196). Cambridge, MA: Harvard University Press.

Brown, B.B., Dolcini, M.M., & Leventhal, A. (1997). Transformations in peer relationships at adolescence: Implications for health-related behavior. In J. Schulenberg, J.L. Maggs, & K. Hurrelmann (Eds.), *Health Risks and Developmental Transitions During Adolescence* (pp. 161–189). New York: Cambridge University Press.

Brown, B.B, & Lohr, M.J. (1987). Peer-group affiliation and adolescent self-esteem: An integration of ego-identity and symbolic-interaction theories. *Journal of Personality and Social Psychology, 52,* 47–55.

Brown, J.D., Childers, K.W., Bauman, K.E., & Koch, G.G. (1990). The influences of new media and family structure on young adolescents' television and radio use. *Communication Research, 17,* 65–82.

Brown, J.D., & Newcomber, S.F. (1991). Television viewing and adolescent sexual behavior. *Journal of Homosexuality, 21,* 77–91.

Brown, P. (1996). Comprehensive neighborhood-based initiatives. *Cityscape: A Journal of Policy Development and Research, 2,* 161–176.

Buhrmester, D. (1990). Intimacy of friendship, interpersonal competence, and adjustment during preadolescence and adolescence. *Child Development, 61,* 1101–1111.

Buhrmester, D. (1996). Need fulfillment, interpersonal competence, and the developmental contexts of early adolescent friendship. In W.M. Bukowski, A.F. Newcomb, & W.W. Hartup (Eds.), *The Company They Keep: Friendship in Childhood and Adolescence* (pp. 158–185). New York: Cambridge University Press.

Buhrmester D., & Furman, W. (1987). The development of companionship and intimacy. *Child Development, 58,* 1101–1113.

Bukowski, W.M., Hoza, B., & Boivin, M. (1994). Measuring friendship quality during pre- and early adolescence: The development and psychometric properties of the Friendship Qualities Scale. *Journal of Social and Personal Relationships, 11,* 471–484.

Bushman, B.J., & Huesmann, L.R. (2001). Effects of television violence on aggression. In D.G. Singer & J.L. Singer (Eds.), *Handbook of Children and the Media* (pp. 223–254). Thousand Oaks, CA: Sage.

Cairns, R.B., Cadwallader, T.W., Estell, D., & Neckerman, H.J. (1999). Groups to gangs: Developmental and criminological perspectives and relevance for prevention. *Handbook of Antisocial Behavior* (pp. 218–233). New York: John Wiley & Sons.

Cairns, R.B. & Cairns, B.D. (1994). *Lifelines and Risks: Pathways of Youth in our Time.* New York: Cambridge University Press.

Cairns, R.B., Cairns, B.D., Neckerman, H.J., Ferguson, L.L., & Gariépy, J. (1989). Growth and aggression: I. Childhood to early adolescence. *Developmental Psychology, 25,* 320–330.

Cairns, R.B., Leung, M., & Cairns, B.D. (1995). Social networks over time and space in adolescence. In L.J. Crockett & A.C. Crouter (Eds.), *Pathways Through Adolescence: Individual Development in Relation to Social Contexts. The Penn State Series on Child & Adolescent Development* (pp. 35–56). Mahwah, NJ: Lawrence Erlbaum Associates.

Centers for Disease Control (1992). Comparison of the cigarette brand preferences of adult and teenage smokers: United States, 1989, and 20 U.S. communities, 1988 and 1990. *Morbidity and Mortality Weekly Report, 41,* 169–181.

Chavis, D.M. & Wandersman, A. (1990). Sense of community in the urban environment: A catalyst for participation and community development. *American Journal of Community Psychology, 18,* 55–81.

Coie, J.D., Dodge, K.A., & Coppotelli, H. (1982). Dimensions and types of social status: A cross-age perspective. *Developmental Psychology, 18,* 557–570.

Cooley-Quille, M., Turner, S., & Beidel, D. (1995). Emotional impact of children's exposure to community violence: A preliminary study. *Journal of the American Academy of Child and Adolescent Psychiatry, 34,* 1362–1368.

Comstock, G. (1991). *Television and the American Child.* Orlando, FL: Academic Press.

Coulton, C., Korbin, J., Su, M., & Chow, J. (1995). Community level factors and child maltreatment rates. *Child Development, 66,* 1262–1276.

Crick, N.R., & Bigbee, M.A. (1998). Relational and overt forms of peer victimization: A multi-informant approach. *Journal of Consulting and Clinical Psychology, 66,* 610–617.

Crick, N.R., Werner, N.E., Casas, J.F., O'Brien, K.M., Nelson, D.A., Grotpeter, J.K. & Markon, K. (1999). Childhood aggression and gender: A new look at an old problem. In D. Bernstein (Ed.), *Nebraska Symposium on Motivation* (vol. 45, pp. 75–141). Lincoln: University of Nebraska Press.

Crick, N.R., & Grotpeter, J.K. (1996). Children's treatment by peers: Victims of relational and overt aggression. *Development and Psychopathology, 8,* 367–380.

Dishion, T.J. & Skaggs, N.M. (2000). An ecological analysis of monthly "bursts" in early adolescent substance use. *Applied Developmental Science, 4,* 89–97.

Dishion, T.J., McCord, J., & Poulin, F. (1999). When interventions harm: Peer groups and problem behavior. *American Psychologist, 54,* 755–764.

Dishion, T., Andrews, D., & Crosby, L. (1995). Antisocial boys and their friends in early adolescence: Relationship characteristics, quality, and interactional process. *Child Development, 66,* 139–151.

Dominick, J.R. (1987). *The Dynamics of Mass Communication.* New York: Random House.

Duncan, G.J. (1994). Families and neighbors as sources of disadvantage in the schooling decisions of Black and White adolescents. *American Journal of Education, 103,* 20–53.

Duncan, G.J., & Raudenbush, S.W. (1999). Assessing the effects of context in studies of children and youth development. *Educational Psychologist, 34,* 29–41.

DuRant, R.H., Cadenhead, C., Pendergrast, R.A., Slavens, G., & Linder, C.W. (1994). Factors associated with the use of violence among urban black adolescents. *American Journal of Public Health, 84,* 612–617.

Elliott, D.S. (1994). Serious violent offenders: Onset, developmental course, and termination—The American Society of Criminology 1993 presidential address. *Criminology, 32,* 1–21.

Ennett, S.T., & Bauman, K.E. (1994). The contribution of influence and selection to adolescent peer group homogeneity: The case of adolescent cigarette smoking. *Journal of Personality & Social Psychology, 67,* 653–663

Fischer, P.M., Schwartz, M.P., Richards, J.W., Goldstein, A.O., & Rojas, T.H. (1991). Brand logo recognition by children aged 3 to 6 years: Mickey Mouse and Old Joe the Camel. *Journal of the American Medical Association, 266,* 3145–3153.

Furman, W., & Buhrmester, D. (1985). Children's perceptions of personal relationships in social networks. *Developmental Psychology, 21,* 1016–1024.

Galbraith, J., Ricardo, I., Stanton, B., Black, M., Feigleman, S., & Kalyee, L. (1996). Challenges and rewards of involving community in research: An overview of the "Focus on Kids" HIV risk reduction program. *Health Education Quarterly, 23,* 383–394.

Gauze, C., Bukowski, W.M., Aquan-Assee, J., & Sippola, L.K. (1996). Interactions between family environment and friendship and associations with self-perceived well-being during adolescence. *Child Development, 67,* 2201–2216.

Gephart, M. (1997). Neighborhoods and communities as contexts for development. In J. BrooksGunn, G. Duncan, & J.L. Aber (Eds.), *Neighborhood Poverty: Vol. 1. Context and Consequences for Children* (pp. 1–43). New York: Russell Sage Foundation.

Gerbner, G., Gross, L., Morgan, M., & Signorielli, N. (1986). Living with television: The dynamics of the cultivation process. In J. Bryant & D. Zillman (Eds.), *Perspectives on Media Effects* (pp. 17–40). Hillsdale, NJ: Lawrence Erlbaum Associates.

Gorman-Smith, D., Tolan, P.H., & Henry, D.B. (2000). A developmental-ecological model of the relation of family functioning to patterns of delinquency. *Journal of Quantitative Criminology, 16,* 169–198.

Graham, S., & Juvonen, J. (1998). Self-blame and peer victimization in middle school: An attributional analysis. *Developmental Psychology, 34,* 587–538.

Grotpeter, J.K., & Crick, N.R. (1996). Relational aggression, overt aggression, and friendship. *Child Development, 67,* 2328–2338.

Hammond, W.R., & Yung, B. (1993). Psychology's role in the public health response to assaultive violence among young African-American men. *American Psychologist, 48,* 142–154.

Harris, L. & Associates (1988). *Sexual Material on American Network Television During the 1987–1988 Season.* New York: Planned Parenthood Federation of America.

Hartup, W.W. (1992). Conflict and friendship relations. In C.U. Shantz & W.W. Hartup (Eds.), *Conflict in Child and Adolescent Development* (pp. 186–215). New York: Cambridge University Press.

Hartup, W.W., & Stevens, N. (1997). Friendships and adaptation in the life course. *Psychological Bulletin, 121,* 335–370.

Hawley, P.H. (1999). The ontogenesis of social dominance: A strategy-based evolutionary perspective. *Developmental Review, 19,* 97–132.

Henggeler, S.W., Schoenwald, S.K., & Pickrel, S.G. (1995). Multisystemic therapy: Bridging the gap between university- and community-based treatment. *Journal of Consulting and Clinical Psychology, 63,* 709–717.

Henrich, C.C., Kuperminc, G.P., Sack, A., Blatt, S.J., & Leadbeater, B.J. (2000). Characteristics and homogeneity of early adolescent friendship groups: A comparison of male and female clique and nonclique members. *Applied Developmental Science, 4,* 15–26.

Hill, H., Levermore, M., Twaite, J., & Jones, L. (1996). Exposure to community violence and social support as predictors of anxiety and social and emotional behavior among African American children. *Journal of Child and Family Studies, 5,* 399–414.

Hodges, E.V.E., & Perry, D.G. (1999). Personal and interpersonal antecedents and consequences of victimization by peers. *Journal of Personality and Social Psychology, 76,* 677–685.

Horn, J., & Trickett, P. (1998). Community violence and child development: A review of the research. In P. Trickett & C. Schellenbach (Eds.), *Violence Against Children in the Family and the Community* (pp. 103–138). Washington, DC: American Psychological Association.

Hudley, C. & Graham, S. (1993). An attributional intervention to reduce peer-directed aggression among African-American boys. *Child Development, 64,* 124–138.

Huston, A.C., Donnerstein, E., Fairchild, H.H., Feshbach, N.D., Katz, P.A., Murray, J.P., Rubinstein, E.A., Wilcox, B.L., & Zuckerman, D. (1992). *Big World, Small Screen: The Role of Television in American Society.* Lincoln: University of Nebraska Press.

Huston, A.C., & Wright, J.C. (1997). Mass media and children's development. In W. Damon, I. Sigel, & K.A. Renninger (Eds.), *Handbook of Child Psychology: Vol. 4. Child Psychology in Practice* (5th ed., pp. 999–1058). New York: Wiley.

Jason, L.A., Pokorny, S.B., Curie, C.J., & Townsend, S.M. (2002). Introduction: Preventing youth access to tobacco. *Journal of Prevention & Intervention in the Community, 24,* 1–13.

Jarrett, R. (1997). Bringing families back in: Neighborhood effects on child development. In J. Brooks-Gunn, G. Duncan, & J. L. Aber (Eds.), *Neighborhood Poverty: Vol. 2. Policy Implications in Studying Neighborhoods* (pp. 48–64). New York: Russell Sage Foundation.

Jenkins, E., & Bell, C. (1997). Exposure and response to community violence among children and adolescents. In J. Osofsky (Ed.), *Children in a Violent Society* (pp. 9–31). New York: The Guilford Press.

Kaiser Family Foundation (2001). *Generation Rx.com: How Young People Use the Internet for Health Information.* Menlo Park, CA: Henry J. Kaiser Family Foundation.

Kandel, D. (1978). Homophily, selection, and socialization in adolescent friendships. *American Journal of Sociology, 84,* 427–436.

Keenan, K. Loeber, R., Zhang, Q., Stouthamer-Loeber, M., & van Kammen, W.B. (1995). The influence of deviant peers on the development of boys' disruptive and delinquent behavior: A temporal analysis. *Development and Psychopathology, 7*, 715–726.

Kiesner, J., Poulin, F., & Nicotra, E. (2003). Peer relations across contexts: Individual-network homophily and network inclusion in and after school. *Child Development, 74*, 1328–1343.

Kindermann, T. (1998). Children's development within peer groups: Using composite social maps to identify peer networks and to study their influences. In W.M. Bukowski & A.H. Cillessen (Eds.), *Sociometry Then and Now: Building on Six Decades of Measuring Children's Experiences with the Peer Group. New Directions for Child Development, 80*, 55–82.

La Greca, A.M., Prinstein, M.J., & Fetter, M.D. (2001). Adolescent peer crowd affiliation: Linkages with health-risk behaviors and close friendships. *Journal of Pediatric Psychology, 26*, 131–143.

Laird, R.D., Jordan, K.Y., Dodge, K.A., Petit, G.S., & Bates, J.E. (2001). Peer rejection in childhood, involvement with antisocial peers in early adolescence, and the development of externalizing behavior problems. *Development and Psychopathology, 13*, 337–354.

Lansford, J.E., Criss, M.M., Pettit, G.S., Dodge, K.A., & Bates, J.E. (2003). Friendship quality, peer group affiliation, and peer antisocial behavior as moderators of the link between negative parenting and adolescent externalizing behavior. *Journal of Research on Adolescence, 13*, 161–184.

Leventhal, T., & Brooks-Gunn, J. (2000). The neighborhoods they live in: The effects of neighborhood residence on child and adolescent outcomes. *Psychological Bulletin, 126*, 309–337.

Luthar, S.S. (2003). The culture of affluence: Psychological costs of material wealth. *Child Development, 74*, 1581–1593.

Lynch, M., & Cicchetti, D. (1998). An ecological-transactional analysis of children and contexts: The longitudinal interplay among child maltreatment, community violence, and children's symptomatology. *Development and Psychopathology, 10*, 235–257.

Maccoby, E.E. (1990). The role of gender identity and gender constancy in sex-differentiated development. *New Directions for Child Development, 47*, 5–20.

Newcomb, A.F., & Bagwell, C.L. (1995). Children's friendship relations: A meta-analytic review. *Psychological Bulletin, 117*, 306–347.

Paik, H., & Comstock, G. (1994). The effects of television violence on anti-social behavior: A meta-analysis. *Communication Research, 21*, 516–546.

Parker, J.G., & Asher, S.R. (1987). Peer acceptance and later personal adjustment: Are low-accepted children "at-risk"? *Psychological Bulletin, 102*, 357–389.

Parker, J.G., & Asher, S.R. (1993). Friendship and friendship quality in middle childhood: Links with peer group acceptance and feelings of loneliness and social dissatisfaction. *Developmental Psychology, 29*, 611–621.

Patterson, G.R., Dishion, T.J., & Yoerger, K. (2000). Adolescent growth in new forms of problem behavior: Macro- and micro-peer dynamics. *Prevention Science, 1*, 3–13.

Paxton, S.J., Schutz, H.K., Wertheim, E.H., & Muir, S.L. (1999). Friendship clique and peer influences on body image concerns, dietary restraint, extreme weight-loss behaviors, and binge eating in adolescent girls. *Journal of Abnormal Psychology, 108*, 255–266.

Peeples, F., & Loeber, R. (1994). Do individual factors and neighborhood context explain ethnic differences in juvenile delinquency? *Journal of Quantitative Criminology, 10*, 141–157.

Peterson, R., & Kahn, J. (1984). Media preferences of sexually active teens: A preliminary analysis. Paper presented at the Annual Meeting of the American Psychological Association. Toronto, Canada.

Prinstein, M.J., Boergers, J., & Vernberg, E.M. (2001). Overt and relational aggression in adolescents: Social-psychological adjustment of aggressors and victims. *Journal of Clinical Child Psychology, 30*, 479–491.

Reppucci, N.D., Woolard, J.L., & Fried, C.S. (1999). Social, community and preventive interventions. *Annual Review of Psychology, 50*, 387–418.

Roberts, D.F., & Christenson, P.G. (2001). Popular music in childhood and adolescence. In D.G. Singer & J.L. Singer (Eds.), *Handbook of Children and the Media* (pp. 395–414). Thousand Oaks, CA: Sage.

Roberts, D.F., Foehr, U.G., Rideout, V.J., & Brodie, M. (1999). *Kids and the Media at the New Millennium: A Kaiser Family Foundation Report.* Menlo Park, CA: Henry J. Kaiser Family Foundation.

Roberts, D.F., Henriksen, L., & Christenson, P.G. (1999). *Substance Use in Popular Movies and Music.* Washington, DC: Office of National Drug Control Policy.

Robinson, T.N., Chen, H.L., & Killen, J.D. (1998). Television and music video exposure and risk of adolescent alcohol use. *Pediatrics, 102*, e54.

Roecker Phelps, C.E. (2001). Children's responses to overt and relational aggression. *Journal of Clinical Child Psychology, 30*, 240–252.

Ryan, A.M. (2001). The peer group as a context for the development of young adolescent motivation and achievement. *Child Development, 72*, 1135–1150.

Sampson, R.J., Raudenbush, S.W., & Earls, F. (1997). Neighborhoods and violent crime: A multilevel study of collective efficacy, *Science, 277*, 918–924.

Schwartz, D., McFadyen-Ketchum, S.A., Dodge, K.A., Pettit, G.S., & Bates, J.E. (1998). Peer group victimization as a predictor of children's behavior problems at home and in school. *Development and Psychopathology, 10*, 87–99.

Selverstone, R. (1992). Sexuality education for adolescents. *Adolescent Medicine: State of the Art Reviews, 3*, 195–205.

Signorielli, N. (1990). Television and health: Images and impact. In C. Atkin & K. Wallack (Eds.), *Mass Communication and Public Health: Complexities and Conflicts* (pp. 96–113). Newbury Park, CA: Sage.

Signorielli, N., & Morgan, M. (Eds.) (1990). *Cultivation Analysis: New Directions in Media Effects Research.* Newbury Park, CA: Sage.

Sly, D.F., Heald, G.R., & Ray, S. (2001). The Florida "truth" anti-tobacco media evaluation: Design, first year results, and implications for planning future state media evaluations. *Tobacco Control, 10*, 9–15.

Sly, D.F., Hopkins, R.S., Trapido, E., & Ray, S. (2001). Influence of a counteradvertising media campaign on initiation of smoking: The Florida "truth" campaign. *American Journal of Public Health, 91*, 233–238.

Spencer, M.B., McDermott, P., Burton, L., & Kochman, T. (1997). An alternative approach to assessing neighborhood effects on early adolescent achievement and problem behavior. In J. Brooks-Gunn, G. Duncan, & J.L. Aber (Eds.), *Neighborhood Poverty: Vol. 2. Policy Implications for Studying Neighborhoods* (pp. 145–163). New York: Russell Sage Foundation.

Steinberg, L., & Morris, A.S. (2001). Adolescent development. *Annual Review of Psychology, 52*, 83–110.

Steinberg, L., Darling, N., & Fletcher, A. (1995). Aurthoritative parenting and adolescent adjustment: An ecological journey. In P. Moen, G.H. Elder, & K. Luscher (Eds.), *Examining Lives in Context: Perspectives on the Ecology of Human Development* (pp. 423–466). Washington, DC: American Psychological Association.

Strasburger, V.C (1997). "Sex, drugs, rock 'n' roll," and the media: Are the media responsible for adolescent behavior? *Adolescent medicine: State of the Art Reviews, 8(3)*, 403–414.

Strasburger, V.C., & Wilson, B.J. (2002). *Children, Adolescents, and the Media.* Thousand Oaks, CA: Sage.

Tate, D.C., Reppucci, N.D., & Mulvey, E.P. (1995). Violent juvenile delinquents: Treatment effectiveness and implications for future action. *American Psychologist, 50*, 777–781.

Thornberry, T.P., & Krohn, M.D. (1997). Peers, drug use, and delinquency. In D.M. Stoff, J. Brieling, & J.D. Maser (Eds.), *Handbook of Antisocial Behavior* (pp. 218–233). New York: John Wiley & Sons.

Underwood, M.K., Kupersmidt, J.B., & Coie, J.D. (1996). Childhood peer sociometric status and aggression as predictors of adolescent childbearing. *Journal of Research on Adolescence, 6*, 201–223.

Urberg, K.A., Degirmencioglu, S.M., & Pilgrim, C. (1997). Close friend and group influence on adolescent cigarette smoking and alcohol use. *Developmental Psychology, 33*, 834–844.

Urberg, K.A., Degirmencioglu, S.M., & Tolson, J.M. (1998). Adolescent friendship selection and termination: The role of similarity. *Journal of Social and Personal Relationships, 15*, 703–710.

Urberg, K.A., Luo, Q., Pilgrim, C., & Degirmencioglu, S.M. (2003). A two-stage model of peer influence in adolescent substance use: Individual and relationship-specific differences in susceptibility to influence. *Addictive Behaviors, 28*, 1243–1256.

Van der Voort, T.H.A. (1986). *Television Violence: A Child's Eye View.* Amsterdam: North-Holland.

Van Evra, J. (1998). *Television and Child Development.* Mahwah, NJ: Lawrence Erlbaum Associates.

Wandersman, A., & Florin, P. (2003). Community interventions and effective prevention. *American Psychologist, 58*, 441–448.

Wilson, W.J. (1991). Studying inner city social dislocations: The challenge of public agenda research. *American Sociological Review, 56*, 1–14.

Wilson, W.J. (1995). Jobless ghettos and the social outcome of youngsters. In P. Moen, G. Elder, & K. Luescher (Eds.), *Examining Lives in Context: Perspectives on the Ecology of Human Development* (pp. 527–543). Washington, DC: American Psychological Association.

Woodard, E., & Gridina, N. (2000). *Media in the Home 2000: The Fifth Annual Survey of Parents and Their Children.* Washington, DC: Annenberg Public Policy Center of the University of Pennsylvania.

Woodruff, K. (1998). Youth and race on local TV news. *Nieman Reports, 52*, 43–44.

Xie, H., Swift, D.J., Cairns, B., & Cairns, R.B. (2002). Aggressive behaviors in social interaction and developmental adaptation: A narrative analysis of interpersonal conflicts during early adolescence. *Social Development, 11*, 205–224.

Chapter 5

Understanding Treatment:
Principles and Approaches

Ronald Jay Werner-Wilson and Kathleen M. Morrissey

In order to understand adolescent treatment, service providers should understand the developmental psychopathology perspective, risk factors associated with problem behavior, aspects of attachment that influence presenting problems and interventions, and diversity issues. Treatment providers should also be able to identify evidence-based treatments (i.e., treatments that have been empirically tested and found to be efficacious and/or effective in ameliorating the mental health issues of adolescents). The present chapter introduces material to provide a context for understanding adolescent treatment.

Developmental Psychopathology Framework

In their critical review of treatments for children and adolescents, Fonagy, Target, Cottrell, Phillips & Kurtz (2002) noted that attention to developmental themes is an emerging trend in youth treatment. Attention to developmental themes is represented by the developmental psychopathology framework that has begun to dominate clinical work with children and adolescents. This approach suggests that psychiatric disorders are "part of a transactional causal chain" that includes "a series of interactions of biological, social, and psychological characteristics across time" (Fonagy et al., 2002, p. 5).

The U. S. Surgeon General's report on mental illness identified five principles associated with a developmental psychopathology perspective. First, it is important to understand the particular history and past experience of youth clients:

> Psychopathology in childhood arises from the complex, multilayered interactions of specific characteristics of the child (including biological, psychological, and genetic factors), his or her environment (including parent, sibling, and family relations, peer and neighborhood factors, school and community factors, and the larger social-cultural context), and the specific manner in which these factors interact with and shape each other over the course of development (U. S. Department of Health and Human Services, 1999, p. 127).

Second, the U. S. Surgeon General's report suggests that children and adolescents have innate tendencies to adapt to their environment, so "some (but not all) 'pathologic' behavioral syndromes might be best characterized as adaptive responses when the child or adolescent encounters difficulty or adverse circumstances" (U. S. Department of Health and Human Services, 1999, p. 128). Third, age and timing factors are associated with problems (e.g., behavior that is considered normal for a two-year-old could be considered immature for an adolescent). Fourth, it is important to understand a child's context, especially the caretaking environment. Finally, normal and abnormal developmental processes "are often separated only by degrees of difference" (U. S. Department of Health and Human Services, 1999, p. 128).

The U. S. Surgeon General's report identified four "virtues" of a developmental perspective (U. S. Department of Health and Human Services, 1999):

1. A developmental perspective provides a broader, "more informed" perspective to understand factors associated with development, maintenance, and recovery from disorders (p. 128).
2. A developmental perspective guards against oversimplified, diagnostic terms.
3. A developmental perspective identifies additional targets (e.g., environmental or contextual factors) for intervention.
4. A developmental perspective identifies "windows of opportunity during a child's development when preventive or treatment interventions may be especially effective" (p. 128).

Risk Factors

Risk factors refer to biological influences, stressful events, or psychosocial risk factors (especially family characteristics) that increase an adolescent's vulnerability to experiencing hardship: "There is now good evidence that *both* biological factors and adverse psychosocial experiences during childhood influence—but not necessarily 'cause'–the mental disorders of childhood" (U.S. Department of Health and Human Services, 1999, p. 129). The U. S. Surgeon General's report on mental health identified the following risk factors (U.S. Department of Health and Human Services, 1999):

- *Biological influence on mental disorders*: intrauterine exposure to alcohol or cigarettes, parental trauma, environmental exposure to lead, malnutrition of pregnancy, traumatic brain injury, specific chromosomal syndromes (p. 130).
- *Stressful life events*: parental death or divorce, economic hardship (p. 132)
- *Psychosocial risk factors*: parental discord, parent psychopathology, large family size, quality of relationship (especially attachment) between children and primary caregiver, child maltreatment, maladaptive peers and siblings (pp. 130–132)

In his book *Raising Children in a Socially Toxic Environment*, James Garbarino describes risk factors affecting youth. "Their risk factors are the stuff of talk shows and headlines and policy seminars: absent fathers, poverty and other economic pressure, racism, addiction, educational failure, poor physical health, family violence, and adult emotional problems that impair parenting" (Garbarino, 1995, p. 6). Garbarino suggests that the accumulation of risk factors is a significant predictor of problems:

> The presence of one or two risk factors does not developmentally disable children, but the accumulation of three, four, or more can overwhelm a child. . . . Once overwhelmed,

children are likely to be highly sensitive to the socially toxic influences surrounding them (1995, p. 151).

Treatment providers should make efforts to screen for the presence of risk factors in adolescent clients. If more than three risk factors are present, treatment planning should incorporate strategies for ameliorating them. The presence of some risk factors will require partnering with social service agencies.

Parent Influence

The parent–child relationship has important implications for treatment, which is why *family therapy* by itself or in conjunction with other therapies is recommended for treatment of several severe mental health disorders. Attachment is an aspect of the parent–child relationship that should be assessed and, when necessary, the target of intervention because "Attachments lie at the heart of family life. They create bonds that can provide care and protection across the life cycle (Ainsworth, 1991), and can evoke the most intense emotions—joy in the making, anguish in the breaking—or create problems if they become insecure" (Byng-Hall, 1995, p. 45). A critical review of attachment research suggests attachment relationships are complex due to three factors: (a) relationships are multi-influential, (b) outcomes are multi-determined, and (c) continuity is complex and multifaceted (Thompson, 1999). For those interested in learning more about attachment, the following edited volume is an excellent resource: *Handbook of Attachment: Theory, Research, and Clinical Applications* (Cassidy & Shaver, 1999). Another resource is *Developmental-Systemic Family Therapy with Adolescents* (Werner-Wilson, 2001), which includes a discussion of different aspects of attachment, assessment recommendations, and treatment implications.

Key Parenting Factors Associated with Psychopathology

It is presumed colloquially and professionally that parents influence psychopathology in children (Cusinato, 1998). Parent influence, according to a review of research, seems to be related to three specific aspects of the parent–child relationship: (a) parental warmth, (b) parental control, and (c) parental consistency (Cusinato, 1998). *Warmth* refers to the balance of supportive (e.g., praise, approval, encouragement, cooperation, expression and demonstration of affection) versus non-supportive (e.g., blame, criticism, punishment, threats, neglect, negative evaluations) behaviors toward the child (Cusinato, 1998). Parental warmth consistently seems to influence self-esteem of children. Parental warmth should be routinely evaluated by helping professionals and a target of intervention if it is lacking in the parent–child relationship.

The *control* factor includes style of parent influence (coercive, democratic, permissive) and frequency of control. Although control is related to warmth (e.g., coercive control is associated with limited parental warmth), it seems to have an independent impact: "when the father's and mother's negative or abusive behaviors add up, the connection to dysfunctional outcomes in offspring becomes stronger and more crucial" (Cusinato, 1998). This conclusion suggests that professionals should assess style and frequency of parental control.

Consistency is the final factor associated with outcomes—especially delinquent behavior. It refers to continuity between parental demands, expectations, and evaluations of children. Agreement on values and expectations between parents seems to be particularly important. As with warmth and control, treatment should include careful assessment of consistency between caregivers in the family.

Now that factors associated with the individuals or families being treated have been described, we will review factors associated with therapeutic relationship since it seems to be a significant predictor of client outcomes.

Therapeutic Relationship

Bordin (1979, 1994) suggested that the therapeutic relationship was influenced by an alliance between therapist and client that transcended theoretical orientation (he referred to it as a "pan-theoretical" perspective). According to Bordin, both the therapist and the client play active roles in therapy. This conceptualization of alliance featured three dimensions: *goals, tasks,* and *bond* (Bordin, 1979, 1994). Therapeutic goals are the negotiated outcomes for therapy; tasks are the behaviors and cognitions which occur during therapeutic process; and bond refers to the quality of attachment between the therapist and client (Bordin, 1979, 1994).

Empirical research seems to support Bordin's (1979, 1994) propositions because therapeutic alliance is associated with positive outcomes in therapy. For example, results from a meta-analysis of 24 studies that evaluated various measures of working alliance to treatment outcome suggested that quality of the working alliance predicted positive therapy outcome (Horvath & Symonds, 1991). Although much of the research on therapeutic alliance has been with adult clients, it seems to be relevant for clinical work with adolescents. For example, adolescents and their families are more likely to drop out of treatment if there is an imbalance (e.g., higher for parent than adolescent) in therapy alliance (Robbins, Turner, Alexander & Perez, 2003).

Influences on Therapeutic Relationship

Carl Rogers was one of the first therapists formally to hypothesize that the degree of client change in therapy was closely related to the client's relationship with the therapist. His call for research in this area began in 1957 and was summarized in his 1965 review of studies of the necessary and sufficient conditions needed for the therapeutic relationship. Rogers (1965) reported that a relationship perceived by the client as having a high degree of genuineness from the therapist with sensitive and accurate empathy on the part of the therapist was related to effective therapeutic bonds and increased growth. Additionally, when clients perceived themselves as unconditionally cared about and respected, they were more likely to rate the therapeutic bond as high. Similar results are found today with clients rating therapists as "most effective" when they are perceived to be more warm, affirming, understanding and helpful (Najavits & Strupp, 1994). Therapists with these qualities are also seen as approachable. The following therapist characteristics continue to be identified by clients as helpful: therapist moderates and controls discussion, therapist provides a safe environment, therapist encourages participation, and therapist helps in resolving problems (Estrada & Holmes, 1999). Gurman (2001) suggested that increased therapist activity in family therapy significantly influenced therapeutic relationship.

Diversity Issues in Assessment and Treatment

Treating clients from different backgrounds requires careful assessment, cultivation of cultural sensitivity, and understanding of acculturation factors. We will review each of these issues in the present section.

Gender Issues

In a classic study published in the *American Psychologist*, Broverman and colleagues (1974) demonstrated that clinicians diagnosed women and men differently. Moreover, they noted that standards for health were based on those consistent with masculine characteristics. They conclude: "The cause of mental health may be better served if both men and women are encouraged toward maximum realization of individual potential, rather than to an adjustment to existing restrictive sex roles" (Broverman et al., 1974, p. 52). Women are also more likely than men to be blamed for their own problems and those of family members (Anderson & Holder, 1989). This has been referred to as mother blaming. "[C]hild guidance clinics have emphasized the involvement of mothers—not fathers—in the child's treatment" (Anderson & Holder, 1989, p. 384).

These expectations about gender roles may influence treatment in three ways: "(1) they limit what we see, (2) they shape how we interpret behaviors, and (3) they influence what we define as important" (Knudson-Martin, 2001, p. 338). This research on differential diagnoses, evaluating clients based on masculine standards, mother-blaming, and expectations about gender have the following implications for adolescents treatment:

- Treatment providers should be especially careful when assessing adolescent girls so that girls are not identified as pathological because they violate gender expectations.
- Since family therapy is a recommended form of treatment for some problems, treatment providers should ensure that fathers are equally engaged in therapy process.
- Assessment of family should include attention to family expectations about gender roles and father involvement.
- Treatment providers should avoid "mother blaming."

Treatment providers should pay attention to difficulties experienced by gay, lesbian, and bisexual youth because their sexuality may be a reason families initiate therapy. Until relatively recently, homosexuality was diagnosed as a disorder and reparative therapy was recommended to treat this diagnoses. Additionally, youth who "come out of the closet" face a variety of stressors:

[These youth] face tremendous challenges to growing up physically and mentally healthy in a culture that is almost uniformly anti-homosexual. . . . [They] face rejection, isolation, verbal harassment and physical violence at home, in school and in religious organizations. Responding to these pressures, many lesbian, gay and bisexual young people engage in an array of risky behaviors" (Center for Population Options, 1992, p. 1).

Gay, lesbian, and bisexual youth may experience any of the following outcomes: (a) school-related problems, (b) running away, (c) conflict with the law, (d) substance abuse, (e) prostitution, and (f) suicide. If adolescents or their families seek treatment for any of these problems, treatment providers should be sensitive to harassment (including internalized homophobia) of gay, lesbian, and bisexual youth (Savin–Williams, 1994).

Multicultural Issues

Factors associated with multicultural treatment are identified in the present section because "[m]any diagnostic formulations tend to reify normative aspects of culture, race, ethnicity, gender, and class membership as forms of psychopathology" (Comas-Díaz, 1996, p. 153).

In the book *Assessing and Treating Culturally Diverse Clients*, Paniagua (1998) suggests that clients from multicultural groups may be overdiagnosed which is referred to as cultivating "false conclusions regarding 'pathology' or mental problems" (p. 14). There seem to be two reasons for overdiagnosing. First, many assessment instruments have not been normed for clients from different groups. Second, misunderstandings about culture can lead treatment providers to diagnose behaviors that are normal for a particular group as pathological (Paniagua, 1998).

We return to the issue of therapeutic relationship—which we noted earlier in the chapter is one of the best predictors of psychotherapeutic outcome—because it seems to be influenced by race and ethnicity. Paniagua (1998) suggests that therapeutic relationship is enhanced if treatment providers demonstrate both *cultural sensitivity* and *cultural competence*. Cultural sensitivity is defined as "awareness of cultural variables that may affect assessment and treatment" (Paniagua, 1998, p. 8). Therapists should be careful that efforts to be culturally sensitive are not influenced by stereotypes because this would represent racism rather than sensitivity. Cultural competence is defined as "translation of this awareness into behaviors leading to effective assessment and treatment of the particular multicultural group" (Paniagua, 1998, p. 8).

Paniagua also suggests that therapist *credibility* influences treatment. Credibility refers to "the client's perception that the therapist is effective and trustworthy" (Paniagua, 1998, p. 8). A treatment provider who operates from stereotyped notions about a particular race/ethnic group toward an individual client will undermine her/his credibility. Dilworth-Anderson, Burton, and Johnson (1993) distinguish between *race* (cultural construction of identity based on social description); *ethnicity* (an experientially based identity that is part of an ongoing process), and *culture* (a subjective and objective expression of self, which includes race and ethnicity, that represents the encompassing aspects of a person's life). Tentative, collaborative questions designed to assess culture increases credibility.

Credibility is also affected if therapists make assumptions about extended family membership. "What is an extended family? The answer should be provided by the client and not by the therapist" (Paniagua, 1998, p. 9). Since family therapy is the recommended treatment for some problems, it seems important to include significant others—even if there is not a biological relationship—identified by clients.

Acculturation should also be considered during assessment and treatment. It refers to "the degree of integration of new cultural patterns into the original cultural patterns" (Paniagua, 1998, p. 8). Acculturation is often used to refer to immigrants from other countries but Paniagua (1998) suggests that this is only one form of acculturation, which he refers to as *external*. There is also an *internal* form of acculturation that refers to someone who moves from one part of a country to another where cultural patterns are different. "For example, when American Indians living in Arizona or New Mexico (or other states with a large number of reservations) move from their reservation to cities, they experience the impact of societal lifestyle quite different from their societal lifestyle experienced on the reservation" (Paniagua, 1998, p. 9). Continuing in the example of American Indians moving from the reservation to a different environment, Paniagua writes, "Competition and individualism are two values with little relevance among American Indians who reside on reservations. These values, however, are extremely important for anyone who resides outside a reservation" (1998, p. 9).

In both forms of acculturation, there may be tension between the original culture and the new culture relative to values, beliefs, and behaviors. This tension between original and new culture could contribute to psychosocial and behavioral problems in adolescents. It could also lead to family systems changes because younger children typically assimilate new cultural behaviors before their elders. This can create tension in the family if elders are threatened by the changes. The family system can also be affected if elders, who are slower to learn new languages or customs (Paniagua, 1998), become dependent on adolescents. Given that family relationships influence adolescents, treatment providers should assess for recent geographic transitions.

Now that conceptual material associated with treating adolescents has been introduced, the next section will review factors associated with providing mental health services to youth.

Perspectives on Therapy Effectiveness

Those who pay for clinical services (e.g., consumers and insurance providers) have demanded better value for their investment, which has resulted in increased attention to the issue of therapy effectiveness (Fonagy, et al., 2002). This increased attention to accountability in the form of therapy effectiveness has revived a long-standing tension between academics who research therapy effectiveness and clinicians who provide treatment (Glenn, 2003). Richard M. McFall (1991), in his "Manifesto for a Science of Clinical Psychology," suggested that all forms of psychotherapy treatment should be empirically investigated. "Well-intentioned clinicians may not be using the most effective approach with their clients, or in some cases may be doing harm" (Ringeisen & Hoagwood, 2002, p. 44). Many interventions are designed through the process of common sense and good intention (Petrosino, Turpin-Petrosino & Finckenhauer, 2000) or by myths and heroic efforts (Bogenschneider, 1996). While these treatments can be popular among service providers, there has been minimal research on the majority of them (Henggler & Sheidow, 2003).

Treatment providers, on the other hand, often complain that clinical research lacks "real-world" relevance since it is conducted in carefully controlled conditions that are difficult or impossible to match under normal treatment conditions (Fonagy et al., 2002; Glenn, 2003). Practicing clinicians worry that insurance companies will mandate specific treatments that underestimate critical aspects of therapy such as therapeutic relationship (Glenn, 2003) which seems to be one of the best predictors of therapeutic outcome (Hanson, Curry & Bandalos, 2002; Horvath, 1994; Horvath & Symonds, 1991). There is also concern that insurance companies will be more likely to pay for psychopharmacological intervention rather than psychotherapies because the former have been investigated more frequently in clinical trials (Glenn, 2003).

The Researcher-Practitioner Model

If these two perspectives remain polarized, clients suffer. If clinicians ignore research, the services they provide could lead to harmful and even fatal outcomes. In some states, licensed therapists are required to obtain continuing education credits that, in theory, are supposed to help therapists remain current about effective treatments. In practice, though, therapists may obtain these credits by attending workshops about treatment that has not been empirically evaluated. Researchers also have responsibilities in this model. In addition to disseminating research regarding therapies to the practitioners using them, they must also take into account the concerns of therapists when both designing treatments and reporting results. The researcher-practitioner model also requires that researchers reach out to clinicians by consulting with practicing therapists on treatment protocols to ensure that treatment procedures have validity. A more recent trend of conducting efficacy studies on therapies (in addition to traditional efficacy studies on pharmacological treatments) is a move toward bridging the researcher-practitioner gap. Studies of treatment should use experimental designs (treatment and control groups), valid and reliable measures, and be replicated by numerous investigators prior to being reported as efficacious. The transformation of efficacy studies conducted in a lab setting to effectiveness studies conducted in community mental health settings aid in the successful treatment of adolescents.

Additionally, the researcher-practitioner model suggests that practicing therapists should be in a position to understand and contribute to the research literature. From this perspective, therapists have a responsibility to remain current about effective therapies from the clinical literature. For those who are working with adolescents, that responsibility includes staying current on basic research associated with adolescent development. In addition to remaining current on the literature, therapists should begin to collect their own outcome research by measuring client progress. It would also seem reasonable for researchers to partner with therapists to conduct more research in the field. This type of research could include process research in which self-report or observational data are collected from therapists and their clients in practice. As part of this field research, investigators should begin to study differences in therapy outcomes across therapy settings (e.g., non-profit service agency versus private practice) while also controlling for community variables in order to provide a more contextual understanding about therapy outcomes.

Measuring therapy outcomes has at least three practical benefits. First, therapists who measure client progress are in a stronger position to negotiate with insurance providers. For example, a therapist could negotiate for more sessions by showing that a client was below a particular threshold (e.g., two standard deviations) for a normal range of behavior. Second, data from systematic measurement can be used to provide information to clients about progress. Finally, therapists could make a contribution to the clinical literature by publishing these findings. There are numerous measures relevant to adolescent outcomes that are easy to obtain and administer for a variety of possible outcomes, including self-esteem, attachment, alcohol and substance abuse, to name just a few (see Werner-Wilson, 2001, for these and other measures). Therapists could also look for opportunities to contribute to the research literature by publishing about interventions.

Evidence-Based Treatment

The American Psychological Association defines efficacious or "well-established" interventions as those that have either (a) two or more well-conducted group-design studies completed by several different researchers or (b) several well-conducted single-case study designs completed by independent investigators showing treatment to be at least as good as if not superior to placebo (Lonigan, Elbert & Johnson, 1998). In keeping with both the APA and the researcher-practitioner model, we define evidence-based treatments as those that have been shown to be at least efficacious and at best both efficacious and effective. We summarized empirical support for a number of therapies and treatment models for adolescents associated with attention-deficit/hyperactivity disorder (ADHD) in Table 1, anorexia and bulimia in Table 2, anxiety disorders in Table 3, conduct disorder (CD) and oppositional defiant disorder (ODD) in Table 4, depression in Table 5, and substance abuse in Table 6. The remainder of this chapter will review literature associated with evidence-based treatments for adolescents.

Table 1. Therapy Outcomes Associated with ADHD

Study	Research Design	Outcomes
Horn, et al. (1991)	Efficacy study using a double-blind, placebo design to compare parent training and self-control therapy to stimulant medication	Parent training and self-control therapy combined with low dosage of methylphenidate was as effective as a high dosage of methylphenidate alone
Pelham, Wheeler & Chronis (1998)	Review of 47 efficacy studies (parent training, behavioral training, and cognitive interventions)	Behavioral parent training and behavioral interventions with the adolescent are efficacious; cognitive interventions are not efficacious
Smith, Waschbusch, Willoughby & Evans (2000)	Review of 29 efficacy studies (stimulants, psychosocial treatments, and other medications)	Methylphenidate has well-established efficacy but some problems with inconvenience and non-compliance; the psychotherapeutic interventions of family therapy and classroom interventions are efficacious and practical; treatment with other types of medications shows promise but is not yet supported empirically; cognitive interventions are neither efficacious nor effective
Cantwell (1995)	Review of books, articles, and chapters published from 1985 to 1995 on the effectiveness of interventions	Multi-modal interventions that combine psychosocial treatments with medication are most effective; interventions must focus on family, school, and child

Table 2. Therapy Outcomes Associated with Anorexia and Bulimia

Study	Research Design	Outcomes
Fairburn, Jones, Peveler, Hope & O'Connor (1993)	Efficacy study using random assignment to compare CBT, IPT, and behavioral therapy (BT) for the treatment of bulimia	CBT and IPT made superior changes in binge eating and purging to BT, although IPT took longer to achieve its effects; Changes produced were maintained at follow-up for both IPT and CBT
Robin, Siegel, Moye, Gilroy, Dennis, & Sikand (1999)	Efficacy study using random assignment comparing behavioral family systems therapy (BFST) with ego-oriented individual therapy (EOIT) for the treatment of adolescents with anorexia nervosa	While both treatments produced improvements in eating attitudes, depression, and eating-related family conflict, BFST produced greater weight gain and higher rates of resumption of menstruation than EOIT

Table 3. Therapy Outcomes Associated with Anxiety Disorders

Study	Research Design	Outcomes
Ollendick (1995)	Controlled study of the efficacy of cognitive behavior therapy (after intervention and at six month follow-up)	The treatment eliminated panic attacks, reduced agoraphobic avoidance and negative mood states, and increased self-efficacy for coping at both waves
Ollendick & King (1998)	Review of 23 efficacy studies	Behavioral treatments such as imaginal desensitization, in vivo desensitization, modeling, and self-instruction training are all superior to wait-list control and as effective or superior as medication; cognitive behavioral therapy is superior to wait-list control and as effective as medication; cognitive behavioral therapy plus family anxiety training increases the effects of traditional CBT
Kendall (1994)	Effectiveness study of a 16-week cognitive behavioral treatment using wait-list control	Cognitive-behavioral intervention was found to be effective in the treatment of anxiety disorder in children with clinical significance continuing at one-year follow-up
Kendall, Flannery–Schroeder, Panichelli–Mindel, Southam-Gerow, Henin & Warman (1997)	Replication of the Kendall (1994) effectiveness study	Cognitive-behavioral intervention was found to be effective in the treatment of anxiety disorder in children with clinical significance continuing at one-year follow-up
Barrett, Dadds, & Rapee (1996)	Efficacy study of cognitive behavioral therapy (CBT) and CBT plus family therapy using waitlist control with random assignment	Both treatment conditions were superior to the wait-list control group in the amelioration of anxiety directly after the interventions and at 12-month follow-up. The CBT plus family therapy treatment was more effective than CBT alone at both end of treatment and 12-month follow-up

Table 4. Therapy Outcomes Associated with CD and ODD

Study	Research Design	Outcomes
Kazdin, Esveldt–Dawson, French & Unis (1987)	Efficacy study examining the effects of a combined parent management training and a cognitive-behavioral problem solving skills training (PMT-PSST) versus traditional psychotherapy	Children in the PMT-PSST treatment showed significantly less aggression and externalizing behaviors at home and school as well as significantly greater pro-social behavior and overall adjustment; results were maintained at one-year follow-up
Alexander, Holtzworth–Monroe & Jameson (1994)	Reviewed several efficacy studies of functional family therapy (FFT)	Changes in conduct-disordered adolescents were significantly greater for those treated with FFT than changes produced by psychodynamically oriented therapies or client-centered therapies; improved family functioning and communication as well as lower rates of court involvement were maintained at two- and three-year follow-ups.
Borduin, Mann, Cone, Henggeler, Fucci, Blaske & Williams (1995)	Efficacy study comparing multisystemic family therapy (MST) to individual therapy	MST was more effective than individual therapy in improving key family correlates of antisocial behavior, preventing future criminal behavior, and in ameliorating adjustment problems in individual family members
Gordon, Graves & Arbuthnot (1995)	Followed delinquent youth treated with functional family therapy (FFT) compared to a traditional probation services control group into adulthood	Youth receiving traditional probation services were five times more likely to be arrested as adults than those ttreated with FFT
Snyder, Kymissis & Kessler (1999)	Efficacy study of brief group therapy for anger control with random assignment	Treatment group participants scores on the MMPI (anger index) were significantly reduced following the treatment intervention, while the control groups' scores increased
Borduin, Schaeffer & Ronis (2003)	Book chapter reporting on several efficacy studies of MST with adolescents	MST is more effective than both usual services and individual therapy in decreasing behavior problems, antisocial peer associations, and arrests, while increasing family communication, positive family relationships, and pro-social peer relationships; follow-up to four years showed continued results
Santisteban, Coatsworth, Perez-Vidal, Kurtines, Schwartz, LaPerriere & Szapocznik (2003)	Efficacy study using random design comparing behavioral systems family therapy (BSFT) to a group treatment control (in a Hispanic sample)	BSFT participants showed significantly greater improvement in adolescent conduct problems, delinquency, marijuana use, and family functioning

Table 5. Therapy Outcomes Associated with Depression

Study	Research Design	Outcomes
Reynolds & Coats (1986)	Efficacy study with random assignment comparing group CBT, group relaxation training, and waitlist control	Both treatments produced statistically and clinically significant changes in depression; neither treatment was superior to the other; additionally, both active group treatments produced improvements in anxiety and school functioning; results were maintained at five-week follow-up
Stark, Reynolds & Kaslow (1987)	Efficacy study with random assignment comparing self-control therapy, behavioral problem solving therapy, and wait-list control	Both treatment conditions produced significantly and clinically significant changes in depression; results were similar for both treatments with neither being superior to the other
Brent et al. (1998)	Efficacy study with random assignment comparing cognitive-behavioral therapy (CBT), systemic-behavioral family therapy (SBFT), and nondirective supportive therapy (NST)	CBT was superior ("more efficacious") to SBFT and NST; SBFT was effective in reducing major depressive disorder and was superior to CBT and NST when mother also had a diagnosis of depression; NST was not effective in any circumstance.
Clarke, Rohde, Lewinsohn, Hops & Seeley (1999)	Efficacy study with random assignment comparing adolescent group CBT, group CBT with parent group, and wait-list control.	Group CBT delivered in 16 two-hour sessions over the span of eight weeks yielded higher depression recovery rates than the wait-list; group CBT plus parent group was not significantly different in results from CBT alone
Diamond, Reis, Diamond, Siqueland & Isaacs (2002)	Efficacy study with random assignment comparing attachment-based family therapy (ABFT) to wait-list control	ABFT was superior to the control with participants showing significantly greater reduction in both depression and anxiety symptoms as well as family conflict; at post-treatment, 81% of participants in treatment no longer met criteria for MDD; treatment effects remained at six-month follow-up
Mellin & Beamish (2002)	Reports on the outcomes of several efficacy studies comparing interpersonal therapy for adolescents (IPT-A), CBT, and wait-list control	IPT-A significantly reduced depressive symptomology and increased global functioning; IPT-A yielded more clinically significant results that CBT
Clarke, DeBar & Lewinsohn (2003)	Reports on the outcomes of four efficacy studies of a specific group CBT for adolescents called "Adolescent Coping with Depression" (CWDA)	Three of the studies showed statistically and clinically significant depression recovery over wait-list control with results maintained at follow-up to two years; the final study did not show a significant difference in outcome between CWDA and traditional psychotherapy

Table 6. Therapy Outcomes Associated with Substance Abuse

Study	Research Design	Outcomes
Stanton & Shadish (1997)	Meta-analysis of 15 controlled, comparative studies of family and couples treatment for drug abuse	Family therapy showed superior results when compared to individual therapy and peer group therapy; family therapy showed superior results compared to parent education or family psycho-education; family therapies were likely to have fewer drop-outs when compared to other types of therapies; no one model of family therapy appears superior to any others
Liddle, Dakof, Parker, Diamond, Barrett & Tejeda (2001)	Efficacy study comparing multidimensional family therapy (MDFT), adolescent group therapy (AGT), and multifamily education (MEI)	There was statistically significant improvement across all three treatments; MDFT showed superior improvement overall with clinical significance in the areas of substance use, academic performance, and family functioning; improvements for the MDFT were maintained at one-year follow-up with academic performance and family functioning increasing at follow-up
Kaminer, Burleson & Goldberger (2002)	Efficacy study comparing CBT to psychoeducational therapy (PT)	Both therapies produced a reduction in substance abuse at post-treatment, three-month follow-up, and nine-month follow-up; CBT was more effective than PT for older youth and males.
Curry, Wells, Lochman, Craighead & Nagy (2003)	Efficacy study on the efficacy of an integrated group CBT with family therapy for adolescents with co-morbid diagnoses of depression and substance abuse dependancy	Significant improvements were obtained in both depression and substance abuse; there was higher retention in the combined intervention than in CBT only group
Latimer, Winters, D'Zurilla & Nichols (2003)	Efficacy study comparing an integrated group CBT with family therapy (IFCBT) with a psychoeducational drug curriculum (DHPE)	IFCBT produced superior results in drug and alcohol use at post-treatment and six-month follow-up; additionally, IFCBT produced superior results for adolescents in the pro-social areas of problem-solving and learning strategy skills, and problem avoidance; improvements in parental communication and norm/value setting were also superior to the DHPE group

Cognitive-Behavioral Therapy (CBT)

Cognitive-behavioral therapy seems to be an effective treatment for attention-deficit/hyperactivity disorder, depression and suicide, and anxiety disorders. Hart and Morgan (1993, p. 6) identified six general considerations associated with cognitive-behavioral therapy:

1. CBT integrates constructs and interventions from cognitive therapies with behavior therapies.

2. Cognitions, which are private events, mediate behavior and learning.
3. Cognitions are a primary focus for intervention.
4. Target behaviors and cognitions should be clearly defined.
5. Cognitions and behaviors are reciprocally related: changes in one are associated with changes in the other.
6. Learning-based techniques are used as interventions for cognitions and behaviors.

CBT TREATMENT FOR DEPRESSION AND SUICIDE. CBT interventions that address coping skills and self-control (also referred to as behavioral problem-solving therapy) have been shown to be effective in the reduction of depression. Multiple studies of the efficacy of CBT as a treatment for depression have found both individual and group CBT to be superior to waitlist control, nondirective supportive therapy, and some forms of family therapy (Brent et al., 1998; Clarke, DeBar & Lewinsohn, 2003; Reynolds & Coats, 1986; Stark, Reynolds & Kaslow, 1987). CBT also seems to be effective in treating depressive symptoms associated with suicidal ideation (U. S. Department of Health and Human Services, 1999).

CBT TREATMENT FOR ANXIETY DISORDERS. Kendall and colleagues (Kendall, 1994; Kendall et al., 1992) developed a CBT treatment for anxiety that includes four factors: (a) recognition of anxious feelings, (b) clarification of cognitions during anxiety-provoking situations, (c) development of a coping plan, and (d) evaluation of the coping strategy. Efficacy studies of Kendall's CBT program have shown the intervention to be both clinically and statistically significant in the treatment of anxiety disorder. Reductions in anxiety continued at 12-month follow-up in both studies (Kendall, 1994; Kendall et al., 1997). Another controlled study of the efficacy of CBT for the treatment of anxiety found similar results, with the treatment condition eliminating panic attacks, reducing agoraphobic avoidance and negative mood states, and increasing self-efficacy for coping (Ollendick, 1995). Barrett, Dadds, and Rapee (1996) also found CBT to be efficacious in the amelioration of anxiety compared to a wait-list control at both post-intervention and 12-month follow-up. Systematic desensitization, modeling, and other CBT approaches are also *"probably efficacious"* (U.S. Department of Health and Human Services, 1999, p. 162; emphasis in original). Research on the effectiveness of CBT treatment for obsessive-compulsive disorder (OCD), which is classified by *DSM-IV* as an anxiety disorder, is inconclusive (U. S. Department of Health and Human Services, 1999).

Parent Skills Training

Parent skills training is often based on principles from cognitive-behavioral therapy. The goal of these psychoeducational programs is to teach effective parenting strategies for behavioral problems. Parent skills training seems to be effective for treating attention-deficit/hyperactivity disorders and disruptive disorders.

PARENT SKILLS TRAINING FOR TREATMENT FOR ATTENTION-DEFICIT/HYPERACTIVITY DISORDER (ADHD). Parents are taught behavioral techniques such as time out, point systems, and contingent attention. These interventions are associated with improvement in "targeted behaviors or skills but are not as helpful in reducing the core symptoms of inattention, hyperactivity, or impulsivity" (U. S. Department of Health and Human Services, 1999, p. 148). Parent skills training combined with self-control therapy for the adolescent was found to be efficacious when combined with a low dose of methylphenidate in a study by Horn et al. (1991). A review of 47 studies of the efficacy of interventions with ADHD disordered youth also found parent training combined with services to the adolescent to be efficacious, and a similar review by Smith, Waschbusch, Willoughby, and Evans (2000) found parent training not only efficacious but practical and safe. Parent training combined with medication is more effective than medication alone.

PARENT SKILLS TREATMENT FOR DISRUPTIVE DISORDERS.   Parent management training combined with CBT problem-solving skills training for adolescents decreased aggression and externalizing behaviors at school and home in a study by Kazdin, Esveldt–Dawson, French, and Unis (1987). This treatment also increased the adolescents' pro-social behaviors. Two specific parent skills programs that are "considered 'well-established' as treatment for disruptive disorders include *Living With Children* (Bernal et al., 1980) and an [untitled] videotape-modeling parent training program (Spaccarelli et al., 1992)" (U. S. Department of Health and Human Services, 1999, p. 166).

Family/Systemic Therapies

Family/systemic therapies seem to be effective treatments for depression and suicide (Brent, et al., 1998; Diamond, Reis, Diamond, Siqueland & Isaacs, 2002; Mellin & Beamish, 2002; Pinsof & Wynne, 1995; U. S. Department of Health and Human Services, 1999), alcohol and substance abuse (Liddle et al., 2001; Pinsof & Wynne, 1995; Stanton & Shadish, 1997; U. S. Department of Health and Human Services, 1999), and behavioral problems associated with conduct disorder and oppositional defiant disorder (Alexander, Holtzworth-Monroe & Jameson, 1994; Borduin et al., 1995; Borduin, Schaeffer & Ronis 2003; Gordon, Graves & Arbuthnot, 1995; Santisteban et al., 2003; Snyder, Kymissis & Kessler, 1999). There is less empirical support, yet some evidence, that family/systemic therapies can be efficacious in the treatment of ADHD (Cantwell, 1995; Smith, Waschbusch, Willoughby & Evans, 2000), anxiety (Barrett, Dadds & Rapee, 1996; Ollendick & King, 1998), and anorexia nervosa/bulima nervosa (Fairburn, Jones, Peveler, Hope & O'Connor, 1993; Robin, Siegel, Moye, Gilroy, Dennis & Sikand, 1999). In a special edition of the *Journal of Marital and Family Therapy* devoted to effectiveness of family intervention, family therapy was defined as "*any psychotherapy that directly involves family members in addition to an index patient and/or explicitly attends to the interaction among family members*" (Pinsof & Wynne, 1995, p. 586).

FAMILY/SYSTEMIC TREATMENT FOR DEPRESSION.   The U. S. Surgeon Generals' report on mental illness suggests that systemic family therapy shows "promise" but has not been investigated adequately to assess effectiveness (USDHHS, 1999, p. 155). Comparisons of family therapy with CBT therapies have shown family-therapy-based treatments to be less effective than CBT but superior to wait-list control groups at post-treatment in the treatment of depression (Clarke, Rohde, Lewinsohn, Hops & Seeley, 1999; Pinsof & Wynne, 1995). There are several notable exceptions, however. Family-based therapy was more effective than CBT when there was parental depression in a study by Brent et al. (1998). A study comparing attachment-based family therapy (ABFT) with wait-list control found ABFT resulted in significant reductions in depression, anxiety, and family conflict with results sustained at two-year follow-up (Diamond et al., 2002). A recent review of the research on family therapy for depression found the effects of family therapy were more likely to be maintained at follow-up than other therapies, with longer term changes in adolescent depression, parental functioning, and behavioral control (Cottrell, 2003). Additionally, family-based therapies were more likely to show specific effects on parent–adolescent relationships/interactions and reduced relapse (Curry, 2001) and were more likely to be effective for youth dealing with co-morbid disorders (Curry, et al., 2003)

FAMILY/SYSTEMIC TREATMENT FOR SUICIDE. "Interpersonal conflicts are important stresses related to the risk of . . . potentially suicidal children and adolescents. Treatment of interpersonal strife may significantly reduce suicidal risk" (U. S. Department of Health and Human Services, 1999, p. 157). The following factors, which can be effectively treated with family therapy, are associated with suicide: (a) experiencing isolation within the family, (b) demonstrating problems associated with independence, and (c) viewing self as expendable in the family (U. S. Department of Health and Human Services, 1999). Empirical investigation of family therapy in the reduction of adolescent suicidal ideation is ongoing, although research to date has shown decreases in suicidal ideation compared to "usual care" (Harrington, Kerfoot, Dyer, McNiven, Gill & Harrington, 1998). Additionally, family therapy appears to have less attrition and increased satisfaction during treatment and at follow-up. Analysis of health-care costs shows that increased participation in family therapy is associated with decreased placements in foster care or residential care resulting in substantial savings (Cottrell, 2003).

FAMILY/SYSTEMIC TREATMENT FOR SUBSTANCE ABUSE DISORDERS. Family therapy by itself or in conjunction with other approaches seems to be the most effective treatment for alcohol and substance abuse. A meta-analysis of 15 controlled, comparative studies of family treatment for drug/alcohol abuse concluded that family therapies were superior to other treatment approaches, enhanced the effectiveness of other treatments, and had fewer drop-outs than other treatment approaches (Stanton & Shadish, 1997). Recent studies continue to show both statistical and clinical significance in the reduction of substance abuse and the improvement of academic performance and family functioning with results maintained at follow-ups (Liddle et al., 2001; Curry et al., 2003).

FAMILY/SYSTEMIC TREATMENT FOR EXTERNALIZING DISORDERS SUCH AS ODD, CD, AND AGGRESSION. Numerous studies have reported the demonstrated efficacy of family therapies for externalizing disorders. Borduin et al. (1995) compared multisystemic family therapy (MST) with individual therapy and found MST to be more effective in improving key family correlates of antisocial behavior, preventing future criminal behavior, and reducing adjustment problems. Further research on MST has continued to find this family therapy to be more effective than both usual services and individual therapy at decreasing behavior problems, criminal behavior, and association with antisocial peers. MST has also shown success in increasing family communication, positive family relationships, and prosocial peer relationships. These improvements are maintained at follow-ups as long as four years (Borduin et al., 2003). Family therapy, either alone or combined with CBT, has been shown to be effective at decreasing behavioral problems, increasing school performance, and improving family functioning at post-treatment, follow-up, and into adulthood for a number of ethnicities (Alexander et al., 1994; Gordon et al., 1995; and Santisteban et al., 2003).

Potentially Ineffective Treatments

Treatments reported on in this section have been found to be ineffective in randomized, controlled studies, have not been found to be efficacious, or lack empirical support.

CBT Treatment for Attention-Deficit/Hyperactivity Disorder (ADHD)

A review of the literature by Pelham, Wheeler, and Chronis (1998) found that cognitive interventions for the treatment of ADHD are not efficacious. A similar review by Smith et al. (2000) reported cognitive interventions to be neither efficacious or effective. Although interventions to improve problem-solving and social skills do not seem to improve behavior or academic performance, CBT may help treat symptoms of accompanying disorders such as oppositional defiant disorder, depression, or anxiety disorders (U. S. Department of Health and Human Services, 1999).

CBT Treatment for Substance Abuse Disorders

Several recent studies have examined CBT treatment for substance abuse disorders. While several of these studies found CBT to be superior to wait-list controls and psychoeducational therapy, they were not as effective as family therapies (Kaminer, Burleson, & Goldberger, 2002; Liddle, et al., 2001; Curry, et al., 2003). Cognitive-behavioral therapy combined with family therapy did show some promise (Curry, et al., 2003; Latimer, Winters, D'Zurilla, & Nichols, 2003) with the combined treatment showing decreases in substance usage as well as improvements in problem-solving skills, family communication and functioning, and school performance.

Inpatient Hospitalization

Inpatient hospitalization—which is the most restrictive form of mental health care provided—is used to treat youth with the most severe disorders. This form of treatment is the most expensive: half of the money paid for treating youth mental health problems is spent on inpatient hospitalizations, which have the weakest empirical support (U. S. Department of Health and Human Services, 1999).

Residential Treatment Centers (RTC)

Residential treatment is less restrictive than inpatient hospitalization and is used by only about 8% of children who are treated, but a significant amount of money is spent for this form of treatment: "nearly one-fourth of the national outlay on child mental health is spent on care in these settings" (U. S. Department of Health and Human Services, 1999, p. 169). Residential treatment centers—which must be licensed—provide twenty-four hour mental health services.

There are concerns about inconsistent admission standards, cost of services, risks associated with treatment, trauma associated with family separation, difficulty returning to family and community, victimization by staff, and learning antisocial behavior because of intensive exposure to other children (U. S. Department of Health and Human Services, 1999). The Surgeon General's report on mental health concludes that "Given the limitations of current research, it is premature to endorse the effectiveness of residential treatment for adolescents. Moreover, research is needed to identify those groups of children and adolescents for whom the benefits of residential care outweigh the potential risks" (U. S. Department of Health and Human Services, 1999, p. 171).

Day Treatment

Day treatment refers to "a specialized and intensive form of treatment that is less restrictive than inpatient care but is more intensive than the usual types of outpatient care (i.e., individual, family, or group treatment)" (U. S. Department of Health and Human Services, 1999, p. 169). This form of treatment typically integrates education, counseling, and family interventions. Family participation during and following treatment is considered "essential" (U. S. Department of Health and Human Services, 1999, p. 169).

Research on day treatment programs suggests that they have a positive influence, but most studies have not included a comparison group. Results from 20 uncontrolled studies suggest that day treatment is associated with improved functioning for youth (and family); three-fourths of the youth are successfully reintegrated into regular school; and day treatment prevents youth from entering residential treatment, which is more costly (U. S. Department of Health and Human Services, 1999). Research from one controlled study that included six-month follow-up also suggested that day treatment was associated with "reducing behavior problems, decreasing symptoms, and improving family functioning" (U. S. Department of Health and Human Services, 1999, p. 169).

Community-Based Treatment

Since the 1980s, services for youth mental health have shifted from institutional to community-based services. Community-based services (sometimes referred to as a "wraparound approach") include "case management, home-based services, therapeutic foster care, therapeutic group home, and crisis services" (U. S. Department of Health and Human Services, 1999, p. 172). Research "evidence for the benefits of some of these services is uneven at best" (U. S. Department of Health and Human Services, 1999, p. 172). Providing integrated treatment across multiple settings—an emerging trend in youth treatment (Fonagy, Target, Cottrell, Phillips & Kurtz, 2002)—is a common thread in these forms of community-based treatments (Grundle, 2002).

Potentially Harmful Treatments

While the lack of evidence regarding certain treatments can and should give therapists pause before using them, there are some treatments that not only lack empirical support, they have been shown to be dangerous to the adolescents experiencing them.

Holding Therapy

Holding therapy, which is sometimes referred to as attachment therapy, was developed to treat for reactive attachment disorder (RAD). Those who practice holding therapy borrow some ideas from research on attachment, but their interventions contradict fundamental concepts from that empirical literature (Werner-Wilson & Davenport, 2003). For example, proponents of holding therapy, who overstate the incidence of RAD, suggest that some children are incapable of forming attachments. This contradicts research which suggests that all children from some type of attachment with their caregiver. Further, those practicing holding therapy use interventions that would undermine development of a secure base. These practices "include three primary treatment components that are directed toward the child: (a) prolonged restraint for purpose other than protection; (b) prolonged noxious stimulation (e.g., tickling, poking ribs); and (c) interference with bodily functions" (Werner-Wilson & Davenport, 2003, p. 182). Holding therapy has been associated with at least two fatalities and lacks empirical support (Hanson & Spratt, 2000; Werner-Wilson & Davenport, 2003). For example, ten-year-old Candace Newmaker died as the result of a treatment referred to as holding therapy (Glenn, 2003). Hanson and Spratt (2000) suggest that "[t]he fact remains that there is simply no empirical evidence at present to support the assertion that attachment therapy is more effective, or even as effective, compared to accepted and conventional approaches" (p. 142).

Conclusion

Professionals who provide services to adolescents have a responsibility to remain current about effective treatments and basic research on adolescent development. At a minimum, those providing treatment to adolescents should understand aspects of adolescent development that influence presenting problems and interventions. In particular, treatment providers should strongly advocate for psychotherapy, recognize which therapies are effective for particular problems, and coordinate closely with other professionals, especially if clients are prescribed medications. Professionals should also cultivate sensitivity to diversity.

References

Ainsworth, M.D.S. (1991). Attachments and other affectional bonds across the life cycle. In C.M. Parkes, J. Stevenson-Hinde & P. Marris (Eds.), *Attachment Across the Life Cycle*. New York: Routledge.

Alexander, J., Holtzworth-Monroe, A., & Jameson, P. (1994). The process and outcome of marital and family therapy research: Review and evaluation. In A. Bergin & S. Garfield (Eds.), *Handbook of Psychotherapy and Behavior Change (4th ed.)* (pp. 595–630). New York, NY: John Wiley & Sons.

Anderson, C.M., & Holder, D.P. (1989). Women and serious mental disorders. In M. McGoldrick, C.M. Anderson, & F. Walsh (Eds.), *Women in Families: A Framework for Family Therapy* (pp. 381–405). New York: Norton.

Barrett, P., Dadds, M., & Rapee, R. (1996). Family treatment of childhood anxiety: A controlled trial. *Journal of Consulting and Clinical Psychology, 64*, 333–342.

Bernal, M.E., Klinnert, M.D., & Schulz, L.A. (1980). Outcome evaluation of behavioral parent training and child-centered parent counseling for children with conduct problems. *Journal of Applied Behavior Analysis, 13*, 677–691.

Bogenschneider, K. (1996). Family related prevention programs: An ecological risk/protective theory for building prevention programs, policies, and community capacity to support youth. *Family Relations, 45*, 127–138.

Bordin, E.S. (1979). The generalizability of the psychoanalytic concept of the working alliance. *Psychotherapy: Theory, Research, and Practice, 16*, 252–260.

Bordin, E.S. (1994). Theory and research on the therapeutic working alliance: New directions. In A.O. Horvath & L.S. Greenberg (Eds.), *The Working Alliance: Theory, Research, and Practice* (pp. 13–37). New York: John Wiley & Sons.

Borduin, C., Mann, B., Cone, L., Henggeler, S., Fucci, B., Blaske, D., & Williams, R. (1995). Multisystemic treatment of serious juvenile offenders: Long-term prevention of criminality and violence. *Journal of Consulting and Clinical Psychology, 63*, 569–578.

Borduin, C., Schaeffer, C., & Ronis, S. (2003). Multisystemic treatment of serious antisocial behavior in adolescents. In C. Essau (Ed.), *Conduct and Oppositional Defiant Disorders* (pp. 299–318). Mahwah, NJ: Lawrence Erlbaum Associates.

Brent, D., Kolko, D., Birmaher, B., Baugher, M., Bridge, J., Roth, C., & Holder, D. (1998). Predictors of treatment efficacy in a clinical trial of three psychosocial treatments for adolescent depression. *Journal of the American Academy of Child and Adolescent Psychiatry, 37*, 906–914.

Broverman, I.K., Broverman, D.M., Clarkson, F.E., Rosenkrantz, P.S., & Vogel, S.R. (1974). Sex-role stereotypes and clinical judgments. In J.M. Neale, G.C. Davison, & K.P. Price (Eds.), *Contemporary Readings in Psychopathology* (pp. 45–53). New York: Wiley.

Byng-Hall, J. (1995). Creating a secure family base: Some implications of attachment theory for family therapy. *Family Process, 34*, 45–58.

Cantwell, D. (1995). Attention Deficit Disorder: A review of the past 10 years. *Journal of the American Academy of Child and Adolescent Psychiatry, 35*, 978–987.

Cassidy, J. & Shaver, P.R. (Eds.). (1999). *Handbook of Attachment: Theory, Research, and Clinical Applications.* New York: Guilford Press.

Center for Population Options. (1992). *Lesbian, Gay, and Bisexual Youth: At Risk and Underserved.* Washington, DC: Author.

Clarke, G., DeBar, L., & Lewinsohn, P. (2003). Cognitive-behavioral group treatment for adolescent depression. In A. Kazdin, (Ed.), *Evidence-Based Psychotherapies for Children and Adolescents* (pp. 120–134). New York, NY: Guilford Press.

Clarke, G., Rohde, P., Lewinsohn, P., Hops, H., & Seeley, J. (1999). Cognitive-behavioral treatment of adolescent depression: Efficacy of acute group treatment and booster sessions. *Journal of the American Academy of Child and Adolescent Psychiatry, 38*, 272–279.

Comas-Díaz, L. (1996). Cultural considerations in diagnosis. In F. Kaslow (Ed.), *Handbook of Relational Diagnosis and Dysfunctional Family Patterns* (pp. 152–168). New York: Wiley.

Cottrell, D. (2003). Outcome studies of family therapy in child and adolescent depression. *Journal of Family Therapy, 25*, 400–416.

Curry, J. (2001). Specific psychotherapies for childhood and adolescent depression. *Biological Psychiatry, 49*, 1091–1100.

Curry, J., Wells, K., Lochman, J., Craighead, W., & Nagy, P. (2003). Cognitive-behavioral intervention for depressed, substance-abusing adolescents: Development and pilot testing. *Journal of the Academy of Child and Adolescent Psychiatry, 42*, 656–665.

Cusinato, M. (1998). Parenting styles and psychopathology. In L.L'Bate (Ed.), *Family Psychopathology: The Relational Roots of Dysfunctional Behavior* (pp. 158–183). New York: Guilford Press.

Diamond, G., Reis, B., Diamond, G., Siqueland, L., & Isaacs, L. (2002). Attachment-based family therapy for depressed adolescents: A treatment development study. *Journal of the American Academy of Child and Adolescent Psychiatry, 41*, 1190–1196.

Dilworth-Anderson, P., Burton, L.M., & Johnson, L.B. (1993). Reframing theories for understanding race, ethnicity, and families. In P.G. Boss, W.J. Doherty, R. LaRossa, W.R. Schumm, & S.K. Steinmetz (Eds.), *Sourcebook of Family Theories and Methods: A Contextual Approach* (pp. 627–649). New York: Plenum Press.

Estrada, A.U., & Holmes, J.M. (1999). Couples perceptions of effective and ineffective ingredients of couple therapy. *Journal of Sex & Marital Therapy, 25*, 151–162.

Fairburn, C., Jones, R., Peveler, R., Hope, R., & O'Connor, M. (1993). Psychotherapy and bulimia nervosa: Longer-term effects of interpersonal psychotherapy, behavior therapy, and cognitive behavior therapy. *Archives of General Psychiatry, 30,* 419–428.

Fonagy, P., Target, M., Cottrell, D., Phillips, J., & Kurtz, Z. (2002). *What Works for Whom? A Critical Review of Treatments for Children and Adolescents.* New York: Guilford Press.

Garbarino, J. (1995). *Raising Children in a Socially Toxic Environment.* San Francisco: Jossey-Bass.

Glenn, D. (2003, October 24). Nightmare scenarios. *The Chronicle of Higher Education, 50 (9),* A14.

Gordon, D., Graves, K., & Arbuthnot, J. (1995). The effect of functional family therapy for delinquents on adult criminal behavior. *Criminal Justice and Behavior, 22,* 60–73.

Grundle, T.J. (2002). Wraparound care. In D.T. Marsh & M.A. Fristad (Eds.), *Handbook of Serious Emotional Disturbance in Children and Adolescence* (pp. 323–333).

Gurman, A.S. (2001). Brief therapy and family/couple therapy: An essential redundancy. *Clinical Psychology: Science and Practice, 8,* 51–65.

Hanson, R.F., & Spratt, E.G. (2000). Reactive attachment disorder: What we know about the disorder and implications for treatment. *Child Maltreatment: Journal of the American Professional Society on the Abuse of Children, 5 (2),* 137–145.

Hanson, W.E., Curry, K.T., & Bandalos, D.L. (2002). Reliability generalization of working alliance inventory scale scores. *Educational and Psychological Measurement, 62,* 659–673.

Harrington, R., Kerfoot, M., Dyer, E., McNiven, F., Gill, J., & Harrington, V. (1998). Randomized trial of a home-based family intervention for children who have deliberately poisoned themselves. *Journal of the American Academy of Child and Adolescent Psychiatry, 37,* 512–518.

Hart, K.J., & Morgan, J.R. (1993). Cognitive-behavioral procedures with children: Historical context and current status. In A.J. Fnch, W.M. Nelson III, & E.S. Ott (Eds.), *Cognitive-Behavioral Procedures with Children and Adolescents.* Boston: Allyn & Bacon.

Henggler, S., & Sheidow, A. (2003). Conduct disorder and delinquency. *Journal of Marital and Family Therapy, 29,* 505–522.

Horn, W., Ialongo, N., Pascoe, J., Greenber, G., Packard, T., Lopez, M., Wagner, A., & Puttler, L., (1991). Additive effects of psychostimulants, parent training, and self-control therapy with ADHD children. *Journal of the American Academy of Child & Adolescent Psychiatry, 30,* 233–240.

Horvath, A.O. (1994). Empirical validation of Bordin's pan theoretical model of the alliance: The working alliance inventory perspective. In A.O. Horvath & L.S. Greenberg (Eds.), *The Working Alliance: Theory, Research, and Practice* (pp. 109–128). New York: John Wiley & Sons.

Horvath, A.O., & Symonds, B.D. (1991). Relation between working alliance and outcome in psychotherapy: A meta-analysis. *Journal of Counseling Psychology, 38,* 139–149.

Kaminer, Y., Burleson, J., & Goldberger, R. (2002). Cognitive-behavioral coping skills and psychoeducation therapies for adolescent substance abuse. *Journal of Nervous and Mental Disease, 190,* 737–745.

Kazdin, A., Esveldt-Dawson, K., French, N., & Unis, A. (1987). Effects of parent management training and problem-solving skills training combined in the treatment of antisocial child behavior. *Journal of the American Academy of Child and Adolescent Psychiatry, 26,* 416–424.

Kendall, P.C. (1994). Treating anxiety disorder in children: Results of a randomized clinical trial. *Journal of Consulting and Clinical Psychology, 62,* 100–110.

Kendall, P.S., Chansky, T.E., Kane, M.T., Kim, R., Kortlander, E., Ronan, K.R., Sessa, F.M., & Siqueland, L. (1992). *Anxiety Disorders in Youth: Cognitive-Behavioral Interventions.* Needham Heights, MA: Allyn & Bacon.

Kendall, P., Flannery-Schroeder, E., Panichelli-Mindel, S., Southam-Gerow, M., Henin, A., & Warman, M. (1997). Therapy for youths with anxiety disorders: A second randomized clinical trial. *Journal of Consulting and Clinical Psychology, 65,* 366–380.

Knudson-Martin, C. (2001). Women and mental health: A feminist family systems approach. In M.M. MacFarlane (Ed.), *Family Therapy and Mental Health: Innovations in Theory and Practice* (pp. 331–359). New York: Haworth.

Latimer, W., Winters, K., D'Zurilla, T., & Nichols, M. (2003). Integrated family and cognitive-behavioral therapy for adolescent substance abusers: A stage I efficacy study. *Drug and Alcohol Dependence, 71,* 303–317.

Liddle, H., Dakof, G., Parker, K., Diamond, G., Barrett, K., & Tejeda, M. (2001). Multidimensional family therapy for adolescent drug abuse: Results of a randomized clinical trial. *American Journal of Drug and Alcohol Abuse, 27,* 651–688.

Lonigan, C., Elbert, J., & Johnson, S. (1998). Empirically supported psychosocial interventions for children: An overview. *Journal of Clinical Child Psychology, 27,* 138–145.

McFall, R.M. (1991). Manifesto for a science of clinical psychology. *The Clinical Psychologist, 44*, 75–88.

Mellin, E., & Beamish, P. (2002). Interpersonal theory and adolescents with depression: Clinical update. *Journal of Mental Health Counseling, 24*, 110–125.

Najavits, L.M., & Strupp, H.H. (1994). Differences in the effectiveness of psychodynamic therapists: A process-outcome study. *Psychotherapy, 31*, 114–123.

Ollendick, T. (1995). Cognitive behavioral treamtment of panic disorder with agoraphobia in adolescents: A multiple baseline design analysis. *Behavior Therapy, 26*, 517–531.

Ollendick, T., & King, N. (1998). Empirically supported treatments for children with phobic and anxiety disorders: Current status. *Journal of Clinical Child Psychology, 27*, 156–167.

Paniagua, F.A. (1998). *Assessing and Treating Culturally Diverse Clients (Second edition)*. Thousand Oaks, CA: Sage.

Pelham, Jr., W., Wheeler, T., & Chronis, A. (1998). Empirically supported psychosocial treatment for Attention Deficit Hyperactivity Disorder. *Journal of Clinical Child Psychology, 27*, 190–205.

Petrosino, Turpin-Petrosino, & Finckenhauer (2000). Well meaning programs can have harmful effects! Lessons from experiments of programs such as Scared Straight. *Crime & Delinquency, 46*, 354–379.

Pinsof, W.M., & Wynne, L.C. (1995). The efficacy of marital and family therapy: An empirical overview, conclusions, and recommendations. *Journal of Marital and Family Therapy, 21*, 585–613.

Reynolds, W., & Coats, K. (1986). A comparison of cognitive-behavioral therapy and relaxation training for the treatment of depression in adolescents. *Journal of Consulting and Clinical Psychology, 54*, 653–660.

Ringeisen, H., & Hoagwood, K. (2002). Clinical research directions for the treatment and delivery of children's mental health services. In D.T. Marsh & M.A. Fristad (Eds.), *Handbook of Serious Emotional Disturbance in Children and adolescents* (pp. 33–55). New York, NY: John Wiley & Sons.

Robbins, M.S., Turner, C.W., Alexander, J.F., & Perez, G.A. (2003). Alliance and dropout in family therapy for adolescents with behavior problems: Individual and systemic effects. *Journal of Family Psychology, 17(4)*, 534–544.

Robin, A., Siegel, P., Moye, A., Gilroy, M., Dennis, A., & Sikand, A. (1999). A controlled comparison of family versus individual therapy for adolescents with anorexia nervosa. *Journal of the American Academy of Child and Adolescent Psychiatry, 38*, 1482–1489.

Rogers, C. (1965). The therapeutic relationship: Recent theory and research. *Australian Journal of Psychology, 17*, 95–108.

Santisteban, D., Coatsworth, J., Perez-Vidal, A., Kurtines, W., Schwartz, S., LaPerriere, A., & Szapocznik, J. (2003). Efficacy of brief strategic family therapy in modifying Hispanic adolescent behaviors and substance abuse. *Journal of Family Psychology, 17*, 121–133.

Savin-Williams, R.C. (1994). Verbal and physical abuse as stressors in the lives of lesbian, gay male, and bisexual youths: Associations with school problems, running away, substance abuse, prostitution, and suicide. *Journal of Consulting and Clinical Psychology, 62(2)*, 261–269.

Smith, B., Waschbusch, D., Willoughby, M., & Evans, S. (2000). The efficacy, safety, and practicality of treatments for adolescents with Attention-Deficit/Hyperactivity Disorder (ADHD). *Clinical Child and Family Psychology Review, 3*, 243–267.

Snyder, K., Kymissis, P., & Kessler, K. (1999). Anger management for adolescents: Efficacy of brief group therapy. *Journal of the American Academy of Child and Adolescent Psychiatry, 38*, 1409–1416.

Spaccarelli, S., Cotler, S., & Penman, D. (1992). Problem-solving skills training as a supplement to behavioral parent training. *Cognitive Therapy and Research, 27*, 171–186.

Stanton, M., & Shadish, W. (1997). Outcome, attrition, and family-couples treatment for drug abuse: A meta-analysis and review of the controlled, comparative studies. *Psychological Bulletin, 122*, 170–191.

Stark, K., Reynolds, W., & Kaslow, N. (1987). A comparison of the relative efficacy of self-control therapy and a behavioral problem-solving therapy for depression in children. *Journal of Abnormal Child Psychology, 15*, 91–113.

Thompson, R.A. (1999). Early attachment and later development. In J. Cassidy & P.R. Shaver (Eds.), *Handbook of Attachment: Theory, Research, and Clinical Applications* (pp. 265–286). New York: Guilford Press.

U.S. Department of Health and Human Services (1999). *Mental Health: A Report of the Surgeon General*. Rockville, MD: U.S. Department of Health and Human Services, Substance Abuse and Mental Health Services Administration, Center for Mental Health Services, National Institutes for Health, National Institute of Mental Health.

Werner-Wilson, R.J. (2001). *Developmental-Systemic Family Therapy with Adolescents*. Binghampton, NY: Haworth Press.

Werner-Wilson, R.J. & Davenport, B.R. (2003). Distinguishing between conceptualizations of attachment: Clinical implications in marriage and family therapy. *Contemporary Family Therapy, 25*, 179–193.

Chapter 6

Evidence-Based Practices

Thomas L. Sexton, Lynn Gilman, and Christine Johnson–Erickson

The last decade has witnessed a dramatic change in the landscape of treatment and prevention programs for adolescents and their families. There is now a wide range of treatment and prevention program choices for service providers and communities hoping to impact at-risk youth positively. Of the prevention and treatment program options currently available, there are a growing number rooted in both clinical trial and community-based outcome research. Other programs also have strong process research that identifies the critical and central mechanism(s) of change that result in successful outcomes. These outcomes have been identified not just by model developers, but as a result of a number of systematic efforts to scrutinize carefully the scientific evidence to ensure that programs work, the outcomes last, and that these outcomes are replicable in local communities (Elliott, 1998; U.S. Public Health Service, 2001, etc). Over the last five years, many evidence-based programs have been successfully implemented in local communities and some across entire statewide systems of care with impressive results (Barnoski, 2004).

The evolution of evidence-based prevention and treatment programs for adolescent behavior problems fits within a broader movement of evidence-based model development in medicine, psychology, and other social services. The impact of evidence-based practices is dramatic in that they are fundamentally changing the way practitioners work, the criteria from which communities choose programs to help families and youth, the methods of clinical training, the accountability of program developers and interventions, and the outcomes that can be expected from such programs. Despite the significant gains made in the development and dissemination of evidence-based programs, many controversies remain. For some, evidence-based programs are viewed as a challenge to well-entrenched traditional means of treatment. EBPs are viewed as simple curricular approaches with *paint by the number*s guidelines that are unresponsive to the needs of youth, families, and communities. While others may agree that such programs are necessary, the definition of what constitutes "evidence based" remains unclear, the criteria for such programs are elusive, and suspicion over science as a basis of human service practice decision making is yet to be universally accepted. In addition, the evidence-based practice movement is increasingly in conflict with other movements also aimed at positively impacting youth (the systems of care movement).

Our goal in this chapter is to provide an overview of the background, the current status, important controversies, and future directions of evidence-based prevention and treatment practices for adolescent behavior problems. Our hope is that a thoughtful analysis of the strengths and future challenges of the evidence-based practices movement can help overcome the continuing suspicion and reluctance of individual practitioners and communities to embrace programs that have the potential to help with a very difficult set of clinical problems. We begin with a consideration of the many forces that have lead to the development of alternative approaches like evidence-based practices. In particular, we focus on the range and nature of adolescent behavior problems, evolution of evidence as criteria for clinical practice, and the traditionally poor outcomes of traditional approaches. Second, we define evidence-based practice and focus on construct definitions of its core elements: evidence and systematic practice. As an illustration we present four prevention and treatment programs that are based in scientific evidence with demonstrated positive outcomes in both clinical and community settings. Finally, we address the emerging problems and future issues related to this movement within the prevention and treatment of adolescent behavior problems in an attempt to set a future agenda for the field.

The Need for Evidence-Based Prevention and Treatment Programs

There is an increasing move to find programs that work for the wide range of problems experienced by adolescents. The search for effective programs is being driven by two factors: the realization that the problems experienced by adolescents are very serious and the inability of traditional prevention and treatment programs to have a significant impact on reducing the negative consequences and impact of these problems on youth, their families, and the communities in which they live.

Adolescent behavior disorders have historically been viewed as one of the most difficult areas of practice for prevention and intervention specialists. The problems experienced by adolescents are significant because of the range of specific difficulties and the prevalence of these issues. Youth and families are often viewed as treatment resistant, lacking motivation, and being untreatable by traditional prevention and intervention programs (Alexander, Sexton & Robbins, 2002). The most public evidence for the seriousness of the problems can be found in the highly publicized consequences of disruptive adolescent behavior problems (e.g., youth violence, school shootings, juvenile crime). These dramatic events are only the most obvious evidence of the seriousness of dysfunctional adolescent behavior problems. Between 1988 and 1994, the juvenile arrest rate for violent crimes (homicide, forcible rape, robbery, and aggravated assault) increased by 62% (Snyder & Sickmund, 1999). Less apparent but equally troubling are the significant number of adolescents in need of mental health treatment. Epidemiological studies suggest that between 17% and 22% of adolescents suffer from a significant developmental, emotional, and/or behavioral problem (Kazdin, 2003). High rates of mental disorders also exist among youth involved in the juvenile justice system (Hogan, 2003; Teplin, Abram, McClelland, Dulcan &

Mericle, 2002; Lyons, Baerger, Quigley, Erlich & Griffin, 2001) with an estimated 50% to 80% of delinquent adolescents meeting the criteria for a mental disorder such as conduct or substance-related disorders (Kazdin, 2000). The economic impact of adolescent behavior problems is significant, with estimates for adolescents in the juvenile justice alone in the millions of dollars each year. Costs for mental health services are equally high (Sexton, Sydnor & Rowland, 2004). These costs do not encompass the other unaccounted psychological costs to the individual, family, and community.

Identifying and describing youth behavior problems (e.g., "dysfunction") is more difficult and complex than one might think. Often, youth with similar behavior problems are identified by way of their involvement in different community systems that give different labels to similar behaviors (e.g., child welfare, juvenile justice, or mental health). Regardless of the system in which they might be involved, adolescents labeled as having "dysfunctional" behavior actually represent complex clinical profiles with a wide range of developmental, emotional, and behavioral problems. Kazdin (2004) distinguishes between psychiatric disorders (diagnosable disorders such as anxiety, mood, substance-related, adjustment, and disruptive behavior disorders, APA, 2000), from problem or at-risk behaviors (such as drug and alcohol use or school suspension and truancy) and delinquency (committing unlawful acts) as adolescent problems that may require intervention. Furthermore, behavior disorders are at times difficult to identify because to some degree they are part of the normal developmental trajectory of youth. For example, fighting, withdrawing, disagreeing, and standing up to authority figures represent behaviors that are often part of normal adolescent development.

Adolescent behavior problems are often described according to two broad categories. *Externalizing disorders* are those directed to others and the environment. They include oppositional, hyperactive, aggressive, and antisocial behaviors. Numerous psychiatric diagnostic categories encompass these areas, including attention-deficit and disruptive disorders. Youth referred to the mental health and juvenile justice systems are most likely to be ones who fall into the externalizing behavior disorders category. This is no surprise given that these behaviors are likely to impact others. *Internalizing disorders* are problems internally directed and include clinical symptoms which as anxiety, withdrawal, and depression. These youth are less likely to be referred for treatment and are easily overlooked in families, schools, and communities. The problems experienced by youth who do not meet the criteria for either internal or externalizing behavior problems may engage in problem behaviors that put them at risk for becoming involved in the mental health or juvenile justice system or to experience future psychiatric problems. These youth might be involved in truancy, vandalism, stealing, drug use, bullying, running away from home, etc. (DiClemente, Hansen & Ponton, 1996). These data led Kazdin (2003) to suggest that prevalence rates for youth behavior problems substantially underestimate the scope of the existing problem.

The need for EBP is further demonstrated by the limited effectiveness and high cost of traditional adolescent treatment and prevention programs. While there are many different prevention and treatment programs in the professional literature (Elliott estimates over 1,000), few are effective. In fact, numerous systematic literature reviews suggest that traditional treatment programs are notoriously unsuccessful at getting youth into treatment and prevention programs, keeping them in programs, and demonstrating successful outcomes (Elliott, 1998; Kazdin, 2003;

Sexton, Alexander & Mease, 2004). It has been estimated that between 40% and 60% of youth in traditional treatment programs drop out prior to program completion (Kazdin, 1996). Using a relatively modest standard, the Blueprint project (Elliott, 1998) found only 1% of reviewed programs (after review of over 1,000 published programs) to have demonstrated effectiveness in community settings. The Surgeon General found only five programs to be effective in successfully preventing and treating violent youth behavior problems (U.S. Public Health Service, 2001). In a systematic review of the research literature, Sexton et al. (2004) found only a few systematic family-based intervention programs to be successful treatments of choice for a wide range of clinical syndromes typically classified as adolescent behavior disorder problems.

The Evolution of "Evidence-Based" Prevention and Intervention Program Models for Adolescent Problems

Given the potentially serious outcomes of adolescent behavior problems and the lack of prevention and treatment programs with demonstrable outcomes, it is no surprise that families, communities, treatment providers, and model developers have searched for programs in which they can have confidence. This search has proved to be more difficult than one might think. In fact, determining what constitutes a clinically "valid" prevention or intervention program has always been difficult. For many years the field relied either on what made sense (face validity), what experts told us (expert validity), or the zeitgeist of the time (consensual validity). The use of scientific evidence in determining a "valid" treatment is a surprisingly new trend in prevention and treatment fields.

Evidence-based prevention and treatment programs for adolescents have evolved in ways similar to that in other areas of professional practice (e.g., medicine). Understanding the evolution of evidence in prevention and treatment of adolescent behavior disorder is best understood within this larger context of evidence-based clinical decision-making across disciplines. The development of EBP in each of these fields has had an important impact on the types of evidence that are viewed as acceptable, the criteria upon which such programs are judged, and the nature of the programs themselves. We present a brief overview of the development of evidence-based medicine, evidence-based psychological treatments, and more specifically, the evolution of evidence-based practices for adolescent prevention and treatment programs, in order to help frame the current status and critical challenges of evidence-based practices within adolescent prevention and treatment.

The Evolution of Evidence-Based Medicine

Evidence-based medicine, a movement established in Canada and Great Britain to address the need to move research into practice, provides a model for the use of systematic research reviews for clinical decision-making with the aim of improving clinical effectiveness. Sackett, Rosenberg, Gray, Haynes, and Richardson (1996) define *evidence-based* medicine (EBM) as "... the conscientious, explicit and judicious use of current best evidence in making decisions about the care of individual patients. The practice of Evidence-based Medicine means integrating individual clinical expertise with the best available external clinical evidence from systematic research." This definition has been broadened to evidence-based health care (EBHC), which encompasses such professional areas as evidence-based mental health and evidence-based nursing, for example. As defined above, the process of making clinical decisions using the evidence-based medicine model relies upon a synthesis of internal and external evidence. Internal evidence is the combination of formal education, general clinical practice, and specific experience from an individual clinician-patient relationship. External evidence is gained from research findings such as those reported from randomized clinical trials of specific treatments or systematic reviews of multiple randomized trials (Porzsolt et al., 2003; Sackett et al., 1996). The decision-making process in evidence-based medicine involves several steps: (1) formation of clinical questions; (2) search for the best external evidence (which may or may not include randomized clinical trials); (3) evaluation of evidence for validity, importance, and relevance; (4) application of research into practice by integrating individual clinical experience with the best available external evidence; and (5) evaluation of decision-making process and outcome (Porzsolt et al., 2003; Rowland & Goss, 2000).

The use of external research findings poses a challenge to clinicians. This challenge requires them to synthesize and critically appraise an enormous volume of information and apply it in their work. In Britain, this challenge is being met through the Cochrane Collaboration and the National Health Service. EBM is having a major impact on health care policy in the UK and other countries. Policy issues aside, the relevance to the present discussion of the Cochrane Collaboration and a related organization in the U.S. called the Campbell Collaboration, is the approach to the management and accessibility of relevant research information for clinicians, patients, and policy-makers. While the Cochrane Collaboration focuses primarily on medical and health-care related studies, the Campbell Collaboration synthesizes research in the areas of social and behavioral interventions, and public policy regarding education, criminal justice, and social welfare. These organizations rely on research synthesis using a rigorous protocol and make the findings available to the public through the Internet and CD-ROM resources. A group of reviewers, editors, and experts at these organizations established guiding principles to follow with regard to avoiding duplication of review efforts, minimizing bias, keeping up to date, striving for relevance, promoting access to information, ensuring quality methodology, and editorial continuity (the Cochrane Collaboration website). These efforts acknowledge the cumulative nature of science and offer a resource for practitioners to consolidate evidence for making treatment decisions (Chalmers, Hedges & Cooper, 2002).

The Use of Evidence in the Treatment of Psychological Problems

The emergence of evidenced-based medicine has been a significant influence on evidence-based practices with adolescents. The health-care-delivery and insurance practices established in the medical field have had an enormous impact on psychosocial treatment approaches. Reimbursement standards and the call for accountability in medical care requires diagnostic specificity to determine effective treatment options. In an effort to achieve parity for consumers of mental health treatment, our field has followed suit to some degree with mixed results. An example is the use of diagnostic codes as categorized in the *Diagnostic and Statistical Manual*. Unfortunately, mental disorders, particularly those of adolescents, are embedded in a complex system that extends far beyond the individual child, and treatment must be matched to more than a single diagnostic label. Furthermore, there are substantially lower levels of consensus on the causes of a particular disorder in the mental health field than in the medical field; hence, there is greater debate on selection of the appropriate treatment (Wampold, 2001).

The evolution of evidence-based psychological practices has been impacted further by the significant rise in the depth, breadth, and clinical relevance of clinical research into the outcomes and change mechanisms of both prevention and treatment programs. In the broader clinical field, initial questions regarding the effectiveness of psychotherapy (Eysenck, 1952) have been replaced by a consistent stream of research evidence that demonstrates the positive effects of a wide range of psychological treatments (Kazdin & Weisz, 2003; Lambert & Bergin, 1994; Lambert & Ogles, 2004; Luborsky, Singer & Luborsky 1975; Shadish et al., 1997; Shadish, Montgomery, Wilson & Wilson, 1993; Smith & Glass, 1977; Wampold, 2001). In the area of family psychology, both outcome and process studies have clearly identified successful treatments (Pinsof & Wynne, 1995, 2000; Sexton, Robbins, Hollimon, Mease & Mayorga, 2003) and the mechanisms of change (Alexander, Holtzworth-Monroe & Jameson, 1994).

These findings have become so robust that in the last ten years the applied psychology profession represented by Division 12 (clinical psychology) and Division 17 (counseling psychology) of the American Psychological Association both developed task forces to guide the evaluation and dissemination of information about treatment effectiveness. Beginning in the early 1990s, Division 12 of the American Psychological Association established the Task Force on the Promotion and Dissemination of Psychological Procedures and the empirically validated treatment movement was born. The model for evaluating treatments put forth by this task force was heavily influenced by Food and Drug Administration (FDA) guidelines for the approval of new drugs and called for standardization, treatment targeted to a specific diagnosis, and replication of results (Task Force on Promotion and Dissemination of Psychological Procedures, 1995). The result of the task force was the establishment of criteria to evaluate treatments and the publication of a list of treatments deemed scientifically "well-established" or "probably efficacious" (Chambless et al., 1996, 1998). In 1996 Division 17 established a special task group (STG) to develop a set of principles to use for evaluating the empirical status of psychosocial interventions for the purposes of informing counseling psychologists, training predoctoral and postdoctoral students, and informing the public about the value of services offered by counseling psychologists. In contrast to the Division 12 task force, Division 17 did not produce a list of empirically supported treatments but instead produced and endorsed seven principles of empirically supported interventions (PESI) to serve as guidance in reviewing research evidence about a particular treatment approach. For a complete description of these principles, please see Wampold, Lichtenburg & Waehler (2002). What both approaches share is that scientific evidence is the primary basis of the determination of a valid treatment and prevention intervention.

Preventing and Treating Adolescent Problems
with Evidence-Based Approaches

There is no field where the rise of evidence-based models of prevention and treatment have had as much impact as within in the area of adolescent behavior disorders. While the "evidence" for adolescent treatment programs has come from the clinical research in family psychology and prevention science, its impetus has been from communities, families, and the broad-based realization that adolescent behavior problems are a behavioral health epidemic. It was after the Columbine school shooting in 1999 that the Centers for Disease Control (CDC) and the Office of Juvenile Justice and Delinquency Prevention (OJJDP) set out to find programs that work, with outcomes that last, and that are replicable in local communities. In 1996, the Center for the Study and Prevention of Violence (CSPV) began a first-ever evaluation of programs for adolescents that work. They assembled a panel of experts in the field who established a set of research-based criteria for determining effective programs. The project became known as the "Blueprint" project for violence prevention in youth (Elliott, 1998). These criteria were intended to serve as a Blueprint for communities choosing programs and for the development of future programs. The criteria for a blueprint program were initially modest at best and included such questions as, Is it a coherent and identifiable program? Does the program work? Are its effects lasting? and Can the program be replicated in local communities? (Elliott, 1998). These criteria were applied more rigorously for what came to be known as "model" Blueprint programs.

Initially CSPV identified approximately 500 published prevention and treatment programs for the broad range of youth behavior problems that might ultimately result in violent behavior of youth. By 2004, the Blueprint staff had reviewed over 1,000 programs. Of the wide range of prevention and intervention programs identified, only 11 met the criteria (about 1%). These 11 programs represent a wide range of both prevention and treatment programs that vary widely in their approach but have all demonstrated results. Of these 11, seven are prevention programs (Midwestern Prevention Project, Big Brothers, Big Sisters of America, Life Skills Training, Bullying Prevention Program, Promoting Alternative Thinking Strategies, The Incredible Years, and Project Towards No Drug Abuse) and four are treatment-based programs (Functional Family Therapy, Nurse–Family Partnership, Multidimensional Treatment Foster Care, and Multisystemic Therapy). Of the treatment programs, two are family-based counseling treatment programs (MST, FFT).

In 2000, the Surgeon General of the United States attempted to identify systematic programs for the prevention and treatment of youth violence. Following a model established by CSPV in the Blueprint project, the Surgeon General identified a number of evidence-based and promising programs. In each category the criteria for effectiveness was scientific research that demonstrated successful outcomes, with lasting effects, with a variety of types of youth (e.g., of different ages and cultures). The Surgeon General's Report on Youth Violence (U.S. Public Health Service, 2001) identified three categories of scientific standards for evaluating the effects of a violence prevention program. Programs were further categorized into Level 1, which are violence prevention programs, and Level 2, which are risk prevention programs. A *model* program had support from rigorous experimental or quasi-experimental research design, significant deterrent effects on violence or serious delinquency (level 1) or deterrence of any risk factor for violence with a large effect (level 2), replication with demonstrated effects, and sustainability of effects. *Promising* programs have similar criteria, but the risk factor prevention effect is smaller and the program may demonstrate either replication or sustainability but not both. Five level 1 programs for violence prevention were identified as meeting the criteria for a model program. These include Functional Family Therapy, Multisystemic Therapy, Multidimensional Treatment Foster Care, Prenatal and Infancy Home Visitation by Nurses, and Seattle Social Development Project. Of these five programs, three are directed at an adolescent population (FFT, MST, and MTFC). The Blueprint project and the Surgeon General's report have had a major impact on the field of prevention and treatment of adolescent behavior problems. The Blueprint project established "research" as the basis of evidence for program choice. It articulated the need for methods of first disseminating and then transporting effective programs to community settings. It has also become a true "blueprint" for the identification and choice of adolescent programs for communities around the nation. The movement has grown to the point that many state mental health and juvenile justice systems now rely on the Blueprint model for identifying programs that will be funded and endorsed for use. For example, Washington mental health officials adopted evidence-based programs as the sole basis for the choice of adolescent prevention and treatment in 1998. Using the Blueprint project findings as an initial starting point they implemented Functional Family Therapy, Multisystemic Therapy, and Aggression Replacement Training throughout the state. Recent studies by the Washington State Institute for public policy found that two of these programs did successfully transport to local Washington communities with remarkable success (Barnoski, 2004). For example, FFT resulted in an over 38% reduction in felony crime and a 50% reduction in violent crime (both rates were statistically significant as compared to a randomly assigned control group) with substantial cost savings ($12.87 return for each $1.00 invested).

Despite the significant impact of evidence-based prevention and treatment programs, many practitioners continue to struggle with their adoption. Some of the practitioner concerns are similar to those expressed by doctors faced with the adoption of an evidence-based medicine approach to treatment (difficulty in accessing evidence, difficulty following specific protocols, etc.). There are additional issues that have complicated the adoption of evidence-based programs. These issues revolve around the definitions of evidence, the criteria for program, and struggles with applying systematic treatment and prevention models. In the next section, we address some of these issues.

What Is Evidence-based Practice?

There is a wide range of specific evidence-based practices in the prevention and treatment field. These models differ in regard to principles and procedures of practice, yet they do share a common philosophy, a common view of what constitutes evidence, and criteria upon which the clinical and prevention models were constructed. Despite the significant body of supporting scientific evidence, these EBP models continue to be viewed with skepticism and uncertainty among prevention and treatment professionals. We suggest that there are three critical components of evidence-based practices that inspire skepticism: the nature and extent of evidence, the nature of a "program," and clinical application of evidence. Like Beutler & Davison (1995), we do not believe that scientific evidence can ever change clinical practice until the myths and mysteries surrounding evidence-based practices are addressed. In the sections that follow, we review each of these issues in order to help clearly define EBP. Our goal is to dispel the myths surrounding each of these areas.

The Philosophical Foundations of EBP

The core philosophical principles of EBP are not unique. In fact, the central guiding principle is likely to be shared by anyone who works with youth and families: every individual has the right to the most effective services available at the time (Hyde, Falls, Morris & Schoenwald, 2003). Through the use of models based in scientific evidence, these approaches attempt to provide clinicians, communities, and families with the opportunity to choose intervention and prevention programs in which they can have confidence. It is the method that EBPs use to achieve this goal that is unique. The basis of the best care is *quality through accountability*. Accountability requires the establishment of programs that when implemented well will result in positive outcomes for youth and families. Accountability is based on scientific evidence to create a standard of quality and reliability that allows the best care possible.

There are two important implications of this definition of accountability. First, it suggests that programs used should be able to demonstrate that they produce positive outcomes with a wide range of youth and families, in different communities, and in a way that the positive outcomes are maintained over time. In addition, it assumes that intervention and prevention programs must maintain a level of quality by insuring fidelity and adherence to the model as it is transported and implemented in local communities. In EBP, accountability and quality are developed and established through the use of systematic, scientific evidence.

One of the most curious myths about EBPs is that they are cold and distant "science" in which numbers and statistical tests of significance outweigh the needs of specific youth and families. What has gone unrecognized is that at the philosophical core, EBPs are about the best interests of youth and families. The goal of the principle of accountability is to help consumers, clinicians, and communities have confidence when choosing to implement or become involved in a prevention or treatment program.

What is the Basis of an EBP?

The basis of most prevention and treatment programs for adolescents is psychological theory. Theoretical models of prevention and treatment have an appealing face validity (they look reasonable and seem logical), have consensual validity (everyone knows they work), and are based on the opinion of authorities in the field (e.g., theory and model developers) (Beutler & Davison, 1995). Unfortunately, the outcomes of the cumulative knowledge research base suggest that many of the common practices often cannot be relied upon to produce reliably positive outcomes (Lambert & Ogles, 2004). Despite the lack of a strong research base, when treatments make sense to the public, are adopted and accepted by large groups of practitioners, and enjoy popular support, the value of scientific evidence is likely to take a back seat when questions of the treatments value arise (Beutler & Davison, 1995). The result of this has been an institutionalization of untested psychological theory as "fact" within the field.

Evidence-based practices have a different foundation. EBPs are those practices that integrate the best research evidence with clinical experiences, the most current and clinically relevant psychological theory, and patient values (Institute of Medicine, 2001; Sexton & Alexander, 2002a). Evidence-based practices are different from "best practices" in that the latter is a clinical or administrative practice that is "best" in the current situation given the client, organizational context, and clinician. Sometimes the term *best practices* is used synonymously with *evidence-based*, but not always. Other times best practices are those derived from clinical wisdom, the common practices of professional guilds, or consensus approaches that do not use evidence as a foundation. What distinguishes evidence-based practices is the use of scientific knowledge in the development, implementation, and use of prevention and treatment programs. The evidence base of current prevention and treatment programs for adolescents is built on a significant body of scientific knowledge verifying the outcomes of programs and identifying the critical mechanisms of change within programs.

Two questions are critical in regard to this definition: What type of evidence is considered most valid? and How much evidence is enough for a program to be considered an EBP? Scientific knowledge is built on two types of outcome studies. *Efficacious* treatments are those that produce positive results in controlled experimental research trials. If efficacious, a treatment/prevention program shows successful outcomes in controlled and usually highly constrained conditions. For example, the clients may be screened to specific and single problems, and the clinicians may be homogeneous and trained to specific treatments. Thus, many of the "real world" complications related to organizations, interventionists, and clients have been removed in order to give the program its best chance at success. However, in the real world, efficacious interventions may be less effective than hoped when the conditions of real practice are introduced. *Effectiveness* studies maintain the same standard of systematic study but in real world settings in which the clinicians, clients, and treatment or prevention activities take place in organizations that provide care in communities. Effective treatments produce positive results in the conditions under which care is usually delivered, or "real world" conditions.

Determining how much evidence is enough is also difficult. As noted above, many attempts have been made in an attempt to establish a "bar" of acceptable evidence. These attempts range from the Division 12 (clinical psychology) approach of establishing a minimum number of a particular type of studies (two efficacy studies with random assignment) to the work of Elliott and colleagues (Elliott, 1998) who had a consensus panel review the evidence and determine if the program met preestablished criteria (worked, worked over time, and could be replicated). Others (Wampold, 2001) argue that the synthesis of research findings through methods such as meta analysis is needed to establish the evidence of an approach. Hyde et al. (2003) suggests that there is a hierarchy of evidence that can be used to determine how much is enough to prove a program is effective and should be implemented. In this approach, the highest level of scientific evidence is the knowledge that comes from controlled clinical trials with random assignment of individuals from similar groups to experimental and routine care conditions.

Sexton and colleagues (Sexton et al., 2003) suggest a *levels of evidence approach* to linking practices with research evidence. They argue that the question of interest (be it a policy question, a broad treatment program decision, or a specific clinical implementation question) should match the research evidence used to answer the question if the knowledge is to be used adequately and successfully. Policy questions, often asked by organizations and large systems, are probably best answered through systematic research reviews (e.g., meta analysis). Intervention and prevention program adoption decisions are probably best made by looking at the cumulative efficacy and effectiveness research over time. Individual clinical decisions are best made by the process research that identifies the operative mechanism of change. It is becoming increasingly clear that while the standards of scientific evidence remain at the core of EBP, issues beyond the traditional markers of "scientific merit" need to be considered if evidence based approaches are to be adopted.

What is an EBP Prevention and Treatment Program?

Current treatment and prevention programs for use with adolescent behavior problems are not broad and general approaches but instead treatment models that target clinically meaningful syndromes or situations with a coherent conceptual framework underlying the clinical intervention, described in sufficient detail to explain the specific interventions and intervention qualities necessary to carry them out (Sexton et al., 2003). In addition, the traditional separation between treatment as therapy and prevention as education no longer holds true (Alexander, Robbins & Sexton & 2000). Many programs traditionally viewed as "therapeutic" are now being used as prevention interventions aimed at interrupting the trajectory of youth behavior problems and preventing them from becoming more deeply involved in the justice system, involved in drug use, or the escalation of family conflict such that more severe mental health problems develop in the future (Alexander, Robbins et al., 2000).

Much of the work defining EBP has come from the treatment literature. Alexander et al. (1994) defined a *clinical intervention program* as one that targets clinically meaningful syndromes or situations with a coherent conceptual framework underlying the clinical intervention, described in sufficient detail to explain the specific interventions and therapist qualities necessary to carry them out. Wampold, Mondin, Moody, Stich, Benson & Ahn (1997) defined a "bona fide" treatment as one in which those providing the program do so within a relationship with the client, using a treatment tailored to the client, in which the treatment is systematically described, with clearly identified psychological change mechanisms, contained within a clinical manual that is used to guide administration of the treatment, in which the active ingredients of the treatment are specified. Both definitions suggest that EBPs have high treatment integrity brought about by clinical supervision, treatment manuals, and/or adherence verification throughout the course of therapy.

Whether we are examining an intervention or treatment program, two highly interdependent components must be in place: *principles* that explain clients, therapy, and change; and a systematic *clinical protocol* followed by the therapist (Sexton & Alexander, 2002a; Sexton, Ridley & Kleiner, 2004). The principles of a model answer the questions How does the client function? and What is the nature of change? while the protocol answers the questions What actions should I take? and When should I take them? The conceptual principles of the model should be comprehensive theoretical articulations that explain how clients function, how psychological problems develop, how to help people change, and the interrelationship among these factors. Principles are the theory and conceptual foundation that form the basis of the therapist's actions and the logic and reasoning behind their moment-to-moment clinical decisions. During the intervention, the principles exist in the background as the basis of specific interventions and therapeutic actions that exist in the foreground. The clinical protocol delineates the specific time and place of therapeutic interventions within the process of therapy. The protocol encompasses the specific therapeutic goals and the clinically based change mechanisms that facilitate the successful delivery of therapy. The protocol remains in the foreground and functions as a map for therapists that guide their clinical activities in a systemic way. The specific protocol is determined by the principles (e.g., the nature of change), which specify and order the activities of the therapist within a temporal process of change.

Current Evidence-Based Models for Dysfunctional Adolescent Behavior

As an illustration, we outline four programs that encompass the current range of evidence-based prevention and treatment programs for adolescent behavior problems. While different each of these approaches share the influence of science upon practice, are evidence-based, and have substantial empirical support, however, the influence of science and the emphasis of the type of research evidence on the model and its development differs. The four programs we will describe are Functional Family Therapy, Multisystemic Therapy, Multidimensional Treatment Foster Care, and Life Skills Training. All four of these programs are "best practices" and are Blueprints model programs as designated by the Center for the Study and Prevention of Violence. Blueprints for violence prevention *model* programs meet rigorous criteria regarding program effectiveness. Three criteria in particular are given the greatest weight in designating a model program: (1) evidence of deterrent effect with a strong research design, (2) sustained effect at least one year beyond the treatment period, and (3) multiple site replications with demonstrated success in diverse settings. It is important to note that these are not the only evidence-based programs for use with adolescents. These programs do, however, represent a range of approaches from family-therapy based (FFT) and family-based (MST) to foster treatment (MTFC) and prevention (Life Skills Training).

Multisystemic Therapy

Multisystemic Therapy (MST) is a family- and community-based treatment model with its roots in family systems, general systems (von Bertalanffy, 1968) and social ecological theories (Bronfenbrenner, 1979) designed to address chronic behavior problems and serious emotional disturbances in adolescents. MST has been used to treat serious emotional disturbances in adolescents, youth violence and criminal behavior, juvenile sex offending behavior, alcohol and drug abuse, and child maltreatment, but the research evidence supporting the model is strongest for youth presenting serious antisocial behavior and their families. The model was developed in the 1970s and drew on the influences of prominent family therapists of the time-period, such as Jay Haley, Salvador Minuchin, Gerald Patterson, and James Alexander as well as the community psychology movement, which acknowledged the interaction between individuals and their environment. This was further articulated and ultimately emphasized in the MST treatment model based on the work of Urie Bronfenbrenner (1979), which posits a social-ecological conceptualization of behavior. MST acknowledges that adolescents live in, and their behavior is influenced by, multiple, interrelated systems, such as the family, neighborhood, school, peer, and cultural environments. In addition, the juvenile justice, child welfare, and mental health systems can be interconnected with the youth and exert influence over his or her behavior (Henggeler & Lee, 2003; Sheidow, Henggeler & Schoenwald, 2003).

The design and implementation of MST is based on several conceptual assumptions. These include (1) the multidetermined nature of serious clinical problems, (2) that caregivers are essential to producing long-term positive outcomes for the youth, (3) the integration of evidence-based practices within the context of MST, (4) intensive services that address barriers to service access, and (5) a rigorous quality assurance program to promote treatment fidelity. With these conceptual assumptions as a foundation, the developers of MST operationalized treatment through adherence to nine core treatment principles that provide direction for treatment planning and implementation (Henggeler & Lee, 2003). The core principles are (1) finding the fit; (2) positive and strength focused; (3) increasing responsibility; (4) present-focused, action-oriented, and well-defined; (5) targeting sequences; (6) developmentally appropriate interventions; (7) continuous effort; (8) accountability and evaluation; and (9) generalization (for a more complete description of the core principles see Henggeler & Lee, 2003; Sheidow et al., 2003).

MST service delivery is based on a model of home-based intervention, which has proven effective at engaging families in treatment and preventing drop-out. The therapists who deliver MST typically have master's level training and carry caseloads of four to six families. The MST therapists work in small teams of three to five full-time therapists, and a supervisor. Services are delivered either at home or some other community-based setting such as school or a neighborhood center to minimize barriers to treatment. The treatment is time-limited, typically lasting between three to six months to promote self-sufficiency and cost effectiveness. Therapists are available 24 hours a day and seven days a week to provide services as needed and to respond to or prevent crises. For a complete description of clinical procedures, please see Henggeler, Schoenwald, Borduin, Rowland & Cunningham (1998).

The primary goal of MST is to help families develop the skills effectively to manage and resolve serious clinical problems that the youth may be experiencing. In addition, MST strives to empower families to prevent potential problems that are likely to occur during adolescence. Acknowledging the multisystemic nature of causal and sustaining factors that affect youth, MST therapists utilize resources within the families' ecologies to develop the families' capacity to cope. Therapists intervene at the family level to reduce conflict, improve communication, improve family cohesion, and increase behavioral monitoring. Treatment may also address parental or marital functioning if it contributes to the youth's problems. In this treatment model, caregivers are considered essential to treatment generalization. MST therapists may also address peer-level factors that contribute to the youth's problems such as association with deviant peers and poor socialization skills. However, much of the therapist's attention is focused on helping the caregiver learn to manage the adolescent's interaction with his or her environment, especially the school environment (Sheidow et al., 2003).

As an evidence-based model of treatment, MST has an extensive research foundation measuring outcomes in clinical trials and community settings. Findings from eight published studies composed of seven randomized clinical trials and one quasi-experimental design provide the evidence that supports the effectiveness of MST. The first MST outcome study was quasi-experimental (Henggeler, Rodick, Borduin, Hanson, Watson & Urey, 1986) and evaluated short-term effectiveness of MST with juvenile offenders. Findings indicated improved family relations, decreased youth behavior problems, and decreased youth association with deviant peers.

This study was followed by three randomized clinical trials with chronic and violent juvenile offenders. Henggeler, Melton & Smith (1992) found that when MST served as a community-based alternative to incarceration, at post-treatment MST was more effective at improving family and peer relations than the usual juvenile justice services. Among the youths treated with MST, recidivism was reduced by 43% and out-of-home placement was reduced by 64% at the 59-week follow-up. In another randomized clinical trial with chronic juvenile offenders, Borduin et al. (1995) reported improved family functioning and decreased psychiatric symptomatology at post-treatment and a 69% decrease in recidivism at four-year follow-up when compared to youths in individual counseling. The third randomized clinical trial with chronic juvenile offenders (Henggeler, Melton, Brondino, Scherer & Hanley, 1997) found that MST was more effective at decreasing youth psychiatric symptomatology at post-treatment and at a 1.7-year follow-up produced a 50% reduction in incarceration compared to the usual juvenile justice services. These studies have also indicated a substantial average net economic gain for MST as a result of reduced placement costs, criminal justice costs, and crime victim benefits according to the Washington State Institute for Public Policy (Aos, Phipps, Barnoski & Lieb, 2001).

A number of other studies related to specific diagnostic groups have produced promising results. Two randomized clinical trials with substance-abusing youth have demonstrated short-term reductions in adolescent substance abuse (Henggeler et al., 1992; Henggeler, Pickrel & Brondino, 1999). Another study has demonstrated long-term reductions in substance-related arrests (Borduin et al., 1995). MST was also found to be successful in treating youth with serious emotional disturbances. In this randomized trial MST was evaluated relative to psychiatric hospitalization for youths who were suicidal, homicidal, or psychotic. When possible youths in this study were stabilized outside the hospital and subsequently participated in a full course of MST. Youths in the comparison group were admitted to an inpatient unit and subsequently received community services upon their release. Outcomes indicated that MST was more effective at improving family relations, improving school attendance, and decreasing externalizing behaviors. Furthermore, at four months post-referral, the youths in the MST treatment group had a 75% reduction in days of hospitalization and a 50% reduction in other out-of-home placements (Henggeler et al., 1999; Schoenwald, Ward, Henggeler & Rowland, 2000). Smaller studies have looked at randomized trials with juvenile sex offenders and child maltreatment with promising results (Borduin, Henggeler, Blaske & Stein, 1990; Brunk, Henggeler & Whelan, 1987) but the strongest research evidence in support of MST effectiveness is with youths with serious antisocial behavior such as criminal activity, violence, and substance abuse.

In addition to randomized clinical trials, MST researchers have developed a quality assurance system designed to maintain the internal validity of the model as it is disseminated to community provider organizations across the country. Several empirical studies have examined the relationship between adherence to MST treatment principles and clinical outcomes (Henggeler et al., 1997, 1999; Huey, Henggeler, Brondino & Pickrel, 2000; Schoenwald, Henggeler, Brondino & Rowland, 2000; Schoenwald, Sheidow & Letourneau, 2004; Schoenwald, Sheidow, Letourneau & Liao, 2003). These studies indicate that therapist adherence and organizational climate predict parent-reported child outcomes immediately post-treatment. Current research is underway regarding recidivism rates in a large sample of approximately 2,000 youths and families participating in a five-year study who are being treated in 41 communities across the country.

Multidimensional Treatment Foster Care

Multidimensional Treatment Foster Care (MTFC), also known as Therapeutic Foster Care, was developed by Patricia Chamberlain and colleagues at the Oregon Social Learning Center in the 1980s as a community-based treatment alternative to corrections facilities and group care for chronic juvenile offenders. This highly cost-effective program places adolescent offenders with foster parents who have been specially trained to care for adolescents with emotional and behavioral problems (Chamberlain, 1998). Foster parents provide a therapeutic living environment with intense supervision, strict discipline, positive reinforcement for positive behaviors, and a supportive relationship. While originally developed for the treatment of antisocial disorder in the juvenile justice system, MTFC has been successfully adapted for use with adolescents referred to mental health and child welfare services (Chamberlain, Moreland & Reid, 1992; Smith, Stormshak, Chamberlain & Bridges-Whaley, 2001).

Multidimensional Treatment Foster Care is grounded in social learning theory (Bandura, 1977) and assumes that individuals learn behaviors through the context in which they live (Chamberlain, 1998; Chamberlain & Mihalic, 1998; Chamberlain & Smith, 2003). Adolescents with delinquency problems are assumed to come from homes in which ineffective parenting methods were routinely utilized with poor child behavior management and reinforcement of negative behaviors. In addition, adolescents are at the age where influence by other peers is paramount over adult influences. The traditional intervention for persistent adolescent delinquency has been residential group care in which adolescents are placed with other youth who have similar problems of delinquency (Elliott, 1998). However, it has been routinely found that adolescents who associate with delinquent peers tend to have higher rates of delinquency than adolescents who do not associate with delinquent peers (Dishion, McCord & Poulin, 1999; Elliott, Huizinga & Ageton, 1985). As such, MTFC attempts to combat this negative peer association effect by separating adolescents from their delinquent peers.

Therapeutic foster parents are recruited from the community and trained in effective parent management skills to provide a structured and consistent therapeutic living environment (Chamberlain, 1998; Chamberlain & Mihalic, 1998; Chamberlain & Smith, 2003). Once the youth is placed with the foster family, foster parents attend weekly supervision meetings and participate in daily phone contact with the program supervisor. Because a goal of the program is the reunification of the adolescent with their biological or adoptive family, the biological (or adoptive) parents also attend family therapy sessions where they are taught parent management skills for maintaining disciple and reinforcing positive behavior. The adolescents participate in home visits, which increase in frequency as the biological (or adoptive) parents learn new skills for behavior management methods. The adolescent also receives individual therapy. Placements are typically six to nine months and most adolescents return to live with their parents following completion of the program.

Multidimensional Treatment Foster Care has been found to be highly effective in the treatment of adolescent delinquency. A series of outcome studies conducted by Chamberlain and colleagues over the past decade have yielded considerable empirical support for the effectiveness of the program. Chamberlain (1990) compared two community-based alternative adolescent treatments to incarceration and found MTFC participants to have spent significantly fewer days incarcerated at a two-year follow-up than those participants receiving a typical community-based treatment. Chamberlain & Reid (1998) compared MTFC to residential group care for male chronic delinquency and found that MTFC participants had significantly fewer arrests, less incarcerations, and higher program completion rates than the group care participants at a one-year follow-up. In addition, Chamberlain & Leve (2002) examined the effectiveness of MTFC versus treatment as usual for female chronic offenders and found significantly fewer arrests and hospitalizations for mental-health related issues for the MTFC female participants than for those participants receiving group care at a one-year follow-up (Chamberlain & Smith, 2003).

Multidimensional Treatment Foster Care has also been found to be effective in the treatment of adolescents leaving state mental hospitals. Chamberlain & Reid (1991) compared MTFC to a typical community treatment and found that a significantly higher number of adolescents in the MTFC condition left the hospital and a higher number where placed with their families at seven-month follow-up than those receiving the typical treatment. Finally, MTFC has also been associated with higher positive outcomes than regular foster care such as less disruptive incidences in the placement as well as greater foster care parent retention (Chamberlain, Moreland & Reid, 1992; Smith, Stormshak, Chamberlain & Bridges-Whaley, 2001).

Functional Family Therapy

Functional Family Therapy (FFT) is a mature clinical model that has evolved over the last 30 years built on a foundation of integrated theory, clinical experience, and empirical evidence. FFT is a well-developed clinical model designed to treat at-risk youth aged 11–18 with a range of maladaptive behaviors, including delinquency, violence, substance use, risky sexual behavior, truancy, conduct disorder, oppositional defiant disorder, disruptive behavior disorder, and other externalizing disorders. The primary focus of treatment is on the family relational system with an emphasis on the multiple domains of client experience (cognition, emotion, and behavior) and the multiple perspectives within and around a family system (individual, family, and contextual/multisystemic). As a treatment program, FFT has produced successful outcomes with at-risk youth and their families. FFT is a short-term family therapy intervention that ranges from 8 to 12 one-hour sessions for mild to moderate cases and up to 30 hours of direct intervention for more serious situations. As stated above the target population is 11–18, along with the younger siblings of referred adolescents. The youths and their families represent multi-ethnic, multicultural populations. The program also works as a preventive measure in diverting the path of at-risk adolescents away from the juvenile justice or mental health systems (Alexander, Pugh, Parsons & Sexton, 2000; Sexton & Alexander, 2002b).

Functional Family Therapy is considered a "mature" clinical model because it represents a comprehensive intervention program consisting of (1) a set of guiding theoretical principles; (2) a systematic therapeutic program based on change mechanisms used in a time-sensitive, phased manner; (3) multi-domain clinical assessment and intervention techniques; (4) an ongoing research program; and (5) a systematic training, supervision, and implementation program. All of these influences converge to help us understand families and the clinical problems they present, to clarify the relational system of the family, and to target fundamental change mechanisms to produce positive outcomes (Sexton & Alexander, 2003).

A number of theoretical, clinical, and research-based constructs guide the intervention program. The clinical model synthesizes a theoretically integrated set of guiding principles and a clearly defined clinical "map" which specifies within-session process goals, linked in a phasic model to guide the therapeutic process. The guiding principles provide a framework for understanding family functioning, the etiology of clinical problems, the driving forces and motivating factors behind change, and direction for how to deal with each family in a way that meets each family's unique needs (Sexton & Alexander, 2003). Functional Family Therapy defines a family as the primary psychosocial system in which the adolescent spends most of his or her "family" time; therefore, the family unit could consist of a wide variety of structural arrangements, including natural or adoptive parents, grandparents, aunts and uncles, single caregivers, etc. The most important feature of FFT is that the model views the family unit in whatever form it takes as the client, rather than the individual adolescent, who may have been referred through the juvenile justice system or for mental health reasons.

From the perspective of the FFT model, clinical problems are multisystemic and occur within the system of the family relational unit and between the family and its environment, including the broader social context. This is not necessarily unique to FFT but is based on evidence that at-risk youth are best understood by looking at their individual behavior, as it exists in the family system, which in turn is part of a broader community system (Robbins, Mayorga & Szapocznik, 2003). The FFT clinical model focuses on the relational patterns that are represented by serious acting-out behaviors as the basis of therapeutic intervention. From this perspective, the specific problem behaviors of the adolescent are the manifestation of enduring family behavioral and relational patterns. While some family relational patterns provide protective factors for the adolescent others represent risk factors and it is these risk and protective factors that are the target of change.

This view of clinical problems allows the intervention to focus on alterable behavior rather than "labeling" the youth or the family as dysfunctional; consequently it suggests that the "problem" behavior is not the source of the family's struggle, but the way in which the problem behavior is handled within the family relational system that creates the struggle. Therefore, FFT therapists do not attempt to change the core relational experiences of the family members, but the means by which they are attained. For example, parents who use violence to gain control over a child are taught to use nurturance and guidance to achieve the same relational outcome of appropriate parental authority over a child. The process of change is guided by four theoretically integrated and clearly articulated principles: (1) change is predicated upon fostering alliance-based motivation; (2) behavior change first requires meaning change, primarily through the relationally based process of reframing which includes validation and a reattribution of meaning; (3) behavioral change goals must be obtainable and appropriate for the culture, abilities, and living context of the family; and (4) intervention strategies match and respect the unique nature of each family.

The FFT model is a phase-based clinical change model consisting of three specific phases of therapeutic intervention: (1) engagement and motivation, (2) behavior change, and (3) generalization. Each phase is marked by specific therapeutic goals and therapist skills that increase the likelihood of success. Each phase also includes assessment components that enhance the therapist's ability to understand the family and intervene effectively. The specificity of the clinical "map" and the accompanying treatment manual requires therapists to be systematic and structured while simultaneously being relational and clinically responsive. This is no "paint by numbers" intervention for the therapist. Rather, it is a complex clinical model informed by a strong theoretical foundation, clinical experience, and substantial research on the process, change mechanisms, and subsequent outcomes of a wide range of families served over the last 30 years.

Both process and outcome research contribute to the scientific knowledge base that supports and informs FFT. There is a long history of systematic and independently replicated series of outcome and process studies. These studies have generated several endorsements regarding the effectiveness of this form of treatment. For example, the Center for Substance Abuse Prevention (CSAP), the Office of Juvenile Justice and Delinquency Prevention (OJJDP), the Center for the Study and Prevention of Violence (CSPV) and the Surgeon General's report have identified FFT as a successful intervention for at-risk adolescents with a variety of problems, including conduct disorder, substance abuse, and violent behavior. The FFT model meets all of the current professional benchmarks of empirically validated, empirically supported interventions (Sexton & Alexander, 2002b). A very brief summary of research results follows.

Process studies have informed the understanding of therapeutic change mechanisms. These studies systematically verified theoretically identified change mechanisms and provided a source of information to improve the treatment model. Published studies as early as 1976 (Alexander, Barton, Schiaro & Parsons) found that the ratio of negative versus supportive statements made by family members was significantly higher in cases that dropped out or terminated treatment prematurely. Termination prior to completion of treatment was then predictive of recidivism. In more recent studies (Newell, Alexander & Turner, 1996) the level of family negativity could successfully predict program dropouts, with higher levels linked to a greater likelihood to drop out. Newberry, Alexander, and Turner (1991) found that therapist supportiveness during the engagement and motivation phase of the treatment model increased the likelihood of a positive response from the family thus reducing negativity in the family system and building the motivating alliance with the therapist. These process studies were critical evidence for substantiating negativity reduction as an essential change mechanism.

Published outcome studies are the "proof" that this treatment works in a range of community settings and with a demographically and culturally varied set of client populations. FFT has proven effective in reducing recidivism between 26% and 73% with status-offending, moderate, and seriously delinquent youths when compared to no treatment and to juvenile court probation services (Alexander et al., 2000). In addition to reduced recidivism rates, other studies have used other dependent measures, such as number of crimes committed and severity of crimes. In a community effectiveness study of violent and drug-abusing youths in a large urban, multicultural setting, the results indicated that adolescents in the FFT treatment condition not only had significantly lower recidivism rates but also committed significantly fewer and less severe crimes even after accounting for pretreatment crime history (Sexton, Ostrom, Bonomo & Alexander, 2000). FFT has also proven cost effective compared to other treatment approaches (see Aos & Barnoski, 1998; Sexton & Alexander, 2000).

Recent studies regarding treatment fidelity and the dissemination of treatment to therapists beyond the clinical research team demonstrate true community effectiveness. In one study moderate- to high-risk adolescent juvenile offenders were randomly assigned to either FFT or treatment as usual (TAU). Notable findings included that nearly 90% of families who attended the first FFT session completed the intervention program, which is dramatically higher than traditional programs, where drop-out rates range from 50% to 75% (Kazdin, 1997; Sexton, Hollimon & Mease, 2002). Furthermore, recidivism rates 18 months after treatment were significantly lower than in the TAU group.

Life Skills Training Program

The Life Skills Training Program (LST) is an effective research-based substance abuse prevention program developed by Gilbert Botvin at the Prevention Research Institute of Cornell University Medical School. The program targets middle and junior high school youth in the prevention of tobacco, alcohol, and marijuana use and abuse through the development of skills that reduce the risk of engaging in high-risk activity (Botvin & Kantor, 2000; Botvin, Mihalic & Grotpeter, 1998). The program consists of three components, drug-related knowledge and skills, personal self-management, and general social skills. The drug-related knowledge and skills component targets knowledge and attitudes related to drug use through drug education, discussion of norm expectations related to drug use, and the teaching of skills to resist media influences as well as peer and social pressures related to drug use. The personal self-management component targets the development of skills in decision-making, problem-solving, self-control, and self-improvement; and the general social skills component targets the development of skills in communication.

The Life Skills Training Program is typically a three-year program conducted in the classroom by teachers or older peers with initial sessions in the first year followed by multiple booster sessions. The program consists of 15 sessions in the first year, 10 sessions in the second year, and 5 sessions in the third year. In school districts with junior high schools, the program can be implemented in seventh grade with booster sessions in eighth and ninth grades. In school districts with middle schools, the program can be implemented in sixth grade, with booster sessions in seventh and eighth grades. The preferred intervention method is through group discussions with a focus on skills training. The skills training consists of instruction and demonstration by the teacher, behavioral rehearsal by the students, feedback to students from the teacher, social reinforcement by the teacher, and continued practice by the students through homework.

The theoretical rationale for the Life Skills Training Program is grounded in social learning theory (Bandura, 1977) and based on a person–environment interactionist model of drug abuse (Botvin & Kantor, 2000; Botvin et al., 1998). This model asserts that the etiology of drug abuse is based on the interaction between the person and the environment through factors that increase a person's risk of drug abuse. This is a complex and dynamic process that is composed of multiple influences (social learning through peer, family, community, and media) and factors (self-esteem, anxiety, excitability) resulting in multiple pathways to drug abuse. As a result, the program focuses on decreasing the number of risk factors as opposed to targeting specific pathways. In addition, due to findings that gateway drugs (tobacco, alcohol, and marijuana) account for the majority of drug-related mortality and findings that drug use generally follows a progression of gateway drugs to other illicit drugs, the program attempts to interrupt the prevalence and progression of drug abuse by targeting these substances (tobacco, alcohol, and marijuana) (Botvin et al., 1998).

Two decades of research has demonstrated the Life Skills Training Program to be highly effective in the prevention of substance abuse for a variety of populations. Across studies, a 50–87% reduction in the prevalence of tobacco, alcohol, and marijuana use has been found relative to adolescent controls who did not participate in the program (Sloboda & David, 1997). Further, several large-scale controlled randomized trials have demonstrated that the program increases drug knowledge and decreases the use of alcohol, tobacco, and marijuana of adolescent participants (Botvin, Baker, Dusenbury, Tortu & Botvin, 1990; Botvin, Schinke, Epstein & Diaz, 1994; Botvin, Baker, Dusenbury, Botvin & Diaz, 1995; Botvin, Schinke, Epstein, Diaz & Botvin, 1995; Botvin, Epstein, Baker, Diaz & Ifill-Williams, 1997; Griffin, Botvin, Nichols & Doyle, 2003).

Early effectiveness studies examined the effects of LST on predominantly white middle-class populations. In these preliminary studies, LST was found to be effective for the prevention of cigarette smoking in seventh through tenth graders with both older peer-led and teacher-led programs (Botvin, Eng & Williams, 1980; Botvin & Eng, 1982; Botvin, Renick & Baker, 1983; Botvin, Baker, Dusenbury, Tortu & Botvin, 1990). In addition, older peer-led LST was shown to be effective in reducing the frequency of alcohol use, including reduction in drinking, heavy drinking, and getting drunk (Botvin, Baker, Renick, Filazzola & Botvin, 1984; Botvin et al., 1990) as well in reducing marijuana use (Botvin et al., 1990).

While preliminary research was conducted with white middle-class adolescents, the Life Skills Training Program has also been demonstrated to be effective with racial and ethnic minority adolescents, as well as with inner-city youth. LST has been found to be effective in the reduction of cigarette smoking in Hispanic adolescents (Botvin, Dusenbury, Baker, James-Ortiz & Kerner, 1989; Botvin, Dusenbury, Baker, James-Ortiz, Botvin & Kerner, 1992) as well as in African American adolescents (Botvin, Batson, Witts-Vitale, Bess, Baker & Dusenbury, 1989). LST was also found to be effective with inner city, predominantly minority (Hispanic and African American) youth, in significantly decreasing cigarette, alcohol, and marijuana use (Botvin et al., 1997; Botvin, Griffin, Diaz & Ifill-Williams, 2001; Griffin et al., 2003). Further, LST was found to be more effective among inner-city minority adolescents in decreasing the frequency and severity of alcohol use when a culturally focused approach was utilized rather than a generic skills approach (Botvin et al., 1994; Botvin et al., 1995).

The significant prevention effects of the Life Skills Training Program also appear to be long-lasting. In a randomized trial of 6,000 students from 56 schools, researchers followed students who began the program in seventh grade (and who received booster sessions in the eighth and ninth grades) through the end of the twelfth grade (Botvin et al., 1995). LST was found to be effective in reducing the frequency of tobacco and marijuana use and in reducing the frequency of excessive drinking (i.e., getting drunk). In addition, the strongest effects were found with participants who received the most complete version of the program (including booster sessions), with 44% fewer participants than controls using tobacco, alcohol, and marijuana one or more times a week and 66% fewer participants than controls using multiple substances one or more times a week.

Critical Issues in Evidence-Based Prevention and Treatment Programs for Adolescent Behavior Problems

EBPs have had a dramatic impact on the development of treatment and intervention approaches, the standards of practice, and the actual prevention and treatment practices of practitioners, systems of care, and large service delivery systems. Evidence-based prevention and treatment programs have the potential to provide reliable and clinically responsive services for a variety of youth. When successfully applied, EBP has the potential to help begin to stem the tide of youth mental health, violence, drug abuse, and at-risk behaviors that significantly impact youth, families, and the communities in which they live. Despite the great potential of EBP, a number of critical issues remain. If they are to be more fully accepted, EBPs need to maintain high standards of science while becoming increasingly relevant to communities through broader dissemination and an increasing range of programs that are clinically responsive and culturally relevant. When implemented beyond the research laboratory, the dynamics of the provider organizations and the ongoing quality assurance become critical. If these issues are addressed adequately, EBPs have the potential to be more widely seen as reasonable interventions for the problems that youth and their families and communities face.

Increasing the Range and Relevance of EBP

While there are a wide range of prevention and intervention programs available, too few communities implement them. One of the obstacles is that many communities are not aware of these programs, do not know where to look to find information, or have misinformation about EBP. Disseminating accurate and relevant information about EBP so that communities, providers, and consumers have access to what is available is seriously lacking. In many settings the "myths" of evidence-based practices remain. For example, EBPs are still considered by many as "cookie cutter" approaches developed by researchers in ways that remove the creativity and clinical responsiveness from prevention and treatment efforts. Even if a community does have accurate knowledge of EBP as a whole, many are not aware of the range and scope of available EBPs that may fit their unique community needs. Systematic dissemination efforts like those undertaken by CSPV through the Blueprints project are examples of how information and standards regarding EBP can be communicated widely. Regardless of the form, the further adoption of EBP will depend upon the dissemination of accurate and easily accessible information.

While there are a number of evidence-based prevention and treatment models currently available, there are many more promising and potentially successful programs in existence or yet to be developed. Certainly, the complexity of problems adolescents face calls for a broad range of programs with demonstrated success. Furthermore, the ultimate acceptance and long-term success of EBP lies in expanding the range of available programs. In doing so, the likelihood of providing programs that have the same "face validity" as some of the traditional theoretical models increases. To support the development and identification of new evidence-based programs it will be critical to clearly articulate and reach consensus on the scope and nature of evidence necessary for a program to be considered evidence based. In earlier sections of this chapter, we describe the criteria shared by the current EBP movement. It is clear that evidence needs to be more than just randomized clinical trial research typically endorsed by the scientific community. It is also vitally important to accept that not all data is equal. Unfortunately, these standards are not universally accepted. As the need to expand the range of EBP increases, there will be pressure to change the definition of evidence. In the end, EBP must maintain high scientific standards of evidence defined by systematic efficacy and effectiveness studies conducted under systematic conditions to ensure that programs demonstrate that they reliably produce the changes sought by youth, communities, and providers.

Disseminating, Transporting, and Implementing EBP

It is increasing clear that treatment fidelity is a critical factor in the delivery of effective programs (Henggeler et al., 1997; Sexton & Alexander, 2002a). When transporting EBP to community settings model adherence is even more important because the tight controls of clinical trial study protocols are not available or practical. Despite its importance, there is a lack of research regarding the role of treatment adherence in successful community replications of efficacious EBPs. The limited range of model adherence studies (Barnoski, 2002; Henggeler et al., 1997; Hogue, Liddle, Rowe, Turner, Dakof & LaPann, 1998; Huey et al., 2000; Sexton & Alexander, 2002a), suggest that that complex, manualized treatments can be implemented with a high degree of fidelity (Barnoski, 2004; Henggeler et al., 1999; Huey et al, 2000; Schoenwald et al., 2000). These studies suggest that acceptable adherence levels require intensive adherence monitoring procedures (i.e., training and supervision of cases by model experts) and that therapist adherence predicted improvements in treatment and prevention outcomes.

More recently, it is becoming clear that EBP, like other activities requiring adherence and competence in specific skill sets, requires systematic programs of ongoing quality improvement. In fact, long-term sustainability of EBP requires model fidelity through ongoing quality improvement. The concept of ongoing quality improvement as an integral part of a prevention or treatment model is somewhat unusual in traditional practice. However, it is more desirable to identify that a program is not being implemented well at either an organizational or an individual interventions level rather than to wait and find poor implementation or inadequate outcomes far down the road. The State of Washington recently implemented a comprehensive quality improvement system for Functional Family Therapy (Barnoski, Aos & Lieb, 2003). The program relies on ongoing quality assurance monitoring and immediate "real time" quality assessment feedback to program implementers. The goal of the program is to support local communities in implementing one EBP in with high fidelity.

Organization and system barriers can also impede the successful implementation of EBP. System barriers include funding streams that allow for prevention and treatment models to be carried out. For example, in the mental health setting, prevention interventions are often not fundable through traditional payment sources. Family-based intervention programs are often difficult to sustain because most mental health settings are focused around individual diagnostic criteria. In other settings, the very nature of the organization in which the EBP is to be implemented may not make the necessary changes in well-established service delivery systems needed to accommodate the EBP with fidelity. In a recent study, Schoenwald, Sheidow, Letourneau & Liao (2003) found that the client outcomes of Multisystemic Therapy were significantly impacted by the climate and structure of the organization in which the intervention was being implemented.

Concluding Remarks

There is little disagreement that the range and the scope of adolescent problems are significant. The psychological and economic costs of these problems are staggering. Youth, families, and communities need and deserve the best possible available treatment with the highest probability of success. Unfortunately, traditional services have not on the whole been successful in either preventing or treating these serious problems. Evidence-based prevention and treatment programs have great potential to help stem the tide of serious adolescent behavior problems. When implemented as designed, these programs provide systematic intervention and prevention programs based on theoretical, clinical, and research-based foundations. There are a wide range of successful prevention and intervention programs that are currently in use in many communities with dramatic outcomes that are changing the lives of youth, families, and communities. Despite their great potential, EBPs struggle with being accepted and often suffer as they are transported from development into community settings. As noted by Beutler & Davison (1995), EBPs will only gain widespread acceptance when they can develop the "face validity" currently enjoyed by traditional treatment and prevention activities. To do so, standards need to remain high, better dissemination needs to take place, and systematic attention to successful implementation and quality assurance and improvement needs to be developed.

References

Alexander, J.F., Barton, C., Schiaro, R.S., & Parsons, B.V. (1976). Behavioral intervention with families of delinquents: Therapist characteristics and outcome. *Journal of Consulting and Clinical Psychology, 44,* 656–664.

Alexander, J.F., Holtzworth-Monroe, A., & Jameson, P. (1994). The process and outcome of marital and family therapy: Research review and evaluation. In A.E. Bergin & S.L. Garfield (Eds.), *Handbook of Psychotherapy and Behavior Change* (pp. 594–630). New York: John Wiley & Sons.

Alexander, J.F., Pugh, C., Parsons, B., & Sexton, T.L. (2000). Functional Family Therapy. In D. Elliott (Series Ed.), Book three: *Blueprints for Violence Prevention (2nd ed.)*. Golden, CO: Venture.

Alexander, J.F., Robbins, M., & Sexton, T.L. (2000). Family-based interventions with older, at-risk youth: From promise to proof to practice. *Journal of Primary Prevention, 21* (2), 185–205.

Alexander, J.F., Sexton, T.L., & Robbins, M. (2002). The developmental status of family therapy in family psychology intervention science. In H.A. Liddle, D. Santisteban, R. Levant, & J. Bray (Eds.), *Family Psychology Science-Based Interventions* (pp. 17–40). Washington DC: APA.

American Psychiatric Association (2000). *DSM-IV-TR: Diagnostic and Statistical Manual of Mental Disorders 4th Edition, Text revision*. Washington, DC: Author.

Aos, S., & Barnoski, R. (1998). *Watching the bottom line: Cost-effective interventions for reducing crime in Washington*. Washington State Institute for Public Policy: RCW 13.40.500.

Aos, S., Phipps, P., Barnoski, R., & Lieb, R. (2001). The comparative costs and benefits of programs to reduce crime. *Washington State Institute for Public Policy*, www.wsipp.wa.gov.

Bandura, A. (1977). *Social Learning Theory*. New York: General Learning Press.

Barnoski, R. (2002). Washington State's implementation of functional family therapy for juvenile offenders: Preliminary findings. *Washington State Institute for Public Policy*, www.wsipp.wa.gov.

Barnoski, R. (2004). Outcome evaluation of Washington State's research-based programs for juvenile offenders. *Washington State Institute for Public Policy*, www.wsipp.wa.gov.

Barnoski, R., Aos, S., & Lieb, R. (2003). Recommended quality control standards: Washington State research-based juvenile offender programs. *Washington State Institute for Public Policy*, www.wsipp. wa.gov.

Beutler, L.E., & Davison, E.H. (1995). What standards should we use? In S.C., Hayes, V.M. Follette, R.M. Dawes, & K.E. Grady, (Eds.), *Scientific Standards for Psychological Practice: Issues and Recommendations* (pp. 11–24). Reno, NV: Context Press.

Borduin, C.M., Henggeler, S.W., Blaske, D.M., & Stein, R.J. (1990). Multisystemic treatment of adolescent sex offenders. *International Journal of Offender Therapy and Comparative Criminology, 34* (2), 105–113.

Borduin, C.M., Mann, B.J., Cone, L.T., Henggeler, S.W., Fucci, B.R., Blaske, D.M., et al. (1995). Multisystemic treatment of serious juvenile offenders: Long-term prevention of criminality and violence. *Journal of Consulting & Clinical Psychology, 63* (4), 569–578.

Botvin, G.J., Baker, E., Dusenbury, L., Botvin, E.M., & Diaz, T. (1995). Long-term follow-up results of a randomized drug abuse prevention trial in a White middle-class population. *Journal of the American Medical Association, 273* (14), 1106–1112.

Botvin, G.J., Baker, E., Dusenbury, L., Tortu, S., & Botvin, E.M. (1990). Preventing adolescent drug abuse through a multimodal cognitive-behavioral approach: Results of a 3-year study. *Journal of Consulting and Clinical Psychology, 58* (4), 437–446.

Botvin, G.J., Baker, E., Renick, N.L., Filazzola, A.D., & Botvin, E.M. (1984). A cognitve-behavioral approach to substance abuse prevention. *Addictive Behaviors, 9*, 137–147.

Botvin, G.J., Batson, H.W., Witts-Vitale, S., Bess, V., Baker, E., & Dusenbury, L. (1989). A psychosocial approach to smoking prevention for urban Black youth. *Public Health Reports, 104* (6), 573–582.

Botvin, G.J., Dusenbury, L., Baker, E., James-Ortiz, S., Botvin, E.M., & Kerner, J. (1992). Smoking prevention among urban minority youth: Assessing effects on outcome and mediating variables. *Health Psychology, 11* (5), 290–299.

Botvin, G.J., Dusenbury, L., Baker, E., James-Ortiz, S., & Kerner, J. (1989). A skills training approach to smoking prevention among Hispanic youth. *Journal of Behavioral Medicine, 12* (3), 279–296.

Botvin, G.J., & Eng, A. (1982). The efficacy of a multicomponent approach to the prevention of cigarette smoking. *Preventive Medicine, 11*, 199–211.

Botvin, G.J., Eng, A., & Williams, C.L. (1980). Preventing the onset of cigarette smoking through Life Skills Training. *Preventive Medicine, 9*, 135–143.

Botvin, G.J., Epstein, J.A., Baker, E., Diaz, T., & Ifill-Williams, M. (1997). School-based drug abuse prevention with inner-city minority youth. *Journal of Child and Adolescent Substance Abuse, 6* (1), 5–19.

Botvin, G.J., Griffin, K.W., Diaz, T., & Ifill-Williams, M. (2001). Drug abuse prevention among minority adolescents: One-year follow-up of a school-based preventive intervention. *Prevention Science, 2*, 1–13.

Botvin, G.J., & Kantor, L.G. (2000). Preventing alcohol and tobacco use through life skills training: Theory, methods, and empirical findings. *Alcohol Research and Health, 24* (4), 250–257.

Botvin, G.J., Mihalic, S.F., & Grotpeter, J.K. (1998). *Blueprints for Violence Prevention, Book Five: Life Skills Training*. Boulder, CO: Center for the Study and Prevention of Violence.

Botvin, G.J., Renick, N., & Baker, E. (1983). The effects of scheduling format and booster sessions on a broad-spectrum psychosocial approach to smoking prevention. *Journal of Behavioral Medicine, 6* (4), 359–379.

Botvin, G.J., Schinke, S.P., Epstein, J.A., & Diaz, T. (1994). Effectiveness of culturally focused and generic skills training approaches to alcohol and drug abuse prevention among minority youths. *Psychology of Addictive Behaviors, 8* (2), 116–127.

Botvin, G.J., Schinke, S.P., Epstein, J.A., Diaz, T., & Botvin, E.M. (1995). Effectiveness of culturally focused and generic skills training approaches to alcohol and drug abuse prevention among minority adolescents: Two-year follow-up results. *Psychology of Addictive Behaviors, 9* (3), 183–194.

Bronfenbrenner, U. (1979). *The Ecology of Human Development: Experiments by Nature and Design*. Cambridge, MA: Harvard University Press.

Brunk, M.A., Henggeler, S.W., & Whelan, J.P. (1987). Comparison of multisystemic therapy and parent training in the brief treatment of child abuse and neglect. *Journal of Consulting & Clinical Psychology, 55* (2), 171–178.

Chalmers, I., Hedges, L.V., Cooper, H. (2002) A brief history of research synthesis. *Evaluation & the Health Professions, 25* (1), 12–37.

Chamberlain, P. (1990). Comparative evaluation of specialized foster care for seriously delinquent youth: A first step. *Community Alternatives: International Journal of Family Care, 2,* 21–36.

Chamberlain, P. (1998). *Family Connections*. Eugene, OR: Northwest Media.

Chamberlain, P., & Leve, L.D. (2002). Preventing health-risking behaviors in delinquent girls. Grant No. R01 DA15208, National Institute on Drug Abuse, National Institutes of Health, U.S. Public Health Service.

Chamberlain, P., & Mihalic, S.F. (1998). *Blueprints for Violence Prevention, Book Eight: Multidimensional Treatment Foster Care*. Boulder, CO: Center for the Study and Prevention of Violence.

Chamberlain, P., Moreland, S., & Reid, K. (1992). Enhanced services and stipends for foster parents: Effects on retention rates and outcomes for children. *Child Welfare League of America, 71,* 387–401.

Chamberlain, P., & Reid, J.B. (1991). Using a specialized foster care community treatment model for children and adolescents leaving the state mental hospital. *Journal of Community Psychology, 19,* 266–276.

Chamberlain, P., & Reid, J.B. (1998). Comparison of two community alternatives to incarceration for chronic juvenile offenders. *Journal of Consulting and Clinical Psychology, 66,* 624–633.

Chamberlain, P., & Smith, D.K. (2003). Antisocial behavior in children and adolescents: The Oregon Multidimensional Treatment Foster Care Model. In A.E. Kazdin & J.R. Weisz (Eds.), *Evidence-Based Psychotherapies for Children and Adolescents* (pp. 282–300). New York: Guilford Press.

Chambless, D.L., Baker, M.J., Baucom, D.H., Beutler, L.E., Calhoun, K.S., Crits-Christoph, P., et al. (1998). Update on empirically validated therapies, II. *The Clinical Psychologist, 51* (1), 3–16.

Chambless, D.L., Sanderson, W.C., Shoham, V., Bennett Johnson, S., Pope, K.S., Crits-Christoph, P., et al. (1996). An update on empirically validated therapies. *The Clinical Psychologist, 49,* 5–18.

DiClemente, R.J., Hansen, W.B., & Ponton, L.E. (Eds.). (1996). *Handbook of Adolescent Health Risk Behavior*. New York: Plenum Press.

Dishion, T.J., McCord, J., & Poulin, F. (1999). When interventions harm: Peer groups and problem behavior. *American Psychologist, 54,* 755–764.

Elliott, D.S. (Series Ed.). (1998). *Blueprints for violence prevention*. University of Colorado, Center for the Study and Prevention of Violence. Boulder, CO: Blueprints Publications.

Elliott, D., Huizinga, D., & Ageton, S. (1985). *Explaining Delinquency and Drug Use*. Beverly Hills, CA: Sage Publications.

Eysenck, H.J. (1952). The effects of psychotherapy: An evaluation. *Journal of Consulting Psychology, 16,* 319–324.

Griffin, K.W., Botvin, G.J., Nichols, T.R., & Doyle, M.M. (2003). Effectiveness of a universal drug abuse prevention approach for youth at high risk for substance abuse initiation. *Preventive Medicine, 36,* 1–7.

Henggeler, S.W., & Lee, T. (2003). Multisystemic treatment of serious clinical problems. In A.E. Kazdin & J.R. Weisz (Eds.), *Evidence-Based Psychotherapies for Children and Adolescents* (pp. 301–322). New York: Guilford Press.

Henggeler, S.W., Melton, G.B., Brondino, M.J., Scherer, D.G., & Hanley, J.H. (1997). Multisystemic therapy with violent and chronic juvenile offenders and their families: The role of treatment fidelity in successful dissemination. *Journal of Consulting & Clinical Psychology, 65* (5), 821–833.

Henggeler, S.W., Melton, G.B., & Smith, L.A. (1992). Family preservation using multisystemic therapy: An effective alternative to incarcerating serious juvenile offenders. *Journal of Consulting & Clinical Psychology, 60*(6), 953–961.

Henggeler, S.W., Pickrel, S.G., & Brondino, M.J. (1999). Multisystemic treatment of substance abusing and dependent delinquents: Outcomes, treatment fidelity, and transportability. *Mental Health Services Research, 1* (3), 171–184.

Henggeler, S.W., Rodick, J.D., Borduin, C.M., Hanson, C.L., Watson, S.M., & Urey, J.R. (1986). Multisystemic treatment of juvenile offenders: Effects on adolescent behavior and family interaction. *Developmental Psychology, 22* (1), 132–141.

Henggeler, S.W., Rowland, M.D., Randall, J., Ward, D.M., Pickrel, S.G., Cunningham, P.B., et al. (1999). Home-based multisystemic therapy as an alternative to the hospitalization of youths in psychiatric crisis: Clinical outcomes. *Journal of the American Academy of Child & Adolescent Psychiatry, 38* (11), 1331–1339.

Henggeler, S.W., Schoenwald, S.K., Borduin, C.M., Rowland, M.D., & Cunningham, P.B. (1998). *Multisystemic Treatment of Antisocial Behavior in Children and Adolescents*. New York: Guilford Press.

Hogan, M.F. (2003). *President's New Freedom Commission on Mental Health*. Washington, DC: Author.

Hogue, A., Liddle, H.A., Rowe, C., Turner, R.M., Dakof, G.A., & LaPann, K. (1998). Treatment adherence and differentiation in individual versus family therapy for adolescent substance abuse. *Journal of Counseling Psychology, 45* (1), 104–114.

Huey, S.J., Jr., Henggeler, S.W., Brondino, M.J., & Pickrel, S.G. (2000). Mechanisms of change in multisystemic therapy: Reducing delinquent behavior through therapist adherence and improved family and peer functioning. *Journal of Consulting & Clinical Psychology, 68* (3), 451–467.

Hyde, P.S., Falls, K., Morris, J.A., & Schoenwald, S.K. (2003). Turning knowledge into practice: A manual for behavioral health administrators and practitioners about understanding and implementing evidence-based practices. *Technical Assistance Collaborative*, www.tacinc.org.

Institute of Medicine (2001). *Crossing the quality chasm: A new health system for the 21st century.* (Executive Summary). Washington, D.C.: National Academy Press.

Kazdin, A.E. (1996). Dropping out of child psychotherapy: Issues for research and implications for practice. *Clinical Child Psychology & Psychiatry, 1* (1), 133–156.

Kazdin, A.E. (1997). Practitioner review: Psychosocial treatments for conduct disorder in children. *Journal of Child Psychology and Psychiatry, 38* (2), 161–178.

Kazdin, A.E. (2000). Adolescent development, mental disorders, and decision making of delinquent youths. In T. Grisso & R. Schwartz (Eds.), *Youth on Trial: A Developmental Perspective of Juvenile Justice* (pp. 33–84). Chicago: University of Chicago Press.

Kazdin, A.E. (2003). Psychotherapy for children and adolescents. *Annual Review of Psychology, 54,* 253–276.

Kazdin, A.E. (2004). Psychotherapy for children and adolescents. In M. Lambert (Ed.), *Bergin and Garfield's Handbook of Psychotherapy and Behavior Change* (5th ed., pp. 543–589). New York: Wiley.

Kazdin, A.E., & Weisz, J.R. (2003). *Evidence-Based Psychotherapies for Children and Adolescents.* New York: Guilford.

Lambert, M., & Bergin, A.E. (1994). The effectiveness of psychotherapy. In A.E. Bergin & S.L. Garfield (Eds.), *Handbook of Psychotherapy and Behavior Change* (pp. 143–189). New York: John Wiley.

Lambert, M.J., & Ogles, B.M. (2004). The efficacy and effectiveness of psychotherapy. In M.J. Lambert (Ed.), *Handbook of Psychotherapy and Behavior Change* (pp. 139–193). New York: Wiley.

Lyons, J.S., Baerger, D.R., Quigley, P., Erlich, J., & Griffin, E. (2001). Mental health service needs of juvenile offenders: A comparison of detention, incarceration, and treatment settings. *Children's Services: Social Policy, Research, and Practice, 4* (2), 69–85.

Luborsky, L., Singer, B., & Luborsky, L. (1975). Comparative studies of psychotherapy: Is it true that "everybody has won and all must have prizes?" *Archives of General Psychiatry, 32,* 995–1008.

Newberry, A.M., Alexander, J.F., & Turner, C.W. (1991). Gender as a process variable in family therapy. *Journal of Family Psychology, 5,* 158–175.

Newell, R.M., Alexander, J.F., & Turner, C.W. (1996). *The effects of therapist divert and interrupt on family members' reciprocity of negativity in delinquent families.* Poster session presented at the Annual Convention of the American Family Therapy Academy, San Francisco.

Pinsof, W.M., & Wynne, L.C. (1995). The efficacy of marital and family therapy: An empirical overview, conclusions, and recommendations. *Journal of Marital and Family Therapy, 21* (4), 585–613.

Pinsof, W.M., & Wynne, L.C. (2000). Toward progress research: Closing the gap between family therapy practice and research. *Journal of Marital and Family Therapy, 26,* 1–8.

Porzsolt, F., Ohletz, A., Gardner, D., Ruatti, H., Meier, H., Scholtz-Gorton, N., et al. (2003) Evidence-based decision making: The 6-Step approach. *The ACP Journal Club, 139* (3), A-11.

Robbins, M.S., Mayorga, C.C., & Szapocznik, J. (2003). The ecosystemic "lens" to understanding family therapy. In T.L. Sexton, G.R. Weeks, & M.S. Robbins (Eds.) *Handbook of Family Therapy* (pp. 21–36). New York: Brunner Routledge.

Rowland, N. & Goss, S. (Eds.). (2000) *Evidence-Based Counseling and Psychological Therapies: Research and Applications.* Philadelphia: Taylor & Francis, Inc.

Sackett, D.L., Rosenberg, W.M.C., Gray, J.A.M., Haynes, R.B., & Richardson, W.S. (1996). Evidence based medicine: What it is and what it isn't; It's about integrating individual clinical expertise and the best external evidence. *British Medical Journal, 312* (7023), 71–72.

Schoenwald, S.K., Henggeler, S.W., Brondino, M.J., & Rowland, M.D. (2000). Multisystemic therapy: Monitoring treatment fidelity. *Family Process, 39* (1), 83–103.

Schoenwald, S.K., Sheidow, A.J., & Letourneau, E.J. (2004). Toward effective quality assurance in evidence-based practice: Links between expert consultation, therapist fidelity, and child outcomes. *Journal of Clinical Child Adolescent Psychology, 33,* 94–104.

Schoenwald, S.K., Sheidow, A.J., Letourneau, E.J., & Liao, J.G. (2003). Transportability of Multisystemic therapy: Evidence for multilevel influences. *Mental Health Services Research, 5* (4), 223–239.

Schoenwald, S.K., Ward, D.M., Henggeler, S.W., & Rowland, M.D. (2000). Multisystemic therapy versus hospitalization for crisis stabilization of youth: Placement outcomes 4 months postreferral. *Mental Health Services Research, 2* (1), 3–12.

Sexton, T.L., & Alexander, J.F. (2000). Functional Family Therapy. *Juvenile Justice Bulletin,* Office of Juvenile Justice and Delinquency Prevention. Washington, DC: Department of Justice.

Sexton, T.L., & Alexander, J.F. (2002a). Family-based empirically supported interventions. *The Counseling Psychologist, 30* (2), 238–261.

Sexton, T.L., & Alexander, J.F. (2002b). Functional Family Therapy for at-risk adolescents and their families. In T. Patterson (Ed.), *Wiley Series in Couples and Family Dynamics and Treatment, Comprehensive Handbook of Psychotherapy, Vol. II: Cognitive-Behavioral Approaches,* (pp. 117–140). New York: Wiley.

Sexton, T.L., & Alexander, J.F. (2003). Functional Family Therapy: A mature clinical model for working with at-risk adolescents and their families. In T.L. Sexton, G.R. Weeks, & M.S. Robbins (Eds.) *Handbook of Family Therapy* (pp. 323–348). New York: Brunner Routledge.

Sexton, T.L., Alexander, J.F., & Mease, A.L. (2004) Levels of Evidence for the Models and Mechanisms of Therapeutic Change in Family and Couple Therapy. In M.J. Lambert (Ed.), *Bergin and Garfield's Handbook of Psychotherapy and Behavior Change* (Fifth Ed.) (pp. 590–646). New York: Wiley.

Sexton, T.L., Hollimon, A.S., & Mease, A.L. (2002). *Family-based interventions in community settings.* Presented at American Association of Marriage and Family Therapy's annual convention, Cincinnati, OH.

Sexton, T.L., Ostrom, N., Bonomo, J., & Alexander, J.F. (2000). *Functional family therapy in a multicultural, multiethnic urban setting.* Paper presented at the annual conference of the American Association of Marriage and Family Therapy, Denver, CO.

Sexton, T.L., Ridley, C.R., & Kleiner, A.J. (2004). Beyond common factors: Multilevel process models of therapeutic change in marriage and family therapy. *Journal of Marriage and Family Therapy, 30* (2), 131–149.

Sexton, T.L., Robbins, M.S., Hollimon, A.S., Mease, A.L., & Mayorga, C.C. (2003). Efficacy, effectiveness, and change mechanisms in couple and family therapy. In T.L. Sexton, G.R. Weeks, & M.S. Robbins (Eds.), *Handbook of Family Therapy* (pp. 229–261). New York: Brunner Routledge.

Sexton, T.S., Sydnor, A.E., & Rowland, M.K. (2004). Identification and treatment of the clinical problems of childhood and adolescence. In R. Coombs (Ed.), *Family Therapy Review: Preparing for Comprehensive and Licensing Exams.* Mahway, New Jersey: Lawrence Erlbaum Associates, Inc.

Shadish, W.R., Matt, G.E., Navarro, A.M., Siegle, G., Crits-Cristoph, P., Hazelrigg, M.D., et al. (1997). Evidence that therapy works in clinically representative conditions. *Journal of Consulting and Clinical Psychology, 65,* 355–365.

Shadish, W.R., Montgomery, L.M., Wilson, P., & Wilson, M.R. (1993). Effects of family and marital psychotherapies: A meta-analysis. *Journal of Consulting and Clinical Psychology, 61,* 992–1002.

Sheidow, A.J., Henggeler, S.W., & Schoenwald, S.K. (2003). Multisystemic therapy. In T.L Sexton, G.R. Weeks, & M.S. Robbins (Eds.), *Handbook of Family Therapy: The Science and Practice of Working with Families and Couples.* Brunner-Routledge: New York, NY.

Sloboda, Z., & David, S.L. (1997). Preventing drug use among children and adolescents: A research-based guide. *National Institute of Drug Addiction.* Washington, DC: NIH Publication no. 97–4212.

Smith, M.L., & Glass, G.V. (1977). Meta-analysis of psychotherapy outcome studies. *American Psychologist, 32*, 752–760.

Smith, D.K., Stormshak, E., Chamberlain, P., & Bridges-Whaley, R. (2001). Placement disruption in treatment foster care. *Journal of Emotional and Behavioral Disorders, 9*, 200–205.

Snyder, H.N., & Sickmund, M. (1999). *Juvenile Offenders and Victims: 1999 National Report.* Washington, DC: U.S. Department of Justice, Office of Justice Programs, Office of Juvenile Justice and Delinquency Prevention.

Task Force on Promotion and Dissemination of Psychological Procedures (1995). Training in and dissemination of empirically validated treatments: Report and recommendations. *The Clinical Psychologist, 48* (1), 3–23.

Teplin, L.A., Abram, K.M., McClelland, G.M., Dulcan, M.K., & Mericle, A.A. (2002). Psychiatric disorders in youth in juvenile detention. *Archives of General Psychiatry, 59* (12), 1133–1143.

U.S. Public Health Service. (2001). *Youth Violence: A Report of the Surgeon General.* Washington, DC: Author.

von Bertalanffy, L. (1968). *General Systems Theory: Foundations, Development, and Applications.* New York: Braziller.

Wampold, B.E. (2001). *The Great Psychotherapy Debate: Models, Methods, and Findings.* Mahway, NJ: Erlbaum.

Wampold, B.E., Lichtenburg, J.W., & Waehler, C.A. (2002). Principles of empirically supported interventions in counseling psychology. *The Counseling Psychologist, 30* (2), 197–217.

Wampold, B.E., Mondin, G.W., Moody, M., Stich, F., Benson, K., & Ahn, H. (1997). A meta-analysis of outcome studies comparing bona fide psychotherapies: Empiricially, "all must have prizes." *Psychological Bulletin, 122* (3), 203–215.

Section II

Disorders

Chapter 7

Anxiety Disorders in Children and Adolescents
Theory, Treatment, and Prevention

Patricia A. Graczyk, Sucheta D. Connolly,
and Feyza Corapci

Introduction

Anxiety disorders represent the most common form of psychopathology in children and adolescents. In community studies including adolescents, approximately 4–19% of young people were found to be suffering from anxiety disorders (Costello & Angold, 1995; Ford, Goodman & Meltzer, 2003; Shaffer et al., 1996). Although rates of anxiety disorders are similar in prepubertal boys and girls, there is a slightly higher occurrence of anxiety disorders in adolescent girls than boys (Costello & Angold, 1995; Shaffer et al., 1996). Anxiety disorders can significantly interfere with a young person's ability to function in interpersonal relationships and at school (Ezpeleta, Keeler, Erkanli, Costello & Angold, 2001), yet they often go unrecognized by parents and teachers.

Anxiety disorders frequently co-occur with other mood disorders, depression, and disruptive behavior disorders (Ford et al., 2003). In addition, anxiety disorders early in life place young people at heightened risk for subsequent anxiety disorders, major depressive disorder, schizophrenia, substance abuse, suicide, and psychiatric hospitalization in adolescence and young adulthood (Kim-Cohen, Caspi, Moffitt, Harrington, Milne & Poulton, 2003; Schuckit & Hesselbrock, 1994). Fortunately, the past decade has witnessed major advances in understanding the development, prevention, and treatment of anxiety disorders in children and adolescents.

This chapter provides an overview of the major anxiety disorders found in children and adolescents, along with several theoretical frameworks for understanding the etiology and maintainance of these disorders. Risk and protective factors for anxiety disorders are discussed according to whether they exist within the individual, family, or broader ecological context. This discussion sets the stage for a review of the treatments and preventive approaches used for anxiety disorders. Because of its major presence in the treatment and prevention area, the cognitive-behavioral theoretical model and treatment approach is described in detail. The chapter concludes with a set of recommendations for best practices in the treatment and prevention of anxiety disorders in children and adolescents.

Description of Anxiety Disorders

The *Diagnostic and Statistical Manual of Mental Disorders IV-TR* (DSM-IV-TR; American Psychiatric Association, 2000) provides a comprehensive categorical system for classifying anxiety disorders. Each of these disorders has distinct features, yet they all share a common foundation of excessive, irrational fear and dread. A brief synopsis of each major anxiety disorder follows.

Children and adolescents with *Separation Anxiety Disorder* (SAD) experience developmentally excessive fear and distress concerning separation from home or significant attachment figures. Frequently these young people worry excessively about their parents' health and safety, have difficulty sleeping without their parents, complain of stomachaches and headaches, and may manifest school refusal.

Generalized Anxiety Disorder (GAD) is characterized by chronic, excessive, and uncontrollable worry. Worries may relate to friends, family, health, safety, and/or the future. A diagnosis of GAD also requires that at least one somatic symptom be present, such as motor tension or sleep difficulty.

Adolescents with *Social Phobia* (SocP) experience excessive fear or discomfort in social or performance situations. These young people fear negative evaluations from others and worry about doing something embarrassing, stupid, or awkward in social settings such as classrooms and restaurants or during sports activities.

Specific Phobia (SP) represents an intense fear of a particular object or situation and frequently is accompanied by avoidance of the focal object or situation. To distinguish between a developmentally normal fear and a specific phobia, one must consider age, severity of symptomatology, and impairment. Compared to normal fears, phobias are excessive, persistent, or maladaptive.

Panic Disorder (PD) involves recurrent and spontaneous attacks or episodes of intense fear. These episodes are accompanied by at least four somatic symptoms such as pounding or racing heart, sweating, shaking, difficulty breathing, chest pain, or fear of dying or going crazy. For many individuals, the onset of PD occurs at some point during adolescence.

Adolescents with *Agoraphobia* (Ag) avoid or are extremely uncomfortable in places they fear they will be unable to get help or escape. Agoraphobia may present independently or accompany panic disorder. Common stressful situations for agoraphobics include crowds, standing in line, shopping malls, traveling (especially via public transportation), enclosed places such as elevators, open spaces such as large parks, and trips or camps away from home.

Other disorders that involve intense anxiety include Obsessive-Compulsive Disorder Post-Traumatic Stress Disorder, and Acute Stress Disorder. *Obsessive-Compulsive Disorder* (OCD) involves recurrent obsessions or compulsive acts that are time-consuming and cause significant impairment or distress for the individual. *Obsessions* are repetitive, intrusive thoughts that often relate to contamination fears, a need for symmetry, excessive doubting, sexual themes, or aggressive or malicious impulses (e.g., to hurt one's parents). *Compulsions* are repetitive acts or mental activities that are performed to assuage the anxiety or distress caused by obsessional thinking (e.g., excessive hand-washing due to contamination fears). *Post-Traumatic Stress Disorder* (PTSD) can occur after a person has experienced or witnessed an extremely traumatic event or has learned that a family member or other significant person in their lives has had such an experience. Individuals with PTSD often experience difficulties sleeping or concentrating, irritability, reexperiencing of the event in dreams or flashbacks, emotional numbing (e.g., restricted range of affect), or avoidance of anything or anyone associated with the event. Individuals with *Acute Stress Disorder* experience similar symptomatology to those with PTSD, but their symptoms typically occur immediately following a traumatic event and abate within four weeks or less.

The typical age of onset varies across the anxiety disorders and approximates the developmental progression of normal fears in childhood. SAD often presents at ages 6–9, GAD at any age but most often at ages 10–12, and social phobia at age 12 and older (Albano & Kendall, 2002). PD with or without agoraphobia typically begins during late adolescence and young adulthood (American Psychiatric Association, 2000). Child and adolescent anxiety disorders progress along a variety of trajectories, including a chronic course with a low remission rate for PD to a high remission rate for SAD (Last, Perrin, Hersen & Kazdin, 1996). SAD in childhood and adolescence also may precede panic disorder and agoraphobia in adulthood (Last et al., 1996). Moreover, the same individual may experience different anxiety disorders at different points in time (Last et al., 1996).

Major Theoretical Models Driving Treatment and Prevention Efforts

Numerous theories have been proposed in the last century to explain the etiology and maintenance of anxiety disorders. Due to space limitations, this section focuses on two types of theoretical perspectives, the behavioral/learning models and the cognitive/behavioral models, because these models serve as the foundation for the majority of treatment and preventive strategies with the most empirical support for their effectiveness at this time.

Behavioral/Learning Models

Early behavioral/learning models of the etiology of phobias and anxiety disorders were grounded in conditioning theory. In *classical conditioning*, a nonaversive stimulus, i.e., the conditioned stimulus or CS, is repeatedly paired with a feared or aversive stimulus, i.e., the unconditioned stimulus or UCS, until the presentation of the CS alone will evoke fear and fear-related behaviors, referred to as the conditioned response, or CR. An early application of this model is reflected in the case study of "Little Albert" conducted by Watson and Rayner (1920). Little Albert was a 9-month-old child who initially did not fear white rats (CS), but did fear loud noises (UCS). Following classical conditioning procedures, Watson and Rayner sounded a loud noise whenever Albert touched the rat. After several such pairings, Albert began to cry when he saw the rat, even when its presentation was no longer followed by a loud noise.

Mowrer (1960) expanded on Watson and Rayner's (1920) work by proposing a two-stage theory to explain how phobias and avoidance behavior developed. In the first stage, a person is classically conditioned to fear a previously nonaversive stimulus, the CS. In the second stage, the person learns that avoiding the CS results in a decrease in anxiety. The drop in anxiety reinforces the person for engaging in avoidance behavior and increases the likelihood that avoidance behavior will occur whenever the CS is presented in the future. Mowrer's two-stage theory not only accounts for the genesis of fears but also the persistence of avoidance behavior in phobic individuals.

These early behavioral models had their limitations. For example, they could not explain why all people who experience a traumatic event do not go on to develop a phobia. They were also unable to account for the role of observational learning in fear acquisition. To address these and other criticisms, Davey and colleagues (Davey, 1997; Field & Davey, 2001) proposed a model of fear acquisition that emphasized the role of cognitions and cognitive processes in developing expectancy evaluations and UCS reevaluation processes. *Expectancy evaluations* refer to an individual's perception of the relationship between the CS and UCS. They can be derived from multiple sources, including the individual's own expectancies and beliefs about the possible consequences associated with the CS. For instance, a person who has had multiple nonaversive experiences in a situation and then experiences a trauma would be less likely to associate the situation with trauma. This could occur, for instance, when a child has had several pleasant or emotionally neutral visits to the dentist and then has a tooth removed. Because of the boy's prior nonaversive experiences with the dentist, this model would predict that he would be less likely to make the association between dentists and pain. In fact, this approach has been applied effectively in the preventive treatment of dental and medical phobias. Expectancy evaluations can also develop from verbally and culturally transmitted information about the relationship between the CS and UCS. For example, the nursery rhyme *Little Miss Muffett* could predispose some children to develop a spider phobia.

Davey's model also postulates that a conditioned fear response could be amplified or attentuated through UCS *reevaluation processes*. These processes refer to an individual's interpretations of the UCS, such as perceiving bodily sensations as signs of threat or minimizing a threat by using adaptive coping strategies. Davey proposed that threat devaluation processes such as adaptive coping strategies could account for the fact that not all people who experience traumatic events go on to develop phobias or PTSD.

In summary, the contemporary conditioning model incorporates a cognitive perspective to augment earlier conditioning models and, in so doing, has increased its power to explain more phenomena related to fears and phobias. The model's emphasis on cognitive and behavioral elements makes it less discernible from cognitive-behavioral models, to be discussed next, than its predecessors that focused solely on behavioral conditioning models.

Cognitive-Behavioral Models

According to Albano and Kendall (2002), anxiety within a cognitive-behavioral framework is viewed as either adaptive or maladaptive. In its adaptive form, anxiety serves a protective function because it signals danger to an individual and motivates her to take action to avoid stress or negative experiences. Anxiety is viewed as consisting of three components: a physiological component, a subjective or cognitive component, and a behavioral component (Lang, 1968). The *physiological component* refers to the activity of the autonomic nervous system that prepares an individual to respond to a threatening situation with "fight or flight" behavior. Such responses include increased rate of respiration, increased heart rate, and blood flow to the muscles, and are activated to enable the person to respond quickly, if necessary. The *cognitive component* of anxiety refers to the selective and focused attention to threat cues and ways to protect oneself, especially through escape. *Behavioral reactions* (e.g., running away) are actions taken to avoid a negative event or encounter. Anxiety in its maladaptive form includes these three components, but develops in response to irrational or unrealistic fears and significantly compromises an individual's ability to function appropriately in circumstances perceived to be unsafe. Therefore, cognitive-behavioral approaches target all three components of anxiety, with the ultimate goal of helping individuals learn to perceive their world less from a "threat" template and more from a "coping" template (Kendall, Aschenbrand & Hudson 2003). Finally, CBT approaches also emphasize how maladaptive cognitions and behaviors are learned through person-environment interactions in which certain behaviors are reinforced, modeled, or both.

Risk and Protective Factors Associated with Anxiety Disorders

Risk factors for anxiety are those that place youth at increased risk of developing an anxiety disorder. *Protective factors* enhance an individual's resilience in the presence of risk factors or emergent pathological anxiety. In this section, risk and protective factors for anxiety disorders are organized according to their reference to characteristics of the individual, the family, or the broader social environment.

Individual Factors

In children and adolescents, temperamental, physiological, and behavioral characteristics have been identified as individual risk factors for anxiety disorders. These characteristics are behavioral inhibition, anxious/withdrawn behavior, and anxiety sensitivity. To date, only one characteristic of the individual has been identified as a protective factor, i.e., problem-focused coping skills.

BEHAVIORAL INHIBITION.   There is evidence of genetic influences in the development of anxiety disorder (Eley, 2001; Thapar & McGuffin, 1995), and it has been suggested that what is inherited is a temperamental predisposition toward behaviorally inhibited behavior (Garcia-Coll, Kagan & Reznick, 1984). Physiological indicators of behavioral inhibition (BI) include high stable heart rates, low vagal tone, and other indicators of high sympathetic arousal or low parasympathetic arousal respectively (Kagan, Reznick & Snidman, 1987). Behavioral manifestations of BI include shyness, caution, and emotional restraint, particularly in response to novel situations (Biederman et al., 1993; Kagan, 1997).

A few longitudinal studies have examined the link between temperamental inhibition and anxiety disorders (Fox, Henderson, Rubin, Calkins & Schmidt, 2001; Kagan,

Snidman, Zentner & Peterson, 1999). For example, Kagan et al. (1999) followed the response of 4-month-old infants extremely high or low in motor activity and negative affect to novel stimuli until the age of seven. Results indicated that 45% of the high reactives, 15% of low reactives, and 21% of the remaining children at four months were classified as having anxious symptoms at seven years of age. This evidence suggests that the four-month high reactive temperamental category reflects a quality that is preserved and can predict later anxiety problems to a modest degree.

A similar behavioral profile to that of BI is a behavioral dimension referred to as anxious/withdrawn. Children and adolescents with elevated scores on the anxious/withdrawn dimension typically exhibit shy, withdrawn, inhibited, and fearful behavior. For example, a recent longitudinal study conducted by Goodwin, Fergusson, and Horwood (2004) found that anxious/withdrawn behavior at age 8 was significantly associated with major depression and anxiety disorders in adolescence and young adulthood, especially SocP and SP.

However, not all children displaying BI or anxious/withdrawn behavior go on to develop anxiety or other disorders. For instance, in the Goodwin et al. (2004) study, only half of the children displaying the highest levels of anxious/withdrawn behavior went on to develop a disorder by age 21. These findings suggest that other risk factors or mechanisms may be involved in the development of anxiety disorders.

ANXIETY SENSITIVITY.   BI and anxious/withdrawn behaviors appear to be risk factors for a variety of anxiety disorders. In contrast, anxiety sensitivity (AS) appears to be a risk factor specific to panic attacks and panic disorder in adolescents and adults. AS refers to a tendency to believe that symptoms of anxiety (e.g., shortness of breath, trembling, increased heart rate) will result in severe negative physical or psychological consequences (Reiss, 1991). Such expectancies then lead to higher levels of anxiety, more intense physical symptoms, and ultimately panic attacks (Reiss, 1991; Reiss & McNally, 1985).

Two studies provide support for the association between panic and AS in a community high school sample (Lau, Calamari & Waraczynski, 1996) and in a clinical sample (Kearney, Albano, Eisen, Allan & Barlow, 1997). Recently, longitudinal investigations have provided evidence of a causal connection between AS and PD for European American, African American, Hispanic, and Asian youth (Ginsburg & Drake, 2002a; Hayward, Killen, Kraemer & Taylor, 2000; Weems, Hayward, Killen & Taylor, 2002). When group differences were investigated, Weems et al. (2002) found the relation between AS and panic was significantly stronger for European American than Hispanic or Asian youth, even though the latter two groups reported more AS overall.

COPING SKILLS.   According to Spence (2001), the ways in which adolescents respond to or cope with unpleasant experiences can influence the extent to which they experience anxiety, distress, and fear. Coping refers to efforts by the individual to mobilize behavioral and cognitive resources when faced with stress, and such efforts can vary in their effectiveness (Compas, Connor-Smith, Saltzman, Thomsen & Wadsworth, 2001). Coping strategies can be categorized as emotion-focused, avoidant, or problem-focused (Donovan & Spence, 2000). *Emotion-focused coping strategies* target the level of distress and *avoidant strategies* emphasize efforts to escape or avoid the problem. In contrast, *problem-focused coping* refers to efforts to deal directly with the problem or to minimize its effect (e.g., seeking information, positive self-talk, doing something to change the situation that is creating stress). Several studies of coping strategies in children and adolescents provide evidence of the benefits of problem-focused activities and the negative impact of emotion-focused and avoidant strategies (for review see Donovan & Spence, 2000).

In conclusion, child characteristics are important factors to consider in the development of anxiety disorders. However, it is important to consider the nature of the adolescent's context to identify additional critical variables that contribute to the development and maintenance of anxiety. Several such factors within the family have been identified and are discussed next.

Family Factors

Some family characteristics are more likely to occur in families of youth with anxiety disorders and have been identified as risk factors for anxiety disorders. They include parental anxiety and negative parent–child interactions.

PARENTAL ANXIETY. Parental anxiety disorder has been associated with increased risk of anxiety disorders in offspring (Merikangas et al., 1998) and high levels of functional impairment in children and adolescents with anxiety disorders (Manassis & Hood, 1998). Donovan and Spence (2000) proposed that parental anxiety might serve as an indirect risk factor and that its effects are moderated or mediated by some other mechanism. They propose that child temperament, such as BI discussed earlier, and parenting behaviors, to be discussed next, may serve as two such mechanisms that link parental anxiety to child anxiety.

ATTACHMENT. The early caregiver–infant relationship that results in an insecure attachment has been proposed as one way that family processes contribute to the development and maintenance of anxiety disorders. According to *attachment theory* (Bowlby, 1988), infants form a trusting and secure attachment if their caregivers are available and responsive to their basic needs for nurturance and support. Unresponsive, rejecting, or inconsistent parenting styles result in insecure attachment. Insecurely attached infants typically show anxious fearfulness in difficult situations because they doubt the availability of caregivers' assistance. These infants also are at increased risk for anxiety disorders.

Findings from two studies (Manassis, 2001; Warren, Huston, Egeland & Sroufe, 1997) suggest that insecure attachment increases the risk of subsequent child and adolescent anxiety disorders. More importantly, some researchers have shown that the link between insecure attachment and anxiety problems is stronger when a child is temperamentally predisposed to fearfulness and inhibition (Fox & Calkins, 1993).

PARENTING BEHAVIOR. Parenting behavior is implicated in the development and maintenance of anxiety disorders in children and adolescents. Parental overcontrol and overprotectiveness have been found to maintain and exacerbate child inhibition (see Wood, McLeod, Sigman, Hwang & Chu, 2003, for reviews). Rubin and colleagues (Rubin, Burgess, Kennedy & Stewart, 2003) have proposed that parents may inadvertently reward and encourage fearful children to avoid challenges by either excessively controlling their child's activities or solving their problems. Several observational studies confirm this hypothesis. Specifically, children who were clinically anxious or temperamentally fearful were observed to have mothers who were overprotective, gave excessive commands, and restricted their child's autonomy during their interactions (Hudson & Rapee, 2001; Krohne & Hock, 1991; Rubin, Burgess & Hastings, 2002). However, there is preliminary evidence to suggest that anxious parents may only display overprotective behavior within situations that are anxiety-provoking (Turner, Beidel, Roberson–Nay & Tervo, 2003).

Several studies also have found that child anxiety was positively correlated with parental rejecting behavior and negatively correlated with parental warmth and sensitivity (Dadds, Barrett, Rapee & Ryan, 1996; Dumas, LaFrenier & Serketich, 1995; Leib, Wittchen, Hofler, Fuetsch, Stein & Merikangas, 2000). Retrospective studies in which adults with anxiety disorders reported on their parents' behavior also revealed a link between lack of warmth in parent–child relations and anxiety disorder (see Wood et al., 2003, for review).

Modeling and vicarious learning of anxiety are two other processes in family interactions that may serve to increase anxious cognitions in children. For example, a recent study by Gerull and Rapee (2002) showed how children use emotional reactions of their caregivers to evaluate the degree of danger/threat in a novel situation. In this study, children were less likely to approach a rubber snake if their mother expressed negative affect toward the snake compared to children whose mothers remained neutral. Still other studies have found that parents' modeling anxiety and/or reinforcing avoidance was higher in children with anxiety disorders compared to their non-anxious peers (Cobham, 1998; Dadds & Roth, 2001; Rapee, 1997; Whaley, Pinto & Sigman, 1999; Wood et al., 2003). Finally, there is growing evidence that anxious children interpret ambiguous situations as threatening and prefer avoidant solutions to these situations just like their parents do (e.g., Barrett, Rapee, Dadds & Ryan, 1996).

In summary, the available evidence highlights the important role of family processes in relation to children's anxiety problems. This is particularly true when parents themselves display high levels of anxiety (Albano, Chorpita & Barlow, 2003; Hirshfeld, Biederman, Brody, Faraone & Rosenbaum, 1997). Parents can encourage anxious behaviors in their children by attending to their child's anxious behaviors, focusing selectively on negative outcomes and threat, modeling poor coping skills such as avoidance of a difficult situation themselves, or by failing to reward their child's brave behaviors.

Social and Community Factors

Events that occur outside the home, such as negative or traumatic life events, community violence, and problematic peer relationships, can place a child or adolescent at increased risk for anxiety disorders. However, social support can come from multiple individuals within the youth's environment and can serve to buffer the effects of other risk factors that may be present.

NEGATIVE LIFE EVENTS. Multiple studies have shown that children and adolescents with mental health needs experience more negative, stressful, or traumatic life events than their healthy counterparts (Boer, Markus, Maingay, Linkhout, Borst & Hoogendijk, 2002), and these events represent risk factors for anxiety disorders as well. Elevated rates of anxiety disorders have been found following natural disasters (Yule & Williams, 1990) and negative life events such as the death of a family member, divorce, or changes in school (Donovan & Spence, 2000). Several studies suggest that youth with anxiety disorders experience a higher incident of negative life events compared to non-anxious children (Benjamin, Costello, & Warren, 1990; Boer et al., 2002; Goodyer & Altham, 1991), even when compared with siblings in the same household (Boer et al., 2002).

Community Violence

Research to understand the risk relationships between child and adolescent anxiety disorders and environmental factors is limited (Spence, 2001), but there is evidence to suggest that minority and economically disadvantaged youth may be at increased risk for anxiety disorders for a variety of reasons. Minority and disadvantaged youth report decreased feelings of safety (Schwab-Stone et al., 1995), are exposed to high rates of community violence (Cooley, Turner & Beidel, 1995; Gladstein, Rusonis & Heald, 1992), and are often victims of violence (Freeman, Mokros & Poznanski, 1993). Violence exposure is consistently linked to symptoms of psychological trauma such as depression, anger, dissociation, anxiety, and posttraumatic stress (Singer, Anglin, Song & Lunghofer, 1995), and minority urban youth exposed to violence in their community have been found to have elevated rates of PTSD (Berman, Kurtines, Silverman & Serafini, 1996; Fitzpatrick & Boldizar, 1993).

PEER RELATIONSHIPS.   In spite of numerous studies demonstrating the association between problematic peer relations and anxiety, the relationship between the two continues to be seriously overlooked. Children with clinically significant anxiety disorders are more likely to be rejected or neglected by their peers compared to non-referred children (Strauss, Lahey, Frick, Frame & Hynd, 1988). Anxious children are at greater risk of becoming actively rejected by their peers in the intermediate grades and beyond when withdrawn, inhibited, and submissive behaviors become viewed as deviant by children and adolescents (e.g., Waas & Graczyk, 2000).

Children with anxiety disorders also appear prone to react to social situations with negative self-appraisals, social skill deficits, and high states of physiological arousal. Spence, Donovan, and Brechman-Toussaint (2000) found that children and adolescents with social phobia demonstrated more social skill deficits and higher levels of negative self-talk when faced with a social-evaluative task than did a nonclinical group. Beidel and Turner (1998) noted that approximately 40% of socially phobic children in their clinic expressed fear of speaking to peers. Such fears may be at least partially grounded in reality because anxious and socially isolated children are more likely to be victimized (Olweus, 1993).

La Greca (2001) proposed that the association between problematic peer relationships and anxiety is mediated by social anxiety. Several studies by La Greca and colleagues and others provide preliminary support in favor of this hypothesis (for review see LaGreca, 2001), but longer-term prospective studies are warranted before more definitive conclusions can be made.

SOCIAL SUPPORT.   Social support may serve as a protective factor for anxious youth despite the presence of risk factors. Social support refers to a person's beliefs about general or specific support that is available from members of their social network to shield him from negative circumstances and/or improve functioning (Demaray & Malecki, 2002). Low levels of family and peer support have been associated with a variety of negative indicators, including anxiety and stress (Demaray & Malecki, 2002). Conversely, multiple investigations provide evidence of the role of social support in promoting psychological and physical well-being (e.g., Levitt, Guacci-Franco & Levitt, 1994; Pryor-Brown & Cowen, 1989) and shielding children and adolescents against psychological and physical adversity (e.g., Compas, Slavin, Wagner & Vannatta, 1986; Dubow, Edwards & Ippolito, 1997). A recent investigation by Demaray and Malecki (2002) evaluated the relationships among social support and a variety of adjustment indicators in a large community sample of children and adolescents. Significant positive correlations were found between social support (provided by parents, teachers, classmates, and close friends) and social skills, self-esteem, adaptive skills, and academic competence.

Evidence-Based Treatment Interventions in Community Settings

In our review of treatment studies, we focus primarily on information derived from carefully controlled investigations that involved random assignment of participants to treatment and comparison conditions. These investigations are referred to as randomized control trials (RCTs). An additional criterion for inclusion in our review is that the studies include at least some adolescent participants, i.e., individuals within the 11–18-year-old-range (Weisz & Hawley, 2002). These decisions were intended to insure greater accuracy in the information provided and relevance to adolescent populations.

In the following sections, treatment and prevention efforts will be classified into three categories: what works, what might work, and what does not work. Interventions categorized under "what works" are those for which a minimum of three studies generated positive outcomes. Interventions categorized under "what might work" are based on solid theory, resulted in positive outcomes in one or two studies, or generated mixed results in multiple studies. The category "what does not work" will include those treatment or prevention efforts for which multiple studies have shown a lack of efficacy at this time.

What Works

Numerous studies provide support for the efficacy of behavioral therapies and cognitive-behavioral therapies for the treatment of anxiety disorders. In the following sections, each approach is briefly described, followed by a summary of supportive treatment outcome studies.

BEHAVIORAL THERAPIES.   Behavioral therapies are grounded in conditioning and learning models and have frequently served as the framework for interventions used to treat SD and SocP. Strategies generated from this perspective include contingency management, systematic desensitization, exposures, modeling, and social skills training, among others.

Contingency management involves the utilization of either positive consequences or punishments contingent on the young person's behavior, for example, providing praise to an adolescent with social phobia for having read aloud to a group of peers. *Systematic desensitization* refers to a counterconditioning technique in which a classically conditioned response (CR), such as a spider phobia, becomes unlearned through repeated pairings of spiders (CS) with a response that is incompatible with anxiety, such as deep muscle relaxation. During *exposure* activities, a youth is presented or exposed to feared stimuli systematically, moving from least to most feared, while she uses relaxation strategies to maintain a calm state. *Extinction,* or the elimination of anxiety as a response to feared stimuli, requires lengthy exposures concurrent with an inability to escape or avoid the situation. Exposures can be conducted imaginally or in vivo (i.e., real life). When conducted in vivo, *modeling* is a critical component of the exposure process. Modeling can be provided in a variety of formats: live (e.g., by the therapist), through videotapes or films, with assistance in approaching the feared stimulus (i.e., participant modeling), or with prompts to display a modeled behavior without assistance (Ollendick & King, 1998).

Social skills training is particularly helpful for children and adolescents with SocP because they often experience significant social skills deficits (Beidel, Turner & Tracy, 1999). Social skills training is often conducted in a group format and covers a wide variety of skills, including making eye contact, handling conflicts, conversational skills, assertion skills, giving corrective feedback, friendship skills, and group skills (Beidel, Turner & Morris, 2000; Spence et al., 2000).

Three RCTs demonstrated the efficacy of modeling, especially participant modeling in the treatment of SP (Bandura, Blanchard & Ritter, 1969; Lewis, 1974; Ritter, 1968). Five RCTs have demonstrated the efficacy of in vivo exposures and systematic desensitization for the treatment of phobias (Barabasz, 1973; Kondas, 1967; Mann & Rosenthanl, 1969; Muris, Merckelbach, Holdrinet & Sijsenaar, 1998; Ost, Svensson, Hellstrom & Lindwall, 2001) when compared to wait-list controls or alternative treatments.

Recently, Beidel and colleagues (Beidel et al., 2000) developed *Social Effectiveness Therapy for Children* (SET-C), a multi-component group treatment for social phobia. The treatment includes psycho-education for the child and parents, social skills training, peer generalization activities, and individual in vivo exposures. SET-C was found superior to a nonspecific intervention, *Testbusters,* in reducing social fears and associated psychopathology, and in enhancing social skills and social interactions. Recovery rates (i.e., percentage of participants who no longer met criteria for their primary disorder) immediately following the interventions were 67% for SET-C compared to 5% for *Testbusters.* Moreover, treatment effects were sustained at six-month follow-up. Thus, SET-C appears to be a promising intervention for SocP that warrants further investigation.

In summary, behavioral interventions have a relatively long history of demonstrated efficacy in the treatment of a variety of phobic conditions. Many of these strategies have been incorporated into cognitive-behavioral treatment protocols.

COGNITIVE-BEHAVIORAL THERAPIES.   CBT has been found efficacious whether treatment is provided individually or in a group, in a clinic or in a school. Due to its relevance to many treatment and prevention efforts, a brief overview of Kendall's (1990) *Coping Cat* treatment protocol is presented next, followed by a summary of CBT treatment outcome studies.

Coping Cat (Kendall, 1990) was the first CBT treatment protocol with demonstrated efficacy for the treatment of child and adolescent anxiety disorders (Kendall, 1994). The protocol is organized such that during the first half of treatment the therapist educates the child about anxiety and teaches him or her somatic management and cognitive coping strategies. Newly learned knowledge and skills are then consolidated and used to develop a FEAR plan. *FEAR* is an acronym that is used to remind the child of steps he or she needs to take when feeling anxious. The *F* refers to frightened feelings and reminds the child to use physical symptoms of anxiety as signals to implement coping strategies. The *E* prompts the child to monitor anxious self-talk that could lead him or her to expect bad things to happen. The *A* serves as a reminder to employ attitudes and actions to counter anxiety. The *R* encourages the child to reflect on results and to reward him- or herself for efforts to cope with her anxiety. Once the FEAR plan is developed, it is applied in graduated and controlled exposure activities, both in and outside of therapy sessions, until eventually the child is able to manage anxiety in response to the most feared or dreaded situations. In the final session of therapy, relapse prevention plans are made with parents to help insure that the child is able to generalize and maintain the skills learned in therapy.

As can be seen, there is considerable overlap between behavioral therapy and CBT. The primary distinction between the two lies in the emphasis they place on cognitive interventions. Whereas cognitive-behavioral therapies focus on changing dysfunctional thoughts directly, behavioral therapies aim to change behavior, which in turn decreases distressing or dysfunctional thoughts and feelings (March & Albano, 2002).

Research conducted by six different groups of researchers in four different countries provides evidence in support of the efficacy of cognitive behavioral interventions for the treatment of child and adolescent anxiety disorders. CBT has been found to be superior to a wait-list or no-treatment control group in multiple randomized studies involving children and adolescents (Barrett, 1998; Barrett, Dadds & Rapee, 1996; Flannery-Schroeder & Kendall, 2000; Hayward, Varady, Albano, Thienemann, Henderson & Schatzberg, 2000; Kendall, 1994; Kendall, Flannery-Schroeder, Panichelli-Mindel, Southam-Gerow, Henin & Warman, 1997; Mendlowitz, Manassis, Bradley, Scapillato, Mietzitis & Shaw, 1999; Muris, Meesters & van Melick, 2002; Rapee, 2000; Shortt, Barrett & Fox, 2001; Silverman, Kurtines, Ginsburg, Weems, Lumpkin & Carmichael, 1999; Spence et al., 2000).

Across the eight CBT studies cited above, that reported recovery rates (Barrett, 1998; Barrett et al., 1996; Flannery-Schroeder & Kendall, 2000; Hayward et al., 2000; Kendall et al., 1997; Shortt et al., 2001; Silverman et al., 1999a; Spence et al., 2000), the average recovery rate for the CBT condition immediately following treatment was 70.4% compared to 24.1% for the control condition. In one study that compared group CBT to an attention control group (Ginsburg & Drake, 2002b), recovery rates at post-intervention were 75% and 20% respectively (Ginsburg & Drake, 2002b) and were comparable to those found when individual-focused CBT is compared with wait-list or no-treatment control groups.

Follow-up recovery rates suggest that treatment gains for CBT interventions can be maintained over time. Across four studies, an average of 72.1% of CBT participants no longer met diagnostic criteria for their pre-treatment primary anxiety disorder diagnosis a year following treatment (Barrett, 1998; Barrett et al., 1996; Hayward et al.,

2000; Spence et al., 2000). There is also evidence to suggest that treatment gains for CBT can be maintained up to six years later (Barrett, Duffy, Dadds & Rapee, 2001).

Several other studies have compared the effectiveness of different delivery formats for CBT (e.g., group format, child-focused format). For the most part, the main effect for format appears equivocal (Barrett, 1998; Barrett et al., 2001; Cobham, Dadds & Spence, 1998; Flannery-Schroeder & Kendall, 2000), with the exception of one study that found individual therapy superior to group in the treatment of socially anxious children (Manassis et al., 2002).

The contributions of a parent component to treatment success appear to vary according to particular child and parent characteristics. Findings from two studies suggest that greater parental involvement may result in enhanced treatment outcomes for younger children, girls, and children with anxious parents (Barrett et al., 1996; Cobham et al., 1998).

The above review suggests that there is ample evidence of the superiority of CBT over no treatment at all. However, studies using no-treatment control groups do not provide information as to the relative superiority of CBT compared to other treatments. Two studies were recently conducted that compared CBT to educational support (ES) and yielded unexpected findings.

Last, Hansen, and Franco (1998) compared CBT to ES in the treatment of school phobia in children and adolescents. Both treatments resulted in a decrease in anxious and depressed symptoms and were equally efficacious in improving school attendance. ES also served as the control condition in a study conducted by Silverman, Kurtines, Ginsburg, Weems, Rabian, and Serafini (1999b). They compared ES to contingency management (CM) and exposure-based cognitive self-control (SC) in the treatment of child and adolescent SD, SocP, and Ag. All three groups demonstrated gains across various outcomes at the end of treatment and at 12-month follow-up. Taken together, these results suggest that treatment studies should move beyond using no-treatment control conditions and include other types of control groups.

The majority of studies related to child and adolescent anxiety disorders have been conducted with European American youth. Thus, a question can be raised as to the extent to which such findings are applicable to youth from other racial and ethnic groups. For those studies that investigated ethnic and racial differences in treatment effects, the overall results appear to suggest that there are more similarities across groups than there are differences. Treadwell, Flannery-Schoeder, and Kendall (1995) found that CBT resulted in equally significant reductions in anxious symptoms and high recovery rates for African American and European American youth. Results from a CBT treatment study conducted by Pina, Silverman, Fuentes, Kurtines, and Weems (2003) indicated that, compared to European American subjects, Hispanic/Latino youth demonstrated similar recovery rates (83.9% and 84.2% respectively) and a similar level of clinically significant change in internalizing symptomatology at post-treatment, and similarly favorable outcomes at 12-month follow-up.

Two other studies investigated factors related to child responsiveness to CBT treatment. Southam-Gerow, Kendall, and Weersing (2001) found that younger age, lower levels of pre-treatment internalizing psychopathology, and lower levels of maternal depressive symptoms were all associated with good treatment response immediately following treatment and at one-year follow-up. However, they found no effects for ethnicity or gender. Similarly, Silverman and colleagues (Berman, Weems, Silverman & Kurtines, 2000) found no association between child responsiveness to treatment and ethnicity or gender for their sample of Hispanic/Latino and European American youth. Instead, the best predictors of treatment outcome were child depression and trait anxiety and parent depression, hostility, and paranoia.

Taken together, these results suggest that CBT appears to be similarly effective for the treatment of anxiety disorders in African American, Hispanic/Latino, and European American youth.

Finally, it should be noted that treatment studies involving CBT have most frequently targeted SAD, GAD, and SocP. Fewer CBT studies have been conducted with children and adolescents suffering from SP, Ag, or PD.

What Might Work

EDUCATIONAL SUPPORT. As discussed earlier, two recent studies (Last et al., 1998; Silverman et al., 1999b) found that treatment effects for educational support (ES) were comparable to those for behavioral and CBT approaches for the treatment of a variety of phobias (school, SD, SocP, and Agora). In both studies, the ES condition utilized a group format and involved the sharing of information and discussions about anxiety disorders.

Similarities between the two studies suggest several possible explanations for the efficacy of ES. First, participants in both studies rated ES as highly credible. In addition, both studies involved a therapist who provided nonspecific therapeutic interventions such as support, empathy, and warmth. These similarities suggest the possibility that credibility and/or nonspecific therapeutic factors might have contributed to the effectiveness of ES. A third possible explanation for the success of ES is that psychoeducation is a major component of CBT approaches. Consequently, the two studies could be viewed as "dismantling" studies in which the efficacy of a treatment package is compared to one or more of its parts to determine which specific components are driving treatment effects. The findings from these two studies suggest that more dismantling studies involving phobias and other anxiety disorders appear warranted to determine if streamlined approaches (i.e., involving fewer components) would prove equally effective to the current, more comprehensive treatment models.

What Does Not Work

A review of the literature at this time did not identify any treatments that were studied in multiple RCTs and were found to be ineffective treatments for anxiety disorders.

Evidence-Based Treatment Interventions in Residential Settings

A review of the literature did not uncover reports of treatment procedures for anxiety disorders specific to residential settings.

Psychopharmacology

The past decade has brought significant advances in the pharmacological treatment of anxiety disorders in children and adolescents. Medication may be combined

**Table 1. Medications Used in the Treatment of Anxiety Disorders
(Controlled Trials Unless Indicated)**

Class	Anxiety Disorder(s)	Medication(s)	References
What works:			
Serotonin reuptake inhibitors (SSRIs)	OCD	Fluoxetine Fluvoxamine Paroxetine Sertraline	Geller et al., 2003 (meta-analysis of controlled trials)
	GAD, social phobia	Fluoxetine	Birmaher et al., 2003
	GAD, SAD, social phobia	Fluvoxamine	RUPP Anxiety Study Group, 2001
	GAD	Sertraline	Rynn et al., 2001
	Social phobia	Paroxetine	Wagner et al., 2002 (preliminary results)
Tricyclic antidepressants (TCAs)	OCD	Clomipramine	Geller et al., 2003 (meta-analysis of controlled trials)
What might work:			
Noradrenergic antidepressants	GAD	Venlafaxine	Rynn et al., 2002 (preliminary results)
SSRIs	Panic disorder	Fluoxetine and other SSRIs	Renaud et al., 1999 (open trial)
Buspirone	GAD	Buspirone	No controlled studies
Benzodiazepines	GAD, SAD	Clonazepam	Labellarte et al., 1999
	Panic disorder	Alprazolam	(review: conflicting results)
TCAs	SAD and others (School phobia)	Imipramine	Labellarte et al., 1999 (review: conflicting results)

Note: OCD = Obsessive-compulsive disorder, GAD = generalized anxiety disorder, SAD = separation anxiety disorder,

with CBT for several reasons, including acute reduction of symptoms in a severely anxious child, management of co-morbid disorders, addressing risk factors that require different interventions, and augmentation of CBT when there is a partial response (March, 2002). Table 1 includes medications used in the treatment of anxiety disorders.

Medications that Work in the Treatment of Anxiety Disorders

SEROTONIN REUPTAKE INHIBITORS (SSRIs). Several RCTs have established SSRIs as the medications of choice for the following anxiety disorders in adolescents: OCD, GAD, SAD, SocP, and possibly PD. SSRIs increase the level of serotonin available in the brain by inhibiting reuptake of serotonin. A low level of serotonin has been hypothesized to be associated with a number of psychiatric disorders, including anxiety, depression, and autism. Side effects with the SSRIs are often transient and mild. The most common side effects include gastrointestinal symptoms (decreased appetite, nausea, stomachache, diarrhea), increased activity level, sleep difficulties (drowsiness or insomnia). Less common side effects include dry mouth, agitation, manic symptoms, or muscle twitching. Decreased libido and sexual function may also occur and can lead to noncompliance with medications if the adolescent is not informed of this. Recently, the FDA has recommended that these medications need to be monitored closely during initiation, dosing changes, and discontinuation, with particular attention to depressive symptoms and suicidal ideation.

CLOMIPRAMINE. Clomipramine is a tricyclic antidepressant (TCA). It has been shown to be effective for adolescent OCD and can be used alone. However, due to frequent side effects (dry mouth, dizziness, constipation, sedation) and need for cardiac monitoring, it is often used at low doses to augment the effect of an SSRI for OCD (Geller et al., 2003).

The efficacy of medications other than SSRIs and clomipramine for the treatment of anxiety disorders (including OCD) in adolescents has not been shown.

Medications that Might Work in the Treatment of Anxiety Disorders

NORADRENERGIC ANTIDEPRESSANTS. In clinical practice, noradrenergic antidepressants such as venlafaxine and tricyclic antidepressants are potential alternatives when SSRIs have not been successful in the treatment of adolescent anxiety disorders. No controlled studies are currently available for medication treatment of PD in adolescents, but SSRIs appear to be promising (Renaud, Birmaher, Wassick & Bridge, 1999). When severe PD is present, adjunct treatment with a benzodiazepine may also be helpful (Renaud et al., 1999) in reducing symptoms.

BENZODIAZEPINES. Benzodiazepines were commonly used to treat anxiety disorders such as GAD, severe SP, and PD prior to the development of SSRIs, but are now often used to supplement other medications in the treatment of anxiety disorders. Benzodiazepines can help to reduce severe anxiety symptoms and avoidance until SSRIs take effect. However, there is risk for dependence after prolonged use of benzodiazepines and they are contraindicated for adolescents with substance abuse disorders (Riddle et al., 1999). Side effects need to be monitored closely and include sedation, disinhibition, cognitive impairment, and difficulty with discontinuation (Labellarte, Ginsburg, Walkup, & Riddle, 1999).

BUSPIRONE. Buspirone is used by clinicians as an alternative to SSRIs for treatment of GAD, but no controlled studies exist to support its efficacy in adolescents. Unlike the benzodiazepines, there is no risk of dependence in the long term. The most common side effects in adolescents are lightheadedness, headache, and upset stomach (Salazar et al., 2001).

Medication Treatment of Anxiety Disorders and Co-Morbid Disorders

It is important to consider treatment of co-occurring conditions in the medication treatment of adolescent anxiety disorders. If severe depression is present along with the anxiety disorder, initiation of antidepressant treatment (preferably an SSRI) may be necessary before the adolescent can benefit from CBT (Labellarte et al., 1999). Careful and regular monitoring for suicidal risk during treatment and recovery from depression is important. Attention-deficit/hyperactivity disorder (ADHD) is another common co-morbid disorder in adolescents with anxiety disorders. Co-morbid anxiety does not seem to diminish the response of core ADHD symptoms to stimulant medication (MTA Cooperative Group, 2001). Clinicians commonly use SSRIs and stimulants together when anxiety disorders and ADHD co-occur, but it is important to monitor for side effects as a subset of anxious children may develop increased insomnia or anxiety on stimulant medications.

The Prevention of Anxiety Disorders

Primary prevention and health promotion encompass those planned activities that help participants prevent predictable problems, protect existing states of health and healthy functioning, and promote desired goals for a specified population. Prevention programs can be classified according to the population targeted for the preventive intervention (Institute of Medicine, 1994). *Universal* prevention activities are intended for all members of a general population. *Selective* prevention activities target subgroups of a population who may be at above-average risk for developing a disorder. Spence (2001) identified several groups of children and adolescents who are at particular risk for anxiety disorders. These groups include children with anxious parents, an anxious/resistant attachment style, temperaments characterized by behavioral inhibition or high negativity combined with low effortful control, and those exposed to traumatic or stress life events. *Indicated* prevention activities are designed for those individuals who are already demonstrating some characteristics of the disorder and are at enhanced risk of increased psychopathology. Children and adolescents appropriate for an indicated prevention intervention would be those who have early symptoms of anxiety but do not meet full criteria for an anxiety disorder.

A primary strategy for many prevention efforts is to target malleable risk and protective factors, i.e., to eliminate or decrease identified risk factors for the targeted disorder and/or introduce or augment protective factors. Although some risk factors may influence a child's development at any point in time (e.g., traumatic life events, parental anxiety), still others may only be influential at particular points in time (e.g., start of formal schooling). During adolescence, Spence (2001) proposed that parental anxiety, the transition to high school, and elevated levels of anxious symptoms serve as risk factors. As will be seen in subsequent sections, most prevention efforts targeting anxiety disorders have taken a developmental perspective and target malleable risk and protective factors.

What Works

Several studies conducted in Australia have demonstrated the benefits of two variations of a group CBT approach: (a) the *FRIENDS* program (Barrett, Lowry-Webster & Holmes, 1999) for use as a universal and selective prevention intervention, and (b) its cousin, *Coping Koala* (Barrett et al., 1996), as an indicated prevention program. These programs are based originally on Kendall's (1990) *Coping Cat* program.

FRIENDS FOR CHILDREN.   Three studies have investigated the benefits of the *FRIENDS* program (Barrett et al., 1999) as a universal prevention strategy. *FRIENDS* consists of ten weekly sessions and two booster sessions, along with four evening sessions for parents. In the Barrett & Turner (2001) study, 489 sixth-graders (10–13-year-olds) were randomly assigned to either a usual care (UC) condition (i.e., standard social studies curriculum), a psychologist-led *FRIENDS* group, or a teacher-led *FRIENDS* group. At the completion of the program, participants in both treatment conditions reported significantly fewer anxious symptoms than those in the UC condition. No significant differences were found between the two treatment groups. When "at-risk" students (i.e., those with elevated symptoms at the start of the program) were compared across conditions, a greater number in the two treatment conditions were found to have moved into the "healthy" category at post-treatment compared to those in UC.

Lowry-Webster, Barrett, and Dadds (2001) also investigated the *FRIENDS* program as a universal prevention program. Study participants included 594 sixth-grade children (10–13-years-olds) who were randomly assigned to either a treatment or wait-list condition. At the end of treatment, both groups showed significant decreases in self-reported anxiety and depression. However, when highly anxious participants (i.e., those who scored above the clinical cut-off) were compared between conditions, only the treatment group showed significant decreases in anxiety and depression at post-treatment. At one-year follow-up, Lowry-Webster, Barrett, and Lock (2003) found that 85% of the treatment group who had originally scored above the clinical cut-off for anxiety and depression were diagnosis-free compared to only 31.2% of the control group. Other intervention gains as measured by self-report and diagnostic interviews were also maintained by both the universal and high-anxiety group in the treatment condition.

Immigrants frequently experience anxiety in conjunction with the stress associated with migration. Thus, adolescents who are immigrants may be appropriate candidates for selective prevention efforts. Barrett, Moore, and Sonderegger (2000) conducted a preliminary investigation of the efficacy of the *FRIENDS* program for use with adolescent girls who had recently immigrated to Australia from Yugoslavia. Teachers referred girls to the program who appeared stressed, worried, or sad. The girls were subsequently assigned to *FRIENDS* or a wait-list condition. Results at post-treatment indicated that girls in the treatment group exhibited significantly fewer anxiety symptoms and that girls in the control group experienced an increase in internalizing symptoms (anxiety, depression, and withdrawn behaviors) over time.

COPING KOALA. Dadds and colleagues (Dadds, Spence, Holland, Barrett & Laurens, 1997) investigated the effectiveness of *The Coping Koala* (Barrett et al., 1996) program as an indicated and early-treatment program. Children and adolescents were randomly assigned to either the treatment or monitoring condition if they either (a) met criteria for a *DSM-IV* anxiety disorder with mild impairment in functioning or (b) did not meet criteria for disorder but had symptoms of anxiety or a "nonspecific sensitivity." *Coping Koala* includes ten group sessions and three parent sessions. Results at post-intervention indicated that both groups showed improvement with nonsignificant differences between groups. At six-month follow-up continued improvement was seen in the treatment group, but some backsliding was found in the control group. At six-month follow-up, significant differences were also found between the percentage of treatment and control groups who met full criteria for an anxiety disorder (16% and 54%, respectively). Dadds, Holland, Laurens,

Mullins, Barrett, and Spence (1999) found that the groups converged at one-year follow-up, but then the intervention group demonstrated significantly better outcomes at two-year follow-up. Pretreatment symptom severity was the sole predictor of chronicity at two-year follow-up (Dadds et al., 1999).

In concert, these results suggest that a group CBT intervention shows promise in preventing anxiety disorders and that durable reductions can occur for those demonstrating high risk or mild severity in diagnosable disorders.

PREVENTING ANXIETY DUE TO MEDICAL PROCEDURES.   Children who undergo painful or stressful medical procedures are at heightened risk for the development of phobias and other anxiety disorders. Selective prevention efforts include a number of techniques that are now widely used to attenuate children's anxiety during medical procedures. These anxiety reduction techniques include sharing information about the procedure, modeling demonstrations, and training in such coping strategies as comforting self-talk, mental imagery (e.g., imagining one's personal hero undergoing the procedure), and cue-controlled relaxation (for review see Spence, 2001).

What Might Work

I CAN DO PROGRAM.   The *I Can Do* program (Dubow, Schmidt, McBride, Edwards & Merk, 1993) is a universal prevention program designed to teach children coping skills to use in response to stressful experiences. The program was evaluated in one RCT in which 88 forth-grade students were randomly assigned to either a treatment or delayed-intervention control group. Results indicated that the treatment group demonstrated significant improvement in their ability to generate effective solutions to stressful situations as well as in their self-efficacy to implement effective solutions to two targeted stressors (i.e., loved one's death, parents' divorce). At follow-up, participants in the treatment condition maintained post-treatment gains in the ability to generate solutions to four out of five stressors and demonstrated continued improvement in their self-efficacy scores. Although preliminary findings are promising, they are based on self-report measures and reactions to hypothetical situations. Thus, this intervention warrants further study involving larger sample sizes, children and adolescents of various ages, and multi-method assessment procedures.

PARENT–CHILD PROGRAM FOR ANXIOUS-WITHDRAWN PRESCHOOLERS.   As discussed earlier, a pattern of anxious-withdrawn behavior places a child at increased risk for anxiety disorders. Recently, LaFreniere and Capuano (1997) conducted an indicated preventive intervention targeting anxious-withdrawn preschool children and their mothers. Parent-child dyads were randomly assigned to either a treatment or no-treatment control condition. The treatment was grounded in attachment, cognitive, and behavioral perspectives. It was home-based and attempted to enhance mothers' understanding of the developmental needs of their preschool child, increase parenting competence, decrease parenting stress, and provide social support. Immediately following the intervention, mothers in the treatment group demonstrated more appropriate control strategies than mothers in the control group. Compared to controls, children in the treatment group also showed an increase in cooperation and enthusiasm in a problem-solving task with their mothers and an increase in teacher-rated social competence. These results suggest that a home-based indicated prevention program for preschoolers and their mothers shows promise and warrants further investigation.

THE MACQUARIE UNIVERSITY PRESCHOOL INTERVENTION PROGRAM (RAPEE, 2002). The Macquarie University Preschool Intervention Program is a selective prevention program for behaviorally inhibited preschoolers, aged 3.5–4.5. According to Rapee (2002), the program targets children with inhibited temperament because several other risk factors (i.e., parental anxiety, modeling and verbal instruction in avoidant behavior, and environmental support of avoidant coping) are likely to be moderated or mediated by this temperament style.

Rapee (2002) provided preliminary data from an ongoing investigation in which inhibited preschoolers were randomly assigned to either a treatment or monitoring condition. The program consisted of six sessions in which parents are educated in techniques to help their children become more social and confident. Parents learned about the nature of anxious-withdrawn behavior, strategies to manage their own anxiety, ways to model competent behavior and promote independence, and proce-dures for developing and implementing an exposure hierarchy with their children. Preliminary results indicated that only 60% of children in both groups were still demonstrating behaviorally inhibited behavior one year after the initial assessment. However, group differences were found in rates of anxiety diagnoses within that time, with significantly fewer anxiety diagnoses in treatment group children com-pared to controls. These findings are particularly noteworthy given the brevity of the intervention.

In summary, preventive interventions for anxiety disorders are beginning to emerge from different sources. Some prevention efforts have been adapted from suc-cessful treatment protocols, while others have been developed from theoretical and empirical findings regarding specific risk factors for anxiety disorders. Although the prevention of anxiety disorders is still in its infancy, efforts to date provide an opti-mistic outlook for the continued success of future work.

Recommendations

Anxiety disorders represent a prevalent and significant form of psychopatholo-gy in youth that can significantly interfere with their current and future well-being and adjustment. Empirical studies support the efficacy of various treatment approaches and have demonstrated the promise of others for the majority of young people who undergo treatment.

- For the treatment of anxiety disorders, behavioral and cognitive-behavioral treatments have the most evidence in support of their efficacy at this time. There is some evidence to suggest that current treatments are efficacious for European American, Latino/ Hispanic, and African American youths. However, further work is needed to determine what treatments work for young people from other racial and ethnic backgrounds.
- Anxiety disorders often co-occur with other mood disorders, depression, and disrup-tive behavior disorders. These co-morbid disorders need to be identified and treated, along with the primary anxiety disorder.

- Medication, such as SSRIs, may be combined with behavioral or cognitive-behavioral treatments when symptoms are severe, co-morbid disorders are present, risk factors exist that require different interventions, or to supplement behavioral or cognitive-behavioral interventions when there is a partial response (March, 2002).
- Social skills training appears to be a promising treatment component for children and adolescents with SocP.
- Far more work has been done to develop treatment interventions for child and adolescent anxiety disorders than preventive interventions, but several prevention trials are underway and are generating promising results. Adaptations of CBT have been used successfully with school-aged youth in universal, selective, and indicated prevention efforts up to this time. However, because most prevention trials have been conducted in Australia with relatively homogenous populations, the validity of these findings for youth from diverse racial or ethnic groups is not yet known.
- There is limited information currently available as to the role of parents in the treatment and prevention of anxiety disorders. Parental involvement in treatment appears most beneficial for younger children, girls, and when parents are anxious themselves. There is some preliminary evidence to suggest that prevention interventions targeting parents or parent–child dyads can be beneficial for preschool-aged children who display inhibited temperaments or a pattern of anxious-withdrawn behaviors.
- Further work is needed to identify effective treatments for the approximately 25–30% of treated youth who do not respond well to current treatments.

Finally, it is important to note that treatment and prevention interventions for anxiety disorders can only be successful if targeted youth are identified and provided access to the interventions. Thus, identification and accessibility represent two of the most pressing needs to be addressed in the future, especially for youth living in disadvantaged and resource-scarce communities.

References

Albano, A.M., Chorpita, B.F., & Barlow, D.H. (2003). Childhood anxiety disorders. In E.J. Mash & R.A. Barkley (Eds.), *Child Psychopathology*, 2nd ed. (pp. 279–329). New York: Guilford Press.

Albano, A.M., & Kendall, P.C. (2002). Cognitive behavioural therapy for children and adolescents with anxiety disorders: Clinical research advances. *International Review of Psychiatry, 14*, 129–134.

American Psychiatric Association (2000). *The Diagnostic and Statistical Manual, Fourth Edition, Text Revision.* New York: Author.

Bandura, A., Blanchard, E.B., & Ritter, B. (1969). Relative efficacy of desensitization and modeling approaches for inducing behavioral, affective, and attitudinal changes. *Journal of Personality and Social Psychology, 13*, 173–199.

Barabasz, A.F. (1973). Group desensitization of test anxiety in elementary school. *The Journal of Psychology, 83*, 295–301.

Barrett, P.M. (1998). Evaluation of cognitive-behavioral group treatments for childhood anxiety disorders. *Journal of Clinical Child Psychology, 27*, 459–468.

Barrett, P.M., Dadds, M.R., & Rapee, R.M. (1996). Family treatment of childhood anxiety: A controlled trial. *Journal of Consulting and Clinical Psychology, 64*, 333–342.

Barrett, P.M., Duffy, A.L., Dadds, M.R., & Rapee, R.M. (2001). Cognitive-behavioral treatment of anxiety disorders in children: Long-term (6-year) follow-up. *Journal of Consulting and Clinical Psychology, 69*, 135–141.

Barrett, P.M., Lowry-Webster, H., & Holmes, J. (1999). *Friends for children group leader manual* (2nd ed.). Brisbane, Australia: Australian Academic Press.

Barrett, P.M., Moore, A.F., & Sonderegger, R. (2000). The FRIENDS program for young former-Yugoslavian refugees in Australia: A pilot study. *Behaviour Change, 17*, 124–133.

Barrett, P.M., Rapee, R.M., Dadds, M.M., & Ryan, S.M. (1996). Family enhancement of cognitive style in anxious and aggressive children. *Journal of Abnormal Child Psychology, 24*, 187–203.

Barrett, P.M., & Turner, C. (2001). Prevention of anxiety symptoms in primary school children: Preliminary results from a universal school-based trial. *British Journal of Clinical Psychology, 40*, 399–410.

Beidel, D., & Turner, S. (1998). *Shy Children, Phobic Adults: Nature and Treatment of Social Phobia*. Washington, DC: American Psychological Association.

Beidel, D.C., Turner, S.M., & Morris, T.L. (2000). Behavioral treatment of childhood social phobia. *Journal of Consulting and Clinical Psychology, 68*, 1072–1080.

Beidel, D.C., Turner, S.M., & Tracy, L. (1999). Psychopathology of childhood social phobia. *Journal of the American Academy of Child an Adolescent Psychiatry, 38*, 643–650.

Benjamin, R.S., Costello, E., & Warren, M. (1990). Anxiety disorders in a pediatric sample. *Journal of Anxiety Disorders, 4*, 293–316.

Berman, S.L., Kurtines, W.K., Silverman, W.K., & Serafini, L.T. (1996). The impact of exposure to crime and violence in urban youth. *American Journal of Orthopsychiatry, 66*, 329–336.

Berman, S.L., Weems, C.F., Silverman, W.K., & Kurtines, W.M. (2000). Predictors of outcome in exposure-based cognitive and behavioral treatment for phobia and anxiety disorders in children. *Behavior Therapy, 31*, 713–731.

Biederman, J., Rosenbaum, J.F., Bolduc-Murphy, E.A., Faraone, S.V., Chaloff, J., Hirshfeld, D.R., et al. (1993). A 3-year follow-up of children with and without behavioral inhibition. *Journal of the American Academy of Child and Adolescent Psychiatry, 32*, 814–821.

Birmaher, B., Axelson, D., Monk, K., Kalas, C., Clark, D., Ehmann, M., et al., (2003). Fluoxetine for the treatment of childhood anxiety disorders. *Journal of American Academy Child & Adolescent Psychiatry, 42*, 415–423.

Boer, F., Markus, M.T., Maingay, R., Lindhout, I.E., Borst, S.R., & Hoogendijk, T.H. (2002). Negative life events of anxiety disordered children: Bad fortune, vulnerability, or reporter bias? *Child Psychiatry & Human Development, 32*, 187–199.

Bowlby, J. (1988). *A Secure Base: Clinical Applications of Attachment Theory*. London: Tavistock-Routledge.

Cobham, V.E. (1998). The case for involving the family in the treatment of childhood anxiety. *Behaviour Change, 15*, 203–212.

Cobham, V.E., Dadds, M.R., & Spence, S.H. (1998). The role of parental anxiety in the treatment of childhood anxiety. *Journal of Consulting and Clinical Psychology, 66*, 893–905.

Compas, B.E., Connor-Smith, J.K., Saltzman, H., Thomsen, A.H., & Wadsworth, M.E. (2001). Coping with stress during childhood and adolescence: Problems, progress, and potential in theory and research. *Psychological Bulletin, 127* (1), 87–127.

Compas, B.E., Slavin, L.A., Wagner, B.A., & Vannatta, K. (1986). Relationship of life events and social support with psychological dysfunction among adolescents. *Journal of Youth and Adolescence, 15*, 205–221.

Cooley, M.R., Turner, S.M., & Beidel, D.C. (1995). Assessing community violence: The children's report of exposure to violence. *Journal of the American Academy of Child and Adolescent Psychiatry 34*, (2), 201–208.

Costello, E.J., & Angold, A. (1995). Epidemiology. In J. March (Ed.), *Anxiety Disorders in Children and Adolescents* (pp. 109–124). New York: Guilford Press.

Dadds, M.R., Barrett, P.M., Rapee, R.M., & Ryan, S. (1996). Family processes and child anxiety and aggression: An observational study. *Journal of Abnormal Child Psychology, 24*, 715–734.

Dadds, M.R., Holland, D.E., Laurens, K,. R., Mullins, M., Barrett, P., & Spence, S.H. (1999). Early intervention and prevention of anxiety disorders in children: Results at 2-year follow-up. *Journal of Consulting and Clinical Psychology, 67*, 145–150.

Dadds, M.R. & Roth, J.H. (2001). Family processes in the development of anxiety problems. In M. Vasey & M. Dadds (Eds.), *The Developmental Psychopathology of Anxiety* (pp. 278–303). New York: Oxford University Press.

Dadds, M.R., Spence, S.H., Holland, D.E., Barrett, P.M., & Laurens, K.R. (1997). Prevention and early intervention for anxiety disorders: A controlled trial. *Journal of Consulting and Clinical Psychology, 65*, 627–635.

Davey, G.C. (1997). A conditioning model of phobias. In G. Davey (Ed.), *Phobias: A Handbook of theory, Research and Treatment* (pp. 301–322). Chichester, UK: Wiley.

Demaray, M.K., & Malecki, C.K. (2002). The relationship between perceived social spport and maladjustment for students at risk. *Psychology in the Schools, 39*, 305–315.

Demaray, M.K., & Malecki, C.K. (2004). Critical levels of perceived social support associated with student adjustment. *School Psychology Quarterly, 17,* 213–241.

Donovan, C.L., & Spence, S.H. (2000). Prevention of childhood anxiety disorders. *Clinical Psychology Review, 20,* 509–531.

Dubow, E.F., Edwards, S., & Ippolito, M.F. (1997). LIfe stressors, neighborhood disadvantage, and resources: A focus on inner-city children's adjustment. *Journal of Clinical Child Psychology, 26,* 130–144.

Dubow, E.F., Schmidt, D., McBride, J., Edwards, S., & Merk, F.L. (1993). Teaching children to cope with stressful experiences: Initial implementation and evaluation of a primary prevention program. *Journal of Clinical Child Psychology, 22,* 428–440.

Dumas, J.E., LaFrenier, P.J., & Serketich, W.J. (1995). Balance of power: A transactional analysis of control in mother-child dyads involving socially competent, aggressive, and anxious children. *Journal of Abnormal Psychology, 104,* 104–113.

Eley, T.C. (2001). Contributions of behavioral genetics research: Quantifying genetic, shared environmental and nonshared environmental influences. In M. Vasey & M. Dadds (Eds.), *The Developmental Psychopathology of Anxiety* (pp. 45–59). London, England: University of London, Institute of Psychiatry.

Ezpeleta, L., Keeler, G., Erkanli, A., Costello, E.J., & Angold, A. (2001). Epidemiology of psychiatric disability in childhood and adolescence. *Journal of Child Psychology & Psychiatry & Allied Disciplines, 42,* 901–914.

Field, A.P., & Davey, G.C. (2001). Conditioning models of childhood anxiety. In W.K. Wilverman & P.D. Treffers (Eds.), *Anxiety Disorders in Children and Adolescents* (pp. 187–211). New York: Cambridge University Press.

Fitzpatrick, K.M., & Boldizar, J.P. (1993). The prevalence and consequences of exposure to violence among African-American youth. *Journal of the American Academy of Child and Adolescent Psychiatry, 32,* 424–430.

Flannery-Schroeder, E.C., & Kendall, P.C. (2000). Group and individual cognitive-behavioral treatments for youth with anxiety disorders: A randomized clinical trial. *Cognitive Therapy and Research, 24,* 251–278.

Ford, T., Goodman, R., & Meltzer, H. (2003). The British child and adolescent mental health survey 1999: The prevalence of DSM-IV disorders. *Journal of the American Academy of Child and Adolescent Psychiatry, 42,* 1203–1211.

Fox, N.A., & Calkins, S. (1993). Social withdrawal: Interactions among temperament, attachment, and regulation. In K.H. Rubin & J.B. Asendorpf (Eds.), *Social Withdrawal, Inhibition, and Shyness in Childhood* (pp. 81–100). Hillsdale, NJ: Erlbaum.

Fox, N.A., Henderson, H. & Rubin, K.H., Calkins, S.D., & Schmidt, L.A. (2001). Continuity and discontinuity of behavioral inhibition and exuberance: Psychophysiological and behavioral influences across the first four years of life. *Child Development, 72,* 1–21.

Freeman, L.N., Mokros, H., & Poznanski, E.O. (1993). Violent events reported by normal urban school-aged children: Characteristics and depression correlates. *Journal of the American Academy of Child and Adolescent Psychiatry, 32,* 419–423.

Garcia-Coll, C., Kagan, J., & Reznick, J.S. (1984). Behavioural inhibition in young children. *Child Development, 55,* 1005–1019.

Geller, D.A., Biederman, J., Stewart, S.E., Mullin, B., Martin, A., Spencer, T., et al. (2003). Which SSRI? A meta-analysis of pharmacotherapy trials in pediatric obsessive-compulsive disorder. *American Journal Psychiatry, 160,* 1919–1928.

Gerull, F.C., & Rapee, R.M. (2002). Mother knows best: The effects of maternal modeling on the acquisition of fear and avoidance in toddlers. *Behavior Research and Therapy, 40,* 169–178.

Ginsburg, G.S., & Drake, K.L. (2002a). Anxiety sensitivity and panic attack symptomatology among low-income African-American adolescents. *Anxiety Disorders, 16,* 83–96.

Ginsburg, G.S., & Drake, K.L. (2002b). School-based treatment for anxious African-American adolescents: A controlled pilot study. *Journal of the American Academy of Child and Adolescent Psychiatry, 41,* 768–775.

Gladstein, J. Rusonis, E.J., & Heald, F.P. (1992). A comparison of inner-city and upper-middle class youths' exposure to violence. *Journal of Adolescent Health, 13,* 275–280.

Goodwin, R.D., Fergusson, D.M., & Horwood, L.J. (2004). Early anxious/withdrawn behaviours predict later internalising disorders. *Journal of Child Psychology and Psychiatry, 45,* 874–883.

Goodyer, I.M., & Altham, P.M. (1991). Lifetime exit events and recent social and family adversities in anxious and depressed school-aged children. *Journal of Affective Disorders, 21,* 219–228.

Hayward, C., Killen, J.D., Kraemer, H.C., & Taylor, C.B. (2000). Predictors of panic attacks in adolescents. *Journal of the American Academy of Child and Adolescent Psychiatry, 39* (2), 207–214.

Hayward, C., Varady, S., Albano, A.M., Thienemann, M., Henderson, L., & Schatzberg, A.F. (2000). Cognitive-behavioral group therapy for social phobia in female adolescents: Results of a pilot study. *Journal of the American Academy of Child & Adolescent Psychiatry, 39,* 721–726.

Hirshfeld, D.R., Biederman, J., Brody, L., Faraone, S.V., & Rosenbaum, J.F. (1997). Expressed emotion toward children with behavioral inhibition and psychopathology: A pilot study. *Journal of the American Academy of Child and Adolescent Psychiatry, 36,* 910–917.

Hudson, J.L., & Rapee, R.M. (2001). Parent—child interactions and anxiety disorders: An observational study. *Behaviour Research & Therapy, 39* (12)1411–1427.

Institute of Medicine (1994). *Reducing Risks for Mental Disorders: Frontiers for Preventive Intervention Research.* Washington, DC: National Academy Press.

Kagan, J., Reznick, J.S., & Snidman, N. (1987). The physiology and psychology of behavioural inhibition in children. *Child Development, 58,* 1459–1473.

Kagan, J. (1997). Temperament and the reactions to unfamiliarity. *Child Development, 68,* 139–143.

Kagan, J., Snidman, N., Zentner, M., & Peterson, E. (1999). Infant temperament and anxious symptoms in school age children. *Development and Psychopathology, 11,* 209–224.

Kearney, C.A., Albano, A.M., Eisen, A.R., Allan, W.D., & Barlow, D.H. (1997). The phenomenology of panic disorders in youngsters: An empirical study of a clinical sample. *Journal of Anxiety Disorders, 11,* 49–62.

Kendall, P.C. (1990). *Coping Cat workbook.* Ardmore, PA: Workbook Publishing.

Kendall, P.C. (1994). Treating anxiety disorders in children: Results of a randomized clinical trial. *Journal of Consulting and Clinical Psychology, 62,* 100–110.

Kendall, P.C., Aschenbrand, S.G., & Hudson, J.L. (2003). Child-focused treatment of anxiety. In A. Kazdin & J. Weisz (Eds.), *Evidence-Based Psychotherapies for Children and Adolescents* (pp. 81–100). New York: The Guilford Press.

Kendall, P.C., Flannery-Schroeder, E., Panichelli-Mindel, S., Southam-Gerow, M., Henin, A., & Warman, M. (1997). Therapy for youths with anxiety disorders: A second randomized clinical trial. *Journal of Consulting and Clinical Psychology, 65,* 366–380.

Kim-Cohen, J., Caspi, A., Moffitt, T.E., Harrington, H., Milne, B.J., & Poulton, R. (2003). Prior juvenile diagnoses in adults with mental disorder: Development follow-back of a prospective-longitudingal cohort. *Archives of General Psychiatry, 60,* 709–717.

Kondas, O. (1967). Reduction of examination anxiety and "stage fright" by group desensitization and relaxation. *Behaviour Research and Therapy, 5,* 275–281.

Krohne, H.W., & Hock, M. (1991). Relationships between restrictive mother-child interactions and anxiety of the child. *Anxiety Research, 4,* 109–124.

Labellarte, M.J., Ginsburg, G.S., Walkup, J.T., & Riddle, M.A. (1999). The treatment of anxiety disorders in children and adolescents. *Biological Psychiatry, 46,* 1567–1578.

LaFreniere, P.J., & Capuano, F. (1997). Preventive intervention as means of clarifying direction of effects in socialization: Anxious-withdrawn preschoolers case. *Development and Psychopathology, 9,* 551–564.

La Greca, A.M. (2001). Friends or foe? Peer influences on anxiety among children and adolescents. In W.K. Silverman and P.D. Treffers (Eds.), *Anxiety Disorders in Children and Adolescents* (pp. 159–186). New York: Cambridge University Press.

Lang, P.J. (1968). Fear reduction and fear behavior: Problems in treating a construct. In J.M. Schlien (Ed.), *The Structure of Emotion* (pp. 18–30). Seattle, WA: Hogrefe & Huber.

Last, C., Hansen, C., & Franco, N. (1998). Cognitive-behavioral therapy of school phobia. *Journal of the American Academy of Child and Adolescent Psychiatry, 37,* 404–411.

Last, C.G., Perrin, S., Hersen, M., & Kazdin, A.E. (1996). A prospective study of childhood anxiety disorders. *Journal of the American Academy of Child and Adolescent Psychiatry, 35,* 1502–1510.

Lau, J.J., Calamari, J.E., & Waraczynski, M. (1996). Panic attack symptomatology and anxiety sensitivity in adolescents. *Journal of Anxiety Disorders, 10,* 355–364.

Lewis, S. (1974). A comparison of behavior therapy techniques in the reduction of fearful avoidance behavior. *Behavior Therapy, 5,* 648–655.

Leib, R., Wittchen, H., Hofler, M., Fuetsch, M., Stein, M., & Merikangas, K. (2000). Parenting psychopathology, parenting styles, and the risk of social phobia in offspring: A prospective, longitudinal community study. *Archives of General Psychiatry, 57,* 859–866.

Levitt, M.J., Guacci-Franco, N., & Levitt, J.L. (1994). Social support achievement in childhood and early adolescence: A multicultural study. *Journal of Applied Developmental Psychology, 15,* 207–222.

Lowry-Webster, H.M., Barrett, P.M., & Dadds, M.R. (2001). A universal prevention trial of anxiety and depressive symptomatology in childhood: Preliminary data from an Australian study. *Behaviour Change, 18,* 36–50.

Lowry-Webster, H.M., Barrett, P.M., & Lock, S. (2003). A universal prevention trial of anxiety symptomatology during childhood: Results at 1-year follow-up. *Behaviour Change, 20,* 35–43.

Manassis, K. (2001). Child-parent relations: Attachment and anxiety disorders. In W. Silverman & P. Treffers (Eds.), *Anxiety Disorders in Children and Adolescents: Research, Assessment, and Intervention* (pp. 255–272). New York: Cambridge University Press.

Manassis, K., & Hood, J. (1998). Individual and familial predictors of impairment in childhood anxiety disorders. *Journal of the American Academy of Child & Adolescent Psychiatry, 37,* 428–434.

Manassis, K., Mendlowitz, S.L., Scapillato, D., Avery, D., Fiksenbaum, L., Freire, M., et al. (2002). Group and individual cognitive-behavioral therapy for childhood anxiety disorers: A randomized trial. *Journal of the American Academy of Child and Adolescent Psychiatry, 41,* 1423–1430.

Mann, J., & Rosenthal, T.L. (1969). Vicarious and direct counter-conditioning of test anxiety through individual and group desensitization. *Behaviour Research and Therapy, 7,* 359–367.

March, J.S. (2002). Combining medication and psychosocial treatments: an evidence-based medicine approach. *International Review of Psychiatry, 14,* 155–163.

March, J.S., & Albano, A.M. (2002). Anxiety disorders in children and adolescents. In D. Stein & E. Hollander (Eds.), *Textbook of Anxiety Disorders* (pp. 415–427). Washington, DC: American Psychiatric Association.

Mendlowitz, S.L., Manassis, K., Bradley, S., Scapillato, D., Miezitis, S., & Shaw, B.F. (1999). Cognitive-behavioral group treatments in childhood anxiety disorders: The role of parental involvement. *Journal of the American Academy of Child and Adolescent Psychiatry, 38,* 1223–1229.

Merikangas, K., Stevens, D.E., Fenton, B., Stolar, M., O'Malley, S., Woods, S.W. et al. (1998). Co-morbidity and familial aggregation of alcoholism and anxiety disorders. *Psychological Medicine, 28* (4), 773–788.

Mowrer, O. (1960). *Learning Theory and Behaviour.* New York: John Wiley & Sons.

MTA Cooperative Group (2001). ADHD comorbidity findings from the MTA study: Comparing comorbid subgroups. *Journal of the American Academy of Child and Adolescent Psychiatry, 40,* 147–158.

Muris, P., Meesters, C., & van Melick, M. (2002). Treatment of childhood anxiety disorders: A preliminary comparison between cognitive-behavioral group therapy and a psychological placebo intervention. *Journal of Behavior Therapy and Experimental Psychiatry, 33,* 143–158.

Muris, P., Merckelbach, H., Holdrinet, I., & Sijsenaar, M. (1998). Treating phobic children: Effects of EMDR versus exposure. *Journal of Consulting and Clinical Psychology, 66,* 193–198.

Ollendick, T.H., & King, N.J. (1998). Empirically supported treatments for children with phobic and anxiety disorders: Current status. *Journal of Clinical Child Psychology, 27,* 156–167.

Olweus, D. (1993). *Bullying at School: What We Know and What We Can Do.* Oxford, England: Blackwell.

Ost, L., Svensson, L., Hellstrom, K., & Lindwall, R. (2001). One-session treatment of specific phobias in youth: A randomized clinical trial. *Journal of Consulting and Clinical Psychology, 69,* 814–824.

Pina, A.A., Silverman, W.K., Fuentes, R.M., Kurtines, W.M., & Weems, C.F. (2003). Exposure-based cognitive-behavioral treatment for phobic and anxiety disorders: Treatment effects and maintenance for Hispanic/Latino relative to European-American Youths. *Journal of the American Academy of Child and Adolescent Psychiatry, 42,* 1179–1187.

Pryor-Brown, L., & Cowen, E.L. (1989). Stressful life events, support, and children's adjustment. *Journal of Clinical Child Psychology, 18,* 214–220.

Rapee, R.M. (1997). Potential role of childrearing practices in the development of anxiety and depression. *Clinical Psychology Review, 17,* 47–67.

Rapee, R.M. (2000). Group treatment of children with anxiety disorders: Outcome and predictors of treatment response. *Australian Journal of Psychology, 52,* 125–129.

Rapee, R.M. (2002). The development and modification of temperamental risk for anxiety disorders: Prevention of a lifetime of anxiety? *Biological Psychiatry, 52,* 947–957.

Reiss, S. (1991). Expectancy model of fear, anxiety, and panic. *Clinical Psychology Review, 11,* 141–153.

Reiss, S. & McNally, R.J. (1985). The expectancy model of fear. In S. Reiss & R.R. Bootzin (Eds.), *Theoretical Issues in Behavior Therapy* (pp. 107–121). New York: Academic Press.

Renaud J., Birmaher, B., Wassick, S.C., & Bridge, J. (1999). Use of selective serotonin reuptake inhibitors for the treatment of childhood panic disorder: a pilot study. *Journal of Child & Adolescent Psychopharmacology, 9,* 73–83.

Research Units on Pediatric Psychopharmacology (RUPP) Anxiety Study Group. (2001). Fluvoxamine for the treatment of anxiety disorders in children and adolescents. *New England Journal of Medicine, 344,* 1279–1285.

Riddle, M.A., Bernstein, G.A. Cook, E.H., Leonard, H.L., March, J.S., & Swanson, J.M. (1999). Anxiolytics, adrenergic agents, and naltrexone. *Journal of the American Academy of Child and Adolescent Psychiatry, 38,* 546–556.

Ritter, B. (1968). The group desensitization of children's snake phobias using vicarious and contact desensitization procedures. *Behaviour Research and Therapy, 6*, 1–6.

Rubin, K.H., Burgess, K.B., & Hastings, P.D. (2002). Stability and social-behavioral consequences of toddlers' inhibited temperament and parenting behaviors. *Child Development, 73*, 483–495.

Rubin, K.H., Burgess, K.B., Kennedy, A.E., & Stewart, S.L. (2003). Social withdrawal in childhood. In E.J. Mash & R.A. Barkley (Eds.), *Child Psychopathology*, 2nd ed. (pp. 372–408). New York: Guilford Press.

Rynn, M., Kunz, N., Lamm, L., Nicolacopoulos, E., & Jenkins, L. (2002). Venlafaxine XR for the treatment of GAD in children and adolescents. *Proceedings of the American Academy of Child Adolescent Psychiatry Meeting, 49*, 91.

Rynn, M.S., Siqueland, L., & Richels, K. (2001). Placebo-controlled trial of sertraline in the treatment of children with generalized anxiety disorder. *American Journal of Psychiatry, 158*, 2008–2014.

Salazar, D.E., Frackiewicz, E.J., Dockens, R., Kollia, G., Fulmor, I.E., Tigel, P.D., et al. (2001). Pharmacokinetics and tolerability of buspirone during oral administration to children and adolescents with anxiety disorder and normal healthy adults. *Journal of Clinical Pharmacology, 41*, 1351–1358.

Schuckit M.A., & Hesselbrock, V. (1994). Alcohol dependence and anxiety disorders: What is the relationship? *American Journal of Psychiatry, 151*, 1723–1734.

Schwab-Stone, M.E., Ayers, T.S., Kasprow, W., Voyce, C., Barone, C. , Shriver, T. et al. (1995). No safe haven: A study of violence exposure in an urban community. *Journal of the American Academy of Child and Adolescent Psychiatry, 34*, 1343–1352.

Shaffer, D., Fisher, P., Dulcan, M.K., Davies, M., Piacentini, J., Schwab-Stone, M.E., et al. (1996). The NIMH Diagnostic Interview Schedule for Children Version 2.3 (DISC-2.3): Description, acceptability, prevalence rates, and performance in the MECA Study. *Journal of the American Academy of Child and Adolescent Psychiatry, 35*, 865–877.

Shortt, A.L., Barrett, P.M., & Fox, T.L. (2001). Evaluating the FRIENDS program: A cognitive-behavioral group treatment for anxious children and their parents. *Journal of Consulting and Clinical Psychology, 30*, 525–535.

Silverman, W.K., Kurtines, W.M., Ginsburg, G.S., Weems, C.F., Lumpkin, P.W., & Carmichael, D.H. (1999a). Treating anxiety disorders in children with group cognitive-behavioral therapy: A randomized clinical trial. *Journal of Consulting and Clinical Psychology, 67*, 995–1003.

Silverman, W.K., Kurtines, W.M., Ginsburg, G.S., Weems, C.F., Rabian, B., & Serafini, L.T. (1999b). Contingency management, self-control, and education support in the treatment of childhood phobic disorders: A randomized clinical trial. *Journal of Consulting and Clinical Psychology, 67*, 675–687.

Singer, M.I., Anglin, T.M., Song, L.Y., & Lunghofer, L. (1995). Adolescents' exposure to violence and associated symptoms of psychological trauma. *Journal of the American Medical Association, 273*(6), 477–482.

Southam-Gerow, M.A., Kendall, P.C., & Weersing, V.R. (2001). Examining outcome variability: Correlates of treatment response in a child and adolescent anxiety clinic. *Journal of Clinical Child Psychology, 30*, 422–436.

Spence, S.H. (2001). Prevention strategies. In M. Vasey and M.R. Dadds (Eds.), *The Developmental Psychopathology of Anxiety* (pp. 325–341). NY: Oxford University Press.

Spence, S.H., Donovan, C., & Brechman-Toussaint, M. (2000). The treatment of childhood social phobia: The effectiveness of a social skills based, cognitive-behavioral intervention, with and without parental involvement. *Journal of Clinical Psychology and Psychiatry, 41*, 713–726.

Strauss, C.C., Lahey, B.B., Frick, P., Frame, C.L., & Hynd, G.W. (1988). Peer social status of children with anxiety disorders. *Journal of Consulting and Clinical Psychology, 56*, 137–141.

Thapar, A., & McGuffin, P. (1995). Are anxiety symptoms in children heritable? *Journal of Child Psychology and Psychiatry, 36*, 439–447.

Treadwell, K.R.H., Flannery-Schroeder, E.C., & Kendall, P.C. (1995). Ethnicity and gender in relative to adaptive functioning, diagnostic status, and treatment outcome in children from an anxiety clinic. *Journal of Anxiety Disorders, 9*, 373–384.

Turner, S.M., Beidel, D.C., Roberson-Nay, R., & Tervo, K. (2003). Parenting behaviors in parents with anxiety disorders. *Behavior Research and Therapy, 41*, 541–554.

Waas, G.A., & Graczyk, P.A. (2000). Child behaviors leading to peer rejection: A view from the peer group. *Child Study Journal, 29* (4), 291–306.

Wagner, K.D., Wetherhold, E., Carpenter, D., Krulewicz, S., & Bailey, A. (2002). The safety and tolerability of paroxetine in children and adolescents. *Proceedings of the American Academy of Child Adolescent Psychiatry Meeting 49*, 91.

Warren, S.L., Huston, L., Egeland, B., & Sroufe, L.A. (1997). Child and adolescent anxiety disorders and early attachment. *Journal of the American Academy of Child and Adolescent Psychiatry, 36*, 637–641.

Watson, J.B., & Rayner, R. (1920). Conditioned emotional reactions. *Journal of Experimental Psychology, 3,* 1–14.

Weems, C.F., Hayward, C., Killen, & J. Taylor, C.B. (2002). A longitudinal investigation of anxiety sensitivity in adolescence. *Journal of Abnormal Psychology, 111,* 471–477.

Weisz, J.R., & Hawley, K.M. (2002). Developmental factors in the treatment of adolescents. *Journal of Consulting and Clinical Psychology, 70,* 21–43.

Whaley, S.E., Pinto, A., & Sigman, M. (1999). Characterizing interactions between anxious mothers and their children. *Journal of Consulting and Clinical Psychology, 67,* 826–836.

Wood, J.J., McLeod, B.D., Sigman, M., Hwang, W., & Chu, B.C. (2003). Parenting and childhood anxiety: Theory, empirical findings, and future directions. *Journal of Child Psychology and Psychiatry, 44,* 134–151.

Yule, W., & Williams, R. (1990). Post-traumatic stress reactions in children. *Journal of Traumatic Stress, 3,* 279–295.

Chapter 8

Attention-Deficit/Hyperactivity Disorder

Melinda Corwin, Kirti N. Kanitkar, Adam Schwebach,
and Miriam Mulsow

Introduction

An association between Attention-Deficit/Hyperactivity Disorder (ADHD) and adolescent behavioral problems has been well established (Lee, Mulsow & Reifman, 2003). For example, adolescents with ADHD have been found to be more likely than adolescents without ADHD to engage in risk-taking behaviors such as substance use and abuse, risky driving, risky sexual behaviors, and behaviors indicative of conduct disorder or oppositional defiant disorder. It is important to note, however, that a meta-analysis of ADHD outcome studies suggests that the contribution of ADHD to problematic behaviors is only small to medium (Lee, Mulsow & Reifman, 2003). This chapter examines those circumstances that may increase or decrease the likelihood of behavioral problems among adolescents with ADHD.

Attention-Deficit/Hyperactivity Disorder is the most commonly diagnosed behavioral disorder of childhood. ADHD has also been called Attention-Deficit Disorder, Hyperactive Child Syndrome, Hyperkinesis, Minimal Brain Dysfunction, Hyperkinetic Syndrome of Childhood, and Hyperkinetic Disorder. In most cases of childhood ADHD, the disorder continues into adolescence. Adolescents with ADHD do not "outgrow" their symptoms and their ADHD status is often a powerful factor influencing every area of development. Adolescents with ADHD face multiple challenges in the academic and social aspects of daily life as a teenager. The direction the adolescent transition takes is often a result of the interplay of individual, family, and social factors that influence risk and resiliency in adolescents with ADHD. A *risk factor* is one that increases the likelihood of a negative outcome, while a *protective factor* is one that ameliorates the effects of adversity and "protects" the individual from deviations in his/her developmental pathway. Protective factors are implied in resilient outcomes. Most of our knowledge about these factors comes from studies of adolescents with ADHD who were diagnosed as children.

Symptoms of ADHD include developmentally inappropriate levels of inattention, hyperactivity, distractibility, and impulsivity (National Institutes of Health, 1998) that appear before age 7, persist longer than six months, and lead to problems in multiple settings (e.g., home, school, work, peer group). However, not all of these symptoms are present in all people with ADHD. For many children with ADHD, hyperactivity diminishes in adolescence, but inattention and impulsivity continue to cause problems throughout the adolescent years.

Inattention symptoms include carelessness, difficulty sustaining concentration, reluctance and difficulty organizing and completing work correctly, failure to follow through, tendency to lose things, excessive forgetfulness, and high distractibility. *Hyperactivity* is excessive movement, restlessness, fidgetiness, or excessive talking. *Impulsivity,* an inability to inhibit behavior, makes it difficult to stop and think before behaving or to delay gratification. *Comorbidity* means the existence of two different conditions in the same person. ADHD is commonly comorbid with *Conduct Disorder (CD)* or *Oppositional Defiant Disorder (ODD)*. These two terms are sometimes used interchangeably, although ODD may be more accurately described as an earlier, less severe disorder similar to CD (Mulsow & Lee, 2003).

Stimulants represent the most common form of medication prescribed for children and adolescents with ADHD, although other drugs have been used with varying degrees of effectiveness, and several new medications have been developed in recent years. Behavioral interventions attempt to increase positive behaviors and decrease negative behaviors by using reinforcement. Cognitive behavioral modification (CBM) involves techniques such as stepwise problem solving and self-monitoring. Multimodal treatment consists of a combination of medication plus other interventions, most commonly some type of behavioral strategy plus educational modifications.

An accurate diagnosis from a professional who is both experienced with ADHD and informed on recent developments in the field is of vital importance. There are several other disorders and circumstances, including environmental factors and other psychological disorders, that can mimic ADHD but are treated very differently (NIH, 1998). For example, both traumatic stress and post-traumatic stress disorder sometimes cause hyperactivity, distractibility, impulsivity, irritability, and aggression (Thomas, 1995). It is important, therefore, for even the experienced diagnostician to rule out other possible causes prior to diagnosis and treatment for ADHD. Information used in diagnosis should include age of onset as well as data on the adolescent's behavior from multiple sources, such as teachers and parents or guardians. Due to the high incidence of the disorder in families of people with ADHD, when ADHD is identified in one family member, other family members should also be screened.

Scale of the Problem

Prevalence estimates for ADHD range from 3% to 10% of the adolescent population (Barkley, 1997; NIH, 1998). Adolescents with ADHD are at elevated risk to repeat a grade, be suspended from school, exhibit conduct disorder and other behavioral problems, have difficulty with written and verbal communication, have memory deficits, make lower grades than they seem to be capable of making, and experience social rejection, depression, anxiety, accidental injuries, risk-taking behavior, poor sense of time, and sleep problems (Barkley, 1998). Family relationships are also impaired, with families of ADHD adolescents reporting more stress, frustration, disappointment, guilt, fatigue, family therapy, marital dysfunction, divorce, and psychological disorders, including ADHD and depression in parents (Fischer, 1990).

Individuals with ADHD consume numerous resources and attention from the health care system, criminal justice system, schools, and other social service agencies (NIH, 1998). "Additional national public school expenditures on behalf of students with ADHD may have exceeded $3 billion in 1995. Moreover, ADHD, often in conjunction with coexisting conduct disorders, contributes to societal problems such as violent crime and teenage pregnancy" (NIH, 1998, p. 4).

A person with ADHD is unable to delay responses to stimuli (Barkley, 1997). The apparent lack of attention in those with ADHD may result from an inability to select important stimuli in the environment versus those that can be ignored. Barkley suggests that this inability is related to a deficiency in behavioral inhibition and that "the problem . . . is not one of knowing what to do but one of doing what you know when it would be most adaptive to do so" (1997, p. 78).

What Causes ADHD?

Although exact causes are not yet known, research strongly suggests the involvement of brain structure or function, with various regions of the brain identified as functioning differently and some subtle structural differences in the brains of those with ADHD (Volkow, 2003). Twin studies support a genetic transmission of ADHD that rivals that of hair or eye color (Gjone, Stevenson & Sundet, 1996; Teeter, 1998), suggesting that ADHD may be one of the most genetically linked of all psychological disorders. Although some consistent findings have emerged in identifying specific gene anomalies associated with ADHD, researchers have not yet clearly identified the full spectrum of anomalies linked to this disorder. We know that genetics play a part in ADHD, but we do not yet know the degree to which environment influences expression of a genetic predisposition to ADHD. It does appear, however, that outcomes for adolescents with ADHD, regardless of the origin of that ADHD, may be influenced by environmental factors, including the parenting they receive, their peer groups, the educational interventions offered, and whether the ADHD is recognized and treated.

What Causes Behavioral Problems Associated with ADHD?

Environmental and Familial Stressors

The child with ADHD who is exposed to repeated environmental stressors becomes more susceptible to adolescent Oppositional Defiant Disorder, Conduct Disorder, Antisocial Behaviors, and Major Depression (Barkley, 2003). Environmental stressors include frequent moves, particularly those that involve changing schools and/or separation from positive peer groups, life events such as parental divorce, and chronic stressors such as high levels of parental anger or conflict. We also know that parenting style can contribute to problematic behaviors among adolescents with ADHD (Hinshaw, Klein & Abikoff, 1998). Because adult ADHD can contribute to parenting problems, we find that a child with ADHD who has a parent with ADHD is up to three times more likely to develop behavioral problems by adolescence (Barkley, 2003) than is an adolescent with ADHD whose parents do not have ADHD. In addition, we know that parenting education for parents with ADHD is less effective than parenting education for parents without ADHD.

Life with ADHD is not easy. People who live with this disorder and its associated costs, in themselves or family members, carry an extra burden of stressors. When an adolescent is stressed or discouraged, we know that one common response is to engage in risky behaviors. Sometimes these adolescents fall into the role of the family scapegoat. Other adolescents who become discouraged may internalize the pain, thus developing problems such as depression or anxiety. In either case, the consequences of living with the stressors and discouragement associated with having ADHD may contribute to problematic behaviors among these adolescents.

Many authors attribute depression and other mood disorders commonly comorbid with ADHD to a lifetime of disappointments and frustrations. However, there is evidence that at least some of the mood disorders associated with ADHD are independent of the ADHD (Barkley, 1998). Thus, it is possible that some of the long-term problems among people with ADHD may be linked to comorbid mood disorders rather than directly to the ADHD.

ADHD and precursors to antisocial personality (conduct disorder and oppositional defiant disorder) commonly coexist. There is some evidence that these conduct problems may be the factors that most strongly predict some problematic outcomes such as criminality and substance abuse (Dulcan et al., 1997). Recent studies, however, suggest that even when conduct problems are controlled, ADHD-linked impulsivity is associated with problematic outcomes (Babinski, Hartsough & Lambert, 1999).

Self-Medication

Some researchers have proposed that people with comorbid ADHD and substance abuse are attempting to self-medicate their ADHD symptoms (Wilens, Biederman, Spencer & Frances, 1994). In fact, the incidence of stimulant use is particularly high among people with ADHD, and studies of substance abusers with ADHD show an increase in self-esteem with the use of substances. Others suggest that the increase in life stressors associated with ADHD (Barkley, 1998) may lead to substance abuse and other negative outcomes.

Impulsivity

The association of hyperactivity and impulsivity, but not inattention, with later criminality lend support to the idea that it is the impulsivity that may lead to some of the most devastating long-term problems associated with ADHD (Babinski et al., 1999). In fact, Barkley (1998) suggests that the key symptom in ADHD is impulsivity and that the inattentive type of ADHD may be a different, and less severe, disorder. He suggests that impulsive people with ADHD lack the ability to stop and consider the consequences before acting. This may lead to risk-taking behaviors, including reckless driving, criminal acts, unsafe sexual activity, substance abuse, and behavior that causes one to be at increased risk for physical injury. Impulsivity also contributes to academic and occupational underachievement. Finally, impulsive behaviors with peers may be perceived as intrusive and cause an adolescent to be rejected by positive peer groups, leaving the adolescent to find friendships where he or she can, often with negative peer groups.

Parenting Practices

Children with ADHD are more likely to experience coercive parenting practices, more physical and non-physical punishment, and more negative communication from their parents than are children from families without ADHD. When researchers examine families of children with ADHD in which parenting styles differ, they find that those children with ADHD whose parents are more coercive (Hinshaw, Klein & Abikoff, 1998) and less protective are more likely to develop aggressive and antisocial behaviors by adolescence than those children with ADHD whose parents are less coercive and more protective.

Gender

Dulcan, Dunne, Ayers, Arnold, Benson, and associates (1997) report a prevalence rate for ADHD of 10.1% in males and 3.3% in females aged 4–11 years in Ontario, Canada. Clinical samples of ADHD overwhelmingly consist of male subjects, leading to a gender bias in existing literature. Although the ratio of males having ADHD is three to one over females, conservative estimates indicate that over one million girls and women are affected by ADHD (Dulcan et al., 1997; NIH, 1998). ADHD in girls tends to be overlooked, not just in studies, but also in diagnosis and treatment. Although girls with ADHD are less likely to develop patterns such as criminal behavior, they do experience increased incidence of unintended pregnancy (NIH, 1998) and depression.

Individual Factors

Certain characteristics of adolescents with ADHD seem to be put them at a greater risk for adverse educational, social, and health outcomes. The latest research also points to some individual level protective factors, which promote resilience.

Comorbidity

Comorbidity is the greatest risk factor. Comorbidity of ADHD with Conduct Disorder (CD) or Oppositional Defiant Disorder (ODD) is particularly difficult to treat successfully. Comorbidity is implicated as a risk factor in all domains of developmental outcomes, impacting educational outcomes, social interactions, emotional difficulties, as well as likelihood of substance use and abuse and juvenile delinquency.

Wilson and Marcotte (1995) conducted a retrospective follow-up study of psychosocial adjustment and educational outcome in 14–18-year-old adolescents with only ADHD, ADHD and comorbid CD, and clinical controls. Participants with comorbid CD had significantly lower academic performance, evidenced deficits in socialization skills, and had more externalizing behavior and emotional difficulties than participants without CD. The presence of CD increased the risk of maladaptive outcomes.

Comorbidity with CD is also implicated in substance use and dependence symptoms in adolescence and young adulthood. Flory, Milich, Lynam, Leukefeld, and Clayton (2003) examined relationships between childhood ADHD and CD symptoms and later alcohol, marijuana, and hard drug use and dependence. Individuals with both ADHD and CD symptoms had the highest level of these outcomes. Molina, Smith, and Pelham (1999) also found significant interactive effects of ADHD and CD on substance use. This finding was replicated by Burke, Loeber, and Lahey (2001). Molina and Pelham (2003) evaluated risk for elevated substance use for ADHD probands and controls. Comorbidity of childhood ODD/CD was predictive of illicit drug use and persistent symptoms of CD. Presence of CD along with ADHD is also a risk factor for later antisocial behavior and juvenile delinquency (Foley, Carlton & Howell 1996).

Some children with ADHD evidence more social deficits than others and can be identified statistically as a separate subgroup of ADHD with social disability (SD) (Greene, Biederman, Faraone, Oullette, Penn & Griffin, 1996). Comorbidity of ADHD with social disability also increases the risk for maladjusted outcomes in adolescence. Examining longitudinal outcomes of boys with initial social disability, Greene, Biederman, Sienna, Garcia-Jetton, and Faraone (1997) found that initial social disability with ADHD was associated with higher rates of mood, anxiety, and disruptive and substance use disorders in adolescence, when compared to socially non-disabled adolescents with ADHD and control participants.

Severity of Inattention Symptoms

Severity of the inattention dimension has often been overlooked as an individual risk factor. Even though the individual dimension of ADHD reflects distinct symptom groupings, very few studies have examined the associations between these and outcomes such as substance use. Burke, Loeber, and Lahey (2001) found that when adolescent inattention was considered independently, it was associated with a 2.2 times greater risk for concurrent tobacco use, even after controlling for CD. Molina and Pelham (2003) found that childhood ADHD, particularly the inattention dimension, predicted adolescent substance abuse, especially prevalent tobacco use, by probands to a greater degree than childhood antisocial behaviors. Adolescent inattention is implied in the self-medication hypothesis for explaining elevated tobacco use in adolescents with ADHD. Nicotine has been demonstrated to enhance vigilance and attentional functioning in general (Levin, Conners, Silva, Hinton, Meck, March & Rose, 1998). Adolescents with ADHD may be drawn to it in an attempt to self-regulate their attention.

In conclusion, the relationship between inattention and nicotine dependence, as well as other outcomes, warrants further investigation. The inattention dimension of ADHD is often neglected in the face of the more obvious hyperactive-impulsive dimension. In fact, it is not measured separately in most studies on ADHD outcomes. However, it may predispose adolescents to unique challenges, and more efforts need to be made to uncover the role it plays in the long term.

Personal Characteristics

Personal characteristics of individuals also contribute to adolescent outcomes of ADHD, though very few have actually been investigated. Hechtman (1991) identifies four child-related factors that contribute to making children at risk resilient: (1) health, (2) temperament, (3) intelligence, and (4) psychosocial factors. The sparse investigation of these factors in adolescents with ADHD has confirmed their role as protective factors, though more research is needed. Lambert (1998) investigated the early-life contributions of biological and psychological characteristics of the children with ADHD to adolescent outcomes. Results indicated that early biological factors such as prematurity, low birth weight, and maternal smoking during pregnancy were predictive of adolescent substance use. Early-childhood symptoms of ADHD were significantly related to educational and social difficulties, as well as mental health difficulties such as depression and aggressiveness at adolescence.

Turning to intelligence and psychosocial factors, Weiss, Minde & Werry (1971) found that children with initial higher IQs fared better academically in later life. Loney, Kramer, and Milch (1981) reported that initial levels of aggression, socioeconomic status, and familial factors all affected adolescent outcomes of aggression, hyperactivity, delinquency, and academic achievement.

Stimulant Therapy of ADHD

Undergoing pharmacotherapy has alternately been viewed as a risk or a protective factor for substance use. Recently, there has been growing concern that stimulant therapy for ADHD may elevate the risk of substance abuse in ADHD adolescents. This gateway hypothesis predicts that exposure to the benefits of these drugs may motivate individuals to adopt other means of chemical coping in the future, thus increasing vulnerability to substance use. Alternatively, the self-medication hypothesis predicts that smoking would decrease in people with ADHD after receiving pharmacotherapy, as they do not have to use nicotine to self-medicate any longer. Empirical data supports the self-medication hypothesis over the gateway one. A meta-analytic review by Wilens, Faraone, Biederman, and Gunawardene (2003) found that stimulant therapy in childhood is associated with a reduction in the risk for subsequent drug and alcohol use disorders. Whalen, Jamner, Henker, Gehricke, and King (2003) found similar results with adolescent cigarette smoking outcomes. Stimulant therapy in childhood is, then, a protective factor against adolescent substance use and abuse problems.

Family Factors

Family environment and processes can moderate the outcomes of ADHD in adolescence. Family factors can increase or reduce the risk of maladaptive outcomes of ADHD in adolescence. Hechtman (1991) reiterates the importance of considering the family context in understanding risk and resiliency in individuals with ADHD. McCleary (2002) recounts theories of parenting stress, the main feature of which is parent–child conflict arising from stress, its impact on the child, plus mediating parent characteristics such as parents' psychological well-being that moderate this process (Abidin, 1990; Mash & Johnston, 1990; Webster-Stratton, 1990).

Parent–Adolescent Interactions

Family relationships among adolescents are commonly characterized by high levels of stress, evident from the study of parent–adolescent interactions. In a sequential analysis of interactions between mothers and adolescents with ADHD, adolescents with ADHD/ODD and a control group, Fletcher, Fischer, Barkley, and Smallish (1996) found that mothers in the ADHD/ODD group were less likely to exhibit warmth and to forgive their teens and more likely to use a tit-for-tat approach when in a conflict interaction. These mothers exhibited greater negativity and seemed less like mothers in the other groups. Most of the conflict between teens with ADHD and their parents seemed to be due to ODD, which stood out as a family characteristic, not just an individual one. Barkley, Anastopoulos, Guevremont, and Fletcher (1992) found that ADHD and ADHD/ODD groups of adolescents and their mothers had greater numbers of topics about which there was conflict and more angry conflict than the control groups. Also, mothers of teens with ADHD/ODD exhibited greater negative interactions during a neutral discussion, greater personal distress, and low marital satisfaction. These findings reveal that stress levels are high in families with adolescents with ADHD and having comorbid ODD compounds the stress.

Family Environment

Family environment has been implicated in adolescent educational as well as psychiatric outcomes. Biederman, Millberger, Faraone, Kiely, Guite, Mick, Ablon, Warburton, and Reed (1995a) found that there is a relationship between family adversity indicators and psychiatric, cognitive, as well as psychosocial impairments in children and adolescents with ADHD. In a related study, Biederman, Milberger, Faraone, Kiely, Guite, Mick, Ablon, Warburton, Reed, and Davis (1995b) reported that exposure to parental conflict and parental psychopathology impacted children and adolescents in negative ways, increasing psychopathology and impairing psychosocial functioning. These findings reiterate the salience of family characteristics as a risk factor for children and adolescents with ADHD.

Educating Parents About ADHD

Families who are affected by ADHD commonly experience anger, guilt, and recriminations concerning the behavior of their members who have the disorder. When families learn that ADHD is biologically based and not caused by parenting, and when they learn about symptoms of ADHD, they are helped to revise their perspectives, diminish accusations and guilt, and understand ways to deal more effectively with their children's problems (Barkley, 1998; Teeter, 1998). This, in itself, can lead to better family relations, which can, in turn, lead to better outcomes for the children.

Although studies show that parenting does not cause this disorder, parent–child interactions can influence long-term outcome for those with ADHD (Hinshaw et al., 1998; Teeter, 1998). Teeter (1998) reviews several different types of parenting education programs, including workbooks that Barkley has published on this topic. In addition, Cunningham, Bremner, and Secord-Gilbert (1993) present a parenting course to be offered through schools.

Family Stability

Another facet of family characteristics is family stability, and adolescents with ADHD seem to fare poorly in this regard. In an eight-year prospective follow-up study, family status of children and adolescents with ADHD was far less stable relative to the control group, with more than three times as many of the children's mothers being divorced from their biological fathers; additionally the adolescents with ADHD had moved four times as often as controls. Fathers of children and adolescents with ADHD also evidenced greater psychiatric disturbances as well as greater involvement in antisocial activities compared to controls, and this was directly related to child outcomes (Barkley, Fischer, Edelbrock & Smallish, 1990).

These findings reflect that a negative and unstable family environment is a risk factor for maladaptive outcomes in adolescents with ADHD. Families can, thus, moderate early risk and afford protection from the adverse outcomes of ADHD. However, hardly any research has been done on parenting practices in resilient adolescents. We know what *not to do*, but we need more empirical research on what *to do*.

Social and Community Factors

A large body of literature exists on peer relationship difficulties in children and adolescents with ADHD and the mechanisms responsible for these difficulties. In a review article, Dumas (1998) reported numerous studies that provided evidence for the social functioning difficulties experienced by adolescents with ADHD, including inadequate social competence, being loners, getting involved in fights, having no steady friends, and having significantly more social problems than controls without ADHD. Litner (2003) also lists peer relationships as one of the major challenges in the transition to high school for adolescents with ADHD. Poor peer relationships in childhood and adolescence has been identified as one of the most powerful predictors of later mental health problems, poor social adjustment, and adolescent antisocial behaviors (Parker & Asher, 1987; Robbins, 1986). Conversely, positive peer relations foster feelings of acceptance, greater resistance to stress, and higher self-esteem (Berndt, 1989). It follows that adolescents with ADHD are at greater risk for negative social outcomes and need positive efforts to maintain good peer relationships that come so easily to many children without ADHD.

The impact of the peer group on adolescents with ADHD has been documented by some researchers. Deviant peer group affiliation has been substantiated as a risk factor in adolescents with a childhood diagnosis of ADHD (Marshal, Molina & Pelham, 2003). Deviant peer affiliation mediated the relationship between ADHD and substance use. Moreover, the relationship between deviant peers and substance use was stronger for adolescents with ADHD than for those without ADHD. Bagwell, Molina, Pelham, and Hoza (2001) reported that friends of adolescents with ADHD were less involved in conventional activities and more involved in unconventional activities than friends of controls without ADHD. Molina, Smith, and Pelham (1999) have demonstrated that ADHD and substance use can result in poor academic achievement and peer difficulties. These findings support the deviance-proneness pathway found in Sher's (1991) model of alcoholism vulnerability, in which initial difficult temperament leads to alcohol involvement through peer influence. Adolescents with ADHD thus seem particularly prone to peer group influences, and a deviant peer group is more of a risk factor for them than for adolescents without ADHD.

On a positive note, Lambert (1998) found that positive rating by peers was a powerful predictor for favorable educational, substance use, and conduct outcomes among adolescents with ADHD. Positive peer relationships can be just the buffer that adolescents with ADHD need in their struggles with their unique set of hassles. It can be difficult to change an adolescent's peer group once this group is established; it may even require that the family move to another school district or town. However, research supports the idea that positive peer relationships are extremely important. As is typical of this literature, more research exists for negative outcomes than positive ones, and this gap needs to be addressed in future studies.

Social relationships can foster hope and resiliency in adolescents with ADHD. More research on positive influences in the lives of adolescents with ADHD is necessary. Positive outcomes need to be highlighted in the search for how to design effective treatments for individuals with ADHD.

Evidence-Based Treatment Interventions in Community Settings

Treatment interventions for ADHD focus on a wide range of behaviors, including academic performance, compliance or role following, social skills/peer interactions, and family interactions (Rapport, Chung, Shore & Isaacs, 2001). Because ADHD varies in type, severity, chronicity, and associated behavioral problems, interventions understandably affect outcomes in a multitude of ways. More studies have been conducted with young children with ADHD compared to adolescents with the disorder. Thus, generalizations must sometimes be made regarding the teen population until further research is conducted specifically with this age group.

What Works

PHARMACOLOGICAL MANAGEMENT.   Pharmacological management with psychostimulants and/or antidepressants, which will be discussed later in this chapter, is typically considered superior to behavioral intervention alone; however, there is widespread agreement that intervention for the adolescent with ADHD should be multimodal and multidisciplinary (Brown, 2000). In addition to psychopharmacological interventions, comprehensive treatment programs involving parent and client education, counseling and training, social skills training, and school interventions are important.

MULTIMODAL TREATMENT.   The National Institute of Mental Health funded a collaborative, six-site multimodal treatment study of children with ADHD (MTA) that involved a four-group parallel design (Conners et al., 2001). Children were randomly assigned to one of four treatment groups for a 14-month period, as follows: medication management (titration followed by monthly medication maintenance), behavioral treatment (including parent training, child-focused summer treatment program, and school-based intervention), combined treatment, or community care. All four groups showed marked reduction in ADHD symptoms over time. Combined medication management and behavioral treatment was statistically superior to behavioral treatment alone and community care but not statistically significant compared to medication management alone. The MTA treatments (i.e., medication management, behavioral treatment, and combined) all offered greater benefits than community care for other areas of function, including oppositional/aggressive behaviors, internalizing symptoms, peer interactions, parent–child relations, and reading achievement. The combined treatment offered the greatest benefit of all, thus supporting a multimodal approach.

PARENTING EDUCATION. One form of behavioral intervention involves parent education and training, based on social learning principles. Weinberg (1999) conducted a study in which parents of 25 children with ADHD participated in a six-week parent training program. The parents attended 90-minute group sessions once per week for six weeks. Programs were presented didactically, and handouts and reading references were provided. Results revealed a significant mean increase in parental knowledge and understanding of ADHD and behavior management skills. Additionally, a significant mean decrease in parental stress occurred, indicating mild stress reduction in managing their child's ADHD. Parents did not, however, observe improvement in the number or severity of behavior problems in their children at the end of the six-week program. Danforth (1998) reported that parenting training improved parenting behavior, reduced maternal stress, and reduced oppositional behavior in children with ADHD. A six-month follow-up revealed that parenting and child behavior remained stable. Cunningham, Bremner, and Secord-Gilbert (1993) reported success in offering parenting courses for parents of ADHD children in large, school-based courses. Parenting training has been used as a successful educational tool to teach and reinforce the use of authoritative methods. Hinshaw and associates (1998) demonstrate that authoritative parenting beliefs predict more positive peer relations among children with ADHD.

SCHOOL-BASED INTERVENTIONS. DuPaul and Eckert (1997) conducted a comprehensive meta-analysis examining the effects of school-based interventions for children and adolescents with ADHD. They reviewed 63 outcome studies conducted between 1971 and 1995. Note that this is a small number compared to the hundreds of studies conducted in the same 24-year period that examined stimulant medication effects. Results indicated that school-based interventions for ADHD lead to significant (moderate to high) behavioral effects regardless of the type of experimental design that was used. Conversely, intervention effects on academic and clinic test performance were less robust (effect sizes ranged from nonsignificant to large, depending on the analysis). Overall, effect sizes for behavior were up to two times greater than effect sizes for academic performance across all three designs. Contingency management and academic interventions were more effective than cognitive-behavioral procedures for improving classroom behavior, and cognitive-behavioral approaches were more effective than contingency management and academic interventions for improving academic performance in within-subjects design studies.

TEACHER TRAINING. Sometimes it is necessary to educate teachers about ADHD prior to involving them in classroom interventions (Teeter, 1998). Barkley (1998) reports that "a positive teacher–student relationship, based on teacher understanding of the student and the disorder, may improve academic and social functioning" (p. 459). Both Barkley (1998) and Teeter (1998) discuss the importance of, and information to be included in, teacher training and support. Teeter (1998) discusses a wide variety of classroom interventions that may be used for children at different developmental stages, whereas Barkley (1998) discusses strategies for the improvement of targeted behaviors in a classroom setting.

What Might Work

FAMILY THERAPY.   Two family therapies were compared involving teens with ADHD and their parents. Problem-solving communication training (PSCT) alone or behavior management training (BMT) followed by PCST (BMT/PSCT) were administered for 18 sessions (Barkley, Edwards, Laneri, Fletcher & Metevia, 2001). Approximately half of the teens in each group were taking medication for ADHD during the study. At the group level of analysis, results suggested that both treatments were associated with significant improvement in participant ratings for various aspects of behavior and on direct researcher observations of mothers' behavior during a parent–teen conflict discussion; however, no significant differences were observed for fathers' or teens' behavior. No significant differences were found between the two treatments. At the individual level of analysis, only 25% or fewer of the participants in each treatment demonstrated reliable change as a result of treatment. It should be noted that 34–70% of the families were brought from "abnormal" to "normal" by treatment and 42–80% were in the "normal" range by the end of therapy.

SOCIAL SKILLS TRAINING.   Antshel and Remer (2003) conducted a study in which 80 children, evenly divided into ten treatment groups, received weekly 90-minute group sessions involving social skills training (SST) intervention over an eight-week period. Their pretest, post-test, and three-month follow-up test scores were compared to control groups matched for age, sex, ADHD subtype, and comorbid conditions. Results revealed that SST led to greater improvements in both parent- and child-perceived assertion skills in the children with ADHD, yet did not affect the other domains of social competence. The results did not strongly support the efficacy of social skills training, especially for children with comorbid ODD.

PEER TUTORING.   DuPaul, Ervin, Hook, and McGoey (1998) investigated the effects of classwide peer tutoring (CWPT) on classroom behavior and academic performance of elementary students with ADHD and ten peer comparison students. Results indicated that CWPT increased active engaged time for students with ADHD and decreased their disruptive, off-task behavior. Fifty percent of students with ADHD exhibited improvements in academic performance in math or spelling with CWPT compared to baseline conditions. In a related single-subject design study, Ervin, DuPaul, Kern, and Friman (1998) found preliminary support for a classroom-based model of functional assessment emphasizing the application of feasible, non-interruptive intervention strategies that are acceptable to both teachers and adolescent students.

NEUROFEEDBACK.   Neurofeedback has shown promise for helping people with ADHD to control their bodies' responses to cognitive stimuli (Fuchs, Birbaumer, Lutzenberger, Gruzelier & Kaiser, 2003; Monastra, Monastra & George, 2002; Nash, 2000). Recent studies indicate that benefits for children with ADHD, as measured in clinical settings, are maintained for the short term even without medication.

Unfortunately, in each of the trials, parents were allowed to choose which treatment was offered to their children. An additional concern exists in that there have not been any follow-ups to see if these skills can be carried over from laboratory settings into the distracting environments of the real world or if effects will be maintained after treatment. Unlike other treatments that also must be continued in order for benefits to be sustained, neurofeedback is too expensive and time-consuming to be maintained for the entire time that benefits are desired. If randomized tests of neurofeedback and follow-up studies are conducted and if they show sustained benefits outside of laboratory or clinical settings, this may be a major breakthrough in the treatment of ADHD. For now, however, neurofeedback remains an expensive option that is not yet recommended for those who are able to use other methods successfully. It has potential for becoming an important component of future interventions.

What Does Not Work

DIET.   One study was reviewed from Harley et al. (1978) which did not provide support for diet modification as a successful intervention for ADHD. The study involved school-age children with ADHD who were randomly assigned to either an experimental (Feingold K-P) or a control diet. Classroom observation ratings were obtained for hyperactivity behaviors, including lack of attention to tasks, restless motor activity, and classroom disruption. Results indicated no significant changes in the hyperactivity indicators attributable to the experimental diet.

Summary of Community-Based Treatments

In sum, psychopharmacology has been proven efficacious in the treatment of ADHD and thus "works" in terms of intervention for the core symptoms of ADHD. Specific medications will be discussed later in this chapter. School-based intervention to modify behavior has also proven to be effective. Additionally, recent studies have supported the use of combined medication management and behavior treatment to address many of the associated behaviors and characteristics of ADHD, such as peer interactions, parent–child relationships, and academic performance. The following interventions have yielded mixed results and thus might work:

1. problem-solving communication therapy combined with behavioral management training for parents and adolescents
2. social skills training, especially if the adolescent does not exhibit comorbid ODD or CD
3. classroom-based intervention, including peer tutoring
4. neurofeedback.

To date, diet modifications have not been empirically proven to work successfully as an intervention for ADHD, although research in this area is continuing.

Evidence-Based Treatment Interventions in Residential Settings

Adolescents are not typically referred to residential settings if ADHD is their primary problem. Thus, no studies were found that specifically evaluated ADHD intervention in residential settings. The closest programs to "residential" were ones that involved intensive, full-day intervention such as a summer therapy program (Abramowitz, Eckstrand, O'Leary & Dulcan, 1992; Conners et al., 2001; Hoza, Mrug, Pelham, Greiner & Gnagy, 2003).) and partial "hospitalization" in the form of a summer treatment and enrichment program (Kolko, Bukstein & Barron, 1999). These studies provided guarded support for improved core symptoms/behaviors, social skills, and peer interactions; however, medication was used in conjunction with behavioral treatment in most of the studies. It should also be noted that adolescents with ADHD who have comorbid ODD or especially CD would more likely be referred to residential treatment centers because of associated risk behaviors such as substance abuse and criminal activity.

Psychopharmacology

History of Medication Use in Treating Children and Adolescents with ADHD

In the late 1930s, the use of *dl*-amphetamine was found to be effective in reducing disruptive behaviors in children (Bradley, 1937). Bradley initially reported that the use of this amphetamine improved compliance, academic performance, and subsequently reduced motor activity in hyperkinetic children. Further reports by Bradley and others continued to demonstrate that stimulant medication decreased oppositional behavior in boys with conduct disorders (Eisenberg, Lachman, Molling, Lockner, Mizelle & Conners, 1961) and also showed improvements in target symptoms of ADHD on a standardized rating form completed by parents and teachers (Conners, Eisenberg & Barcai, 1967). Since these initial observations, stimulant medications have now become the most commonly prescribed medication for children and adolescents with ADHD (American Academy of Child and Adolescent Psychiatry, 2002).

Today there are a variety of stimulant medications, such as methylphenidate (Ritalin®), amphetamine (Dexedrine® and Adderall®) and pemoline (Cylert®), commonly used to treat symptoms related to ADHD. Over the past decade there has been a dramatic increase in the rate of prescriptions written for stimulant medication. Individuals receiving outpatient care by a primary practitioner for ADHD-related symptoms increased from 1.6 to 4.2 million per year during the years 1990 to 1993 (Swanson, Lerner & Williams, 1995). During these visits, 90% of the children received a prescription, 71% of which were for methylphenidate. More than 10 million prescriptions for methylphenidate were written in 1996 (Vitiello and Jensen, 1997) and epidemiological surveys estimate that 12-month prescription rates range from 6% in urban Baltimore (Safer, Zito & Fine, 1996) to 7.3% in rural North Carolina (Angold, Erkanli, Egger & Costello, 2000). One survey found that up to 20% of white boys in the fifth grade in one location were receiving medication for ADHD (LeFever, Sawson & Morrow, 1999) and another study reported a 2.5-fold increase in methylphenidate use between 1990 and 1995 (National Institute of Mental Health, 2000).

Many speculate that the increase in stimulant use may be related to individuals' requiring longer periods of medication for symptom relief. Others hypothesize that the increased usage of stimulant medication may be related to the fact that more girls and adults now receive medication treatment for ADHD, to an improved awareness of the condition by physicians, or even to an increase in prevalence rates of the disorder (Goldman, Genel, Bezman & Slanetz, 1998). Regardless, the increase use of stimulant medication is a source of concern for both parents and professionals and has been highly scrutinized by the media.

Stimulant Medications and Their Effectiveness in the Treatment of Adolescents with ADHD

Although psychostimulant medications are the primary treatment for individuals with ADHD, little is known about the central mechanisms of these medications. However, sufficient data is available demonstrating that stimulant medications primarily impact central dopamine and norepinephrine neurotransmitters in the prefrontal cortex part of the brain. Stimulants act on the striatum by binding to the dopamine transporter, resulting in an increase in synaptic dopamine. This reaction may enhance the functioning of executive control processes, overcoming deficits in inhibitory control and working memory reported in children with ADHD (Douglas, Barr, Amin, O'Neill & Britton, 1988; Barkley 1997). Psychostimulants are absorbed rapidly in the gut, usually within the first 30 minutes following ingestion. Thus, effects on behavior are quick and noticeable by both parents and teachers.

There has been extensive research conducted on the short-term effectiveness of stimulant medications in the treatment of ADHD. However, the primary focus of this research involved investigating stimulant use in school-aged children with little emphasis being placed on stimulant use with adolescents, preschoolers, and adults. A review by Spencer, Biederman, Wilens, Harding, O'Donnell, and Griffin (1996) reported 161 randomized control studies investigating the effectiveness of psychostimulants. The studies encompassed 5 with preschool-aged children, 140 with school-aged children, 7 with adolescents, and 9 with adults. All of the studies demonstrated robust short-term improvements in ADHD symptoms when treated with stimulant medication. Improvement occurred in 65–75% of the 5,899 patients assigned stimulant treatment when compared to only 4–30% of those assigned placebo. Other short-term and well-controlled double-blind studies have further demonstrated improvements in inattentive and hyperactive symptoms when treated with stimulants. Several meta-analyses have also demonstrated robust effects of stimulant use with effect sizes on behavior of .8–1.0 standard deviations (Kavale, 1982; Ottenbacher & Cooper, 1983; Thurber & Walker, 1983).

Perhaps the most well known study investigating the effectiveness of stimulant medication in the treatment of ADHD is the NIMH Collaborative Multisite Multimodal Treatment Study of Children with Attention-Deficit/Hyperactivity Disorder (MTA study), which concluded that stimulant medication (when taken either by itself or in combination with behavioral treatments) leads to stable improvements in ADHD symptoms as long as the medication continues to be taken. Similar results were replicated across six sites in various geographical locations, involving diverse groups of individuals, indicating that stimulant medications can be beneficial for many groups of children.

Besides the MTA study, there have only been three long-term randomized controlled studies on the effectiveness of stimulant medications for the treatment of ADHD (Abikoff & Hechtman, 1998; Gillberg, Melander, von Knorring, Janols, Thernlund, Hagglof, Eidevall-Wallin, Gustafsson & Kopp 1997; Schachar, Tannock, Cunningham, & Corkum 1997). Although various findings were observed, in general all of these studies continued to demonstrate superior benefits of medication treatment lasting for more than a 12-month period.

Although little research has been done on stimulant medication use in adolescent populations, the benefits of stimulants in children are well documented. In general, stimulant medications are beneficial in ameliorating disruptive ADHD behaviors across multiple settings (e.g., classroom, home, playground) when taken throughout the day (Greenhill, 2002). Stimulants also are beneficial in inhibiting impulsive responding on cognitive tasks; they also increase accuracy of performance and improve short-term memory, reaction time, seat-work completion, and attention. Improvement in both behavior and attention has been demonstrated with greater results being noted in behavior effects (Greenhill, 2002).

Stimulant medication treatment may pose greater challenges with adolescent populations. Adolescents are more aware of the effects stimulants have on them and can report the benefits of their use. However, only some adolescents may report benefits of taking stimulant medication, while others may rebel against frequent administration or the social stigma associated with such treatment. Compliance in taking the medication is no longer the sole responsibility of the parent. Now the adolescent is responsible for complying with treatment. It may be vitally important to work directly with the adolescent and parent together in regard to medication management to ensure optimal compliance. Adolescents should be informed about the risks and benefits of medication treatment and the importance of compliance. If the adolescent is concerned about taking multiple doses of medication throughout the day, a longer-lasting or extended release medication may be beneficial to increase compliance. Concerta® may be a good selection because it cannot be ground or snorted and has longer-lasting effects (American Academy of Child and Adolescent Psychiatry, 2002).

Non-Stimulant Medications and the Treatment of ADHD

Although there are a number of stimulant medications available to treat ADHD in adolescents, there have also been promising results shown for the usefulness of non-stimulant interventions. Some adolescents may not tolerate stimulant medications well or may have a condition that is contraindicated for the use of stimulants (e.g., cardiovascular defects, or Tourette's disorder) (American Academy of Child and Adolescent Psychiatry, 2002). Tricyclic antidepressants (TCAs) have been the most widely researched non-stimulant medication for the treatment of ADHD. Their long half-life (approximately 12 hours) and decreased potential for abuse make TCAs a positive alternative for treating adolescents with ADHD. There are a number of randomized controlled studies demonstrating that TCAs, such as imipramine and desipramine, are effective in eliminating various ADHD symptoms in children and adolescents (Biederman & Spencer, 2002). Beta-blockers have also been well studied and have demonstrated robust effects for the treatment of ADHD. In contrast, however, little benefit has been shown for the use of traditional antidepressants affecting serotonin, such as Prozac® and Zoloft®, in treating ADHD. Pharmaceutical companies appear to have recognized the need for developing a non-stimulant medication for the treatment of ADHD. Elli Lilly Corporation, for example, recently released Straterra® as a new non-stimulant intervention for the treatment of ADHD.

Does Treatment with Stimulant Medication Predict Later Substance Abuse in Adolescents with ADHD?

Originally it was hypothesized that the treatment of ADHD with stimulant medications early in childhood may predispose youth and adults to later substance abuse problems. In fact, the opposite has been demonstrated in the literature. A number of well-controlled longitudinal studies have found that adolescents with ADHD who were treated with stimulant medication were less likely to engage in cigarette smoking or abuse illegal drugs when compared to adolescents who were untreated (Biederman, 2003; Fischer, & Barkley, 2003; Whalen, Jamner, Henker, Gehricke & King, 2003). Biederman (2003) concluded that stimulant medication treatment acted as a protective factor against later substance use, which occurred at rates three or four times greater among those individuals who did not receive stimulant medications as a treatment.

Childhood factors that appear to predict adolescent substance use are severe childhood inattentive symptoms, affiliation with deviant peer groups, and childhood oppositional/conduct disorder symptoms (Marshal, Molina & Pelham, 2003; Molina & Pelham, 2003). Marshal and colleagues (2003) demonstrated that children with ADHD are more likely to become involved in deviant peer relationships, in turn increasing the risk that they will become substance abusers. Further, they found that adolescents involved in deviant peer groups were more vulnerable to the negative social influences of those groups. Marshal and colleagues suggest it is important to assist adolescents with ADHD who may become or are at risk to become engaged in deviant social groups as a primary focus of intervention to prevent later substance abuse by such individuals.

The Prevention of Problematic Behavior in Adolescents with ADHD

Prevention of behavior problems among adolescents with ADHD must start in childhood, in order to catch such problems as they originate. There are few well-controlled studies demonstrating specific treatments useful in preventing behavior problems among adolescents having ADHD. Typically, preventive actions focus on alleviating symptoms associated with ADHD. There has been an assumption that effective treatment for ADHD symptoms and reduction of stressors in the lives of children with ADHD will prevent many of the behavioral problems seen in adolescence. However, these assumptions have not been adequately tested in most domains of problematic adolescent behavior. Therefore, with the exception of the prevention of substance abuse, there is no preventive measure that has been shown in three or more studies to be effective.

What Works

As discussed in the treatment section of this chapter, there are many ways in which ADHD symptoms are treated, with the assumption that such treatment prevents later behavior problems. However, only one domain of adolescent behavior problems has been examined in three or more well-designed studies and found to be effective in preventing those problems. This domain is that of adolescent drug, alcohol, and cigarette use disorders. Stimulant treatment in children with ADHD has been clearly linked to a reduction in the risk for adolescent substance use disorders (Biederman, 2003; Fischer & Barkley, 2003; Whalen, Jamner, Henker, Gehricke & King, 2003; Wilens, Faraone, Biederman & Gunawardene, 2003).

What May Work

Typically, treatments focus on alleviating symptoms associated with ADHD. Such interventions may include components such as helping to improve social skills or assisting with academic problems (e.g., disorganization), cognitive problems (e.g., inattention), or behavior problems (e.g., hyperactivity, non-compliance). However, medication has dominated the literature as the most effective symptom relief intervention for ADHD.

As previously discussed, current treatment standards support the superiority of a combination of medication and behavioral interventions (multimodal treatment) over the use of stimulants alone. However, not enough time has elapsed for long-term outcomes of these combination (multimodal) treatments to be tested. It is very likely that even stronger support will be found for the use of multimodal treatment beginning in childhood to prevent adolescent behavioral problems, especially those involving substance use.

The MTA study, funded by the National Institute of Mental Health, clearly demonstrated that impairments related to ADHD (e.g, poor attention, hyperactivity, etc.) are dramatically reduced through education about the condition, medication intervention, parent training, and behavior management. Further analysis of the data reveals that the most robust effects in treating ADHD come when closely monitored medication and behavior management interventions are used collaboratively instead of using medication alone. Furthermore, adolescents with ADHD who were treated with a combination of medication and behavior management interventions improved performance on academic tasks such as note taking, daily assignments, and quiz scores. Other interventions specifically focused on helping children with ADHD to develop appropriate social skills are also necessary, given the fact that children with ADHD who demonstrate poor social relatedness often carry such behaviors into their adolescence, in turn becoming even more socially rejected (Bagwell, Molina, Pelham & Hoza, 2001).

Such interventions may help to reduce impairments in adolescents having ADHD, but is simply reducing symptoms enough to help such adolescents' transitions into adulthood? Some adolescents who may respond well to a symptom-focused treatment approach do not necessarily become well-functioning adults. Brooks and Goldstein (2001) propose that more has to be done than just alleviating the symptoms of ADHD.

First, Brooks and Goldstein propose that the treatment for adolescents with ADHD must include research-validated tools such as medication, behavior management, and classroom interventions. Such interventions are critical because of their usefulness in helping adolescents function better in daily life. However, the second component to treating adolescents with ADHD is providing such individuals the opportunity to develop a resilient mindset. Adolescents who possess a resilient mindset are empathetic, they communicate well with others, can problem solve, have a social conscience, and are self-disciplined. With the help of parents and teachers, these skills can be reinforced and modeled, so that the adolescent with ADHD can incorporate them in daily life. These skills may, in turn, help adolescents as they transition into adult life. If adolescents with ADHD are better able to see their strengths rather than their weaknesses, they may be able to function more effectively in their future lives.

What Does Not Work

As with the treatment of existing behavioral problems among children and adolescents with ADHD, much work has been done on the use of diet to prevent later behavioral problems among children with ADHD. Researchers have explored the addition of various nutrients as well as the reduction of various food additives or sugars. Although work is continuing in this area, to date no dietary modifications have been identified that are effective in preventing adolescent behavioral problems among those diagnosed with ADHD.

Another area that has received attention is the use of sensory integration treatment to prevent behavioral problems among adolescents with ADHD. This, too, has not been found to be an effective way to prevent such problems. There are people who experience sensory integration problems and, for them, this treatment may well be effective. However, sensory integration treatment has not been shown to work on current symptoms or later behavioral problems in people with ADHD.

Recommendations

As with other issues in adolescence, early prevention may be more effective than interventions initiated after behavioral problems are established in adolescents. However, both prevention and intervention methods have primarily been tested on boys with combined-type ADHD. There are few studies that include adequate numbers of girls and not enough studies that focus on the inattentive or hyperactive types of ADHD. With these limitations in mind, we know that the most important preventive method is for the child with ADHD to be diagnosed by a qualified practitioner; given a combination of behavioral and psychopharmacological treatments (this is referred to as multimodal treatment); and, probably most important, for the family to be educated about the disorder. The family should identify a health care professional who has stayed current with the literature and is knowledgeable about ADHD. After diagnosis, careful medication management is needed, with attention to identifying an appropriate dose for the individual child, keeping in mind that dosages commonly change and may be smaller after puberty. Treatment should occur before adolescence to prevent adolescent behavioral problems.

Behavioral methods include the modification of aspects of the child's environment (e.g., classroom, parenting practices, stressors, social support) to prevent or reduce the likelihood of later behavioral problems in adolescence. For example, when parents have symptoms of ADHD, they, too, should be screened and, when ADHD exists, treated. Parenting education that is specific to children with ADHD is an important part of this process, as is educating the child's teachers about ADHD, when necessary. Reducing stressors and providing prosocial sources of support are important ways to "inoculate" a child with ADHD against risky choices that he or she may face. An environment that allows for regular physical activity with positive peer groups is important for many children and adolescents with ADHD. Again, the earlier this starts, the more likely it is to work.

However, many of the families with whom we interact come to us seeking help for behavioral problems that are already established in their adolescents with ADHD. The method that has been evaluated and found successful in decreasing oppositional and aggressive behaviors and internalizing symptoms, and improving peer and parent–child interactions is multimodal treatment of the adolescent. This should be offered by a health care professional who is familiar with the latest ADHD treatment, using medication (for most adolescents, time-release stimulant medication) plus behavioral interventions. These behavioral interventions may include parent and client education, child-focused summer treatment programs, and school-based intervention (contingency management and academic interventions), keeping in mind the need to educate the adolescent's teachers about the disorder and the child's needs prior to the initiation of the school-based intervention. Peer tutoring has been effective for reducing disruptive behaviors in school for some students. Family therapy may help with overcoming some of the problems created in the family by the adolescent's behaviors, thus reducing overall stress levels.

There are other interventions that have shown mixed results or have not been adequately tested to date. For example, neurofeedback may hold promise for future intervention, but still needs more testing before its expense can be justified for most families. Problem-solving communication therapy, combined with behavioral management training for parents and adolescents has shown positive effects for some families. Social skills training has been somewhat controversial, given that many people with ADHD know what to do but do not take the time to draw on that knowledge before acting impulsively. However, social skills training has shown positive results for some adolescents without comorbid oppositional defiant disorder or conduct disorder.

General intervention methods include reduction of stress levels in families of adolescents with ADHD. Again, when parents have ADHD, it is important to get them diagnosed and treated in order to give them more resources to use in parenting their adolescents with ADHD. The entire family may need to be educated about ADHD. Studies indicate that this education about the disorder may be one of the most important parts of treatment for many families. Russel Barkley, a noted researcher in ADHD, gave a keynote address at the 2002 meeting of the organization, CHADD (Children and Adults with ADHD) in which he addressed methods reported by clinicians for use with adolescents who have ADHD and who exhibit behavioral problems.

The most common behavioral problem reported by Barkley for adolescents with ADHD is in the area of driving. We know that an adolescent with ADHD tends to be developmentally delayed by at least three years. This means that a 16-year-old with ADHD has a developmental age of about 13. Barkley (2002) recommends protecting adolescents with ADHD from the dangers associated with driving by delaying the initiation of independent driving as long as possible, then introducing independent driving in stages, with no distractions allowed (e.g., no friends in the car; cell phones stay in the trunk, to be used only in emergencies) in the early stages. Adolescents who take medications for ADHD should not be allowed to drive without those medications (Cox, Merkel, Kovatchev & Seward (2000).

Another area of difficulty arises when adolescents with ADHD are involved in peer groups that engage in antisocial behaviors. It is vitally important to separate adolescents with ADHD from these peer groups, even if it means that the family has to move to another school district or town. In the area of substance use and abuse, we know that this behavior is easier to prevent than to stop, but studies indicate that educating parents and adolescents about ADHD and providing appropriate treatment for ADHD is linked to more successful recovery from substance use disorders.

On a societal level, studies have uncovered a severe deficiency among many health care professionals concerning knowledge and practice of appropriate diagnosis and treatment of ADHD (Conners et al., 2001; MTA Cooperative Group, 1999). This was made apparent when the least effective means of treating ADHD was the community standard of treatment in the six locations of the MTA study. It is evident that widespread education of health care professionals is needed.

Adolescents with ADHD do not always exhibit major behavioral problems. In fact, most adolescents with ADHD do not have these problems. When these issues do arise, we know that ADHD may be only a small to moderate contributor to problem behaviors (Lee, Mulsow & Reifman, 2003). However, ADHD is consistently linked in studies to problematic behaviors. More research is needed into "what went right" in the lives of the many adolescents who avoid these problems. In addition careful attention is needed to do what we know, at this time, can be done to help more children with ADHD grow into successful adolescents and adults.

References

Abidin, R.R. (1990). Introduction to the special issue: The stresses of parenting. *Journal of Clinical Child Psychology, 9*, 298–301.

Abikoff, H., & Hechtman, L, (1998). *Multimodal treatment for children with ADHD: Effects on ADHD and social behavior and diagnostic status.* Unpublished manuscript.

Abramowitz, A.J., Eckstrand, D., O'Leary, S.G., & Dulcan, M.K. (1992). ADHD children's responses to stimulant medication and two intensities of a behavioral intervention. *Behavior Modification, 16:2*, 193–203.

American Academy of Child and Adolescent Psychiatry, (2002). Practice parameters for the use of stimulant medications in the treatment of children, adolescents, and adults. *Journal of the American Academy of Child and Adolescent Psychiatry, 41(2)*, 27s–49s.

Angold, A., Erkanli, A., Egger, H.L., & Costello, E.J. (2000). Stimulant treatment for children: a community perspective. *Journal of the American Academy of Child and Adolescent Psychiatry, 39*, 975–984.

Antshel, K.M., & Remer, R. (2003). Social skills training in children with attention deficit hyperactivity disorder: A randomized-controlled clinical trial. *Journal of Clinical Child and Adolescent Psychology, 32:1*, 153–165.

Babinski, L.M., Hartsough, C.S., & Lambert, N.M. (1999). Childhood conduct problems, hyperactivity-impulsivity, and inattention as predictors of adult criminal activity. *Journal of Child Psychology & Psychiatry & Allied Disciplines, 40*, 347–355.

Bagwell, C., Molina, B.S.G., Pelham, W.E., & Hoza, B. (2001). Attention-deficit hyperactivity disorder and problems in peer relations: Predictions from childhood to adolescence. *Journal of the American Academy of Child and Adolescent Psychiatry, 40(11)*, 1285–1299.

Barkley, R. (1997). Behavioral inhibition, sustained attention, and executive functions: Constructing a unifying theory of ADHD. *Psychological Bulletin, 121*, 65–94.

Barkley, R.A. (1998). *Attention Deficit Hyperactivity Disorder: A Handbook for Diagnosis and Treatment.* New York: Guilford Press.

Barkley, R.A. (October, 2002). Keynote address. Children and Adults with Attention Deficit Disorder (CHADD) Annual Meeting, Miami, FL.

Barkley, R.A. (2003). Attention-Deficit/Hyperactivity Disorder. (pp. 75–143) in E.J. Mash & R.A. Barkley (Eds.), Child psychopathology (2nd ed.). New York: Guilford Press.

Barkley, R.A., Anastopoulos, A.D., Guevremont, D.C., & Fletcher, K.E. (1992). Adolescents with attention deficit hyperactivity disorder: Mother-Adolescent interactions, family beliefs and conflicts, and maternal psychopathology. *Journal of Abnormal Psychology, 20(3),* 263–288.

Barkley, Edwards, Laneri, Fletcher, & Metevia, (2001). The efficacy of problem-solving communication training alone, behavior management training alone, and their combination for parent-adolescent conflict in teenagers with ADHD and ODD. *Journal of Consulting Clinical Psychology.69,* 926–941.

Barkley, R.A., Fischer, M., Edelbrock, & Smallish, L. (1990). The adolescent outcomes of hyperactive children diagnosed by research criteria: I. An 8-year prospective follow-up study. *Journal of the American Academy of Child and Adolescent Psychiatry, 29(4),* 546–557.

Berndt, T.J. (1989). Contributions of peer relationships to children's development. In T.J. Berndt, & G.W. Ladd (Eds.), *Peer Relationships in Child Development.* New York: Wiley.

Biederman, J. (2003). Pharmacotherapy for attention-deficit/hyperactivity disorder (ADHD) decreases the risk for substance abuse: Findings from a longitudinal follow-up of youths with and without ADHD. *Journal of Clinical Psychiatry,* 64(suppl11). 3–8.

Biederman, J., Milberger S., Faraone, S.V., Kiely, K., Guite. J, Mick, E., Ablon, S., Warburton, R., & Reed, E. (1995 a). Family-environment risk factors for attention-deficit hyperactivity disorder. A test of Rutter's indicators of adversity. *Archives of General Psychiatry, 52(6),* 464–70.

Biederman, J., Milberger S., Faraone, S.V., Kiely, K., Guite. J, Mick, E., Ablon, S., Warburton, R., Reed, E., & Davis, S.G. (1995b). Impact of adversity on functioning and comorbidity in children with attention-deficit hyperactivity disorder. *Journal of the American Academy of Child and Adolescent Psychiatry, 34(11),* 1495–503.

Biederman, J., & Spencer, T.J. (2002). Nonstimulant treatment for ADHD. In P.S. Jensen, & J.R. Cooper (Eds.), *Attention Deficit Hyperactivity Disorder. State of the Science. Best Practices.* New Jersey: Civic Research Institute.

Bradley, C. (1937). The behavior of children receiving benzedrine. *American Journal of Psychiatry,* 94, 577–585.

Brooks, R., & Goldstein, S. (2001). *Raising Resilient Children.* Chicago Illinois: Contemporary Books.

Brown, M.B. (2000). Diagnosis and treatment of children and adolescents with attention-deficit/hyperactivity disorder. *Journal of Counseling & Development,* 78:2.

Burke, J.D., Loeber, R., & Lahey, B.B. (2001). Which aspects of ADHD are associated with tobacco use in early adolescence? *Journal of Child Psychology and Psychiatry, 42(4),* 493–502.

Conners, C.K., Eisenberg, L., & Barcai, A. (1967). Effect of dextroamphetamine on children: studies on subjects with learning disabilities and school behavior problems. *Archives of General Psychiatry,* 17, 478–485.

Conners, C.K., Epstein, J.N., March, J.S., Angold, A., Wells, K.C., Klaric, J., et al. (2001). Multimodal treatment of ADHD in the MTA: An alternative outcome analysis. *Journal of the American Academy of Child and Adolescent Psychiatry, 40,* 159–167.

Cox, D.J., Merkel, R.L., Kovatchev, B., Seward, R. (2000) Effect of stimulant medication on driving performance of young adults with attention-deficit hyperactivity disorder: A preliminary double-blind placebo controlled trial. *Journal of Nervous and Mental Disorders, 188,* 230–234.

Cunningham, C.E., Bremner, R., & Secord-Gilbert, M. (1993) Increasing the availability, accessibility, and cost efficacy of services for families of ADHD children: A school-based systems-oriented parenting course. *Canadian Journal of School Psychology, 9,* 1–15.

Danforth, J.S. (1998). The outcome of parent training using the Behavior Management Flow Chart with mothers and their children with oppositional defiant disorder and attention-deficit hyperactivity disorder. *Behavior Modification, 22,* 443–473.

Douglas, V.I., Barr, R.G., Amin, K., O'Neill, M.E., & Britton, B.G. (1988). Dose effects and individual responsivity to methylphenidate in attention deficit disorder. *Journal of Child Psychology and Psychiatry,* 29, 453–475.

Dulcan, M., Dunne, J.E., Ayers, W., Arnold, V., Benson, S., Bernet, W., et al. (1997). Practice parameters for the assessment and treatment of children, adolescents, and adults with attention-deficit/hyperactivity disorder: AACAP Official Action. *Journal of the American Academy of Child and Adolescent Psychiatry, 36,* Supplement, 85S–121S.

Dumas, M.C. (1998). The risk of social interaction problems among adolescents with ADHD. *Education and Treatment of Children, 21(4),* 447–460.

DuPaul, G.J., & Eckert, T.L. (1997). The effects of school-based interventions for attention deficit hyperactivity disorder: A meta-analysis. *School Psychology Review,* 26:1.

DuPaul, G.J., Ervin, R.A., Hook, C.L., & McGoey, K.E. (1998). Peer tutoring for children with attention deficit hyperactivity disorder: Effects on classroom behavior and academic performance. *Journal of Applied Behavior Analysis, 31:4,* 579–592.

Eisenberg, L., Lachman, R., Molling, P., Lockner A, Mizelle, J., & Conners, C. (1961). A psychopharmacologic experiment in a training school for delinquent boys: methods, problems and findings. *American Journal of Orthopsychiatry, 33,* 431–437.

Ervin, R.A., DuPaul, G.J., Kern, L., & Friman, P.C. (1998). Classroom-based functional and adjunctive assessments: Proactive approaches to intervention selection for adolescents with attention deficit hyperactivity disorder. *Journal of Applied Behavior Analysis, 31:1,* 65–78.

Fischer, M, & Barkley, R.A. (2003) Childhood stimulant treatment and risk for later substance abuse. *Journal of Clinical Psychiatry. 64,* 19–23.

Fischer, M. (1990). Parenting stress and the child with Attention Deficit Hyperactivity Disorder. *Journal of Clinical Psychology, 19,* 337–346.

Fletcher, K.E., Fischer, M., Barkley, R.A., & Smallish, L. (1996). A sequential analysis of the mother-adolescent interactions of ADHD, ADHD/ODD, and normal teenagers during neutral and conflict discussions. *Journal of Abnormal Child Psychology 24 (3),* 271–297.

Flory, K., Milich, R., Lynam, D.R., Leukefeld, C., & Clayton, R. (2003). Relation between childhood disruptive behavior disorders and substance use and dependence symptoms in young adulthood: Individuals with symptoms of attention-deficit/hyperactivity disorder and conduct disorder are uniquely at risk. *Psychology of Addictive Behaviors, 17(2),* 151–158.

Foley, H.A., Carlton, C.O., & Howell, R.J. (1996). The relationship of attention deficit hyperactivity disorder to juvenile delinquency: Legal implications. *Bulletin of the American Academy of Psychiatric Law, 24(3),* 333–345.

Fuchs, T., Birbaumer, N., Lutzenberger, W., Gruzelier, J.H., Kaiser, J. (2003) Neurofeedback Treatment for Attention-Deficit/Hyperactivity Disorder in Children: A Comparison with Methylphenidate. *Applied Psychophysiology & Biofeedback, 28,* 1–12.

Gillberg, C., Melander, H., von Knorring, A., Janols, L.O., Thernlund, G., Hagglof, B., Eidevall-Wallin, L., Gustafsson, K., & Kopp, S. (1997). Long-term central stimulant treatment of children with attention-deficit hyperactivity disorder. A randomized double-blind placebo-controlled trial. *Archives of General Psychiatry, 54,* 857–864.

Gjone, H., Stevenson, J., & Sundet, J.M. (1996). Genetic influence on parent-reported attention-related problems in a Norwegian general population twin sample. *Journal of the American Academy of Child and Adolescent Psychiatry, 35,* 588–596.

Goldman, L.S., Genel, M., Bezman, R.J., & Slanetz, P.J. (1998). Diagnosis and treatment of attention-deficit/hyperactivity disorder in children and adolescents. *Journal of the American Medical Association, 279,* 1100–1107.

Greene, R., W., Biederman, J., Faraone, S.V., Ouellette, C. Penn, C., & Griffin, S. (1996). Toward a new psychometric definition of social disability in children with attention deficit hyperactivity disorder. *Journal of the American Academy of Child and Adolescent Psychiatry, 35,* 571–578.

Greene, R.W., Biederman, J., Sienna, M., Garcia-Jetton, J., & Faraone, S.V. (1997). Adolescent outcomes of boys with attention-deficit/hyperactivity disorder and social disability: Results from a 4-year longitudinal follow-up study. *Journal of Consulting and Clinical Psychology, 65(5),* 758–767.

Greenhill, L. (2002) Stimulant medication treatment of children with attention deficit hyperactivity disorder. In P.S. Jensen, & J.R. Cooper (Eds.), *Attention Deficit Hyperactivity Disorder. State of the Science. Best Practices.* New Jersey: Civic Research Institute.

Harley, J.P., Ray, R.S., Tomasi, L., Eichman, P.L., Matthews, C.G., Chun, R., Cleeland, C.S., & Traisman, E. (1978). Hyperkinesis and food additives: Testing the Feingold hypothesis. *Pediatrics, 61:6,* 818–828.

Hechtman, L. (1991). Resilience and vulnerability in long-term outcome of attention deficit hyperactive disorder. *Canadian Journal of Psychiatry, 36,* 415–421.

Hinshaw, S.P., Klein, R.G., & Abikoff. H. (1998). Childhood Attention Deficit Hyperactivity Disorder: Non-pharmacological and combination treatment. In P.E. Nathan & J.M. Gorman, (Eds.), *A Guide to Treatments that Work* (pp. 26–41). New York: Oxford University Press.

Hoza, B., Mrug, S., Pelham, W.E. Jr., Greiner, A.R., & Gnagy, E.M. (2003). A friendship intervention for children with attention-deficit/hyperactivity disorder: Preliminary findings. *Journal of Attention Disorders, 6,* 87–98.

Kavale, K. (1982). The efficacy of stimulant drug treatment for hyperactivity: A meta-analysis. *Journal of Learning Disabilities, 15,* 280–289.

Kolko, D.J., Bukstein, O.G., & Barron, J. (1999). Methylphenidate and behavior modification in children with ADHD and comorbid ODD or CD: Main and incremental effects across settings. *Journal of the American Academy of Child and Adolescent Psychiatry, 38:5,* 578–586.

Lambert, N.M. (1998). Adolescent outcomes of hyperactive children. *American Psychologist, 43,* 786–799.

Lee, J.R., Mulsow, M., & Reifman, A. (2003) Long-term correlates of Attention Deficit Hyperactivity Disorder: A meta-analysis. *Journal of Family and Consumer Sciences.*

LeFever, G., Sawson, K.V., & Morrow, A.L. (1999). The extent of drug therapy for attention deficit-hyperactivity disorder among children in public schools. *American Journal of Public Health, 89,* 1359–1364.

Levin, E.D., Conners, C.K., Silva, D., Hinton, S.C. Meek, W.H., March, J., & Rose, J.E. (1998). Transdermal nicotine effects on attention. *Psychopharmacology, 140,* 135–141.

Litner, B. (2003). Teen with ADHD: The challenge of high school. *Child and Youth Care Forum, 32(3),* 137–158.

Loney, J., Kramer, J., & Milich, R.S. (1981). The hyperactive child grows up: Predictors of symptoms, delinquency and achievement at follow-up. In K.D. Gadow & J. Loney (Eds.), *Psychological Aspects of Drug Treatment in Hyperactivity* (pp. 381–416). Boulder, CO: West-view Press.

Marshal, M.P., Molina, B.S.G., & Pelham, W.E. (2003). Childhood ADHD and adolescent substance use: An examination of deviant peer group affiliation as a risk factor. *Psychology of Addictive Behaviors, 17(4),* 203–302.

Mash, L., & Johnston, C. (1990). Determinants of parenting stress: Illustrations from families of hyperactive children and families of physically abused children. *Journal of Clinical Child Psychology, 19,* 313–328.

McCleary, L. (2002). Parenting adolescents with attention deficit hyperactivity disorder: Analysis of the literature for social work practice. *Health and Social Work, 27(4),* 285–292.

Molina, B.S.G., & Pelham, W.E. (2003). Childhood predictors of adolescent substance use in a longitudinal study of children with ADHD. *Journal of Abnormal Psychology, 112(3),* 497–507.

Molina, B.S.G., Smith, B.H., & Pelham, W.E. (1999). Interactive effects of attention deficit hyperactivity disorder and conduct disorder on early adolescent substance use. *Psychology of Addictive Behaviors, 13,* 348–358.

Monastra, V.J., Monastra, D.M., & George, S. (2002). The Effects of Stimulant Therapy, EEG Biofeedback and Parenting Style on the Primary Symptoms of Attention-Deficit/Hyperactivity Disorder. *Applied Psychophysiology and Biofeedback, 27,* 249–260.

MTA Cooperative Group (1999). A 14-month randomized clinical trial of treatment strategies for Attention Deficit/Hyperactivity Disorder. *Archives of General Psychiatry, 56,* 1073–1086.

Mulsow, M., & Lee, J.R. (2003) The prevention of long-term problems associated with Attention Deficit/Hyperactivity Disorder in childhood, in M. Bloom & T.P. Gullotta (Eds.), *Encyclopedia of Primary Prevention and Health Promotion.* New York: Kluwer/Plenum Academic Press, 207–212.

Nash, J.K. (2000). Treatment of attention deficit hyperactivity disorder with neurotherapy. *Clinical Electroencephalography, 31,* 30–37.

National Institutes of Health (NIH) Consensus Statement Online 16 (1998, Nov. 10) Diagnosis and Treatment of Attention Deficit Hyperactivity Disorder. Accessed Nov 16–18, 1999, pp. 1–37. Available at: http://odp.od.nih.gov/ consensus/cons/110/110_statement.htm.

National Institute of Mental Health (2000). Information obtained from http://www.nimh.nih.gov.

Ottenbacher, J., & Cooper, H. (1983). Drug treatment of hyperactivity in children. *Developmental Medicine and Child Neurology, 25,* 358–366.

Parker, J.G., & Asher, S.A. (1987). Peer relations and later personal adjustment: Are low accepted children at risk? *Psychological Bulletin, 102,* 357–389.

Rapport, M.D., Chung, K., Shore, G., & Isaacs, P. (2001). A conceptual model of child psychopathology: Implications for understanding attention deficit hyperactivity disorder and treatment efficacy. *Journal of Clinical Child Psychology, 30:1.*

Robbins, L.N (1986). *Deviant children grown up.* Baltimore: Williams & Wilkins.

Safer, D., Zito, J., & Fine, E. (1996). Increased methylphenidate usage for attention deficit hyperactivity disorder in the 1990's. *Pediatrics, 98,* 1084–1088.

Schachar, R.J., Tannock, R., Cunningham, C., & Corkum, P.V. (1997). Behavioral, situational, and temporal effects of treatment of ADHD with methylphenidate. *Journal of the American Academy of Child and Adolescent Psychiatry, 36(6),* 754–763.

Sher, K.J. (1991). *Children of Alcoholics: A Critical Appraisal of Theory and Research.* Chicago: University of Chicago Press.

Spencer T., Biederman J., Wilens T., Harding M., O'Donnell D., & Griffin S. (1996) Pharmacotherapy of attention-deficit hyperactivity disorder across the life cycle. *Journal of the American Academy of Child and Adolescent Psychiatry, 35(4),* 409–432.

Swanson, J., Lerner, M., & Williams, L. (1995). More frequent diagnosis of attention deficit hyperactivity disorder. *New England Journal of Medicine, 333,* 944.

Thurber, S., & Walker, C. (1983). Medication and hyperactivity: a meta-analysis. *Journal of General Psychiatry, 108,* 79–86.

Teeter, P.A. (1998). *Intervention for ADHD: Treatment in Developmental Context.* NY: Guilford.

Thomas, J.M. (1995) Traumatic stress disorder presents as hyperactivity and disruptive behavior: Case presentation, diagnoses, and treatment. *Infant Mental Health Journal,* 16, Special Issue: Posttraumatic stress disorder (PTSD) in infants and young children, 306–317.

Vitiello and Jensen, (1997) Medication development and testing in children and adolescents. Current problems, future directions. *Archives of General Psychiatry, 54(9),* 871–876.

Volkow, N.D. (2003) PET imaging in adults with AD/HD. Research symposium: From the Laboratories of NIH Directors, CHADD annual conference, October, 2003.

Weinberg, H.A. (1999). Parent training for attention-deficit hyperactivity disorder: Parental and child outcome. *Journal of Clinical Psychology, 55 (7),* 907–913.

Webster-Stratton, C. (1990). Stress: A potential disruptor of parent perceptions and family interactions. *Journal of Clinical Child Psychology, 19,* 302–312.

Weiss, G., Minde, K., & Werry, J. (1971). The hyperactive child. VIII: five-year-old follow-up. *Archives of General Psychiatry, 24,* 409–414.

Whalen, C.K., Jamner, L.D., Henker, B., Gehricke, J., & King, P.S. (2003). Is there a link between adolescent cigarette smoking and pharmacotherapy for ADHD? *Psychology of Addictive Behaviors, 17(4),* 332–335.

Wilens, T.E., Faraone, S.V., Biederman, J., Gunawardene, S. (2003). Does stimulant therapy of attention-deficit/hyperactivity disorder Beget later substances abuse? A meta-analytic review of the literature. *Pediatrics, 111,* 179–185.

Wilens, T.E., Biederman, J., Spencer, T., & Frances, R.J. (1994). Comorbidity of attention-deficit hyperactivity and psychoactive substance use disorders. *Hospital & Community Psychiatry, 45,* 421–423, 435.

Wilson, J.M., & Marcotte, A.C. (1995). Psychosocial adjustment and educational outcome in adolescents with a childhood diagnosis of attention deficit disorder. *Journal of the American Academy of Child and Adolescent Psychiatry, 35(5),* 579–587.

Chapter 9

Pediatric Bipolar Disorder

Mani N. Pavuluri, Michael W. Naylor, and John A. Sweeney

Introduction

Pediatric Bipolar Disorder (PBD) is one of the most common serious disorders among child psychiatry referrals (Geller and Luby, 1997; Wozniak et al., 1995). It is associated with high rates of suicide, school failure, and aggression, as well as high-risk behaviors such as sexual promiscuity and substance abuse (Wilens et al., 1999). High incidence of relapse and low recovery rates are common to the disorder (Geller et al., 2001; Craney and Geller, 2003). PBD is frequently misdiagnosed as attention-deficit/hyperactivity disorder (ADHD) and/or anxiety or depression, which often results in inappropriate treatment and worsening of symptoms (Biederman et al., 1999, 2000; DelBello et al., 2001a; Mota–Castillo et al., 2001; Soutullo et al., 2002). While the prevalence of bipolar disorder is estimated to be 1% in the adolescent population (Lewinsohn et al., 1995), there is a lack of solid epidemiological data on the prevalence of bipolar disorder in younger age groups.

One of the initial steps in recognizing this disorder is developing a comprehensive understanding of how it presents in children and early adolescents. Older adolescents tend to have a more typical presentation, similar to that of adult bipolar disorder (Pavuluri et al., 2002a). This chapter focuses on the presentation of bipolar disorder in childhood and early adolescence, and within this context the term PBD is used.

Conceptualizing PBD

There are four critical dimensions in understanding PBD. They include (1) the specific features of PBD that set it apart from adult bipolar disorder, (2) differentiation between PBD and ADHD, (3) descriptions of each of the key symptoms of PBD as they present in children, and (4) classifying subtypes within the bipolar spectrum.

UNIQUE FEATURES OF PBD. The five specific features are (1) rapid cycling, (2) predominantly mixed episodes, (3) prominent irritability, (4) comorbid ADHD and oppositional defiant disorder (ODD), and (5) chronicity (Geller et al., 1998; Findling et al., 2001; Wozniak et al., 1995). This presentation in children resembles the most severe variant of adult bipolar disorder where rapid cycling is seen in 20% and mixed episodes in 40% of patients defined as treatment resistant (Goodwin and Jamison, 1990; Craney and Geller, 2003).

DIFFERENTIATION BETWEEN PBD AND ADHD.   Geller et al. (1998, 2002) compared PBD with ADHD and found that five symptoms of mania in the *DSM IV* criteria (American Psychiatric Association, 1994) differentiated the two disorders. The presence of elated mood, grandiosity, hypersexuality, flight of ideas or racing thoughts, and decreased need for sleep signify PBD. Geller et al. (1998, 2002) recommends ensuring the presence of either elated mood or grandiosity before making a diagnosis of PBD. Irritability, an accompanying key feature along with elated or expansive mood (according to *DSM IV*), was considered nonspecific. The authors recommend that at least two of the three key features of elated mood, grandiosity, and irritability be present among the cluster of defining symptoms. A child may be grandiose, but without at least one of the two accompanying features of affect disinhibition (elated mood or irritability) there may be a room for misinterpretation. Therefore, we recommend adhering to *DSM IV* criteria with additional value to grandiosity.

CHARACTERISTIC CLINICAL DESCRIPTION OF MANIA IN PBD.   The clinical picture in this group can be very confusing, since healthy children can be active, imaginative, boastful, sensitive to the environment, and will "act out" periodically. Experienced clinicians, however, can differentiate the abnormal from the normal based on qualitative changes from baseline, persistence and severity of dysfunction in multiple contexts, and a typical clustering of symptoms. For example, it is critical for the clinician to assess grandiosity by taking into account the context and the developmentally appropriate level of judgment given the consequences for grandiose statements or behaviors. The following clinical description in children and adolescents illustrates PBD.

- *Elated mood* is often excitable, silly, giddy, feeling invincible, and "overwhelmed," with behavior such as laughing fits and excessive joking. Often, these episodes of elated mood are couched amidst other feelings of jealousy, love, anger, and sadness, and present a picture of extreme emotional lability.
- *Irritability* presents as intense and inconsolable affective responses that are out of proportion to the psychosocial situation that may result in aggression. Behaviors indicating irritability can include throwing things, slamming doors, being hostile or acidic, kicking, and screaming. An extreme example of this is illustrated by one preschool-aged boy who presented with scars on his face due to scratching himself in a state of rage until he bled. He would apologize to his parent later, "I said 'no, no, no' to my brain, but it can not stop being mad." Parents of bipolar children often report that they are "walking on eggshells." One adolescent described the anger he felt as an "invisible fist." At times, symptoms of irritability can be mixed with symptoms of grandiosity in PBD.
- *Inflated self-esteem and grandiosity* are characterized by unsupported statements such as "I will teach the coach how to swim, "He has no clue," "I am absolutely sure that I will get an Oscar before I am 35," "I am going to make millions through E Trade," and "I do not need to go to school." For example, a 9-year-old reported that she would beat

up her brother if he did not call her "princess." Sometimes, parents will describe grandiose behaviors in their children without giving it a name, as they are new to the concept of grandiosity. One parent reported that her daughter called herself: "Queen of the Universe." In fact, the daughter's email address was *QOU@XXX*.com. As with adults, psychosis is often seen in the manic phase. Delusions of grandiosity are the most common delusions in this age group. These children frequently act on their delusions, as they often lack an "age-appropriate reality check" system for monitoring their own behaviors.

- *Decreased need for sleep* is often illustrated by parents' descriptions of their children refusing to go to bed, getting little sleep, and still not feeling tired in the morning. Reports frequently include instances of playing, singing, and/or watching television into the early morning hours. Children often describe their subjective experience as feeling like an "Energizer Bunny™."

- *Pressure to keep talking* is often illustrated by statements like "My mind is like a Ferrari, a million thoughts are racing" and "No stoppers." Parents describe these children as rambling constantly. One 6-year-old child described his experience as "My mind is like a ship with too many passengers." One child developed what he referred to as "Twin language" (he did not have a twin), a conglomeration of grandiosity, creativity, and pressured speech.

- *Constant goal-directed activity* is illustrated by continued activity such as fiddling with objects and making messes at home that looks like disorganization. Often when parents confront the child about the mess or spill, they become defensive, denying that they were responsible. In our experience, parents often report this behavior as "lying," and it can take considerable effort to piece together the history of these "frenzied episodes." One child described himself as going through "crazy maniacal spells." Another child reported, "I ran for class president, and I lost, but I am fund-raising for 'N Sync to organize a concert."

- *Excessive pleasurable activities, poor judgment, and risk-taking* can be described with factual details. Youngsters may call 1-900 sex lines; suddenly start dressing inappropriately; get on sexually oriented chat lines; masturbate excessively; cut, hoard, or carry pornographic pictures; simulate sexual activity with animals; use their parents' credit cards to pay for mail-ordered sex items; or pressure parents to buy expensive/inappropriate clothing or other items. A history of sexual abuse is often considered in the differential diagnosis in these poorly socialized, sexually disinhibited children. In an ongoing phenomenological study, only 1.1% of the PBD sample had a history of sexual abuse or overstimulation, while 43% exhibited hypersexuality (Geller et al., 2002), supporting hypersexuality as a critical symptom in PBD.

- *Features of depression* are often described in age-specific terms. Children with PBD may report feeling crabby, whine excessively, cry for no reason, look unhappy, spend hours in a dark room, change moods rapidly from irritable to tearful, engage in skin-pinching and self-scratching at a young age, or complain of somatic symptoms. These children often develop intense rejection sensitivity after years of negative response from others due to their prickly and cyclic behavior. Even very young, prepubertal children may report suicidal behavior, stating a desire to hang or choke themselves. This usually represents desperate attempts to regulate or escape from these affective swings. Suicidal behavior has been reported to be on the order of 25% in PBD (Pavuluri et al., 2002a; Geller et al., 2002). In psychotic depressive episodes, mood-congruent delusions of doom, disaster, and nihilism are common. For example, one child drew pictures of a black ghost trying to take over the world.

CLASSIFICATION INTO SUBTYPES OF PBD SPECTRUM.   Leibenluft et al. (2003) suggested defining PBD into narrow, intermediate, and broad phenotypes. The narrow phenotype is attributed to those that meet the full *DSM IV* diagnostic criteria for mania or hypomania, including the duration criterion of seven and four days, respectively, and also have hallmark symptoms of elevated mood or grandiosity. Intermediate phenotypes are two categories that include those with (1) hallmark symptoms of short duration, i.e., one to three days, and (2) episodic irritable mania or hypomania meeting the duration criteria without elation. The broader phenotype consists of nonepisodic chronic illness without the hallmark symptoms of elated mood or grandiosity but with the severe irritability and hyperarousal associated with the narrow phenotypes. Bipolar NOS category in *DSM IV* corresponds to the intermediate and broad phenotypes (NIMH Roundtable on Bipolar NOS, 2001). This phenotyping is critical in research studies of neuropsychopharmacology and neurophysiology to examine underlying biological variables. At this stage of clinical practice, however, it has minimal significance in choosing treatment options.

Assessment Measure for Use in the Community to Screen for Bipolar Disorder

We developed the first mania rating scale specifically designed for children and adolescents, the Child Mania Rating Scale-Parent Version (CMRS-P). CMRS-P has excellent test re-test reliability (0.96), internal consistency (.96), and both the sensitivity and specificity of 0.92 with a cut-off for determining the presence of PBD at 35 out of 63 (the scale has 21 items with a range from 0 to 3) (Pavuluri et al., 2004a). Factor analysis yielded a single factor of mania. The Young Mania Rating Scale (YMRS; Young et al., 1978) is a clinician-rated scale that distinguished children with bipolar disorder and ADHD in a small sample and in an open trial (Fristad et al., 1992). To suit our clinical and research application of YMRS, wording that is suitable for the child was added to the existing items and it became customary to rely on parent reports over a week than merely on child observation in the clinic (personal communication, Kowatch, 2000). Gracious et al. (2002) tested YMRS in parents and found it to be reliable. But the scale relies heavily on items that are not well described or child-friendly if used as a parent report, especially with items such as lacking in insight and appearance. ADHD rating scales are not useful in differentiating the two disorders (Wilens et al., 2002).

Individual Factors

There are no clear neuroendocrine, biochemical, genetic, or neuroimaging findings that confirm or rule out PBD. However, there are several emerging findings in neuropsychology and neuroimaging.

Dickstein et al. (2003) administered a computerized neuropsychological test battery known as the Cambridge Neuropsychological Test Automated Battery (CANTAB) to a sample of 21 children and adolescents with PBD and compared them with 21 age- and gender-matched controls. In comparison to controls, children with PBD were impaired on measures of attentional set-shifting and visuospatial memory. Post hoc analyses in individuals with PBD subjects did not show significant associations between neuropsychological performance and acute mania or ADHD comorbidity. Meyer et al. (2003) found similar executive dysfunction using the Wisconsin Card Sorting Test (WCST) not explained by preexisting attentional disturbance. In fact, executive function deficits preceded formal diagnosis and treatment of bipolar disorder, even when controlling for intelligence, age, gender, and premorbid attentional deficits.

Davanzo et al. (2003) used magnetic resonance spectroscopy to show that myoinositol levels were higher in the anterior cingulate in PBD compared to intermittent explosive disorder. Preliminary functional magnetic resonance imaging (fMRI) results suggested decreased activation of dorsolateral prefrontal cortex and increased activation of right cerebellar hemisphere in chronic PBD compared to first-episode mania in adolescents (DelBello et al., 2003). Additionally, youth experiencing their first manic episode demonstrated greater activation of the DLPFC and the limbic cortex in response to the Continuous Performance Test than normal controls. A similarly high activation was found in DLPFC and anterior cingulate and subgenual cingulate cortex in PBD compared to normal controls in response to viewing positively and negatively valenced pictures using fMRI (functional Magnetic Resonance Imaging) methods (Adleman et al., 2001). Structural magnetic resonance imaging studies have shown subcortical white matter hyperintensities in mania (Botteron et al.,1995; Pillai et al., 2002). Smaller amygdala volume was found in adolescents with PBD (Karchemskiy et al., 2003) compared to increased size reported in adult studies (Strakowski et al., 1999). These preliminary findings need replication in larger sample studies.

Family factors

Familial Genetic Studies

Faraone et al. (1997) examined ADHD probands (with and without bipolar disorder), non-ADHD controls, and their first-degree biological relatives. Relatives of ADHD probands with bipolar disorder had an equal risk of manifesting ADHD as did relatives of ADHD without bipolar disorder. In contrast, relatives of ADHD probands with bipolar disorder were at a higher risk for bipolar disorder and major depression than those of the non-bipolar ADHD and control groups. One study based on detailed interviews with parents of an outpatient population of bipolar I children or adolescents found that roughly 80% had at least one parent diagnosed with a mood disorder (Findling et al., 2001).

Psychosocial Risk Factors

Psychosocial factors are relevant in PBD compared to ADHD and control populations. While their exact role is unknown, they do play a critical role when planning psychosocial interventions. Geller et al. (2002) reported that more than half of those diagnosed with PBD had no friends, were teased by other children, and had poor social skills. They had poor relationships with siblings and conflictual relationships with their parents. Specifically, there was a high degree of hostility and low warmth in maternal–child relationships, poor agreement between parents on child-rearing practices, and minimal problem-solving skills.

Social and Community Factors

The most serious risk factors, given the biological nature of PBD, are iatrogenic in nature. As noted, there is a high incidence of PBD in the offspring of bipolar subjects (Chang et al., 2000). The incidence of PBD in the offspring of bipolar parents was much lower in a similar Dutch study (Wals et al., 2001), however. One of the reasons offered for the higher incidence in the USA was the increased prescription of stimulants and antidepressants (Magno-Zito et al., 2003) that are likely to precipitate a predisposed condition (Biederman et al., 1999, 2000; DelBello et al., 2001a; Mota-Castillo et al., 2001; Soutullo et al., 2002).

Environmental factors appear to have a greater impact on clinical course than the incidence of illness. One critical factor related to poor clinical outcome appears to be lack of early recognition and appropriate treatment. A majority of patients in Geller et al.'s (2002) psychopathology studies were recruited from the community where they were not treated with mood stabilizers. While they did not analyze the results to show that lack of appropriate treatment in the community is indeed a significant factor, only 37.1% recovered at the end of one year and 65.2% recovered at the end of 2 years. We showed a much higher recovery at 84.2% in preschool-onset bipolar disorder at the end of one year with a closer and tailored treatment follow-up (Pavuluri et al., 2004b).

Evidence-Based Treatment Interventions in Community Settings

Given the restrictions of reimbursement and pediatric psychiatric bed availability, the majority of the severe PBD patients are being treated in the community. Prior to initiating definitive treatment, the baseline evaluation should include a comprehensive psychiatric evaluation; recent physical examination; electrocardiogram (ECG); complete blood count; comprehensive metabolic profile, including liver and thyroid function tests; urine pregnancy test in teenage girls; and a drug screen.

Psychopharmacology

Table 1 summarizes the key medication trials. Information from these trials helped in formulating a pharmacotherapy algorithm for PBD (Pavuluri et al., 2003). An emerging theme is the need for combination pharmacotherapy given a limited response to monotherapy. Response rates vary based on definition of outcome criteria. Significantly, the majority of the studies of pharmacotherapy in PBD allowed rescue medications; primarily the continuation of stimulant medication to address ADHD.

Table 1. Pharmacotherapy Studies in Pediatric Bipolar Disorder

Author/Study Title	Diagnosis/Age	Design/Setting/Duration	Outcome Measures	Definition of Outcome/Complete Responders/Complete Remitters
Geller et al., 1998 "Double-Blind and Placebo Controlled Study of Lithium for Adolescent Bipolar Disorders with Secondary Substance Dependency"	BP I (n = 12), BP II (n = 5), MDD with BP predictors (n = 8)/state not specified;comorbid substance abuse (alcohol and marijuana mostly)/ 16.3 ± 1.2 years	Double-blind, placebo-controlled, pharmacokinetically dosed/ outpatient/6 weeks	Weekly random lithium levels and urine samples for drug assays, CGAS ≥ 65	Out of 13 on active drug, 6 were active responders (46.2%)/ 10% positive urine drug screen in those on lithium and 40% in those on placebo
Kowatch et al., 2000 "Effect Size of Lithium, Divalproex Sodium and Carbamazepine in Children and Adolescents with Bipolar Disorder"	BP I and II (35)/mixed, manic, or hypomanic/ 8–18 years, mean age 11.4 years	Open-label, randomized to 3 arms/outpatient/ 2-week screening + 6-week trial period	Weekly YMRS, CGI-Improvement score	50% reduction in YMRS from baseline +CGI ≤ 2; effect sizes/response rate: DVPX, 53%; Li, 38%; CBZ, 38%; ES, 1.63-DVPX; 1.06-Li, 1-CBZ
Wagner et al., 2002 "An Open-Label Trial of Divalproex in Children and Adolescents with Bipolar Disorder"	Bipolar I and II (n = 40)/ manic, hypomanic, mixed MRS score ≥ 14/7–19 years; mean age 12.1 (3.62) years	Open-label study (2–8 weeks) depending on clinical response followed by double-blind placebo-controlled trial (8 weeks)/outpatient	MRS, Manic Syndrome Scale (MSS) and Behavior Ideation Scale (BIS), Endicott and Spitzer, 1978), BPRS, CGI-Severity Scale, HAM-D	Pre-post scores are compared on all outcome measures (reported p-values eg, 0.001 on all measures); 22 of 36 (61%) showed ≥50% improvement from baseline in MRS score; effect size for change in base line to final score on MRS was 1.12
DelBello et al., 2002a A "Double-Blind, Randomized, Placebo-Controlled Study of Quetiapine as Adjunctive Treatment for Adolescent Mania"	BP type I (30)/manic or mixed/12–18 years	DVPX open trial, with randomized double-blind placebo-controlled strategy for augmentation/inpatients followed later as outpatients/ 6 weeks	YMRS, PANSS-P, CDRS, CGAS	Response was change of ≥50% from baseline to end point on YMRS; secondary response measures of change from baseline—CGAS, PANSS-P, CDRS (P-values, ANOVAS between groups)/87% in combination vs. 53% in monotherapy; no difference in CDRS, PANSS-P, C-GAS

(continued)

Table 1. (*continued*)

Author/Study Title	Diagnosis/Age	Design/Setting/Duration	Outcome Measures	Definition of Outcome/Complete Responders/Complete Remitters
Findling et al., 2003 "Combination Lithium and Divalproex sodium in Pediatric Bipolarity"	B I and II (n = 90)/ heterogenous cohort- episode can be mixed, manic, depressed, hypomanic, euthymic/ 5–17 years	Initial phase of stabiliza- tion(of a multiphase study)/outpatient/1–20 weeks and an average of 11.3 ± 5.3 weeks	YMRS, CDRS-R, CGI- Severity Scale, CGI- Improvement Scale, CGAS	Symptom response: YMRS ≥ 50% change from baseline; remitters are those who scored ≤12.5 at end point and CGI-I ≤2 and CGAS ≥ 51/remitters = 46.7%; using Kowatch crite- ria, complete response = 70.6%; using Frazier's criteria, complete response = 75.3%
Kafantaris et al., 2001a "Adjunctive Antipsy- chotic Treatment of Adolescents with Bipolar Psychosis"	BP I(n = 35)/acute mania with psychosis/12–18 years	Open trial of combination therapy of Li+antipsy- chotic followed by Li monotherapy/88.1% were inpatients at enrollment/ 4 weeks of open combination trial + 4 weeks of Li monotherapy	YMRS CGI-I HAM-D C GAS	YMRS score 33% decrease from baseline and CGI-Improvement 1 or 2/see numbers retained; 64% improved on combination; few remained stable on monotherapy; predictors of response to monotherapy correlated with short duration of psychosis, first episode, and baseline thought disorder
Kafantaris et al., 2001b "Adjunctive Antipsy- chotic is Necessary for Adolescents with Psychotic Mania"	Bipolar type I(n = 10)/ manic episode with YMRS ≥16/12–18 years; mean 15.40 ± 1.14 years in psychotic group and 14.20 ± 0.84 in nonpsy- chotic group	Combination therapy in psychotic patients for 1 week; otherwise, 4-week open Li monotherapy for all (followed by double- blind discontinuation)/ inpatient/6 weeks	YMRS, HAM-D, BPRS	YMRS score 33% decrease from baseline and CGI-Improvement 1 or 2/Psychotic mania = all got better on combination therapy, but none responded (3 needed combination again and two completed 4-week Li monotherapy); nonpsychotic mania = 3 out of 5 responded to Li monotherapy

Study	Sample/Diagnosis/Age	Design/Setting/Duration	Measures	Results
DelBello et al., 2002b "Adjunctive Topiramate Treatment for Pediatric Bipolar Disorder: A Retrospective Chart Review"	Bipolar I and II (n = 26)/mania, hypomania, mixed episodes/14 ± 3.5 years	Chart review/outpatient/4.1 ± 6.1 months	CGI-Mania, CGI-Overall, CGAS	CGI-Improvement ≤2 at end point/73% for mania and 62% for overall illness; G GAS improved from 40 ± 12 to 59 ± 16
Frazier et al., 1999 "Resperidone Treatment for Juvenile Bipolar Disorder: A Retrospective Chart Review"	BP/mixed and hypomanic/10.4 ± 3.8 years	Chart review/outpatient/6.1 ± 8.5 months	CGI-BP	CGI-Improvement ≤2/82% on mania and aggression subscales, 69% on psychosis subscale, and 8% on ADHD subscale; mean CGI-Severity scores reduced significantly ($P < 0.01$) on mania (5.4 to 2.9), aggression (5.1 to 3) and psychosis (3.6 to 1.5) scales; modest yet significant change on ADHD scale (5.0 to 4.3)
Masi et al., 2002 "Clozapine in Adolescent Inpatients with Acute Mania"	BP (n = 60)/treatment-resistant manic and mixed episodes that did not adequately respond to mood stabilizers or risperidone, olanzapine, or haloperidol 12–17 years or 14.8 ± 1.9 years	Chart review over 3 years from being inpatient for 15–28 days to 12–24-month outpatient follow-up	CGI MRS BPRS C-GAS	CGI-Improvement ≤2 and pre-post comparisons on all measures with P-values/ All 10 score 1 or 2 on CGI-I scale; improvement was $P < 0.001$ on MRS, BPRS, C-GAS and CGI-Severity
Frazier et al., 2001 "A Prospective Open-Label Treatment Trial of Olanzapine Monotherapy in Children and Adolescents with Bipolar Disorder"	BP I or II(n = 23)/mixed, manic, hypomanic/5–14 years/10.3 ± 2.9 years	Open trial/outpatients/8 weeks	YMRS CGI-S BPRS CDRS	YMRS decrease in score by 30% from baseline +CGI-S score ≤3/using the YMRS decrease in score by 30%, 61% improved/there was significant change in all scales when baseline and end point scores are compared ($P < 0.001$)

(continued)

193

Table 1. (*continued*)

Author/Study Title	Diagnosis/Age	Design/Setting/Duration	Outcome Measures	Definition of Outcome/Complete Responders/Complete Remitters
Pavuluri et al., 2004 "A Prospective Trial of Combination Therapy of Risperidone with Lithium or Divalproex Sodium in Severe Pediatric Mania"	BP I and YMRS > 20/ 12.1 ± 3.5 years	Open trial of sequential assignment of Li + Risperidone or DVPX + risperidone/ outpatient/6 months	YMRS CGI-BP CDRS-R C-GAS	YMRS 50% improvement from baseline /80% for DVPX + Risp and 82.4% for Li + Risp; using an outcome criteria for remission of ≥50% change from baseline on YMRS, CGI-BP-Improvement subscale of ≤2, and ≥51 CGAS score, the response rate in the Li + Risp group was 64.7% and in the DVPX + Risp group it was 60.0%
Kowatch et al., 2003 "Combination Pharmacotherapy in Children and Adolescents with Bipolar Disorder"	BP/types I (n = 17)and II(n = 18)/ mean age of 11 ± 2.8 years	Seminaturalistic follow-up or extension phase of acute trial/outpatient/ an extension of 16 weeks (6–8 weeks of acute trial + 16 weeks of follow up study phase = 24 weeks altogether)	YMRS CGI-BP CGAS	YMRS 50% improvement from baseline/80% among the 20 subjects requiring combination therapy
Pavuluri et al., 2003 "A Pharmacotherapy Algorithm for Stabilization and Maintenance of Pediatric Bipolar Disorder"	BP I (n = 64 + 17 matched controls receiving treatment as usual (TAU))/ 11.74 years (SD = 3.36 years)	Open trial of algorithm TAU versus TAU/18.6 months follow-up	CGI-BP CGAS	CGI-BP-Improvement scale score of 1 or 2/complete response was seen in 68.75% (n = 44/64) in the overall sample that received algorithm treatment; there was 94.1% response in matched algorithm group (n = 17), while none improved in TAU group; patient satisfaction on an overall scale of 1–5 (1 = worst and 5 = best) that defines acceptability, availability, and efficacy was at 4.6 (± 0.83)

Study	Diagnosis / Sample	Design / Duration	Measures	Results
Kafantaris et al., 2003 "Lithium Treatment of Acute Mania in Adolescents: A Large Open Trial"	BP/Acute manic episode/12–18 years	Open trial/77% were inpatients at enrollment with mean length of hospitalization 35.10 days ± 31.64 days / 4 weeks	YMRS CGI-BP HAM-D C-GAS BPRS	YMRS score 33% decrease from baseline and CGI-Improvement 1 or 2/63 patients responded; effect size = 1.48; on all measures, improvement was noted at $P < 0.001$; 50% met response criteria if based on 50% decrease in YMRS score; 26 patients achieved remission based on YMRS score ≤6; suicidal ideation decreased in all but 4 out of 23 at baseline
Chang et al., 2003 "Divalproex Monotherapy in the Treatment of Bipolar Offspring with Mood and Behavioral Disorders and at Least Mild Affective Symptoms"	Bipolar offspring (n = 24)/one parent with bipolar disorder/MDD, ADHD, dysthymia or cyclothymia past or current + YMRS score of 12 or HAM-D score of 12/n = 24, 17 boys and 7 girls/11.3 years = mean, 6–18 years	Open trial/outpatient/12 weeks	CGI-Improvement scale score of 1 or 2—primary efficacy measure; secondary measures are YMRS or HAM-D score change of 50% or more	YMRS change = $P < 0.001$ HAM-D change = $P = 0.0002$; 100% (7/7)females and 69%(11/16) males met the criteria for response

Note: MDD; ADHD; BP; HAM-D; YMRS; CGAS; CGI; PANSS-P; BPRS; CDRS-R; TAU; DVPX; Li; CBZ.

Medication Algorithm for PBD

It is critical to extrapolate a potentially useful treatment plan based on the findings from various studies and the pharmacotherapy algorithm study (Pavuluri et al., 2004). Essential steps in mood stabilization are the following: (1) eliminate destabilizing agents such as stimulants and antidepressants, (2) stabilize primary mood with monotherapy using lithium or divalproex sodium, (3) augment with second-generation antipsychotics (SGAs) if mood is still unstable, and (4) address associated symptomatology such as ADHD, sleep difficulties, hyperarousal, breakthrough symptoms of psychosis, depression, and medication-induced weight gain. If *depression* is the primary symptom, lithium is the choice for mood stabilization. The adult literature indicates that lithium may reduce the suicide rate associated with PBD (Baldessarini et al., 2003). In addition to a mood stabilizer, bupropion or venlafaxine may be viable additions, in view of their possible decreased propensity to switch mood states in comparison to other antidepressants (Kahn, 2000).For *concurrent PBD and ADHD*, a psychostimulant may be necessary. It is important, however, to stabilize mood symptoms before embarking on such a course. Methylphenidate (Ritalin, Concerta), dextroamphetamine (Dexedrine), or dextroamphetamine and amphetamine sulfate (Adderall XR) are all reasonable choices. We start at low doses of methylphenidate (e.g., 10 to 15 mg) and titrate up as needed, seldom prescribing doses higher than 60 mg. Likewise, excessive doses of dextroamphetamine may trigger psychosis or mania (Janicak et al., 2001). For a subgroup of bipolar children, symptoms of inattention may worsen on stimulants even after mood stabilization. Bupropion SR (150 mg per day) may effectively treat cognitive symptoms of ADHD (inattention and impulsivity), especially in the presence of depressed symptoms (Daviss et al., 2001). For excessive motoric symptoms, clonidine may be an appropriate choice (Pliszka et al., 2000). Of note, emergent symptoms of inattention may be due to pharmacotherapy with a mood stabilizer or residual symptoms. While atomoxetene is available for use in ADHD, its safety and efficacy has not been established in PBD with comorbid ADHD. For *sleep difficulties*, the initial step is to prescribe the primary medication at night. If inadequate, trazodone (25–50 mg) or clonidine (0.05 mg qhs) may be effective adjuncts (Prince et al., 1996). Pharmacotherapy for insomnia should be time limited, especially if using benzodiazepines or other agents that can cause habituation and rebound insomnia upon discontinuation (Janicak et al., 2001). If *arousal and aggression* are prominent, the dose of the mood stabilizer is maximized as tolerated, and a novel antipsychotic initiated at low doses (Schur et al., 2003). If there is clear but only partial response with a primary mood stabilizer plus novel antipsychotic, the addition of clonidine or guanfacine (1 mg qd or bid) may be useful to reduce arousal and increased activity (Pliszka et al., 2000; Prince et al., 1996). *Weight gain* is often an issue with olanzapine, risperidone, or valproate. If significant weight gain occurs, alternative medications should be considered. Frequently, topiramate is used in adults to stabilize mood and reduce weight (Janicak et al., 2001). This raises the question of whether it can be used for a similar indication in children (Lessig et al., 2001; Pavuluri et al., 2002b). We urge caution in this regard, given the cognitive side effects associated with topiramate. Reviewing healthy eating habits, consulting a nutritionist, and providing information on weight management may be effective. *Breakthrough symptoms or emerging psychosis* with the maximum tolerated dose of mood stabilizer may require intermittent, short adjunctive courses of a novel antipsychotic. Since the hepatic enzyme system in *preschoolers* may not be mature, lithium is the drug of choice. Total T_3, T_4, free T_4, and TSH should be obtained periodically. If thyroid abnormalities occur, referral to an endocrinologist is appropriate. If gastrointestinal symptoms occur with one preparation (e.g., Synthroid), an alternative (e.g., Levothroid) may be as effective and better tolerated.

What Works

Combination therapy for severe mania and antipsychotic medication as an adjuvant to a mood stabilizer for psychosis or severe illness were shown to be helpful. It is effective and safe to treat residual comorbid ADHD with stimulants, although there may be worsening of symptoms in a subgroup of children or adolescents.

What Might Work

Antidepressants in very low doses, used in combination with a mood stabilizer, may help alleviate treatment-resistant depression mixed with manic symptoms in PBD. Pharmacotherapy algorithm may be effective in outpatients with PBD. Often, it is not adequate just to treat "mood dysregulation," and co-existing problems such as sleep difficulties need

What Does Not Work

Antidepressants or stimulants as first-line medications are potentially harmful without prior mood stabilization.

Psychosocial Therapy

There are no proven psychosocial treatment methods for PBD. Fristad et al. (1998) employ a manual-driven, adjunctive, *multiple family group treatment* for youths aged 8–12 years with bipolar and depressive spectrum disorders. This method includes psychoeducation about the disorder, the role of medications, reducing self-blame, improving communication between parents and children, stress management, and helping the youth to develop coping strategies.

Miklowitz (2001) is developing a manual for adolescents (ages 13–17 years) with bipolar I disorder. This is based on the success of a *family-focused psychoeducation model* in bipolar adults. The program involves psychoeducation, family problem-solving, improving communication (communication enhancement training, CET) to reduce expressed emotion, managing crises, and helping the patient rehearse and develop coping strategies in the event of a future relapse.

Finally, Greene (2001) has developed a *"collaborative problem-solving"* model that focuses on parents as a "surrogate frontal lobe" so children can develop appropriate skills. The main focus is to help parents avoid engaging their children when they are raging and not ask, "why is he/she doing this?" or give up passively but to let the rage pass. Only after a rage attack subsides can the parent encourage collaborative problem-solving. This approach is controversial, since this group emphasizes "no consequences" for the rage behavior or actions related to it.

We have developed a treatment program called *"child- and family-focused cognitive behavior therapy (CFF-CBT)"* that involves parent and child sessions for 8–12-year-olds with bipolar disorder (Pavuluri et al., 2004). An Article Plus Section on treatment protocol is available on the web to complement the empirical data and can be accessed at www.jaacap.org. Central to this approach is building the youth's self-esteem and helping all involved parties to understand that PBD is a neuropsychiatric problem of affect dysregulation, rather than willful misbehavior. Over 12 sessions, parents are trained as coaches, while engaging in parallel therapy to address their own affect regulation in dealing with their children, restructuring their thoughts regarding their effectiveness as parents, and learning to resolve interpersonal conflicts through empathy.

In this approach, both the parents and children are instructed in the use of *RAINBOW*:

- R = the importance of a routine (includes sleep hygiene)
- A = affect regulation/anger control (includes knowledge about the disorder, medication, life charts)
- I = "I can do it" (positive self-statements)
- N = no negative thoughts (restructuring negative thinking)/living in the "now"
- B = be a good friend/balanced lifestyle (also for parents)
- O = "Oh, how can 'we' solve it?" (letting the rages pass, interpersonal and situational problem-solving)
- W = ways to ask and get support (build a "support tree")

The school receives the work folder of the child documenting what has been accomplished in the individual sessions. In addition, we also have a teleconference with the school to educate them in the use of the RAINBOW program. Additional support and psychoeducation can be obtained from the Child and Adolescent Bipolar Foundation (CABF, via www. bpkids.org).

What Works

Involving parents, positive reinforcement, empathy, and measured feedback are potentially useful in psychosocial therapy.

What Does Not Work

Using negative consequences and punishment without collaboration with the patients can be disruptive to the parent–child relationship and recovery.

Evidence-Based Treatment Interventions in Residential Settings

Studies of the prevalence of bipolar disorder and psychopathology in the bipolar spectrum indicate that behavioral problems in the bipolar spectrum are common. Hunt et al. (2003) reported a prevalence rate of PBD of 18.8% in residential setting. While their sample scored high on the K-SADS Mania Rating Scale (KSADS-MRS,

Axelson et al., 2003), the majority were irritable, evinced poor judgement, and were hyperactive and labile in affect. Very few had hallmark symptoms of elated mood or grandiosity. Therefore, it is critical to interpret the results in light of sample characteristics. Carlson and Kelly (1998) examined psychiatrically hospitalized prepubertal children aged 5–12 years with multiple disorders and reported clinically significant Child Behavior Checklist (CBCL) factor scores on the social, thought, and aggressive behavior factors. Based on the parents' report, four or more manic symptoms were present in 80%. These results indicate that manic symptoms must be recognized, since they are a marker for more severe psychopathology, even if they do not always meet the criteria for a full episode. They also warn against the diagnosis of mania if there is no clear change from premorbid functioning or if symptoms of irritability and aggression are explained by a lack of limit setting. There are no published studies of PBD in residential settings as opposed to the hospitalized inpatient population.

What Works

Prevalence of "mania-like" symptoms were found to be high in the inpatient units, regardless of the diagnosis. It is important to identify and attempt symptomatic treatment.

What Might Work

A pharmacotherapy algorithm proposed in outpatient study may be effective also in inpatient population with "mania-like" symptoms.

What Does Not Work

Antidepressants or stimulants as first-line medications without a mood stabilizer on board is detrimental to the affective stability.

The Prevention of PBD

Early identification of prodromal symptoms is critical for prevention and early intervention. To identify behavioral and other problems that predict the future emergence of bipolar disorder in children, Egeland et al. (2000) coded medical record data from the first hospital admission for treatment of bipolar disorder in an Amish population. The most frequently reported symptoms were episodic changes in mood (depressed and irritable) and anger dyscontrol with no gender differences in symptom presentation. Many of these children were reported to be very sensitive and seemed "hyperalert" to the feelings of others. Rapid "extreme changes" from silence to bold, loud, and hostile behavior were also noted in many. Symptoms increased by 13–15 years of age, with a time interval of 9–12 years between first symptoms and the first documented manic episode. Chang et al. (2000) found a similar symptom profile (i.e., increased severity of depressed and irritable mood, lack of affect modulation and rejection sensitivity) in the offspring of bipolar patients. These prodromal symptoms may be more accurately termed "symptoms of high risk," since not all children develop PBD. DelBello and Geller (2001b) reviewed studies of child and adolescent offspring of bipolar parents and found that rate of mood disorders was 5–67% compared with rates in offspring of healthy volunteers of 0–38%, underlining that bipolar offspring are a high-risk cohort.

Early recognition can be facilitated by screening for bipolar symptomatology using CMRS (Pavuluri et al., 2004a). This facilitates early intervention and prevention using a mood stabilizer (Chang et al., 2003). However, one needs to exercise caution in subsyndromal cases with regard to intervening with pharmacotherapy, as several factors causing affect dysregulation may be at play and may not progress into bipolar disorder. There are no published studies of psychosocial intervention for prodromal symptoms of bipolar disorder.

What Works

Screening high-risk populations such as offspring of parents with bipolar disorder will result in early identification of PBD.

What Might Work

Early intervention with mood stabilizers to treat affect dysregulation may decrease the risk of developing full-blown disorder.

What Does Not Work

No data is available on harmful or ineffective strategies.

Recommendations

Characteristics of PBD include chronic persistence of symptoms with poor remission rates, ultradian cycling, and a mixed picture with manic and depressive symptoms. Central features of a manic episode are elated mood, grandiosity, and irritability. Without intervention, on follow-up, outcome is poor (37% recovery at the end of one year without tailored intervention compared to 84.2% with targeted treatment plan). Findings on biological and psychosocial risk factors are inconclusive given that the field is relatively young. A parent screening measure, the CMRS (Pavuluri et al., 2004a), is in development for early recognition of mania and appears to be an effective screening instrument based on our preliminary analysis. A pharmacotherapy algorithm and several psychosocial interventions are available and are effective tools to achieve clinical remission. It is the combination of the right medications at appropriate doses and continuing titration in response to the changing needs of the patient based on the illness state that is the "name of the game" in treating PBD. Despite a diversity of names and some differences in strategies, there is an overlapping theme of providing children with PBD and their families with practical skills to facilitate affect regulation. Future neuroscience research is needed to enhance understanding of the pathophysiology of PBD and to grasp the mechanisms of action underlying successful affect remediation. Identification of pathophysiology at the bio-psycho-social risk level and translating it into treatment and early interventions designed to enhance clinical outcome is an overarching broader goal.

References

Adleman N., Chang K.D., Dienes, K. (2001). FMRI of emotional processing in pediatric bipolar disorder. Poster presented at the 48th annual meeting of the American Academy of Child and Adolescent Psychiatry, Honolulu.

American Psychiatric Association (1994). *Diagnostic and Statistical Manual of Mental Disorders* (4th ed.). Washington, DC: Author.

Axelson, D., Birmaher, B., Brent, D., Wassick, S., Hoover, C., Bridge, J., et al. (2003). A preliminary study of the KSADS mania rating scale for children and adolescents. *Journal of Child & Adolescent Psychopharmacology, 13* (4), 463–470.

Baldessarini, R.J., Tondo, L., & Hennen, J. (2003). Lithium treatment and suicide risk in major affective disorders: Update and new findings. *Journal of Clinical Psychiatry, 64*, 44–52.

Biederman, J., Mick, E., Prince, J., Bostic, J.O., Wilens, T.E., Spencer, T., et al. (1999). Systematic chart review of the pharmacological treatment of comorbid attention deficit hyperactivity disorder in youth with bipolar disorder. *Journal of Child & Adolescent Psychopharmacology, 156*, 1931–1937.

Biederman, J., Mick, E., Spencer, T., Wilens, T.E., & Faraone, S.V. (2000). Therapeutic dilemmas in the pharmacotherapy of bipolar depression in the young. *Journal of Child & Adolescent Psychopharmacology, 10*(3), 185–192.

Botteron, K.N., Vannier, M.W., Geller, B., Todd, R.D., & Lee, B.C.P. (1995). Preliminary study of magnetic resonance imaging characteristics in 8- 16-year-olds with mania. *Journal of the American Academy of Child & Adolescent Psychiatry, 34*, 742–749.

Carlson, G.A., & Kelly, K.L. (1998). Manic symptoms in psychiatrically hospitalized children-what do they mean? *Journal of Affective Disorders, 51*(2), 123–135.

Chang, K.D., Dienes, K., Blasey, C., Adleman, N., Ketter, T., Steiner, H., et al. (2003). Divalproex monotherapy in the treatment of bipolar offspring with mood and behavioral disorders and at least mild affective sypmtoms. *Journal of Clinical Psychiatry, 64*(8), 936–942.

Chang, K.D., Steiner, H., & Ketter, T., A. (2000). Psychiatric phenomenology of child and adolescent bipolar offspring. *Journal of the American Academy of Child & Adolescent Psychiatry, 39*, 453–460.

Craney, J.L., & Geller, B. (2003). A prepubertal and early adolescent bipolar disorder-I phenotype: Review of phenomenology and longitudinal course. *Bipolar Disorders, 5*, 243–256.

Davanzo, P., Yue, K., Thomas, M.A., Belin, T., Mintz, J., Venkatraman, T.N., et al. (2003). Proton magnetic resonance spectroscopy of bipolar disorder versus intermittent explosive disorder in children and adolescents. *American Journal of Psychiatry, 160*(8), 1442–1452.

Daviss, W.B., Bentivoglio, P., Racusin, R., Brown, K.M., Bostic, J.Q., & Wiley, L. (2001). Bupropion sustained release in adolescents with comorbid attention-deficit/hyperactivity disorder and depression. *Journal of the American Academy of Child & Adolescent Psychiatry, 40*, 307–314.

DelBello, M.P., Carlson, G.A., Tohen, M., Bromet, E.J., Schwiers, M., & Strakowski, S.M. (2003). Rates and predictors of developing a manic or hypomanic episode 1 to 2 years following a first hospitalization for major depression with psychotic features. *Journal of Child & Adolescent Psychopharmacolgy, 13*(2), 173–185.

DelBello, M.P., & Geller, B. (2001b). Review of studies of child and adolescent offspring of bipolar parents. *Bipolar Disorders, 3*, 325–334.

DelBello, M.P., Kowatch, R.A., Warner, J., Schwiers, M.L., Rappaport, K.B., Daniels, J.P., et al. (2002b). Adjunctive topiramate treatment for pediatric bipolar disorder: A retrospective chart review. *Journal of Child & Adolescent Psychpharmacology, 12*(4), 323–330.

DelBello, M.P., Schwiers, M.L., Rosenberg, H.L., Strakowski, & S.M. (2002a). A double-blind, randomized, placebo-controlled study of quetiapine adjunctive treatment for adolescent mania. *Journal of the American Academy of Child & Adolescent Psychiatry, 41*(10), 1216–1223.

DelBello, M.P., Soutullo, C.A., Hendricks, W., Niemeier, R.T., McElroy, S.L., & Strakowski, S.M. (2001a). Prior stimulant treatment for adolescents with bipolar disorder: Association with age at onset. *Bipolar Disorders, 3*(2), 53–57.

Dickstein, D.P., Treland, J.E., Snow, J., McClure, E.B., Mehta, M.S., Towbin, K.E., et al. (2003). *Neuropsychological performance in pediatric bipolar disorder*. Poster presented at the National Institute of Mental Health, Bethesda, MD.

Egeland, J.A., Hostetter, A.M., Pauls, D.L., & Sussex, J.N. (2000). Prodromal symptoms before onset of manic-depressive disorder suggested by first hospital admission histories. *Journal of the American Academy of Child & Adolescent Psychiatry, 39*, 1245–1252.

Faraone, S.V., Biederman, J., Mennin D, Wozniak, J., & Spencer, T. (1997). Attention-deficit hyperactivity disorder with bipolar disorder: A familial subtype? *Journal of the American Academy of Child & Adolescent Psychiatry, 36*, 1387–1390.

Findling R.L., Gracious, B.L., McNamara N.K., Youngstrom, E.A., Demeter C.A., Branicky, L.A., et al. (2001). Rapid, continuous cycling and psychiatric co-morbidity in pediatric bipolar I disorder. *Bipolar Disorders, 3*, 202–210.

Findling, R.L, McNamara, N.K., Gracious, B.L., Youngstrom, E.A., Stansbrey, R.J., Reed, M.D., et al. (2003). Combination lithium and divalproex sodium in pediatric bipolarity. *Journal of the American Academy of Child & Adolescent Psychiatry, 42*(8), 895–901.

Frazier, J.A., Biederman, J., Tohen, M., Feldman, P.D., Jacobs, T.G., Toma, V., et al. (2001). A prospective open-label treatment trial of olanzapine monotherapy in children and adolescents with bipolar disorder. *Journal of Child & Adolescent Psychopharmacology, 11*(3), 239–250.

Frazier, J.A., Meyer, M.C., Biederman, J, Wozniak, J., Wilens, T.E., Spencer T.J., et al. (1999). Risperidone treatment for juvenile bipolar disorder: A retrospective chart review. *Journal of the American Academy of Child & Adolescent Psychiatry, 38*, 960–965.

Fristad, M.A., Weller, E.B., & Weller, R.A. (1992). The Mania Rating Scale: Can it be used in children? A preliminary report. *Journal of the American Academy of Child & Adolescent Psychiatry, 31*, 252–257.

Fristad, M.A., Gavazzi, S.M., Soldano, K.W. (1998). Multi-family psychoeducation groups for childhood mood disorders: A program description and preliminary efficacy data. *Contemporary Family Therapy, 20*, 385–402.

Geller, B., Craney, J.L., Bolhofner, K., DelBello, M.P., Williams, M., & Zimerman, B. (2001). One-year recovery and relapse rates of children with a prepubertal and early adolescent bipolar disorder phenotype. *American Journal of Psychiatry, 158*, 303–305.

Geller, B., Craney, J.L., Bolhofner, K., Nickelsburg, M.J., Williams, M., & Zimerman, B. (2002). Two-year prospective follow-up of children with a prepubertal and early adolescent bipolar disorder phenotype. *American Journal of Psychiatry, 159*(6), 927–933.

Geller, B., Cooper, T.B., Sun, K., Zimerman, B., Frazier, J., Williams, M., et al. (1998). Double-blind and placebo-controlled study of lithium for adolescent bipolar disorders with secondary substance dependency. *Journal of the American Academy of Child & Adolescent Psychiatry, 37*, 171–178.

Geller, B., & Luby, J. (1997). Child and adolescent bipolar disorder: A review of the past 10 years. *Journal of the American Academy of Child & Adolescent Psychiatry, 36*(9), 1168–1176.

Goodwin, F.K., & Jamison, K.R. (1990). *Manic-Depressive Illness*. New York: Oxford University Press.

Gracious, B.L., Youngstrom, E.A., Findling, R.L., & Calabrese, J.R. (2002). Discriminative validity of a parent version of the Young Mania Ratings Scale. *Journal of the American Academy of Child & Adolescent Psychiatry, 41*(11), 1350–1359.

Greene, R.W. (2001). *The Explosive Child: A New Approach for Understanding and Parenting Easily Frustrated, "Chronically Inflexible" Children* (2nd ed.). New York: Harper Collins.

Hunt, I.M., Robinson, J., Bickley, H., et al. (2003). Suicides in ethnic minorities within 12 months of contact with mental health services. National clinical survey. *British Journal of Psychiatry, 183*, 155–60.

Janicak, P.G., Davis, J.M., Preskorn, S.H., & Ayd, F.J. (2001). *Principles and Practice of psychopharmacotherapy* (3rd ed.). Philadelphia: Lippincott Williams & Wilkins.

Kahn, D.A., Sachs, G.S., Printz, D.J., et al. (2000) Medication treatment of bipolar disorder 2000: A summary of the expert consensus guidelines. *Journal of Psychiatry Practice, 6*, 197–211.

Kafantaris, V., Coletti, D.J., Dicker, R., Padula, G., & Kane, J.M. (2003). Lithium treatment of acute mania in adolescents: A large open trial. *Journal of the American Academy of Child & Adolescent Psychiatry, 42*(9), 1038–1035.

Kafantaris, V., Coletti, D.J., Dicker, R., Padula, G., & Pollack, S. (2001a). Adjunctive antipsychotic treatment of adolescents with bipolar psychosis. *Journal of the American Academy of Child & Adolescent Psychiatry, 40*, 1448–1456.

Kafantaris, V., Dicker, R., Coletti, D.J., & Kane, J.M. (2001b). Adjunctive antipsychotic treatment is necessary for adolescents with psychotic mania. *Journal of Child & Adolescent Psychopharmacology, 11*(4), 409–413.

Karchemskiy, A., Chang, K., Barnea-Goraly, N., Simeonoa, D.I., Garret, A., Adleman, N., et al. (2003). *Structural MRI reveals bilateral amygdala decrease in familial pediatric bipolar disorder.* Poster presented at the American Academy of Child & Adolescent Psychiatry (AACAP) conference, Miami, FL.

Kowatch, R.A., Sethuraman, G., Hume, J.H., Kromelis, M., & Weinberg, W.A. (2003). Combination pharmacotherapy in children and adolescents with bipolar disorder. *Biological Psychiatry, 53*(11), 978–984.

Kowatch, R.A., Suppes, T., Carmody, T.J., Bucci, J.P., Hume, J.H., Kromelis, M., et al. (2000). Effect size of lithium, divalproex sodium and carbamazepine in children and adolescents with bipolar disorder. *Journal of the American Academy of Child & Adolescent Psychiatry, 39*, 713–720.

Leibenluft, E., Charney, D.S., Towbin, K.E., Bhangoo, R.K., & Pine, D.S. (2003). Defining clinical pheno-types of juvenile mania. *American Journal of Psychiatry, 160*(3), 430–437.

Lessig, M.C., Shapira, N.A., Murphy, & T.K. (2001). Topiramate for reversing atypical antipsychotic weight gain. *Journal of the American Academy of Child & Adolescent Psychiatry, 40*, 1364.

Lewinsohn, P.M., Klein, D.N., & Seeley, J.R. (1995). Bipolar disorders in a community sample of older ado-lescents: Prevalence phenomenology, comorbidity, and course. *Journal of the American Academy of Child & Adolescent Psychiatry, 34*, 454–463.

Magno-Zito, J., Safer, D.J., dosReis, S., Gardner, J.F., Madger, L., & Soken, K. (2003). Psychotropic practice patterns for youth: A 10-year perspective. *Archives of Pediatric & Adolescent Medicine, 157*(1), 17–25.

Masi, G., Mucci, M., & Millepiedi, S. (2002). Clozapine in adolescent inpatients with acute mania. *Journal of Child & Adolescent Psychopharmacology, 12*(2), 93–99.

Meyer, S.E., Carlson, G.A., Wiggs, E.A., Martizez, P.E., Ronsaville, D.S., Klimes-Dougan, B., et al. (2003). A prospective study of the relation among impaired executive functioning, attentional deficits, and early onset bipolar illness, NIMH Pediatric Bipolar Disorder Conference, April 2003, Washington DC.

Miklowitz, D.J. (2001, November). *Coping with bipolar disorder during the transition to young adulthood.* Pre-sented at the Jean Paul Ohadi Conference on Children and Adolescents with Bipolar Disorders.

Mota-Castillo, M., Torruella, A., Engels, B., Perez, J., Dedrick, C., Gluckman, M., et al. (2001). Valproate in very young children: An open case series with a brief follow-up. *Journal of Affective Disorders, 67*(1–3), 193–197.

National Institute of Mental Health (2001). National Institute of Mental Health research roundtable on pre-pubertal bipolar disorder. *Journal of the American Academy of Child & Adolescent Psychiatry, 40*, 871–878.

Pavuluri, M.N., Grayczyk, P., Carbray, J., & Heidenreich, J. (2004). Child and Family Focused Cognitive Behavior Therapy in Pediatric Bipolar Disorder. *Journal of American Academy of Child and Adolescent Psychiatry.*

Pavuluri, M.N., Henry, D., Carbray, J.A., Devineni, B., Shaw, R.J., Sampson, G., & Birmaher, B. (2004a). Child Mania Rating Scale (CMRS): Development, Reliability and Validity, NIMH Pediatric Bipolar Disorder Conference, Boston.

Pavuluri, M., Henry, D., Carbray, J., Sampson, G., Naylor, M., & Janicak, P.G. (2004b). Risperidone Aug-mentation of Lithium in Preschool- onset Bipolar Disorder. Oral presentation, Society for Biological Psychiatry, NewYork.

Pavuluri, M.N., Henry, D., Naylor, M., Carbray, J., Sampson, G., & Janicak, P.G (2004). A Pharmacothera-py Algorithm for Stabilization and Maintenance of Pediatric Bipolar Disorder. *Journal of American Academy of Child and Adolescent Psychiatry.*

Pavuluri, M.N., Henry, D., Naylor, M., Sampson, G., Carbray, J., & Janicak, P.G. (2004). A Prospective Trial of Combination Therapy of Risperidone with Lithium or Divalproex Sodium in Pediatric Mania. *Journal of Affective Disorders, Special issue.*

Pavuluri, M.N., Janicak, P.G., & Carbray, J. (2002b). Topiramate plus Risperidone for Preschool Mania. *Journal of Child and Adolescent Psychopharmacology, 12*, 271–273.

Pavuluri, M.N., Kraus, M., & Sweeney, J.A. (2003). fMRI: Clinical Applications. *Contemporary Psychiatry, 2*(2), 1–8.

Pavuluri, M.N., Naylor, M.W., & Janicak, P.G. (2002a). Recognition and Treatment of Pediatric Bipolar Dis-order, *Contemporary Psychiatry, 1*(1), 1–10.

Pillai, J.J., Friedman, L., Stuve, T.A., Trinidad, S., Jesberger, J.A., Lewin, J.S. et al. (2002). Increased presence of white matter hyperintensities in adolescent patients with bipolar disorder. *Psychiatry Research Neu-roimaging, 114*, 51–56.

Pliszka, S.R., Greenhill, L.L., Crismon , M.L., Sedillo, A., Carlson, C., Conners, C.K., et al. (2000). The Texas children's medication algorithm project: Report of the Texas consensus conference panel on medica-tion treatment of childhood attention-deficit/hyperactivity disorder. *Journal of the American Academy of Child & Adolescent Psychiatry, 39*, 909–919.

Prince, J.B., Wilens, T.E., Biederman, J., Spencer T.J., & Wozniak, J.R., (1996). Clonidine for sleep distur-bances associated with attention-deficit hyperactivity disorder: A systematic chart review of 62 cases. *Journal of the American Academy of Child & Adolescent Psychiatry, 35*, 599–605.

Schur, S.B., Sikich L., Findling, R.L., Malone, R.P., Crimson, M.L., Derivan, A., MacIntyre, J.C., Pappadop-ulos, E., Greenhill, L., Schooler, N., Van Orden, K., & Jensen, P.S., (2003). Treatment Recommendations for Use of Antipsychotics for Aggressive Youth (TRAAY). Part I: A Review. *Journal of the American Academy of Child & Adolescent Psychiatry, 42(2)*, 599–605.

Soutullo, C.A., DelBello, M.P., Ochsner, J.E., McElroy, S.L., Taylor S.A., Strakowski, et al. (2002). Severity of bipolarity in hospitalized manic adolescents with history of stimuland or antidepressant treatment. *Journal of Affective Disorders, 70(3)*, 323–327.

Strakowski, S.M., DelBello, M.P., Sax, K.W., Zimmerman, M.E., Shear, P.K., Hawkins, J.M., et al. (1999). Brain magnetic resonance imaging of structural abnormalities in bipolar disorder. *Archives of General Psychiatry, 56*, 254–260.

Wagner, K.D., Weller, E.B., Carlson, G.A., Sachs, G., Biederman, J., Frazier, J.A., et al. (2002). An open-label trial of divalproex in children and adolescents with bipolar disorder. *Journal of the American Academy of Child & Adolescent Psychiatry, 41(10)*, 1224–1230.

Wals, M., Hillegers, M.H., Reichart, C.G., Ormel, J., Nolen, W.A., & Verhulst, F.C. (2001) Prevalence of psychopathology in children of a bipolar parent. *Journal American Academy of Child & Adolescent Psychiatry, 40(9)*: 1094–102.

Wilens, T.E., Biederman, J., Millstein, R.B., Wozniak, J., Hahesy, A.L., & Spencer, T.J. (1999). Risk for substance use disorders in youths with child- and adolescent-onset bipolar disorder. *Journal of the American Academy of Child & Adolescent Psychiatry, 38(6)*, 680–685.

Wilens, T.E., Biederman, J., & Spencer, T.J. (2002). Attention deficit/hyperactivity disorder across the lifespan. *Annual Review of Medicine.* 2002; 53: 113–131.

Wozniak, J., Biederman, J., Kiely, K., Ablon, J.S., Faraone, S.V., & Mundy, E. (1995). Mania-like symptoms suggestive of childhood-onset bipolar disorder in clinically referred children. *Journal of the American Academy of Child & Adolescent Psychiatry, 34(7)*, 867–876.

Young, R.C., Biggs, J.T., Ziegler, V.E., & Meyer, D.A. (1978). A rating scale for mania: Reliability, validity, and sensitivity. *British Journal of Psychiatry, 133*, 429–435.

Chapter 10

Depression

Clare Roberts and Brian Bishop

Introduction

Adolescent depression is characterized by mood, thoughts, and behaviors that range from a mild reactive despondency or sadness to more extreme feelings of dysphoria, hopeless thoughts, withdrawn or irritable behavior, and even suicidal thoughts or behavior. This chapter focuses on Major Depressive Disorder (MDD), which is episodic and often recurrent, and Dysthymic Disorder (DD) involving more chronic mood disturbance.

Definitions

Depressed mood, defined as an unhappy or sad mood, is common in adolescence. High levels of depressive mood and symptoms increase the risk for future depressive disorders in adolescence (Lewinsohn, Clarke, Seeley & Rohde, 1994). *Depressive syndrome* is defined as a sad mood plus other emotional symptoms, such as anhedonia, low self-esteem, worry, pessimism, guilt, and loneliness. Clinical cut-offs based on empirically validated levels of symptom clusters are used to identify syndromes. *Depressive disorders* are defined by clinically derived standard diagnostic criteria of emotional, behavioral, cognitive, and somatic symptoms, and associated with functional impairment. They are assessed through structured clinical interviews and observation. *The Diagnostic and Statistical Manual of Mental Disorders* (*DSM-IV*; American Psychiatric Association, 2000) and *International Classification of Diseases 10* (ICD-10; World Health Organization, 1992) use the same criteria to diagnose depressive disorders in children, adolescents, and adults. Symptoms for adolescents and adults are similar, with increased anhedonia and psychomotor retardation with age, and more depressed appearance, somatic complaints, and poor self-esteem occurring at younger ages. More hypersomnia and slightly more weight loss have been observed in depressed adolescents (Roberts, Lewinsohn & Seeley, 1995).

Prevalence and Incidence

Estimates of the point prevalence of MDD in adolescence range from 0.4% to 8.3%. Lifetime prevalence rates across adolescence range from 15% to 20%. Point prevalence rates for DD range from 1.6% to 8.0% with a small proportion having both disorders (Roberts & Bishop, 2003). These rates are nearly twice those of childhood and are comparable to adult prevalence rates by late adolescence. Studies of depressive syndromes report differential prevalence rates depending on the informants. Sawyer et al. (2000) found that parents reported 3.6% of 13–17-year-old males and females had clinical levels anxiety and depression. However, adolescents reported nearly double these rates, 6.7% for males and 6.8% for females. A total of 29.5% of adolescents reported depressive mood and symptoms, and 2.6% of these had a clinical disorder in Roberts et al.'s (1995) study.

Lewinsohn, Hops, Roberts, Seeley, and Andrews (1993) reported a first incidence rate for depressive disorders of 6.32% for females and 4.25% for males in adolescence. The breakdown for MDD and DD were 7.14% and 0.13%, respectively, for females, and 4.35% and 0%, for males. An increased rate of first incidence of depressive disorders occurs in adolescence. Hankin et al. (1998) showed incidence at age 11 was 1.79% for males and 0.31% for females compared to 0.56% for males and 4.39% for females at age 15, and 9.58% for males and 20.69% for females at age 18. Adolescent depression has a poor prognosis—increasing the risk for adult depressive symptoms and disorders (Lewinsohn, Rohde, Klein & Seeley, 1999).

Individual Risk and Resiliency Factors

Genetics

Twin and adoptive studies in children and adolescents have indicated that approximately 50% of mood disorders could be attributed to genetic predispositions (Pike, McGuire, Hetherington, Reiss & Plomin, 1996). In a study of adopted children, Eley, Deater-Deckard, Fombonne, Fulker, and Plomin (1998) provided evidence for the importance of both shared and non-shared environmental effects on depressive disorders, with less strong genetic association for depressive symptoms. In a study of twins aged 8–16 years, Thaper and McGuffin (1994) indicated that the hereditability of depression symptomology was estimated at 79%. However, symptoms in children could be explained by environmental factors alone, while in adolescents heredity was still the main explanation. Thus, genetics and shared family environment are risk factors for depression, with some evidence that the genetic risk is stronger in adolescents.

Gender and Age Differences

More female adolescents have depressive disorders and elevated depressive symptoms (Hankin et al., 1998; Wichstrom, 1999). Gender differences in the prevalence of depressive disorders in New Zealand adolescents emerged between 13 and 15 years, and were most pronounced at age 18. Severity and the reoccurrence of depression was not gender related (Hankin et al., 1998). Also, Ge, Lorenz, Conger,

Elder, and Simmons (1994) found that after the age of 13, females showed greater levels of depressive symptoms than males. Wichstrom's (1999) cross-sectional study of 12,000 Norwegian school children, reported little difference between boys and girls at age 13, but more girls showed depressed mood at age 18, while boys showed relatively stable levels across adolescence. Explanations for these gender differences include biological changes associated with puberty, cognitive coping styles, family support, gender role socialization, and parenting style (Roberts & Bishop, 2003). Hence, female gender and the adolescent developmental period are both risk factors for depression.

Comorbidity and Previous Psychological Problems

Depression is comorbid with anxiety and attention deficit/hyperactivity (ADHD), disruptive behavior, substance abuse, and eating disorders in adolescence. Angold, Costello, and Erkanli's (1999) meta-analysis indicated that depression was most commonly comorbid with anxiety, then conduct/oppositional defiant disorder, and ADHD. The comorbidity of depression and anxiety is more common for girls, while boys are more likely to have depression with externalizing disorders (Kessler, Avenevoli & Merkingas, 2001). Comorbidity has been associated with more severe and more recurrent depressive episodes (Lewinsohn et al., 1994).

A history of clinical levels of depressive symptoms increase the risk for depressive disorders in adolescents (Ge, Best, Conger & Simons, 1996; Lewinsohn et al., 1994). Similarly, anxiety frequently occurs before depression in children and adolescents (Cole, Peeke, Martin, Truglio & Seroczynski, 1998). Reinherz et al. (1989) reported that anxiety at age 9 significantly increased the risk for depression at age 15. Hence, childhood depression and anxiety are risk factors, and comorbid disorders increase risk for more severe and reoccurring depression in adolescence.

Cognitive Factors

Cognitive factors have been associated with depression, particularly in association with stressful life events. Muris, Schmidt, Lambrichs, and Meesters (2001) showed a negative explanatory style was associated with depression in adolescents. Lewinsohn et al. (1994) found that attributions, particularly pessimism, was a strong risk factor for depression in adolescents over a 12-month period. Turner and Cole (1994) indicated that a pessimistic attribution style for negative events and negative cognitive errors strengthened the relationship between negative life events and depression in young adolescents but not in children. Schwartz, Kaslow, Seeley, and Lewinsohn (2000) found that maladaptive attributions were associated with depressive symptoms, suicidal ideation, and associated psychosocial problems concurrently and prospectively.

Self-worth/self-esteem have been described as both risk factors and protective factors in times of stress. Renouf and Harter (1990) showed that poor self-worth predicted depressive symptoms in adolescents over time. Reinherz et al. (1993) reported poor self-worth in females at 9 years was associated with depression at 18 years. Lewinsohn et al. (1994) found that self-esteem and to a lesser extent self-consciousness were both predictive of and associated with depressive symptoms over 12 months. Further, Lewinsohn et al. (1997) identified low self-worth as specifically predictive of depressive disorder, rather than other non-affective disorders. Robinson, Garber, and

Hillsman (1995) showed that low self-esteem and pessimistic attributions moderated depressive symptoms in adolescents moving on to high school. In contrast, Piko and Fitzpatrick (2003) found that high self-esteem and being happy offered protection from depression. Thus, pessimistic attribution style, cognitive errors, and low self-worth are risk factors for adolescent depression, while, high self-esteem may be protective.

Physical Health

Lewinsohn et al. (1996) found that physical health problems and diseases with functional impairments were associated with and predicted elevated depressive symptoms. Reinherz et al. (1993) identified serious preschool illness as a risk factor for MDD at age 18. Further, Lewinsohn, Gotlib, and Seeley (1997) showed that changes in physical activity due to physical injury or illness predicted depression in adolescents, but not other mental illnesses. Physical health problems, particularly those with functional impairments, are risk factors for depression.

Social Factors

Perceptions of incompetence, peer relationship difficulties and unpopularity, and poor problem-solving have been associated with and predictive of depression in adolescents (Cole, Martin & Powers, 1997; Roberts & Bishop, 2003). However, poor social skills, perceptions of poor peer support, and self-rated social competence are more symptomatic of adolescent depression, rather than predictive risk factors (Lewinsohn et al., 1998; Lewinsohn et al., 1994). Goodyer and Altham (1991) concluded that friendship difficulties exerted a direct effect, of similar magnitude to aversive life events, on the probability of any emotional disorder in childhood. The cumulative effects of multiple lifetime exit events represented an increasing risk for the development of later depressive disorder. Puskar, Tusaie-Mumford, Sereika, and Lamb (1999) reported significant associations between depressive symptomology and losing a close friend, arguments with parents, and trouble with classmates in rural adolescents.

Negative Life Events

Negative life events and chronic daily stress have been implicated as risk factors for many adolescent disorders (Lewinsohn et al., 1994). Rudolph et al. (2000) indicated that high levels of interpersonal stress often overwhelmed young people's coping resources and contributed to a sense of helplessness. This is supported by Hammen, Adrian, and Hiroto's (1988) observations that stressful life events predicted depression in adolescents of depressed mothers. Reinherz et al. (1993) identified the death of a parent before age 15 years and teenage pregnancy as predictive of major depression by 18 years in females. However, Lewinsohn et al. (1994) found that early parental death was not associated with depression in their community sample of adolescents. Goodyer and Altham (1991) showed that the impact of negative life events is increased by the effect of chronic friendship difficulties and maternal depression in children and adolescents. However, negative life events may only account for a small amount of variance (Garrison, Jackson, Marsteller McKeown & Addy, 1990).

The accumulation of family stressors such as parental conflict, divorce, parental depressive mood, parental physical health problems, and conflictual parent/adolescent relationships, rather than a single life stressor predicted adolescent adjustment problems (Forehand, Biggar & Kotchick, 1997). This interaction produced a multiplicative effect, with an increase from three to four stressors identified as a trigger point for the development of later depression. Rudolph et al. (2000) contends that negative life events that are meaningful to self-esteem influence depression, and that depressed individuals actually generate more stress in their lives, particularly interpersonal conflict. This hypothesis is consistent with the research on cognitive and social factors reviewed above.

Resiliency Factors

The review of individual risk factors above indicates that high self-worth can act as a protective factor. Conrad and Hammen (1993) identified the child's self-worth, good academic performance, social competence, positive perceptions of mother, and maternal social competence as significant resource factors for children and adolescents living the depressed or medically ill mothers. Reinherz et al. (1993) found family cohesiveness, social supports, and high self-worth protectively mediated depression in 18-year-old adolescents. In addition, Baumgartner (2002) indicated that hardy or resilient people prefer active coping solutions to avoidance in stressful situations. Adolescents with higher IQs and greater educational aspirations have been identified as more resilient (Tiet et al., 1998).

Family Risk and Resiliency Factors

Parental Depression

Parental affective disorders have been associated with greater risk of adolescent depression. The offspring of depressed parents are six times more likely to develop depression than other children (Beardslee, Versage & Gladstone, 1998). Hops (1992) demonstrated that fluctuations in maternal depression were associated with depression in female adolescents, while the effect of paternal depression on male adolescents was weaker. Depressed mothers and their children participate in negative interactions, reciprocally contributing to each other's unhappiness, and they experience temporally related episodes of depression (Hammen, Burge & Adrian, 1991). Ferguson, Horwood, and Lynsky (1995) showed that mothers' depression was more associated with depression in adolescent females than in adolescent males. Genetic contributions to the relationship between parental and offspring depression may be substantial. However, Ge et al. (1996) argued that the impact of parental depression is indirect, mediated by parenting styles. Downey and Coyne's (1990) review indicated that the effect was mediated through marital discord. Family functioning may also be a mediator.

Family Functioning and Relationships

Nilzen and Palmérus (1997) found that families of depressed adolescents had a higher frequency of major family problems, life events, parent symptoms, and parental overprotection. They were also less cohesive and more unhappy. Reinherz et al. (1993) identified family arguments and violence between 10 and 15 years as predictive of depression at 18 years in males, and a poor perception of role in the family at 9 years as a predictor of MDD by 18 years for both genders. Lewinsohn et al. (1994) showed that conflict with parents was predictive of depressive symptoms and disorders in adolescents. Sheeber, Hops, Alpert, Davis, and Andrews (1997) found that family support and conflict were predictive of depression concurrently and prospectively over one year, but the reverse relationship was not apparent. Hence, family conflict and poor perceptions of role in the family are risk factors for adolescent depression. Family conflict is an ongoing stressor that prevents the development of protective resources, while compounding existing stress levels. In time these processes overwhelm adolescent coping capacities.

Parenting Style

Rapee's (1997) review of this area concluded that parental rejection and control were associated with child and adolescent depression, particularly rejection. Lack of rewards and having high criteria for obtaining maternal rewards were more common among adolescents with depression than among controls (Cole & Rhem, 1986). Finkelstein, Donenberg, and Martinovich (2001) found that a controlling maternal parenting style was not associated with depression in Caucasian and Latino girls, but was important for African American girls (in contrast to Rapee's findings that high maternal control was associated with low levels of depressive symptoms). This study indicates the importance of not generalizing studies of Caucasian youth to other ethnic groups.

Family Context

Families with high levels of expressed emotion, such as critical and emotionally overinvolved attitudes, are more likely to have depressed children and adolescents (Nelson, Hammen, Brennan & Ullman, 2003). Garrison et al. (1990) found that family cohesion rather than life events predicted lower levels of depressive symptomology within any given year across the seventh through ninth grades. Boyce Rodgers and Rose (2002) indicated a small effect for adolescents from intact families having fewer internalizing problems, including depressed mood, compared to adolescents from blended, divorced, or single families. For adolescents experiencing marital transitions, internalizing problems were buffered by parental support, parental monitoring, perceiving peers as supportive, high school attachment, and having a neighbor to confide in. Amato and Keith's (1991) meta-analysis on the impact of divorce on children and adolescents found a moderated negative effect of divorce on the depression. McMahon, Yarcheski, and Yarcheski (2003) also found greater depression among adolescents from divorced families. However, poor family context variables appear to be risk factors associated with the onset of depression and characteristics of currently depressed adolescents, rather than distal risk factors.

Resiliency Factors

Walsh (2003) developed a model of family resilience. Key processes identified in her model included family belief systems, e.g., a shared construction of reality, finding meaning in adversity, positive outlook or optimism, transcendence and spirituality—the sense that life has meaning beyond ourselves, and support through religious connections. Walsh cites Werner's (1993) longitudinal research with children living in poverty on the Hawaiian island of Kauai in support of her model. Two-thirds of the sample showed poor adjustment in adolescence with high levels of teenage pregnancy and mental health problems, but the other third, who experienced the processes noted above, were functioning well at follow-ups.

Family support, parental monitoring, perceiving peers as supportive, high school attachment, and having a neighbor to confide in have been identified as a significant protective factors for adolescent (Boyce Rodgers & Rose, 2002; Puskar et al., 1999). Garrison et al. (1990) and Nilzen & Palmérus (1997) showed that adolescents from adaptively cohesive families evidenced fewer mental health problems and depressive symptomatology. Adolescent reports of good attachment and relationships with parents have been related to lower levels of depression (Nada Raja, McGee & Stanton, 1992), consistent with research on insecure attachment as a specific risk factor for adolescent depression (Sund & Wichstrom, 2002). There has been a lack of research on risk and resilience factors for minority groups (Sagrestano, Paikoff, Holmbeck & Fendrich, 2003). It is unclear how risk and protective factors, mapped for white adolescents, function for minority and multicultural youth (Smokowski, Mann, Reynolds & Fraser, (2004).

Social and Community Factors

The literature in this area focuses on general well-being rather than specific psychological disorders. A number of social and community risk factors have been identified as predictors of poor well-being, such as poverty, war (Luthar, 1991), living in a high crime area (Felsman & Vaillant, 1987), experiencing a disaster (Reijneveld, Crone, Verhulst & Verloove-Vanhorick, 2003) and ethnicity (Wolkow & Ferguson, 2001). Cultural background is a risk factor for depression. Roberts, Roberts, and Chen (1997) reported that Chinese American adolescents had the lowest levels of depression (2.9%), whites had rates of 6.3% and Mexican Americans had the highest rate of 12.0%. Siegel, Aneschensel, Taub, Cantwell, and Driscoll (2001) also reported that Hispanic Americans had higher rates of depressed mood than Caucasians. However, different rates of depression in different cultural groups, may indicate larger issues of social disadvantage.

Evidence-Based Treatment Interventions in Community Settings

Treatments available in community settings include both psychosocial and somatic interventions. This section reviews psychosocial interventions. Skaer, Robinson, Sclar, and Galin (2000) investigated depression treatments in the United States, by sampling office-based physician-patient visits from 1990 to 1995. They found that 19.4% of children and adolescents with a diagnosis of depression received neither psychotherapy nor pharmacotherapy, while 34.8% received psychotherapy alone, 11% received pharmacotherapy alone, and 34.8% received both psychotherapy and antidepressants. Community practitioners providing treatment to depressed children and adolescents in the United States indicated that therapists favor eclectic and psycho-dynamic approaches over cognitive and behavioral interventions (Weersing, Weisz & Donenberg, 2002).

What Works

PSYCHOSOCIAL TREATMENTS.   Contrary to psychodynamic practices in many out-patient mental health clinics (MHCs), research into psychosocial interventions has focused cognitive-behavioral therapy (CBT), interpersonal (IPT), or family therapy (FT) models (Curry, 2001). Michael and Crowley's (2002) meta-analysis found a large effect size of .93 for psychosocial interventions for adolescent depression tested in random-ized controlled trials (RCTs), and 1.35 derived from pre-post uncontrolled studies that were completed from 1980 to 1999. If we compare this with the small effect size of .28 derived from randomized placebo-controlled trials (RPCT) of pharmacological interventions, we can conclude that psychosocial treatments for adolescent depres-sion work.

COGNITIVE-BEHAVIORAL THERAPY.   CBT is based on the theory that negative cog-nitions and/or maladaptive coping behaviors are the cause of depression by them-selves or in association with stressful life events. Adolescent treatments include strategies to build behavioral skills and manage negative cognitions and affect (Curry, 2001). A meta-analysis by Reinecke, Ryan, and DuBois (1998) found overall effect sizes of 1.02 for post-treatment and .61 for follow-up of CBT with depressed adolescents. Narrative reviews conclude that interventions based on CBT are effec-tive in treating depressive symptoms and disorders in clinical and non-clinical sam-ples of adolescents (Curry, 2001; Kaslow & Thompson, 1998). Of nine RCTs, seven showed CBT to be more effective than wait-list control groups or alternative treat-ments. Further, Weersing and Weisz's (2002) benchmarking study comparing CBT outcomes from 13 trials with the outcomes of outpatient health clinics (MHCs) in the US showed that depressed adolescents treated with CBT had steep declines in symp-toms within three months, with maintenance up to two years. Adolescents treated at MHCs took twice as long to achieve symptom relief. Hence, CBT-based psychosocial treatments work for adolescent depression.

ADOLESCENTS COPING WITH DEPRESSION PROGRAM.   The Adolescents Coping with Depression program (CWDA) is a group program based on Lewinsohn's social learn-ing model of depression, which suggests that the cause and maintenance of depression is a deficit in positive reinforcement, and negative cognitions (Clarke, DeBar & Lewinsohn, 2003). This program is described as probably efficacious according to the Task Force on Promotion and Dissemination of Psychological Procedures guidelines (1995). The treatment uses a psycho-educational group approach with 16 twice-weekly, two-hour sessions for adolescents and 8 weekly one-hour sessions for parents. The content comprises mood monitoring, social skills training, scheduling pleasant events, relaxation, cognitive restructuring, communication skills, problem-solving, and maintenance strategies.

Three RCTs of this intervention have confirmed that the CWDA group program is significantly better than wait-list control groups for adolescents with MDD (Clarke, Rohde, Lewinsohn, Hops & Seeley, 1999; Lewinsohn, Clarke, Hops & Andrews, 1990) and significantly better than lifeskills tutoring for delinquent youth with MDD (Rohde et al., 2001, cited in Clarke et al., 2003). Adolescent-only groups were just as effective as adolescent-plus-parent interventions (Clarke et al., 1999; Lewinsohn et al., 1990). Response rates for remission of MDD were 46–67% for CBT compared to 5–48% for wait-listed adolescents, with two-year follow-up remission rates of 83–100% (Clarke et al., 1999; Lewinsohn et al., 1990). Recovery rates are lower for delinquent adolescents, 26% for CBT versus 14% for the attention placebo condition, plus no group differences at 12-months follow-up (Rohde et al., 2001, cited in Clarke et al., 2003). Clarke et al. (2002) found no group differences in response rates, at post-treatment, or 24-months follow-up for depressed adolescent children of depressed parents who had received the CWDA program plus usual care (brief psychotherapy and/or antidepressant medication) or a usual care condition in Health Management Organizations. Hence, the CWDA group program works. However, it effectiveness in the regular health care systems requires further research.

What Might Work

Brent et al. (1997) and Wood, Harrington, and Moore's (1996) individual CBT interventions are promising and have been evaluated in RCTs, but have not yet been tested in three evaluations. In addition, interventions based on interpersonal (Mufson & Pollack Dorta, 2003) and family theories (Cottrell, 2003) of depression have shown promise and efficacy in at least one trial.

INDIVIDUAL COGNITIVE-BEHAVIORAL THERAPY. Brent et al. (1997) based their individual CBT treatment for adolescent depression on *Beck's cognitive model*, emphasizing the impact of negative automatic thoughts, systematic distortions in underlying beliefs, and perceptual biases. The 12–16 individual weekly sessions included cognitive restructuring, regulation of mood and impulsivity for risky and suicidal behavior, problem-solving, pleasant events scheduling, and relapse prevention. This intervention was compared to *Systemic Behavioral Family Therapy* (SBFT), which was based on theories of *Functional Family Therapy* and strategies from *Behavioral Family Therapy*. This treatment engaged families and aimed at increasing interfamilial support and changing interpersonal and family triggers for depression. A control group of adolescents received *Nondirective Supportive Therapy* (NST) as an attention placebo condition. Significantly more adolescents from the CBT (60%) condition experienced post-treatment remission of disorders compared to SBFT (38%) and NST (39%). The CBT program resulted in more rapid symptom reduction compared to the other conditions. By two-year follow-up, there were no group differences in rates of diagnosis (CBT—6%; SBFT—23%; NST—26%). Depression recurrence in all groups was associated with parent–child conflict and family discord (Birmaher et al., 2000). Post-treatment and follow-up CBT outcomes were associated with fewer cognitive distortions, while SBFT outcomes at follow-up only were associated with improved parent–child relationships (Kolko, Brent, Baugher, Bridge & Birmaher, 2000).

A brief individualized CBT program that involved emotional recognition, self-regulation, social problem-solving, cognitive restructuring, and reduction of somatic depressive symptoms was evaluated by Wood et al. (1996) in a RCT. This five- to eight-session intervention was compared with a relaxation attention placebo control group. At post-treatment CBT was associated with fewer depressive symptoms than relaxation and more adolescents with MDD had remitted with

CBT (54%) versus relaxation (21%). At six-month follow-up there were no group differences on depression measures, but the CBT group reported lower levels of anxiety and higher self-esteem. Kroll, Harrington, Jayson, Fraser & Gowers (1996) continued the brief CBT intervention with 17 adolescents with MDD, using biweekly to monthly sessions for an additional 6 months (CBT-C). Compared to a historical control group, the cumulative relapse rate for CBT-C was 0.2 versus 0.5 for the historical control group. Jayson et al. (1998) reported that younger participants with less severe problems were more likely to respond. However, a small pilot study comparing this intervention to an attention placebo control, found that CBT was no group differences at post-treatment or 9-months follow-up (Vostanis, Feehan, Grattan & Bickerton, 1996).

Individual and brief versions of CBT may work in the acute treatment of adolescent depression. They are more effective than family therapy, supportive counseling, and relaxation. However, by follow-up group differences are less apparent, and continued treatment may be required to achieve better follow-up results.

COGNITIVE BIBLIOGRAPHY.   This innovative CBT-based intervention has shown efficacy in one RCT (Ackerson, Scogin, McKendree-Smith & Lyman, 1998). Adolescents with mild to moderate depressive symptoms read the book *Feeling Good* (Burns, 1980) over a four-week period and received weekly phone calls to check on their progress. The book provides a description of the cognitive theory of depression plus interactive exercises to assess and treat depressive symptoms. The 12 adolescents who received this treatment reported significant reductions in depressive symptoms compared to a wait-list group at post-treatment, with maintenance up to one-month follow-up. This treatment may be useful for depressive syndromes and mood, which are risk factors for clinical disorders (Lewinsohn et al., 1994).

INTERPERSONAL PSYCHOTHERAPY.   IPT is a brief time-limited therapy originally developed for adults with depression. It is based on the theory that interpersonal conflicts and transitions both trigger and maintain depression (Mufson & Pollack Dorta, 2003). ITP-A, an adaptation for adolescents, uses 12 weekly individual sessions and telephone contact in the first month, plus parent contact as required, to enlist their assistance in supporting the adolescent's progress. Seven potential problem areas are addressed in therapy—grief, separation, illness, interpersonal disputes, role transitions, interpersonal deficits, and single-parent family issues (Mufson & Pollack Dorta, 2003). In an early open trial of IPT-A with 14 adolescent females with MDD, all outpatients remitted at post-treatment. Also, there were significant symptom reductions and enhanced general functioning in the home and at school (Mufson et al., 1994). A 12-month follow-up study of ten of these adolescents found that only one had relapsed, and all were experiencing better relationships with their parents, albeit with poorer general functioning (Mufson & Fairbanks, 1996).

A RCT comparing the efficacy of IPT-A to clinical monitoring with clinically referred adolescents with MDD found adolescents in the ITP-A condition reported fewer depressive symptoms, and better social functioning and problem-solving (Mufson, Weissman, Moreau & Garfinkel, 1999). Significantly more ITP-A adolescents (88%) were diagnosis-free compared to the clinical monitoring condition (58%). A second RCT of this intervention conducted by independent researchers Rossello and Bernal (1999) with Puerto Rican adolescents with MDD, DD, or both compared IPT-A with CBT and a wait-list control condition. Both IPT-A and CBT resulted in significant reductions in depressive symptoms. However, the IPT-A group also increased in self-esteem and social adaptation. An open trial of IPT-A with moderately to severely depressed adolescents assessed it efficacy for use with therapists who were had no previous experience in this model (Santor & Kusumakar, 2001). Therapists who had received three days of training achieved significant post-treatment reductions in depressive symptoms and enhanced global functioning. Individual IPT-A administered in outpatient settings is likely to be an effective treatment for adolescent depression.

FAMILY THERAPY.   Variants of FT include systemic, structural, functional, and behavioral, and attachment-based therapies (Cottrell, 2003; Diamond, Reis, Diamond, Siqueland & Isaacs, 2002). Family therapy interventions share the underlying theory that interactions and communication patterns within families are associated with the onset and maintenance of depression. Where families have been provided with intervention aimed at supporting adolescent group CBT treatment, promoting parental acceptance of change, and giving parents strategies for coping with family problems, treatment is equally as effective as adolescent CBT groups, and better than wait list control groups (Clarke et al., 2003). The gains are maintained up to two years, and Lewinsohn et al.'s (1990) reported that an adolescent plus parent treatment condition showed greater reductions in parent ratings of adolescent symptoms than the condition without parental involvement. In Brent et al.'s (1997) study, SBFT did not perform any better than the control condition on depression, general family functioning, or parent's marital satisfaction at post-intervention. However, this treatment did result in specific positive effects on parent–adolescent relationships at follow-up. Hence, despite the important role that family variables play in adolescent depression, family treatments that are based primarily on behavioral and functional models of therapy are at best equivalent to CBT.

Diamond et al. (2002) reported on an attachment-based family therapy (ABFT). This therapy is based on the theory that suggests poor attachment bonds, high conflict, harsh criticism, and low affective attunement can create a negative family environment, which inhibits children from developing stress-buffering skills. The treatment involved 12 weekly sessions plus phone calls, and included various family and extra-familial members, depending on the evolving treatment plan. The content of therapy included relational reframing, alliance building, parent education, reattachment to re-build trust and respect, and strategies to promote competency. A RCT showed that more ABFT adolescents with MDD (81%) were diagnosis-free at post-treatment compared to a wait-list control group (47%). The ABFT group had significant reductions in depressive and anxious symptoms and family conflict. In addition, 87% of the ABFT-treated adolescents continued in remission at a 6-month follow-up. Hence, ABFT-treatment may work, but more research is required.

CONCLUSIONS.   Both CBT and IPT administered individually may be effective in treating depressive disorders and symptoms. CBT administered as bibliotherapy may be effective for reducing depressive symptoms. The evidence for FT is less promising; however, it may work in some cases. ABFT may work, but further studies with larger samples are required to draw firm conclusions.

What Does Not Work

Non-directive supportive counseling is not an effective treatment for adolescent depression (Brent et al., 1997). Treatments received as part of the usual care in outpatient mental health clinics may not work, given that Weersing and Weisz (2002) reported that outcomes for depressed adolescents in MHCs were similar to outcomes under control conditions of CBT trials, and similar to the natural course of youth depression. This may be the result of differences in therapy. Therapists reported that MHC services were predominantly psychodynamic, whereas the treatments reviewed that work above are based on pure CBT (Weersing & Weisz, 2002). Only one narrative review that included psychodynamic approaches was located (Kutcher & Marton, 1996). This review indicated that there has been little empirical investigation of this approach and that it lacked theoretical and procedural thoroughness in the area of adolescent depression.

Evidence-Based Treatment Interventions in Residential Settings

Few reports of the effectiveness of residential/inpatient treatments could be found in the literature, despite the fact that such treatments are regularly used to treat adolescent problems (Lyman & Wilson, 2001). Sawyer et al (2000) indicated that approximately 3% of Australian adolescents with clinical scores on the Child Behavior Checklist received inpatient psychiatry services, while 2% of children and adolescents with clinical disorders attended such services. Residential and inpatient services may include combinations of treatments, such as medication, other somatic treatments, e.g., electroconvulsive therapy (ECT), and psychosocial group, individual, and/or family interventions (Lyman & Wilson, 2001).

What Works

No published studies that have been subjected to any sort of methodological rigor could be found relating to residential treatments for adolescent depression.

What Might Work

Given that group CBT has been found to work and individual CBT and IPT treatments show promise for adolescent depression, there is every chance that these interventions may work in a residential setting either with medication or independently. However, the outcomes have not been documented. Lyman and Wilson (2001) indicate that residential treatments based on behavioral, psycho-educational, and wilderness therapy have shown effectiveness in enhancing competencies, but specific application to adolescent depression outcomes has not been investigated.

Electroconvulsive therapy is always carried out in inpatient residential settings. However, it is not commonly used to treat children or adolescents (Duffett, Hill & Lelliott, 1999). Findling, Feeny, Stansbrey, DelPorto-Bedoya, and Demeter (2002) found no controlled trials of this treatment. Uncontrolled trials and retrospective case reports indicate that when administered to children or adolescents with very severe symptoms or drug-resistant depression, the rate of symptom improvement across studies is 63% in the short term (Rey & Walter, 1997). A retrospective case report study found that 58% of adolescents, four with MDD, achieved acute remission from depression (as rated by their treating physicians) with ECT, while 33% were re-hospitalized within one year (Bloch, Levcovitch, Bloch, Mendlovic & Ratzoni, 2001). Concerns relate to the acute and long-term side effects of this treatment, particularly with regard to cognition, verbal fluency, and memory, at least in the short term (Cohen et al., 2000). ECT may be effective for adolescents with very severe depression or treatment–resistant depression. However, it is not recommended as a first-line treatment (Rose, Wykes, Leese, Bindman & Freishmann, 2003).

What Does Not Work

No published studies could be found relating to residential treatments for adolescent depression that do not work. Supportive counseling is unlikely to work in a residential setting, given its lack of outpatient efficacy (Brent et al., 1997).

Psychopharmacology

Skaer et al.'s (2000) study found that 48.2% of physician office visits for depressed children or adolescents resulted in the prescription of an antidepressant medication—50.1% of these were for serotonin-selective reuptake inhibitors (SSRIs) and 41.9% for tricyclic antidepressants (TCAs). Other drugs used include monoamine oxidase inhibitors (MAOIs) and other nontricyclic antidepressants, such as trazodone, bupropion, and nefazodone, and lithium (Findling et al., 2002).

What Works

Recent reviews and meta-analyses have been conducted into the effectiveness of psychopharmacological treatments (Emslie & Mayes, 2001; Emslie, Walkup, Pliszka & Ernst, 1999; Findling et al., 2002; Geller, Reising, Leonard, Riddle & Walsh, 1999; Hazell, O'Connell, Heathcote, Robertson & Henry, 1995; Michael & Crowley, 2002; Varley, 2003). These reviews and the Consensus Conference Panel on Medication Treatment of Childhood Major Depressive Disorder (Hughes et al., 1999) concluded that the SSRI drugs, in particular, fluoxetine (Prozac), paroxetine (Paxil), and sertraline (Zoloft) should be the first-line pharmacological treatment for child and adolescent depression. However, there are currently no pharmacotherapies that meet the criteria of three successful randomized controlled trials.

What Might Work

SEROTONIN-SELECTIVE REUPTAKE INHIBITORS. SSRIs are antidepressant compounds that act specifically and selectively to inhibit the reuptake of seretonin at the synaspe (Findling, et al., 2002). Drugs in this class include fluoxetine (Prozac), sertraline (Zoloft), paroxetine (Paxil), fluvoxamine (Luxov), and citalopram. More research has been completed on fluoxetine than any other SSRI, including three randomized, double-blind, placebo-controlled trials (RCPTs) (Emslie et al., 2002; Emslie et al., 1997; Simeon, Dinicola, Ferguson & Copping, 1990). Fluoxetine has received United States

Food and Drug Administration (FDA) labeling as safe and effective for the treatment of MDD in children and adolescents (Varley, 2003).

A small study by Simeon et al. (1990) using 60 mg of fluoxetine daily found no differences in response rates between adolescents receiving placebo or the active treatment. Using larger samples, Emslie et al. found that 56% (1997) and 65% (2002) of children and adolescents treated with fluoxetine (20 mg daily) reported symptom reduction, compared to 33% (1997) and 30% (2002) of the placebo group. There were no significant group differences in aversive side effects in either study. In a 12-month follow-up of the 1997 study, Emslie et al. (1998) found that 85% of those who received acute treatment were recovered. However 39% of these had experienced a recurrence of MDD in the follow-up period, a rate higher than that found in adults. Hence, fluoxetine may be a successful acute treatment for adolescent depression.

In open-label trials with children and adolescents sertraline was effective in more than 65% of cases (Findling et al., 2002). The pooled results of two multicenter double-blind RCPTs indicated that flexible daily doses of sertraline (50–200 mg) resulted in significantly greater symptom reduction than placebo in 6–17-year-old outpatients (Wagner et al., 2003). A total of 69% of treated patients responded compared to 59% given a placebo. Adolescents showed slightly greater symptom reduction than children. However, 9% of treated and 3% of placebo patients discontinued due to aversive side effects such as diarrhea, vomiting, anorexia, and agitation.

Similarly, in open-label trials paroxetine is effective and well tolerated by children and adolescents (Findling et al., 2002). Keller et al. (2001) have conducted a large double-blind RCPT of paroxetine (20–40 mg daily) compared to the TCA imipramine. Adolescents who received paroxetine showed significant reductions in depressive symptoms (63%), compared to imipramine (50%) and placebo (40%). However, discontinuation due to aversive events occurred in 9.7% of the paroxetine, 31.5% of imipramine, and 6.9% of the placebo groups. Eleven paroxetine patients experienced serious adverse events, including headaches, emotional lability, suicidal ideation and gestures, worsening depression, conduct problems or hostility, and euphoria, compared to two placebo group patients. Hence, the US Food and Drug Administration (2003) has recommended that paroxetine not be used for children or adolescents.

Reports of trials with other SSRIs are limited. Two small open-label trials of fluvoxamine with depressed adolescents have reported significant reductions in depressive symptomology and good tolerance of the drug (Findling et al., 2002). Citalopram treatment for adolescents with MDD, DD, or bipolar disorder was effective in 76% of cases investigated in a retrospective case review study from a community mental health centre (Bostic, Prince, Brown & Place, 2001). Fluoxetine, sertraline, and paroxetine currently may be effective treatments for acute adolescent depression. However, in the case of seretraline and paroxetine, further investigation is required into adverse side effects.

MONOAMINE OXIDASE INHIBITORS.   MAOIs inhibit the oxidative degradation of monoamine neurotransmitters. Older MAOIs such as phenelzine and tranylcypromine are not recommended for adolescents because strict dietary restrictions in foods that are rich in tyramine (e.g., ripe cheese) are necessary to reduce the risk of hypertensive crises. Ryan et al. (1988) completed a chart review study of 23 depressed adolescents unresponsive to TCAs who were subsequently treated with either phenelzine or tranylcypromine, alone or adjunctively. Fair to good results were achieved in 70%

of all cases, but 30% did not comply with the dietary restrictions. Two case reports identified phenelzine as effective for adolescents with severe, melancholic depression with psychotic features, unresponsive to TCAs or SSRIs (Strober, Pataki & DeAntonio, 1998). Although the more recently developed MAOIs, such as moclobemide and brofaromine, are not associated with hypertensive risks or dietary restrictions, there have been no published studies of their effects with adolescents (Emslie, Walkup, Pliszka & Ernst, 1999; Findling et al., 2002).

OTHER NONTRICYLIC ANTIDEPRESSANTS. Bupropion (Wellbutrin) inhibits the reuptake of norepinephrine and dopamine. The sustained-release form of this drug has been effective in treating adults with depression (Findling et al., 2002). One open-label study by Daviss and colleagues (2001) showed that bupropion was associated with reductions in depressive symptomology in 16 adolescents with comorbid attention-deficit/hyperactivity disorder (ADHD) and MDD/DD. Controlled trials have indicated the effectiveness of this drug in reducing inattentive and hyperactive symptoms (Emslie et al., 1999). Hence, it may be a useful treatment for cormorbid depression and ADHD.

Nefazodone (Serzone) blocks postsynaptic serotonin and inhibits the reuptake of both serotonin and norepinephrine. It had been effective in treating adult depression (Findling et al., 2002). A retrospective case review study found that four out of seven children and adolescents with treatment-resistant depression were "much" or "very much" improved with this treatment (Wilens, Spencer, Biederman & Schleifer, 1997). An open-label study of adolescents showed significant improvements in depressive symptomology after an eight-week treatment period (Findling et al., 2002).

Lithium is most commonly used in the treatment of biolar disorder (Emslie & Mayes, 2001). However, it has been used in adults to prevent recurrence of MDD episodes and to augment other drugs in treatment-resistant cases. There is some evidence for a similar role in adolescence. Two retrospective case reports found lithium to enhance treatment responsiveness in adolescents who did not respond to TCAs or venlafaxine, and one open-label trial found that lithium was a helpful adjunctive treatment (Findling et al., 2002). However, no RCPTs have been completed.

CONCLUSIONS. The SSRIs have the strongest empirical support, and of these drugs, fluoxetine appears to be the most promising. Other pharmacological treatments may work directly or as adjuncts to other interventions.

What Does Not Work

The TCAs are a group of drugs that impact on the noradrenergic system by blocking the reuptake of monamine neurotransmitters. Depending on the particular compound, they also have effects on other neurotransmitter systems. TCAs that are commonly used for adolescents include imipramine (Tofranil), amitriptyline (Elvil), nortriptyline (Pamelor, Aventyl), desimipramine (Norpramin, Pertofrane), and clomipramine (Anafranil). Reviews have concluded that no RCPTs of TCAs with child and adolescent samples find superiority of TCAs over placebo conditions (Findling et al., 2002; Geller et al., 1999). In addition, meta-analyses (Hazell et al., 1995; Thurber, Ensign, Punnett & Welter, 1995) indicate that the effect size for TCAs was nonsignificant. Use of TCA in adolescents has been associated with side effects such as dry mouth and cardiovascular problems, including reports of four unexplained sudden deaths of children receiving desipramine (Hazell et al. 1995). Also, TCAs have sedating effects and can be associated with mild confusion, which interferes with learning and school activities (Geller et al., 1999). The lack of significant treatment effects and the side effects indicate that TCAs do not work in adolescents.

The Prevention of Depression

Adolescent depression prevention programs include interventions that target adolescents with known risk factors as well as universal interventions, usually implemented in school settings (Gillham, Shatte & Freres, 2000; Greenberg, Domitrovich & Bumbarger, 2001; Roberts & Bishop, 2003). Michael and Crowley's (2002) meta-analysis indicated a small effect size of .17 based on three controlled trials published up to 1999.

What Works

PENN OPTIMISM PROGRAM. The Penn Optimism Program (POP) is a 12-session school-based intervention program based on CBT, teaching skills to reduce cognitive errors, promote optimistic attribution styles, and enhance social problem-solving and coping skills (Jaycox et al., 1994). The program has been implemented with groups of 10–13-year-olds with elevated levels of depressive symptoms and parental conflict (Jaycox et al., 1994), children of divorce (Zubernis, Cassidy, Gillham, Reivich & Jaycox, 1999), low-income minority group children (Cardemil, Reivich & Seligman, 2002), Chinese children (Yu & Seligman, 2002), Australian rural children (Roberts, Kane, Thompson, Bishop & Hart, 2003), as well as universally (Patterson & Lynd–Stevenson, 2001; Quayle, Dziurawiec, Roberts, Kane & Ebsworthy, 2001).

In a targeted controlled trial of this intervention, significant intervention group differences in depressive symptoms were found at post-intervention, six-month follow-up (Jaycox et al., 1994), and two-year follow-up (Gillham, Reivich, Jaycox & Seligman, 1995), but were no longer significant at a three-year follow-up (Gillham & Reivich, 1999). The intervention group made fewer pessimistic attributions compared to the control group at all follow-ups. Analysis of effects for children of divorce from this study found that the program was effective with this at-risk sample, but that the effects diminished over time (Zubernis et al., 1999). Four targeted RCTs of this program and two small RCTs of universal applications of this prevention program have been published. Cardemil et al. (2002) showed that significant intervention effects for depressive symptoms, negative automatic thoughts, and hopelessness occurred immediately after treatment, and at three- and six-month follow-ups, compared to a no-intervention control group, for low-income Latino children, but not for African American children. A RCT of a Chinese version of POP with children with elevated depressive symptoms and parental conflict found that the program was effective in reducing depressive symptoms and enhancing optimistic explanatory styles at post-intervention and three- and six-month follow-ups (Yu & Seligman, 2002). Conversely, an effectiveness trial of POP with Australian rural school children with elevated levels of depression, showed no immediate or six-month follow-up effects on depressive symptoms (Roberts et al., 2003). Instead, an effect on anxiety symptoms was apparent. Two small RCTs of universal applications of POP have been conducted in Australia. Patterson and Lynd-Stevenson (2001) found no immediate or follow-up effect of POP compared to an attention control condition. However, Quayle et al. (2001), using a shorter eight-session adaptation of POP, showed six-month follow-up effects for depression and self-esteem in girls after their high school transition.

The Penn Optimism Program works to prevent adolescent depressive symptoms when run in small groups in schools with pre-adolescents targeted because of increased risk factors. It has not been shown to work for African Americans or when used with non-selected groups of Australian children, and is only effective for anxiety symptoms when implemented under regular service delivery conditions. Effects on MDD and DD are unknown.

What Might Work

COPING WITH STRESS COURSE.   In an RCT of prevention of MDD and DD in high-risk adolescents, Clarke et al. (1995) identified adolescents with depressed mood. The *Coping with Stress Course* (CWSA) consisted of fifteen, 45-minute group sessions and involved techniques to identify and challenge negative thoughts, social skills training, activity scheduling, problem-solving, and education about feelings and interpersonal behavior. Survival analysis revealed that those in the intervention group were less likely to develop a depressive disorder (14.5%) compared to the control group (25.7%) at a 12-month follow-up. More recently, Clarke, Hornbrook, Lynch, and Polen (2001) reported on an RCT of the CWSA intervention with the adolescent offspring of adults treated for depression in a health maintenance organization. All adolescents had elevated levels of depressive symptoms and different levels of intervention were offered to adolescents with different symptoms severity. The intervention group experienced an incidence of 9.3% at 12-month follow-up compared to 28.8% for the usual-care control condition. The risk of depression in the control group was five times that of the intervention group. Hence, this CBT-based prevention program holds significant promise as a targeted prevention program for both adolescent depressive symptoms and disorder.

FAMILY-BASED PREVENTION.   Gladstone and Beardslee (2000) review a program of research that targets youngsters whose parents have affective disorders. They compared two interventions, a family–based therapy that uses CBT and a psycho-educational approach. The six- to ten-session individual family intervention helped families to develop a shared perspective of the depressive illness, to change parents' behavior toward their children, and to promote resilience in children by providing information about the parent's illness and ways of coping and encouraging supportive relationships outside the home. The psycho-educational approach involved two short group lectures. Post-intervention and at 18-month follow-up, family intervention parents reported significantly more changes in behavior and attitudes about their illness than did families that received the psycho-educational intervention only (Beardslee et al., 1993, 1997a). Children of families in the family intervention group experienced better understanding of their parent's disorder, improved communication with parents, and enhanced global functioning at 18-month follow-up (Beardslee et al., 1997b). Depressive disorders occurred in 9% of the children and adolescents in the family-based intervention, compared to 25% in the lecture-based condition at follow-up. Thus, family-based intervention may work.

THE RESOURCEFUL ADOLESCENT PROGRAM.   Shochet et al. (2001) developed a universal school-based program for young adolescents, the *Resourceful Adolescent Program* (RAP-A) plus an adjunctive parent component (RAP-P). RAP-A is an 11-session program based on cognitive-behavioral, interpersonal, and family theories. The program content includes cognitive and interpersonal strategies. In a controlled trail of RAP-A versus RAP-A plus RAP-P and a monitored control group with 12–15 year-olds, Shochet et al. found that depression and hopelessness symptoms were lower in both RAP groups than the controls at post-intervention and ten-month follow-up. Rates of clinically significant symptom levels were significantly lower in the intervention groups compared to the control condition. This program was easily integrated into the school and may be the first universal intervention program to work.

FRIENDS.   *The Friends Program* (Lowry-Webster, Barrett & Dadds, 2001) is an anxiety prevention program that has recently been used universally with children and young adolescents in schools. The program involves ten sessions run in school time and an adjunctive three-session parent program. Given that anxiety frequently coexists or predates depression, anxiety prevention may act as a prevention strategy for depression (Cole et al., 1998). Lowry-Webster et al. showed that children and adolescents with elevated anxiety scores at pre-intervention reported improvements in depression symptoms at post-interventions and 12-month follow-up (Lowrey–Webster, Barrett & Lock, 2003). Hence, anxiety prevention programs that are implemented in late childhood period may work to prevent adolescent depression.

CONCLUSIONS.   Targeted CBT-based depression prevention programs may work to prevent depressive symptoms and disorders in adolescents with elevated levels of depressive symptoms, as well as in the offspring of depressed adults. Of the targeted interventions Clarke et al.'s (1995) CWSA program shows the most promise. Universal school-based depression and anxiety prevention programs may also be effective in preventing depressive symptoms.

What Does Not Work

Information on depression prevention strategies for adolescents that do not work comes mostly from trials of universal applications of depression prevention programs. Clarke, Hawkins, Murphy, and Sheeber (1993) studied two short, low-intensity interventions incorporated into mandatory health classes for ninth- or tenth-grade students based on a behavioral theory of depression, and designed to encourage adolescents to increase their rates of pleasant activities. The results of an RCT indicated no effect on depression for girls, a short-term effect for boys at post-test, but no effects at 12-week follow-up. A second study involved a five-session skills development program targeting pleasant events and irrational thinking styles. The results indicated that the program was ineffective in the short-term and at 12-week follow-up. The programs may have been too brief to impact on symptomology.

Petersen, Leffert, Graham, Alwin, and Ding (1997) report on a universal 16-session psycho-educational program, based on stress and coping skills models of adolescent depression. The intervention resulted in better coping in both girls and boys and reductions in depressive symptoms in girls in the short-term, compared to the control group. However, depressive symptoms were increased among boys in the intervention and intervention effects did not persist over time. The authors suggested that the intervention was too brief. A recent RCT of the *Problem-Solving for Life Program,* conducted by Spence, Sheffield, and Donovan (2003) found no effects at 12-month follow-up on depressive symptoms or depressive disorders in 12–14-year-olds, after teachers implemented the eight-week universal depression prevention program. Finally, Hains and Ellmann (1994) reported a trial of a targeted school-based stress inoculation program for adolescents with high levels of arousal. The 13-session group and individual program involved a variety of CBT strategies. No effects on depression or anxiety symptoms at post-intervention or follow-up were identified in a RCT.

CONCLUSIONS.   Strategies that involve brief interventions, whether targeted or universal, are unlikely to have lasting preventive effects. Further, brief interventions that are based on stress and coping models have not demonstrated maintenance.

Recommendations

Adolescent depression is a serious problem that is affecting more youngsters than ever before. It creates a significant burden for adolescents, their families, and teachers. In addition, it leaves adolescents vulnerable to a lifetime of poor mental health. Treatment and prevention programs have been developed with an emphasis on individual risk and resilience factors. However, family and community risk and resilience variables are also important in the development and maintenance of adolescent depression treatment.

The research literature indicates that psychosocial treatments, in particular CBT-based treatments for adolescent depression, work, for example, the CWDA group program (Clarke et. al., 2003). However, there is still some way to go to ensure that such interventions are implemented effectively as part of regular health care systems. Both CBT and IPT administered individually may be effective in treating adolescent depressive disorders and symptoms, and CBT administered by way of bibliotherapy may be effective for reducing symptoms. The evidence for FT is less promising, but it may work in some cases. The current research base suggests that the variety of treatments received as part of usual care in outpatient mental health clinics in the United States may not work (Weersing & Weisz, 2002).

Group and individual CBT and IPT treatments may work in a residential setting either with medication or independently. Other effective residential treatments have not been specifically applied to adolescent depression Lyman & Wilson (2001). ECT carried out in residential settings may be an effective treatment for adolescents with very severe depression or treatment-resistant depression, but there remain concerns about aversive effects and it is not recommended as a first-line treatment (Rose, Wykes, Leese, Bindman & Freishmann, 2003). SSRIs may work, and of these drugs, fluoxetine appears to be the most promising. Other pharmacological treatments may work directly or as adjuncts to other interventions. Lack of treatment effects and associated side effects indicate that TCAs do not work in adolescents (Findling et al., 2002).

Psychosocial CBT-based interventions, for example, the POP program (Jaycox et al., 1994), work to prevent adolescent depressive symptoms when run in small groups in schools with pre-adolescents targeted because of increased risk factors. Targeted CBT-based depression prevention programs, for example, the CWSA program (Clarke et al., 1995), may work to prevent depressive disorders in adolescents in school-based settings, as well as in the offspring of depressed adults. Universal school-based depression and anxiety prevention programs may be effective in preventing depressive symptoms. However, their effects on the incidence of depressive disorders are as yet unknown. Strategies that involve brief interventions, whether targeted or universal, are unlikely to have lasting preventive effects.

The evidence base for the effectiveness of treatments and preventions for adolescent depression is promising. Psychosocial treatments, in particular CBT and IPT approaches, currently hold the most promise. The SSRI fluoxetine may be the most effective pharmacological treatment. Further research is needed in the area of family-based interventions and interventions for treatment-resistant adolescent depression. More RCTs of promising interventions will be important in the future.

References

Ackerson, J., Scogin, F., McKendree-Smith, N., & Lyman, R.D. (1998). Cognitive bibliotherapy for mild and moderate adolescent depressive symptomatology. *Journal of Consulting and Clinical Psychology, 66,* 685–690.

Amato, P.R. & Keith, B. (1991). Parental divorce and well-being of children: A meta analysis. *Psychological Bulletin, 110,* 26–46.

American Psychiatric Association. (2000). *Diagnostic and Statistical Manual of Mental Disorders* (4th ed.) text revision. Washington, DC: Author.

Angold, P.R., Costello, E.J., & Erkanli, A. (1999). Comorbidity. *Journal of Child Psychology and Psychiatry, 40,* 57–87.

Baumgartner, F. (2002). The effect of hardiness in the choice of coping strategies in stressful situations. *Studia and Psychologica, 44,* 69–74.

Beardslee, W.R., Salt, P., Porterfield, K., Rothberg, P.C., van der Velde, P., Swatling, S., Hoke, L., Moilanen, D.L., & Wheelock, I. (1993). Comparison of preventative interventions for families with parental affective disorder. *Journal of the American Academy of Child and Adolescent Psychiatry, 32,* 254–263.

Beardslee, W.R., Salt, P., Veersage, M.A., Gladstone, T.R.G., Wright, E.J., & Rothberg, P.C. (1997a). Sustained change in parents receiving preventive interventions for families with depression. *American Journal of Psychiatry, 154,* 510–515.

Beardslee, W.R., Versage, E.M., & Gladstone, T.R.G. (1998). Children of affectively ill parents: A review of the past 10 years. *Journal of the American Academy of Child and Adolescent Psychiatry, 37,* (11), 1134–1144.

Beardslee, W.R., Wright, E.J., Salt, P., Drezner, K., Gladstone, T.R.G., Versage, E.M., & Rothberg, P.C. (1997b). Examination of children's responses to two prevention intervention strategies over time. *Journal of the American Academy of Child and Adolescent Psychiatry, 36,* 196–204.

Birmaher, B., Brent, D.A., Kolko, D., Baugher, M., Bridge, J., Iyengar, S., & Ulloa, R.E. (2000). Clinical outcome after short-term psychotherapy for adolescents with major depressive disorder. *Archives of General Psychiatry, 57,* 29–36.

Bloch, Y., Levcovitch, Y., Bloch, A.M., Mendlovic, S., & Ratzoni, G. (2001). Electroconvulsive therapy in adolescents: similarities and differences from adults. *Journal of the American Academy of Child and Adolescent Psychiatry, 40,* 1332–1336.

Bostic, J.Q., Prince, J., Brown, K., & Place, S. (2001). A retrospective study of citalopram in adolescents with depression. *Journal of Child and Adolescent Psychopharmacology, 11,* 159–166.

Boyce Rogers, K., & Rose, H.A. (2002). Risk and resiliency factors among adolescents who experience marital transitions. *Journal of Marriage and Family, 64*, 1024–1037.

Brent, D.A., Holder, D., Kolko, D., Birmaher, B., Baugher, M. Roth, C., & Johnson, B. (1997). A clinical psychotherapy trial for adolescent depression comparing cognitive, family, and supportive treatments. *Archives of General Psychiatry, 54* 877–885.

Burns, D. (1980). *Feeling Good*. New York: Signet.

Cardemil, E.V., Reivich, K.J., & Seligman, M.E.P. (2002). The prevention of depressive symptoms in low-income minority middle school students. *Prevention & Treatment, 5*, Atricle 8.

Clarke, G.N., DeBar, L.L., & Lewinsohn, P.M. (2003). Cognitive-behavioual group treatment for adolescent depression. In A.E. Kazdin & J.R. Weisz (Eds.), *Evidence-Based Psychotherapies for Children and Adolescents* (pp. 120–147). New York: Guildford Press.

Clarke, G.N., Hawkins, W., Murphy, M., & Sheeber, L. (1993). School-based primary prevention of depressive symptomology in adolescents: Findings from two studies. *Journal of Adolescent Research, 8*, 183–204.

Clarke, G.N., Hawkins, W., Murphy, M., Sheeber, L.B., Lewinsohn, P.M., & Seeley, J.R. (1995). Targeted prevention of unipolar depressive disorder in an at-risk sample of high school adolescents: A randomized trial of a group cognitive intervention. *Journal of the American Academy of Child Adolescent Psychiatry, 34*, 312–321.

Clarke, G.N., Hornbrook, M.C., Lynch, F.L., & Polen, M. (2001). A randomised trial of a group cognitive intervention for preventing depression in adolescent offspring of depressed parents. *Archives of General Psychiatry, 58*, 1127–1136.

Clarke, G.N., Hornbrook, M.C., Lynch, F.L., Polen, M., Gale, J., O'Connor, E.A., Seeley, J., & DeBar, L.L. (2002). Group cognitive behavioural treatment for depressed adolescent offspring of depressed parents in a HMO. *Journal of American Academy of Child and Adolescent Psychiatry, 41*, 305–313.

Clarke, G.N., Rohde, P., Lewinsohn, P.M., Hops, H., & Seeley, J.R. (1999). Cognitive-behavioural treatment for adolescent depression: Efficacy of acute group treatment and booster sessions. *Journal of the American Academy of Child and Adolescent Psychiatry, 38*, 252–279.

Cohen, D., Taieb, O., Flament, M., Benoit, N., Chevret, S., Corcos, M., Fossati, P., Jeammet, P., Allilaire, J., & Basquin, M. (2000). Absence of cognitive impairment at long term follow-up in adolescents treated with ECT for severe mood disorders. *The American Journal of Psychiatry, 157*, 460–462.

Cole, D.A., Martin, J.M., & Powers, B. (1997). A competency-based model of child depression: A longitudinal study of peer, parent, teacher and self-evaluations. *Journal of Child Psychology and Psychiatry, 38*, 505–514.

Cole, D.A., Peeke, L.G., Martin, J.M., Truglio, R., & Seroczynski, A.D. (1998). A longitudinal look at the relation between depression and anxiety in children and adolescents. *Journal of Consulting and Clinical Psychology, 66*, 451–460.

Cole, D.A., & Rehm, L.P. (1986). Family interaction patterns and childhood depression. *Journal of Abnormal Child Psychology, 14*, 297–314.

Conrad, M., & Hammen, C. (1993). Protective and resource factors of high- and low-risk children: A comparison of children with unipolar, bipolar, medically ill, and normal mothers. *Development and Psychopathology, 5*, 593–607.

Cottrell, D. (2003). Outcome studies of family therapy in child and adolescent depression. *Journal of Family Therapy, 25*, 106– 416.

Curry, J. (2001). Specific psychotherapies for childhood and adolescent depression. *Biological Psychiatry, 49*, 1091–1100.

Daviss, W.B., Bentivoglio, P., Racusin, R., Brown, K.M., Bostic, J.Q., & Wiley, J. (2001). Bubropion sustained release for adolescents with comorbid addtentin-deficit/hyperactivity disorder and depression. *Journal of the American Academy of Child and Adolescent Psychiatry, 40*, 307–314.

Diamond, G.S., Reis, B.F., Diamond, G.M., Siqueland, L., & Isaacs, L. (2002). Attachment-based family therapy for depressed adolescents: a treatment development study. *Journal of the American Academy of Child and Adolescent Psychiatry, 41*, 1190–1197.

Downey, G., & Coyne, J.C. (1990). Children of depressed parents: An integrative review. *Psychological Bulletin, 108*, 50–76.

Duffett, R., Hill, P., & Lelliott, P. (1999). Use of electroconvulsive therapy in young people. *British Journal of Psychiatry, 175*, 228–230.

Eley, T.C., Deater-Deckard, K., Fombonne, E., Fulker, D.W., & Plomin, R. (1998). An adoption study of depressive symptoms in middle childhood. *Journal of Child Psychology and Psychiatry, 39*, 337–345.

Emslie, G.J., Heiligenstein, J.H., Wagner, K.D., Hoog, S.L., Ernest, D.E., Brown, E., Nilsson, M., & Jacobson, J.G. (2002). Fluoxetine for acute treatment of depression in children and adolescents: A placebo-controlled, randomised clinical trial. *Journal of the American Academy of Child and Adolescent Psychiatry, 41*, 1205–1215.

Emslie, G.J., & Mayes, T.L. (2001). Mood disorders in children and adolescents: psychopharmacological treatment. *Biological Psychiatry, 49*, 1082–1090.

Emslie, G.J., Rush, A.J., Weinberg, W.A., Kowatch, R.A., Carmody, T., & Mayes, T.L. (1998). Fluoxetine in child and adolescent depression: Acute and maintenance treatment. *Anxiety Depression, 7*, 32–39.

Emslie, G.J., Rush, A.J., Weinberg, W.A., Kowatch, R.A., Hughes, C.W., & Carmody, T. (1997). A double-blind, randomised, placebo-controlled trial of fluoxetine in children and adolescents with depression. *Archives of General Psychiatry, 54*, 1031–103.

Emslie, G.J., Walkup, J.T., Pliszka, S.R., & Ernst, M. (1999). Nontricyclic antidepressants: Current trends in children and adolescent. *Journal of the American Academy of Child and Adolescent Psychiatry, 38*, 517–528.

Felsman, J.K., & Vaillant, G.E. (1987). Resilient children as adults: A 40 year study. In E.J. Anthony & B.J. Cohler (Eds.), *The Invulnerable Child* (pp. 289–314). New York: Guilford Press.

Ferguson, D.M., Horwood, L.J., & Lynsky, N.T. (1995). Maternal depressive symptoms and depressive symptoms in adolescents. *Journal of Child Psychology and Psychiatry, 36*, 1161–1178.

Findling, R.L., Feeny, N.C., Stansbrey, R.J., DelPorto-Bedoya, D., & Demeter, C. (2002). Somatic treatment for depressive illnesses in children an adolescents. *Child and Adolescent Psychiatric Clinics of North America, 11*, 555–578.

Finkelstein, J.S., Donenberg, & Martinovich, Z. (2001). Maternal control and adolescent depression: Ethnic differences among clinically referred girls. *Journal of Youth and Adolescence, 30*, 155–171.

Food and Drug Administration. (2003). FDA statement regarding the antidepressant Paxil for pediatric depression. FDA Talk Paper. June 19, 2003. Available at: http://www.fda.gov/bbs/topics/ANSWERS/2003/ANSO1230.html

Forehand, R., Biggar, H., & Kotchick, B.A. (1997). Cumulative risk across family stressors: Short- and long-term effects for adolescents. *Journal of Abnormal Child Psychology, 26*, 119–128.

Garrison, C.Z., Jackson, K.L., Marsteller, F., McKeown, R., & Addy, C. (1990). A longitudinal study of depressive symptomatology in young adolescents. *Journal of the American Academy of Child and Adolescent Psychiatry, 29*, 581–585.

Ge, X., Best, K.M., Conger, R.D., & Simons, R.L. (1996). Parenting behaviors ands the occurrence and co-occurrence of adolescent depressive symptoms and conduct problems. *Developmental Psychology, 32*, 717–731.

Ge, X., Lorenz, F.O., Conger, R.D., Elder, G.H., & Simmons, R.L. (1994). Trajectories of stressful life events and depressive symptoms during adolescence. *Developmental Psychology, 30*, 467–483.

Geller, B., Reising, D., Leonard, H.L., Riddle, M.A., & Walsh, B.T. (1999). Critical review of tricyclic antidepressant use in children and adolescents. *Journal of Academy of Child and Adolescent Psychiatry, 38*, 513–516.

Gillham, J.E. & Reivich, K.J. (1999). Prevention of depressive symptoms in school children: Update. *Psychological Science, 10*, 461–462.

Gillham, J.E., Reivich, K.J, Jaycox, L.H., & Seligman, M.E.P. (1995). Prevention of depressive symptoms in school children: Two-year follow-up. *Psychological Science, 6*, 343–351.

Gillham, J.E., Shatte, A.J., & Freres, D.R. (2000). Preventing depression: A review of cognitive-behavioural and family interventions. *Applied & Preventative Psychology, 9*, 63–88.

Gladstone, T.R.G. & Beardslee, W.R. (2000). The prevention of depression in at-risk adolescents: Current and future directions. *Journal of Cognitive Psychotherapy: An International Quarterly, 14*, 9–23.

Goodyer, I.M., & Altham, P.M. (1991). Lifetime exit events and recent social and family adversities in anxious and depressed school-age children and adolescents: II. *Journal of Affective Disorders, 21*, 229–238.

Greenberg, M.T., Domitrovich, C. & Bumbarger, B. (2001). The prevention of mental disorders in school-aged children: State of the field. *Prevention and Treatment, 4*, Article 1.

Hains, A.E. & Ellmann, S.W. (1994). Stress inoculation training as a preventative intervention for high school youths. *Journal of Cognitive Psychotherapy: An International Quarterly, 8*, 219–232.

Hammen, C., Adrian, C., & Hiroto, D. (1988). A longitudinal test of the attributional vulnerability model in children at risk for depression. *British Journal of Clinical Psychology, 27*, 37–46.

Hammen, C., Burge, D., & Adrian, C. (1991). Timing of mothers and child depression in a longitudinal study of children at risk. *Journal of Consulting and Clinical Psychology, 59*, 341–345.

Hankin, B.L., Abramson, L.Y., Moffitt, T.E., Silva, P.A., McGee, R., & Angell, K.E. (1998). Development of depression from pre-adolescence to young adulthood: Emerging gender differences in a 10-year longitudinal study. *Journal of Abnormal Psychology, 107,* 128–140.

Hazell, P., O'Connell, D., Heathcote, D., Robertson, J., & Henry, D. (1995). Efficacy of tricyclic drugs in child and adolescent depression: a meta-analysis. *British Medical Journal, 3,* 897–901.

Hops, H. (1992). Parental depression and child behavior problems: Implications for behavioral family interventions. *Behavior Change, 9,* 126–138.

Hughes, C.W., Emslie, G.J., Crismon, M.L., Wagner, K.D., Birmaher, B., Geller, B., Pliszka, S.R., Ryan, N.D., Strober, M., Trivedi, M.H., Topric, M.G., Sedillo, A., Llana, M.E., Lopez, M., & Rush, A.J. (1999). The Texas Children's Medication Algorithm Project: Report of the Texas Consensus Conference Panel of Medication Treatment of Childhood Major Depressive Disorder. *Journal of the American Academy of Child and Adolescent Psychiatry, 38,* 1442–1454.

Jaycox, L.H., Reivich, K.J., Gillham, J., & Seligman, M.E.P. (1994). Preventing depressive symptoms in school children. *Behaviour Research and Therapy, 32,* 801–816.

Jayson, D., Wood, A., Kroll, L., Fraser, J., & Harrington, R. (1998). Which depressed patients respond to cognitive-behavioural treatment? *Journal of the American Academy of Child and Adolescent Psychiatry, 37,* 35–39.

Kaslow, N.J., & Thompson, M.P. (1998). Applying the criteria for empirically supported treatments to studies of psychosocial interventions for child and adolescent depression. *Journal of Clinical Child Psychology, 27,* 146–155.

Keller, M.B., Ryan, N.D, Strober, M., Klein, R.G., Kutcher, S.P., Birmaher, B., Hagino, O.R., Koplewicz, H., Carlson, G.A., Clarke, G.N., Emslie, G.J., Feinberg, D., Geller, B., Kusumakar, V., Papatheodorou, G., Sack, W.H., Sweeney, M., Wagner, K.D., Weller, E.B., Winters, N.C., Oakes, R., & McCaffery, J.P. (2001). Efficacy of Paroxetine in the treatment of adolescent major depression: A randomized controlled trial. *Journal of the American Academy of Child and Adolescent Psychiatry, 40,* 762–772.

Kessler, R.C., Avenevoli, S., & Merkingas, K.R. (2001). Mood disorders in children and adolescents: An epidemiological perspective. *Biological Psychiatry, 49,* 1002–1014.

Kolko, D., Brent, D., Baugher, M., Bridge, J., & Birmaher, B. (2000). Cognitive and family therapy for adolescent depression: treatment specificity, mediation and moderation. *Journal of Consulting and Clinical Psychology, 68,* 603–614.

Kroll, L., Harrington, R., Jayson, D., Fraser, J., & Gowers, S. (1996). Pilot study of continuation cognitive–behavioural therapy for major depression in adolescent psychiatric patients. *Journal of the American Academy of Child and Adolescent Psychiatry, 35,* 1156–1161.

Kutcher, S.P., & Marton, R. (1996). Treatment of adolescent depression. In K. Shulman, M. Tohen, & S.P. Kutcher (Eds.), *Mood Disorders Across the Life Span.* (pp. 101–126). New York: John Wiley.

Lewinsohn, P.M., Clarke, G.N., Hops, H., & Andrews, J.A. (1990). Cognitive-behavioural treatment for depressed adolescents. *Behaviour Therapy, 21,* 385–401.

Lewinsohn, P.M., Clarke, G.N., Seeley, J.R., & Rohde, P. (1994). Major depression in community adolescents: Age at onset, episode duration, and time to recurrence. *Journal of the American Academy of Child and Adolescent Psychiatry, 33,* 714–722.

Lewinsohn, P.M., Gotlib, I.H., & Seeley, J.R. (1997). Depression-related psychosocial variables: Are they specific to depression in adolescents? *Journal of Abnormal Child Psychology, 106, (3),* 365–375.

Lewinsohn, P.M., Hops, H., Roberts, R.E., Seeley, J.R., & Andrews, J.A. (1993). Adolescent psychopathology: I. Prevalence and incidence of depression and other DSM-III-R disorders in high school students. *Journal of Abnormal Psychology, 102,* 133–144.

Lewinsohn, P.M., Roberts, R.E., Seeley, J.R., Rohde, P., Gotlib, I.H., & Hops, H. (1994). Adolescent psychopathology: II. Psychosocial risk factors for depression. *Journal of Abnormal Psychology, 103,* 302–315.

Lewinsohn, P.M., Rohde, P., Klein, D.N., & Seeley, J.R. (1999). Natural course of adolescent major depressive disorder: I. Continuity into young adulthood. *Journal of the American Academy of Child & Adolescent Psychiatry, 38,* 56–63.

Lewinsohn, P.M., Rohde, P., & Seeley, J.R., (1998). Major depressive disorder in older adolescents: prevalence, risk factors, and clinical implications. *Clinical Psychology Review, 18, (7),* 765–794.

Lewinsohn, P.M., Seeley, J.R., Hubbard, J., Rohde, P., & Sack, W.H. (1996). Cross-sectional and prospective relationships between physical morbidity and depression in older adolescents. *Journal of the Academy of Child and Adolescent Psychiatry, 35,* 1120–1129.

Lowry-Webster, H., Barrett, P.M., & Dadds M.R. (2001). A universal prevention trial of anxiety and depression symptomatology in childhood: Preliminary data from an Australian Study. *Behaviour Change, 18,* 36–50.

Lowrey-Webster, H., Barrett, P.M., & Lock, S. (2003). A universal prevention trial of anxiety symtomology during childhood: Results at 1-year follow-up. *Behaviour Change, 20*, 25–43.

Luthar, S.S. (1991). Vulnerability and resilience: A study of high risk adolescents. *Child Development, 62*, 600–616.

Lyman, R.D., & Wilson, D.R. (2001). Residential and inpatient treatment of emotionally disturbed children and adolescents. In C.E. Walker & M.C. Walker (Eds.), *Handbook of Child Clinical Psychology. (3rd ed.)* (pp. 495–894). New York: John Wiley & Sons.

McMahon, N.E., Yarcheski, A., & Yarcheski, T.J. (2003). Anger, anxiety, and depression in early adolescents from intact and divorced families. *Journal of Paediatric Nursing, 18*, 267–273.

Michael, K.D., & Crowley, S.L. (2002). How effective are treatments for child and adolescent depression? A meta-analytic review. *Clinical Psychology Review, 22*, 247–269.

Mufson, L., & Fairbanks, J. (1996). Interpersonal psychotherapy for depressed adolescents: A one-year naturalistic follow-up study. *Journal of the American Academy of Child and Adolescent Psychiatry, 35*, 1145–1155.

Mufson, L., & Pollack Dorta, K. (2003). Interpersonal psychotherapy for depressed adolescents. In A.E. Kazdin & J.R. Weisz (Eds.). *Evidence-based psychotherapies for children and adolescents.* (pp. 148–164). New York: Guildford Press.

Mufson, L., Moreau, D., Weissman, M.M., Wickramaratne, P., Martin, J., & Samoilov, A. (1994). The modification of interpersonal psychotherapy with depressed adolescents (IPT-A): Phase I and Phase II studies. *Journal of the American Academy of Child and Adolescent Psychiatry, 33*, 695–705.

Mufson, L., Weissman, M.M., Moreau, D., & Garfinkel, R. (1999). Efficacy of interpersonal psychotherapy for depressed adolescents. *Archives of General Psychiatry, 56*, 573–579.

Muris, P., Schmidt, H., Lambrichs, & Meesters, C. (2001). Protective and vulnerability factors of depression in normal adolescents. *Behavior Research and Therapy, 39*, 555–565.

Nada Raja, S. McGee, R., & Stanton, W.R. (1992). Perceived attachments to parents and peers and psychological well-being in adolescence. *Journal of Youth and Adolescence, 21*, 471–485.

Nelson, D.R., Hammen, C., Brennan, P.A., & Ullman, J.B. (2003). The impact of maternal depression on adolescent adjustment: The role of expressed emotion. *Journal of Consulting and Clinical Psychology, 71*, 935–944.

Nilzen, K.R., & Palmérus, K. (1997). The influence of familial factors on anxiety and depression in childhood and early adolescence. *Adolescence, 32*, 935–943.

Nelson, D.R., Hammen, C., Brennan, P.A., & Ullman, J.B. (2003). The impact of maternal depression on adolescent adjustment: The role of expressed emotion. *Journal of Consulting and Clinical Psychology, 71*, 935–944.

Patterson, C., & Lynd-Stevenson, R. (2001). The prevention of depressive symptoms in children: The immediate and long-term outcomes of a school-based program. *Behaviour Change, 18*, 92–102

Petersen, A.C., Leffert, N., Graham, B., Alwin, J., & Ding, S. (1997). Promoting mental health during the transition into adolescence. In J. Schulenberg, J.L. Maggs, & K. Hurrelmann (Eds.). *Health Risks and Developmental Transitions During Adolescence* (pp. 471–497). Cambridge: Cambridge University Press.

Pike, A., McGuire, S., Hetherington, E.M., Reiss, D., & Plomin, R. (1996). Early environmental and adolescent depressive symptoms and antisocial behavior: A multivariate genetic analysis. *Journal of Child Psychology & Psychiatry and Allied Disciplines, 37*, 695–704

Piko, B.F., & Fitzpatrick, K.M. (2003). Depressive symptomatology among Hungarian youth: A risk and protective factors approach. *American Journal of Orthopsychiatry, 73*, 44–54.

Puskar, K.R., Tusaie-Mumford, K., Sereika, S.M., & Lamb, J. (1999). Screening and predicting adolescent depressive symptoms in rural settings. *Archives of Psychiatric Nursing, 13*, 3–11.

Quayle, D., Dziurawiec, S., Roberts, C., Kane, R., & Ebsworthy, G. (2001). The effect of an optimism and lifeskills program on depressive symptoms in preadolescence. *Behaviour Change, 18*, 194–203.

Rapee, R.M. (1997). Potential role of childrearing practices in the development of anxiety and depression. *Clinical Psychology Review, 17*, 47–67.

Reijneveld, S.A., Crone, M.R., Verhulst, F.C., & Verloove-Vanhorick, S P. (2003). The effects of severe disaster on the mental health of adolescents: A controlled study. *The Lancet, 362*, 691–696.

Reinecke, M.A., Ryan, N.E., & DuBois, D.L. (1998). Cognitive-behavioual therapy of depression and depressive symptoms during adolescence: A review and meta-analysis. *Journal of the American Academy of Child and Adolescent Psychiatry, 37*, 26–34.

Reinherz, H.Z., Giaconia, R.M., Pakiz, B., Silverman, A.B., Frost, A.K., & Lefkowitz, E.S. (1993). Psychosocial risks for major depression in late adolescence: a longitudinal community study. *Journal of the American Academy of Child and Adolescent Psychiatry, 32, (6)*, 1159–1164.

Reinherz, H.Z., Stewart-Berghauer, G., Pakiz, B., Frost, A.K., Moeykens, B.A., & Holmes, W.M. (1989). The relationship of early risk and current mediators to depressive symptomatology in adolescents. *Journal of the American Academy of Child and Adolescent Psychiatry, 28,* 942–947.

Renouf, A.G., & Harter, S.U. (1990). Low self-worth and anger as components of depressive experience in young adolescents. *Development and Psychopathology, 2,* 293–310.

Rey, J.M., & Walter, G. (1997). Half a century of ECT use in young people. *The American Journal of Psychiatry, 154,* 595–602.

Robinson, N.S., Garber, J., & Hillsman, R. (1995). Cognitions and stress: Direct and moderating effects on depressive versus externalising symptoms during the junior high school transition. *Journal of Abnormal Psychology, 104,* 453–463.

Roberts, C., & Bishop, B. (2003). Depression, adolescents. In T. Gullotta & M. Bloom (Eds.). *Encyclopedia of Primary Prevention and Health Promotion* (pp. 403–410). Kluwer Academic/Plenum Press.

Roberts, C., Kane, R., Thompson, H., Bishop, B., & Hart, B. (2003). The prevention of depressive symptoms in rural school children: A randomised controlled trial. *Journal of Consulting and Clinical Psychology, 71,* 622–628.

Roberts, R.E., Lewinsohn, P.M., & Seeley, J.R. (1995). Symptoms of DSM-III-R major depression in adolescence: Evidence from an epidemiological survey. *Journal of the American Academy of Child Adolescent Psychiatry, 34,* 1608–1617.

Roberts, R.E., Roberts, C.R., & Chen, Y.R. (1997). Ethnocultural differences in prevalence of adolescent depression. *American Journal of Community Psychology, 25,* 95–110.

Rose, D., Wykes, T., Leese, M. Bindman, J., & Freishmann, P. (2003). Patient's perspectives on electroconvulsive therapy: Systematic review. *British Medical Journal, 326,* 1363–1366.

Rossello, J., & Bernal, G. (1999). The efficacy of cognitive-behavioral and interpersonal treatments for depression in Puerto Rican adolescents. *Journal of Consulting and Clinical Psychology, 67,* 734–745.

Ryan, N.D., Puig-Antich, J., Rabinovich, H., Fried, J. Ambrosini, P., Meyer, V., Torres, D., Dachille, S., & Mazzie, D. (1988). MAOIs in adolescent major depression unresponsive to tricyclic antidepressants. *Journal of the American Academy of Child and Adolescent Psychiatry, 27,* 755–758.

Rudolph, K.D., Hammen, C., Burge, D., Lindberg, N., Herzberg, D., & Daley, S.E. (2000). Toward an interpersonal life-stress model of depression: The developmental context of stress generation. *Development and Psychopathology, 12,* 215–234.

Sagrestano, L.M., Paikoff, R.L., Holmbeck, G.N., & Fendrich, M. (2003). A longitudinal examination of familial risk factors for depression among inner-city African American adolescents. *Journal of Family Psychology, 17,* 108–120.

Santor, D.A., & Kusumakar, V. (2001). Open trial of interpersonal therapy for adolescents with moderate to severe major depression: Effectiveness of novice IPT therapists. *Journal of the American Academy of Child and Adolescent Psychiatry, 40,* 236–240.

Sawyer, M.G., Kosky, R.J., Graetz, B.W., Arney, F., Zubrick, S.R., & Baghurst, P. (2000). The national survey of mental health and well being: The child and adolescent component. *Australian and New Zealand Journal of Psychiatry, 34,* 214–220.

Schwartz, J.A., Kaslow, N.J., Seeley, J., & Lewinsohn, P. (2000). Psychological, cognitive and interpersonal correlates of attributional change in adolescents. *Journal of Clinical Child Psychology, 29,* 188–198.

Sheeber, L., Hops, H., Alpert, A., Davis, B., & Andrews, J. (1997). Family support and conflict: Prospective relations to adolescent depression. *Abnormal Child Psychology, 25,* 33–344.

Shochet, I.M., Dadds, M.R., Holland, D., Whitefield, K., Harnett, P.H., & Osgarby, S.M. (2001). The efficacy of a universal school-based program to prevent adolescent depression. *Journal of Clinical Child Psychology, 30,* 303–315.

Siegel, J.M., Aneschensel, C.S., Taub, B., Cantwell, D.P., & Driscoll, A.K. (2001). Adolescent depressed mood in a multiethnic sample. *Prevention Research, 8,* 4–6.

Simeon, J.G., Dinicola, V.F., Ferguson, H.B., & Copping, W. (1990). Adolescent depression: A placebo-controlled fluoxetine treatment study and follow-up. *Progress in Neuropsychopharmacology & Biological Psychiatry, 14,* 791–795.

Skaer, T.L., Robinson, L.M., Sclar, D.A., & Galin, R.S. (2000). Treatment of depressive illness among children and adolescents in the United States. *Current Therapeutic Research, 61,* 692–705.

Smokowski, P.R. Ecological risk and resilience: A mixed-method analysis of disadvantaged, minority youth. [Dissertation Abstract] *Dissertation Abstracts International Section A: Humanities & Social Sciences. Vol 60(5-A), Dec 1999, 1769.* US: Univ Microfilms International.

Spence, S.H., Sheffield, J.K., & Donovan, C.L. (2003). Preventing adolescent depression: An evaluation of the Problem Solving for Life Program. *Journal of Consulting and Clinical Psychology, 71*, 3–13.

Strober, M., Pataki, C., & DeAntonio, M. (1998). Complete remission of *treatment resistant* severe melancholia in adolescents with phenelzine: Two case reports. *Journal of Affective Disorders, 50*, 55–58.

Sund, A.M., & Wichstrom, L. (2002). Insecure attachment as a risk factor for future depressive symptoms in early adolescents. *Journey of American Academy of Child and Adolescence Psychiatry, 41*, 1478–1486.

Task Force on Promotion and Dissemination of Psychological Procedures. (1995). Training in and dissemination of empirically-validated psychological treatments: Report and recommendations. *The Clinical Psychologist, 8*, 3–24.

Thaper, A. & McGuffin, P. (1994). A twin study of depressive symptoms in childhood. *British Journal of Psychiatry, 65*, 259–265.

Tiet, Q.Q., Bird, H.R., Davies, M., Hoven, C., Cohen, P., Jenson, P., & Goodman, S. (1998). Adverse life events and resilience. *Journal of the American Academy of Child and Adolescent Psychiatry, 37*, 1191–1200.

Thurber, S. Ensign, J., Punnett, A.F., & Welter, K. (1995). A meta-analysis of antidepressant outcome studies that involved children and adolescents. *Journal of Clinical Psychology, 51*, 340–345.

Turner, J.E., & Cole, D.A. (1994). Developmental differences in cognitive diatheses for child depression. *Journal of Abnormal Child Psychology, 22*, 15–32.

Varley, C.K. (2003). Psychpharmacological treatment for major depressive disorder in children and adolescents. *Journal of the American Medical Association, 290*, 1091–1093.

Vostanis, P., Feehan, C., Grattan, E., & Bickerton, W. (1996). A randomised controlled out-patient trial of cognitive–behavioural treatment for children and adolescents with depression: 9-month follow-up. *Journal of Affective Disorders, 40*, 105–116.

Wagner, K.D., Ambrosini, P., Ryan, M., Wohlberg, C., Yang, R., Greenbaum, M.S., Childress, A., Donnelly, C., & Deas, D. (2003). Efficacy of sertraline in the treatment of children and adolescents with major depressive disorder. *Journal of the American Medical Association, 290*, 1033–1041.

Walsh, F. (2003). Family resilience: A framework for clinical practice, theory and practice. *Family Process, 42*, 1–18.

Weersing, V.R., & Weisz, J.R. (2002). Community care treatment of depressed youth: Benchmarking usual care against CBT clinical trials. *Journal of Consulting and Clinical Psychology, 70*, 299–310.

Weersing, V.R., Weisz, J.R., & Donenberg, G.R. (2002). Development of the Therapy Procedures Checklist: A therapist-report measure of technique use in child and adolescent treatment. *Journal of Clinical Child and Adolescent Psychology, 31*, 168–180.

Werner, E.E. (1993). Risk, resilience and recovery: Perspectives from the Kaui longitudinal study. *Development and Psychopathology, 5*, 503–515

Wichstrom, L. (1999). The emergence of gender difference in depressed mood during adolescence: The role of intensified gender socialization. *Developmental Psychology, 35*, 232–245.

Wilens, T.E., Spencer, T.J., Biederman, J., & Schleifer, D. (1997). Case study: nefazodone for juvenile mood disorder. *Journal of the American Academy of Child and Adolescent Psychiatry, 36*, 481–485.

Wood, A., Harrington, R., & Moore, A. (1996). Controlled trial of a brief cognitive behavioural intervention in adolescent patients with depressive disorders. *Journal of Child Psychology and Psychiatry, 37*, 737–746.

Wolkow, K.E., & Ferguson, H.B. (2001). Community resilient factors in the development of resiliency: Considerations and future directions. *Community Mental Health Journal, 37*, 489–498.

World Health Organization. (1992). *The ICD-10 Classification of Mental and Behavioral Disorders*. World Health Organization, Geneva.

Yu, D.L., & Seligman, M.E.P. (2002). Preventing depressive symptoms in Chinese children. *Prevention & Treatment, 5*, Article 9.

Zubernis, L.S., Cassidy, K.W., Gillham, J.E., Reivich, K.J., & Jaycox, L.H. (1999). Prevention of depressive symptoms in pre-adolescent children of divorce. *Journal of Divorce & Remarriage, 30*, 11–35.

Chapter 11

Suicide

John Kalafat

Introduction

Theoretical Perspectives

The organization of this handbook and other texts on adolescent dysfunctional behaviors reflects the predominant state of the field, which is characterized by research and practice that is categorical or addresses specific dysfunctions. However, in one sense, such categorization is at variance with recent developments in the prevention and, to a lesser degree, treatment of adolescent dysfunctional behaviors. Current reviews of the prevention of youth problem behaviors conclude that they are mediated—increasing the likelihood or positively associated with common risk factors—and moderated—decreasing the likelihood or negatively associated with common protective factors (Biglan, Mrazek, Carnine & Flay, 2003). Moreover, as implied by the common chapter headings in this volume, adolescent dysfunctional behaviors are associated with risks and protections at every ecological level, including individual, peer, family, school, and community or society (Durlak, 1998). For example, substance abuse and other problem behaviors are associated with problem-solving and learning problems (individual); negative norms/modeling (peers); family pathology and punitive child-rearing (family); low expectations and poor relationships among students, faculty, and parents (school); and lack of resources (community). Suicide is no exception, as it has long been characterized as multiply determined (Goldsmith, Pellmar, Kleinman & Bunney, 2002; Gould, Greenberg, Velting & Shaffer, 2003; Rudd & Joiner, 1998). These findings have substantial implications for prevention programming and have led to the development of programs that have been variously described as comprehensive and multilevel (Silverman & Felner, 1995), ecological (Felner & Felner, 1989), and systemic (Kalafat, 2001; Sanddal, Sanddal, Berman & Silverman, 2003). They are described in subsequent sections of this chapter.

In regard to treatment, the categorical treatment of dysfunctions, reinforced by categorical or dysfunction-specific funding, has contributed to youth service systems that have been characterized as fragmented, inaccessible, and duplicative (Saxe, Cross & Silverman, 1988). This has resulted in calls for wraparound, integrated services (Illback, Cobb & Joseph, 1997).

In this context, prevention and treatment are conceived of as complementary components of a systemic continuum of care. In fact, whether using the traditional concepts of primary, secondary, and tertiary prevention or the more recent concepts of universal, selective, and indicated interventions, treatment occupies the secondary and indicated niches, respectively.

While adolescent dysfunctional behaviors share many risk and protective factors and appear to be most effectively addressed by broad, multilevel prevention programs and integrated services, there are risk and protective factors and concomitant prevention and treatment approaches that are unique to given dysfunctions. For example, at the societal level, suicidal behavior does not arise in a context that encourages such behavior as is the case with interpersonal violence and substance abuse where powerful media and business interests foster violence and chemical solutions to problems. In addition, there are individual risk factors that appear to be particularly, if not uniquely, associated with suicide as described in the next section.

For suicide, the framework outlined above yields a formulation of prevention and treatment that addresses the unfolding process or developmental trajectory of youth suicide that leads to the emergence of suicidal behavior (Silverman & Felner, 1995). As one moves along that trajectory, the risk and protective factors targeted initially are distal, broad-based, and shared with other dysfunctional behaviors (e.g., problem solving, social bonding) and are addressed in universal approaches (e.g., Positive Youth Development Programs, Catalano et al., 2002). Then, moving closer to the emerging phenomenon of the suicidal state, the risk and protective targets become progressively more proximal, severe, and specific to suicide (e.g., help negation) and are addressed by selective and indicated approaches (e.g., cognitive-behavioral therapy for suicidal depression). The prevention and treatment approaches reviewed in this chapter reflect this formulation.

Definitional Issues

Progress in the field of suicide prevention and treatment has been hampered by a lack of universally accepted definitions of suicide and suicidal behavior. Research-based definitions have been developed (O'Carroll et al., 1996) and accepted by the Institute of Medicine (Goldsmith et al., 2002). A *suicide completion* is defined as death from injury where there is explicit or implicit evidence that the injury was self-inflicted and that the decedent intended to kill him/herself. A *suicide attempt* is defined as an action resulting in nonfatal injury, or potentially self-injurious behavior with a nonfatal outcome, where there is explicit or implicit evidence that the injury was self-inflicted and that the decedent intended at some (nonzero) level to kill him/herself. *Suicidal ideation* consists of thoughts of harming or killing oneself; and, frequency, intensity, and duration are all posited as important to determining the severity of ideation. *Suicidality* refers to all suicide-related behaviors and thoughts, including completing or attempting suicide, and suicidal ideation.

Incidence Rates[1]

In 2000, the national suicide rate for 15–19-year-olds was 8.2 per 100,000. Suicide ranks as the third leading cause of death among adolescents, after accidents and homicides (although, across all age groups, more people die in the United States by suicide than homicide). Rates for 15–19-year-olds increased by 11% between 1980 and 1987 and 99% for those between the ages of 10 and 14. Both age groups have shown small declines in rates in 2001 and 2002. Rates for ages 15–19 in 2000 for different groups are as follows: all males (13.2), all females (2.8), all whites (8.6), all blacks (6.3), American Indian/AK Native (18.4), Hispanic (6.2). Rates for black females of all ages are consistently the lowest of any group (generally lower than 2 per 100,000). While rates for black males are lower than for white males, black male rates increased 80% between 1980 and 2000. Firearms remain the most common suicide method among youth, regardless of race or gender, accounting for almost three of five completed suicides. Since 1993, the Centers for Disease Control and Prevention (CDC) has conducted the Youth Risk Behavior Survey (YRBS) with a representative sample of high school students in grades 9–12 every two years. Within this survey there is information on suicide attempts and ideation. In the 2001 survey, 19% of students "seriously considered attempting suicide," 14.8% made a specific plan for suicide, 8.8% had attempted suicide at least once in the 12 months preceding the survey, and 2.6% made a suicide attempt that had to be treated by a doctor or nurse (Grunbaum et al., 2002). For every completed suicide among adolescents it is estimated that there may be over 100 attempts. While more males complete suicide, females attempt suicide four to five times more than males. Within a typical high school classroom, it is likely that three students (one boy and two girls) have made a suicide attempt in the past year. In regard to suicide rates among gay, lesbian, and bisexual youths, most studies document an elevation of risk for attempts among males with mixed findings for females. Findings are also not clear regarding suicide completion for these groups (McDaniel et al., 2001). Finally, a recent comprehensive report by the Institute of Medicine (Goldsmith et al., 2002) pointed out that official suicide statistics are fraught with inaccuracies due to regional differences in definitions of suicide, classifications of deaths, training and background of coroners and medical examiners, the extent to which cases are examined, and the quality of data management. Most of these problems result in underreporting of suicide. Suicide remains stigmatized in our society and, particularly for youth, there are pressures from families, secondary schools, and colleges to report deaths as accidents.

Individual Factors[2]

Risk Factors

Risk factors for suicide include vulnerabilities such as psychopathology and psychological variables, and characteristics specific to the suicidal state, including help negation, prior attempts, and characteristics of current suicidal ideation.

---

[1] Note: unless otherwise specified, data come from the National Center for Injury Prevention and Control (NCIPC), 2003.

[2] Unless otherwise specified, the primary sources for the sections on risk and resiliency are Goldsmith et al., 2002; Gould et al., 2003; Rudd & Joiner, 1998.

PSYCHOPATHOLOGY. Depressive disorders are the most prevalent disorders among adolescent suicide completions, and female victims are more likely than males to have affective disorders. Substance abuse is also a significant risk factor, particularly among older adolescent males. There is also a high prevalence of comorbidity between affective and substance abuse disorders. Conduct disorder is a risk factor for males, often comorbid with depression and substance abuse. Bipolar disorders among youth contribute to risk for suicide, and these are often diagnosed as conduct disorders. Studies have also found a 40–50% prevalence rate of personality disorders, mainly borderline disorders, among youth suicide victims. Recent research also implicates anxiety and panic disorders as risk factors.

There appears to be some differences in determinants of risk for black and white youths. For whites, antisocial behavior is positively associated with suicide. For blacks, this association is curvilinear in that low levels of antisocial behavior are associated with greater risk than no antisocial behavior, but those with high antisocial behavior were not at greater risk. This pattern requires further investigation, as it may be an artifact of the phenomenon of suicide by black male youths through risky antisocial behavior that prompts lethal responses from peers or police. Also, problem drinking appears to be less associated with suicide in blacks than whites (Castle, et al., 2002).

PSYCHOLOGICAL VARIABLES. Characteristics such as cognitive rigidity, ineffective problem solving/coping styles, negative attributional style, and hopelessness have been found in various combinations among youth who attempt or complete suicide. *Cognitive rigidity* refers to inability to generate alternate views of or solutions to problems. Poor problem-solving is characterized by less active and more avoidant (e.g., suppressive, blame) approaches, and impulsive problem-solving, which includes unrealistic expectations as to the effort or amount of time needed to arrive at a resolution. Explanatory style in depressed and suicidal individuals has been characterized as hapless and helpless in that negative events are attributed to internal, stable, global causes, while positive events are attributed to unstable, external causes. Hopelessness can arise independently from mood disorders and occurs across diagnostic categories.

These characteristics may be trait-like, perhaps mediated by family characteristics and chronic negative life events. Or, they may interact or mediate each other. Thus, hopelessness may arise within the context of depression or negative attributions interacting with negative life events; and, in turn, such hopelessness predicts suicide in adults and adolescents. Likewise, cognitive rigidity may be mediated by depression or anxiety, which may be reactive to acute stressors. Two trait-like variables that have a degree of heritability have been associated with suicidality. These are impulsive/aggressive (which includes risk-taking) and depressive/withdrawn temperament.

HELP NEGATION. This is a refusal to accept or access available helping resources as a way of dealing with one's pathology or problems. Research has shown significant positive correlations between help negation and suicidal ideation and behavior (Carlton & Deane, 2000; Rudd, Joiner & Rajab, 1995). Few adolescents experiencing stress or personal problems consider seeking help, particularly from adults or mental health services; and troubled or at-risk adolescents prefer peers to adults if they seek help at all (Lindsey & Kalafat, 1998).

PRIOR ATTEMPTS.   A history of a prior suicide attempt is one of the strongest predictors of completed suicide, particularly for boys (probably because girls attempt suicide six to seven times more often than boys). Recent research (Joiner, Walker, Rudd & Jobes, 1999) indicates that any more than one attempt significantly increases the risk over a single attempt.

CHARACTERISTICS OF CURRENT SUICIDAL IDEATION.   The frequency, intensity, and duration of suicidal thoughts, as well as the subjective sense of control over the thoughts, contribute to the level of risk. The presence of plans, as well as their lethality, availability, or specificity increase the level of risk. Also, specific preparatory behaviors, such as acquiring means or giving away prized possessions, suggest increased risk. There appears to be a continuum of increased risk from thoughts, plans, and preparation to attempts. However, during assessments, individuals may deny thoughts and acknowledge plans or preparation. Thus, each of these must be inquired about.

SEXUAL ORIENTATION.   Recent epidemiological studies found a significant two- to sixfold increased risk for suicide attempts, but not completions, for homosexual and bisexual youths. The association between same-sex sexual orientation and suicide behavior appear to be substantially mediated by depression, alcohol abuse, family history of attempts, and victimization.

Resilience or Protective Factors

Even more so than risk factors, a common set of protective factors moderates the risk for many youth problem behaviors. Moreover, protective factors appear to be more powerful predictors of outcomes with youth than risk factors (Jessor et al., 1995). Many protective factors at all ecological levels are the converse of risk factors. Thus, at the individual level, positive outlook or hopefulness and the related sense of self-efficacy and internal locus of control can attenuate the risk for suicide. Likewise, effective problem-solving, characterized as proactive and flexible as to alternatives, is a protective factor.

Family Factors

Risk Factors

SUICIDE.   A family history of suicidal behavior greatly increases the risk for suicide attempts and completions. While suicide and psychopathology almost always co-occur, suicide in families appears to confer risk independent of pathology. Learning or imitation of poor problem-solving may play a role, but adoption and twin studies indicate heritability plays a role independent of learning.

PSYCHOPATHOLOGY.   High rates of parental psychopathology, particularly substance abuse and depression, have been found to be associated with ideation, attempts, and completed suicide in adolescents.

FAMILY DISCORD AND PARENT–CHILD RELATIONSHIPS. Discord among family members, including between parents, appears to be more prevalent in families of suicide victims. Related to discord, witnessing violence contributes to the risk of suicide. Impaired parent–child relationships are associated with increased risk of suicide. However, this may not be independent of the impact of youths' psychological problems on these relationships. More research is needed to disentangle these variables.

CHILDHOOD TRAUMA. Physical and sexual abuse are both associated with suicide in adolescents. Sexual abuse appears to impact boys more than girls; and the relationship between childhood trauma and suicide is stronger when the trauma has been of long duration, the perpetrator is known to the victim, and force and penetration have taken place. The effects of trauma are cumulative, as the risk for suicide increases with additional trauma. Longitudinal studies depict a pathway from trauma to suicide such that childhood trauma induces a range of effects that, over time, coalesce into mental disorders and suicidal ideation and attempts by adolescence and young adulthood.

Protective Factors

Cohesive families and adolescents' sense of connection to family and parents are associated with less risk for suicide in white and minority youth (Castle, Duberstein, Nelson & Conwell, 2002).

Social and Community Factors

Risk Factors

COMMON RISK FACTORS. Several community risk factors have demonstrated relationships with multiple problem outcomes in youth such as substance abuse, problem pregnancy, delinquency, and interpersonal violence (Durlak, 1998). Their relationship to suicide has not been investigated. However, given that other problem behaviors often co-occur with suicide, it is likely that these characteristics contribute to suicide risk in vulnerable populations characterized by other suicide risk factors. These common risk factors include resource-poor communities and ineffective schools, which are characterized by low expectations and poor relationships among administration, faculty, and students. The relationship between resource-poor communities and suicide may be one of the reasons (along with greater prevalence of firearms and isolation) for the higher suicide rates of rural versus urban communities. Also, there is evidence that low school involvement is associated with suicidal ideation (Dubow et al., 1989) and that improving opportunities for bonding and participation in schools may attenuate suicidal behavior (McBride et al., 1995; Thompson, Eggert, Randell & Pike, 2001).

INACCESSIBLE SERVICES. Services for youth have been described as fragmented and inaccessible. Studies of barriers to adolescent help-seeking reveal that adolescents consider psychological services in schools and communities to be psychologically (because of a perceived stigma associated with psychotherapy), culturally (not responsive to or knowledgeable about adolescent culture and concerns), financially, or geographically inaccessible to them (Lindsey & Kalafat, 1998). This is supported by adolescents' low compliance and high drop-out from psychotherapy (Piacentini et al., 1995; Trautman, Steart & Morishima, 1993).

ACCESS TO FIREARMS.   Firearms are the most common method of committing suicide in the United States, among youth of both genders. Over half of the almost 2,000 youth under 19 who died by suicide in 2000 used firearms (NCIPC, 2003). The dramatic increase in youth suicide since 1960, including the recent increase in the black male suicide rate, is primarily attributable to increase in the use of firearms. The presence of firearms in the home is a significant risk factor for suicide in youths (Brent & Bridge, 2003), and there is strong evidence that firearms used for both suicides and unintentional injuries by adolescents are disproportionately obtained from the home environment (Shah, Hoffman, Wake & Marine, 2000). Of note, youth who use firearms for suicide reportedly have fewer identifiable risk factors, such as expressing suicidal thoughts, suicidal intent, psychopathology, and substance abuse, compared to those using other means; and firearms suicides appear to be more impulsive and spontaneous (Miller, Azrael & Hemenway, 2001). Thus, to at least some extent, means availability appears to function as a contributing factor to youth suicide, independent of other factors.

However, this area also illustrates another community level risk factor: ineffective social policies. In 1996, the House of Representatives slashed $2.6 million from the National Center for Injury Control and Prevention, the branch of the CDC that had planned to use the funds for research on firearm-related injuries. Republican lawmakers accused the injury center of promoting research that advocates gun control (Walker, 1996).

Contagion/Imitation

There is considerable evidence for increases in youth suicidal behavior after media coverage of suicides that includes graphic descriptions and pictorial coverage. The magnitude of the suicide increase is proportional to the amount, duration, and prominence of media coverage (Gould, 2001). This has prompted the development of guidelines for responsible media coverage (American Foundation for Suicide Prevention, 2001). However, with the exception of a program in Austria (Sonneck et al., 1994), there is little evidence that media guidelines have a direct effect on suicide rates (Goldsmith et al., 2002). Moreover, recent events in local school districts indicate that news of youth suicides is now being rapidly and widely spread among adolescents through instant messaging on the internet. These messages often include unfounded speculation about the reasons for and circumstances of the death.

In addition to media exposure, imitative suicidal behavior among adolescents can follow exposure to suicide among peers (Brent et al., 1992). Brent's research indicates that the effects are greater for those who were less acquainted with the suicidal adolescent. This may be because they were not exposed to the severe impact of the loss, and this raises concerns about the possible impact of exposure through instant messaging. Even more menacing, there are websites that youth can access that depict suicide, provide instructions for suicide, and offer opportunities for group suicide.

STRESSFUL EVENTS.   Life stressors, including interpersonal losses, legal or disciplinary problems, setbacks such as rejection from the military or college choice, and school drop-out are associated with suicide attempts and completions in vulnerable youth (Gould et al, 2003; Kalafat, 1997).

Protective Factors

Two major community level factors attenuate the risk for suicide among adolescents and young adults. These are contact with a caring adult and bonding or connection with school and/or community, which is mediated by opportunities to participate and contribute (Evans et al., 1996; McBride et al., 1995; Castle, Duberstein, Nelson & Conwell, 2002).

Evidence-Based Treatment Interventions in Community Settings

What Works

At the present time, interventions that meet the required standard could not be identified.

What Might Work

The field of evidence-based treatment interventions for suicidal adolescents consists of a small amount of good news and a preponderance of bad news. The good news primarily involves research on psychotherapy for children and adolescents. In his comprehensive review, Kazdin (2003) reported that there is firm evidence that therapy for children and adolescents is effective, and that the magnitude of this effect, when treatment is compared to no treatment, is rather large (effect sizes $\cong$ 0.70). In addition, he describes effective evidence-based treatments for anxiety, depression, and conduct disorders. However, it has not been established why treatment works, for whom, or what the key conditions that optimize change are. Moreover, the research establishes the efficacy, not effectiveness, of these treatments. That is, treatment in practice departs in many respects from treatment in research studies. This will be explicated below through a description of the current context for therapy with adolescents.

There is considerably less research on treatment of suicidal individuals, as several reviews have identified fewer than two dozen studies that approach sound research criteria for randomness or control (Berman et al., in press; Rudd, Joiner, Jobes & King, 1999; Links, Bergmans & Cooks, 2003; Zemetkin, Alter & Yemini, 2001). Most of these studies exclude patients at high risk for suicide, and only a handful of studies specifically address adolescents. Thus, as Berman et al. (in press) point out, clinicians who are treating suicidal patients in ongoing therapy are often forced to rely on literature that is principally case-based and largely anecdotal.

Due to the paucity of research in this area, studies involving adults will be reviewed and their potential applicability to adolescents will be considered. Following this, treatment research on suicidal adolescents will be reviewed.

In a review focusing on randomized controlled studies in which outcome was suicidal behavior and interventions were targeted to adults at risk, Links et al. (2003)

reported the following promising results. Problem-solving interventions improve problem-solving skills, depression, and loneliness, but may not prevent repeated suicidal behavior. Interventions can effectively decrease hopelessness, but these may not prevent subsequent suicidal behavior. Dialectical behavior therapy (DBT) (Linehan et al., 1991) appears to reduce suicidal behavior in individuals with borderline personality disorders, but this is a complex approach that requires considerable training and needs dismantling studies to identify its active ingredients. A multifaceted approach that is organized around partial hospitalization has reduced suicidal behavior and subsequent hospitalization of borderline personality disordered patients (Bateman & Fonagy, 1999). Again, this approach has several components that requires dismantling studies. In a well-designed study involving regression analyses, Joiner et al. (2001) found that higher positive emotions such as joy, interest, and contentment mediated gains in problem-solving attitudes, which in turn led to fewer suicidal symptoms in young adults. Rudd et al. (1999) identified six controlled studies that provided evidence that time-limited cognitive therapy that includes a core of problem-solving skills development yields reductions in ideation and related symptoms such as depression, hopelessness, and loneliness. They suggested that longer-term treatment may be necessary to reduce attempts. Two controlled studies found that adjuncts to therapy reduced subsequent attempts. Van Heeringen et al. (1995) found that home visits by community nurses increased compliance with treatment and subsequent attempts by moderately suicidal outpatients. Morgan, Jones & Owen (1993) found that increasing ease of access to 24-hour emergency services for one year following a suicide attempt significantly reduced subsequent suicide attempts in the experimental group relative to those receiving management as usual. Improved ease of access was accomplished by providing a green card with emergency numbers and encouraging the use of emergency room or telephone services in crises. Interestingly, service demand was also significantly reduced in this group. Finally, reports by Linehan et al. (1991) on DBT with borderline personality disorder and cognitive-behavior therapy with young adults by Rudd et al. (1996) indicate that outpatient treatment of high-risk patients is safe and can be effective for reducing suicidality when acute hospitalization is also available.

In sum, the limited available evidence indicates that cognitive-behavior therapy and DBT show promise for treating suicidal patients. The specific change mechanisms of these approaches have not been identified. Additional interventions to increase compliance and access to emergency services may help to reduce subsequent attempts. Reasonable, conceptually grounded treatment models have been developed that incorporate rapport building strategies, appropriate crisis intervention, cognitive and problem-solving skills development, and appropriate risk management practices (Rudd, Joiner & Rajab, 2001; Bongar, 2002).

The applicability of these approaches and findings to adolescents remains an open question. Rathus and Miller (2002) compared an adolescent adaptation of CBT to treatment as usual for suicidal adolescents with borderline personality features. They found that patients receiving DBT showed reductions in suicidal ideation, general psychiatric symptoms, and borderline personality symptomatology. Brent and Poling (1997) developed a CBT approach for adolescents that emphasized guided discovery to monitor cognitive distortions, encouraged more assertive and direct communication, and increased teens' ability to conceptualize alternate solutions to problems. The intervention was reported to be as effective as family therapy and nondirective supportive therapy in reducing suicidal ideation in depressed adolescents.

In general, reviews of the literature on treatment of suicidal adolescents have agreed with Rudd & Joiner (1998), who stated, "The gap in the existing treatment outcome literature addressing adolescent suicidal behavior is considerable" (p. 496). For example, in their review, Zemetkin, Alter & Yemini (2001) reported that no treatment approach has reduced subsequent suicide attempts and no controlled studies have demonstrated that treatment of conduct disorders or substance abuse decreases the number of future suicide attempts. In addition, several features of adolescent development, contexts, and attitudes complicate the treatment of adolescents.

First, adolescents are beginning to assert their independence from adult support and are reluctant to seek help from adults rather than their peers (Lindsey & Kalafat, 1998). In part due to their increasing involvement with peers, they are concerned about the stigma of using mental health services. Most adolescents come to therapy at the behest of some adult, and the majority do not comply with referrals or remain in treatment. Second, in spite of their movement toward independence, adolescents are still substantially affected by their family context and families of at risk youth may also exhibit pathology, concern about the stigma of suicide, and/or a reluctance to comply with treatment recommendations for their offspring (Berman et al., in press). Third, practitioners today are confronted with the dilemma of how to provide effective psychotherapeutic services for high-risk patients within the constraints of managed care and escalating liabilities (Rudd et al., 1999). Managed care has limited the length of outpatient and inpatient treatment, and, along with the pharmaceutical industry, has promoted an exponential use of psychotropic medication over psychotherapy or psychosocial interventions. Evidence-based research in the provision of mental health care has consistently shown that a combination of psychotherapy and medication is more effective than either approach by itself (Berman et al., in press). Given the sometimes dysfunctional family dynamics of suicidal adolescents and the protective impact of a caring adult, it has been argued that a positive outpatient alliance may be an important component of treatment for suicidal youth (Berman et al., in press).

The fragmentation and inaccessibility of community-based services for youth has led to a substantial movement to provide mental health services in schools (Adelman & Taylor, 1999). These services are often combined with health services and their staff are familiar with and to the students, thus reducing their stigma (Nabors & Reynolds, 2000). In fact, schools may be the "de facto mental health system for children and adolescents" (Burns et al., 1995, p. 147). There is evidence for the effectiveness of school-based mental health services in treating youth's mental health concerns (Dryfoos, Brindis & Kaplan, 1996; Hoagwood & Erwin, 1997; Nabors & Reynolds, 2000). While there is no published research on the treatment of suicidal youth in school-based mental health services, well-controlled studies of an indicated school-based program for suicidal youth has demonstrated reductions in suicidal ideation and favorable attitudes toward suicide (Thompson, Eggert, Randell & Pike, 2001). This program involves classes for identified suicidal youth that include social and communication skills training, peer support, and school bonding activities. Interestingly, a comparison group that was provided brief contact with a school-based consultant who provided support, referral, and involvement of parents also evidenced reductions in suicide ideation over a shorter follow-up period. Another program that consisted of classes addressing youth's depression, hopelessness, and suicidal urges, as well as coping and alternative solutions, found significant reductions in suicidal feelings for class participants as compared to controls (Orbach & Bar-Joseph, 1993).

Finally, while evidence-based data on family therapy of suicidal adolescents is lacking, the established role of the family in the etiology of and protection against youth suicide dictates that family involvement be included in the standards for treatment of suicidal adolescents (Berman et al., in press; Wagner, Silverman & Martin, 2003).

In sum, research on community-based treatment for suicidal adolescents remains in its infancy. Promising cognitive and DBT approaches, as well as reasonable treatment models (Berman et al., in press), are available. School-based mental health services are spreading, though they are not firmly established; and communities have increased the accessibility of services for youth. Indicated suicide programs show promise for addressing at-risk youth. These indicated school-based suicide programs are best complemented by universal school programs, to be described below, and coordinated community emergency and mental health services.

What Does Not Work

Not enough is known at the present time to identify ineffective practices.

Evidence-Based Treatment Interventions in Residential Settings

What Works

At the present time, interventions that meet the required standard could not be identified.

What Might Work

There is no evidence-based data that hospitalization prevents immediate or eventual suicide (Zemetkin et al., 2001). However, this may be because hospitalization is best thought of as an adjunct to school or community outpatient treatment rather than as an independent treatment modality. The effectiveness of hospitalization for stabilizing acutely suicidal youth may be attenuated by briefer stays mandated by managed care (Berman et al., in press) and lack of coordination with families and school systems during admission and discharge (Kalafat & Mackey, 1994).

What Does Not Work

Not enough is known at the present time to identify ineffective practices.

Psychopharmacology

What Works

At the present time, interventions that meet the required standard could not be identified.

What Might Work

Drug treatment can play a role in the therapy of suicidal adolescents. While there is no drug that has demonstrated direct effects on suicide, medication may be helpful in cases where a diagnostic condition and related symptoms associated with suicide can be targeted with certain medicines. It should be noted, however, that only a few well-controlled drug studies with adolescent subjects have appeared to date in the literature, without much support for effectiveness. One possible reason for this outcome is that adolescents tend to respond well to placebo treatment, thereby masking differences between drug and placebo treatments. Also, many studies exclude patients who are at high risk for suicide and most clinical drug trials exclude children and adolescents. This does not necessarily mean that pharmacological treatment is useless. The current standard of care in the treatment of the suicidal condition calls for consideration of possible beneficial effects of medication (Berman et al., in press). Major psychiatric disorders associated with suicide in adolescents include depression, bipolar disorder, and anxiety disorders.

MEDICATIONS FOR DEPRESSIVE DISORDERS.   Antidepressants have been shown to be clearly effective for the treatment of major depressive disorders. There are well over 20 antidepressants on the market, only a few of which are selective serotonin reuptake inhibitors (SSRIs). Hence, global statements about causal mechanisms cannot be made, because rigorous studies have not been undertaken. Furthermore, there is a controversy as to whether certain classes of antidepressants can be associated with the worsening, or even the emergence, of suicidal ideation or behavior in the early weeks of treatment (Mann & Kapur, 1991; Montgomery et al., 1995). In July 2003, both the FDA and its British equivalent, the Medicines and Healthcare Products Regulatory Authority (MHRA) published warnings about the use of paroxetine for those patients in the under-18 age group, because of a possible increased risk of suicidal impulses. New data from various clinical trials showed episodes of self-harm and potentially suicidal behavior were between 1.5 and 3.2 times higher in patients younger than 18 taking the medication vs. those receiving a placebo. As with many other drugs in this class, paroxetine does not have a license for use in the under-18 age group, but physicians have widely prescribed it (and other psychopharmaceuticals) for this age group. SSRIs are the preferred psychpharmacological treatment for adolescent depression, with caution that suicidal youth on SSRIs must be watched for any increase in agitation or suicidality, especially in the early phase of treatment (Montgomery, 1997). In general, when medications are prescribed, careful monitoring of their administration to a suicidal adolescent is essential. Dosage levels must be carefully considered and caution with regard to hoarding of pills and access to medications in general by suicidal adolescents is required. While medications may be essential in stabilizing and treating the suicidal child and adolescent, all administration must be carefully monitored by a trustworthy third party who can report any unexpected change of mood, increase in agitation or emergency state, or unwanted side effects, and who can regulate dosage (Shaffer & Pfeffer, 2001). The majority of time a non-physician clinician/therapist will be working with a general practitioner or pediatrician in the treatment of youths with psychotropic medications. Open lines of communication must be maintained among these providers and the adolescent's caretakers.

In sum there are reasons to believe that SSRIs might reduce suicidality, including their potential to reduce irritability, affective response to stress, hypersensitivity, depression and anxiety. SSRI's may be effective at reducing suicidal ideation (Berman et al., in press).

BIPOLAR DISORDERS.   Not only has lithium been shown to be effective in the treatment of bipolar disorder and recurrent major depressive disorder, but it also has been shown to significantly reduce suicide attempt rates (Tondo et al., 1997). Other studies suggest that lithium may exert antisuicidal effects independent of its mood-stabilizing properties (Müller-Oerlinghausen et al., 1992; Schou, 1999). Exactly what is the mechanism is unknown, although there is some speculation that the antisuicidal effect goes beyond the action of lithium alone, and relates to the increased contact and monitoring that occurs when patients are prescribed lithium.

ANXIETY DISORDERS.   Patients with primary anxiety disorders (generalized anxiety disorder, panic disorder, phobias, obsessive-compulsive disorder, and post-traumatic stress disorder) have increased risk for suicide, independent of a comorbid depressive disorder. Fawcett has shown that the suicide risk is higher in patients with both anxiety symptoms and affective disorders, compared to patients who only suffer from affective disorders without anxiety. Fawcett et al. (1997) have concluded that prompt and adequate treatment of severe anxiety with anxiolytics and/or sedating antidepressants will lower agitation, impulsivity and the acute risk of suicide. Nevertheless, clinicians should be cautious about prescribing medications that may reduce self-control, such as the benzodiazepines. Montgomery (1997) noted that benzodiazepines may disinhibit some individuals who then exhibit aggression and suicide attempts.

Fawcett (2001) has postulated that SSRI's stimulate serotonin-2 receptors, resulting in a worsening of a patient's perception of anxiety during the first few weeks of treatment. The combination of increased anxiety and simultaneous relaxation of psychomotor inhibition elevates the risk of self-destructive acts such as suicide attempts and suicide. Fawcett argues for a need for extra vigilance on the part of physicians, therapists, and family members during the first weeks of treatment for depression with marked anxiety.

What Does Not Work

Not enough is known at the present time to identify ineffective practices.

The Prevention of Youth Suicidal Behavior

What Works

While there are many promising approaches to the prevention of adolescent suicide, at the present time no approach has been tested three times successfully.

What Might Work

The primary approach to youth suicide prevention is school-based prevention programs. Prevention has been attempted to a lesser degree through gatekeeper training and means (firearms) restriction.

GATEKEEPER TRAINING.   The primary assumption underlying training programs for gatekeepers is that the key people who come into contact with youth at risk for suicide—teachers, counselors, physicians, mental health workers, parents, and community leaders—frequently lack the knowledge and skills necessary to identify such youth and respond to them effectively. These programs generally aim to increase suicide awareness and intervention skills among one or more caregiver groups.

Several gatekeeper training programs have reportedly been successful in improving participants' knowledge and awareness of youth suicide, and increasing their intentions to make appropriate intervention. For example, QPR Gatekeeper Training (Quinnett, 1995) was provided as part of the Washington State Youth suicide Prevention Program. A pre-post evaluation of the program found significant increases in participants' knowledge about suicide and willingness to act (get help) on behalf of a suicidal individual (Hazel & McDonell, 2002). Other disseminated programs include LivingWorks (Turley & Tanney, 1998) and Suicide Options, Awareness, and Relief (SOAR) (King & Smith, 2000). Most such programs are relatively brief, however, and have not included long-term follow-up of participants to determine actual behavioral changes. Although evaluations of the LivingWorks and QPR program suggest that gatekeepers who receive the training report using the skills learned, and that the training has resulted in an increase in referrals to treatment, there are currently no data on the impact of training programs on suicidal behavior among youth.

MEANS RESTRICTION.   The key assumption underlying programs that encourage restriction of access to firearms is that accessibility is a primary risk factor for suicide. Programs of this type have been directed primarily to parents. A core strategy of firearms restriction programs has involved firearm safety counseling to parents that encourages removal or safe storage of firearms from homes where children reside. One such effort, entitled Love our Kids: Lock your Guns, was developed by Coyne-Beasley, Schoenbach and Johnson (2001). The intervention aimed essentially to reach male gun owners who lived with children, and thus was implemented in an outdoor community setting. Program developers provided firearm safety counseling, distributed free gunlocks and demonstrated their use on a community-wide basis. A six-month follow-up evaluation found improved safe storage habits among gun owners who had participated in the program. Participants with children, who overall were more likely than other gun owners to store weapons unlocked and loaded at baseline, were found in the post-test to be more likely to have removed guns from the home and to lock the guns that remained. Those who had participated in the counseling were also more likely to report talking with friends about safe storage practices.

The policy statement on firearm safety of the American Academy of Pediatrics (AAP, 2000) has urged parents to remove guns from the environment where children live and visit, and if guns remain in the home, to store them unloaded and locked, with ammunition stored separately. One attempt to apply this policy in an intervention program is the Steps to Prevent Firearms Injury Program (STOP) of the American Academy of Pediatrics and the Center to Prevent Handgun Violence, which provides a counseling intervention to parents in primary care clinics. Evaluations have not found the program to be effective in reducing firearm safety and removal (Oatis et al., 1999; Grossman et al., 2000), possibly because it has primarily reached mothers, while fathers and other males in the household are more responsible for the presence and storage practices of the guns in the home.

Community-based programs targeting males within households in which children and youth live appear to hold the highest potential for effective firearms restriction education. Although the program developed by Coyne-Beasley and her colleagues represents an important step in this direction, more widespread implementation and evaluation is needed before definitive findings of impact can be reached.

School Programs

In North America there are published reports of a variety of universal programs, no selective programs, and a single indicated program addressing suicide prevention.

UNIVERSAL PROGRAMS.   The overall goal of universal programs is to create competent (Iscoe, 1974) school communities in which all members accept responsibility for the safety of each other and can provide an appropriate initial response to those at risk. The specific conceptual and empirical base for such programs is that suicidal youth are more likely to tell a peer about their thoughts or plans and the majority of these peer confidents do not tell an adult about their troubled peer. In addition school-based adults are usually the last choice for youth to turn to for their concerns (Kalafat, 2003). Therefore, current comprehensive universal school based suicide prevention programs are designed to increase the likelihood that school gatekeepers (administrators, faculty, and staff) and peers who come into contact with at-risk youth can more readily identify them, provide an appropriate initial response to them, will know how to obtain help for them, and are consistently inclined to take such action. The role of schools in this endeavor is critical, but limited to the identification and referral to specialized school or community-based mental health services.

In order to meet these goals, model comprehensive universal suicide prevention programs include the following components, usually implemented in this order: (a) administrative consult to ensure appropriate policies and procedures for responding to suicidal youth and to ensure linkages between the school and local community services; (b) training for all faculty and staff on school procedures and resources, warning signs, and appropriate initial responses to at-risk students; (c) parent training, which covers the same material as school personnel training, with the addition of guidelines for means restriction and monitoring their offspring's internet use; (d) classroom lessons for students, usually as part of a health curriculum, that provide the knowledge, attitudes and skills for responding to at risk peers and obtaining adult help. Programs can also include the development of school-and community-based crisis teams, as well as training for community gatekeepers.

Comprehensive universal prevention programs fit within the school's resources and culture because they have an educational rather than clinical focus; the classroom curriculum consists of packaged, self-contained lesson plans designed to be provided by teachers rather than external consultants; and, they fit within the existing curriculum structure without requiring pull-out activities. The student curriculum also uses appropriate instructional principles such as participatory activities, skills practice and feedback, and reinforcement and acknowledgement of students' experience (in this case, dealing with troubled peers).

Examples of programs that include these components are Adolescent Suicide Awareness Program (ASAP; now called SafeTeen) (Ryerson, 1990) and Lifelines (Kalafat & Underwood, 1989), each of which has been evaluated and widely disseminated. Similar comprehensive programs have also been developed in Florida (Zenere & Lazarus, 1997) and Washington (Eastgard, 2000). The Washington program features substantial involvement of students in the development of local peer support/involvement messages and the provision of classroom lessons, which may represent a mediational process superior to the predominant teacher-to-student process.

Evaluations of universal suicide prevention classes have found significant increases in suicide knowledge and intent to seek help on behalf of troubled peers (Kalafat, 2003). A meta-analysis of 13 school-based suicide prevention programs found moderate average effect sizes of suicide knowledge, and ideation, and small positive effect size for attitudes for seven programs (Konick, Brandt, & Gutierrez, 2002).

It must be noted that changes in knowledge and attitudes do not necessarily translate into behavior. Research needs to be done that provides evidence for the relationship between these proximal outcomes and such intermediate behavioral outcomes as increased identification and referral of at risk youth by school based adults and students. Recently, a school-based program, the *SOS Suicide Prevention Program,* was developed that combines brief classroom lessons to raise awareness about depression and suicide and promote help seeking with screening for depression and other risk factors associated with suicide. Initial evaluations indicate that the program is well received by students and staff, is not perceived as burdensome by staff, and resulted in 60% increases in help seeking among students who participated in the program (Aseltine, 2003). An outcome evaluation in which 2,100 students from five schools were randomly assigned to intervention and control conditions found significantly lower self-reported attempts among he intervention group three months after the program was implemented (Aseltine & DeMartino, 2004). No differences between groups were found for help-seeking. Small but significant differences favoring the intervention group were found for knowledge and adaptive attitudes about depression and suicide, and these changes were significantly associated with the reported reduction in suicide attempts.

Programs that focus on the identification and referral of at-risk youth must be complemented by effective treatment and follow up of identified youth (Kalafat, 2001). As noted earlier, there is a dearth of research in this area. Moreover, in order to assess distal program effects (reduction of suicide rates) programs must be (a) carefully implemented with fidelity; (b) address multiple levels of school and community contexts (i.e., administrative policies & procedures; education for all school staff; classroom curricula; parent education; connections between school & community gatekeepers); (c) disseminated to enough sites to obtain large population samples for epidemiological impact assessment; and (d) institutionalized or sustained over sufficient length of time to detect epidemiological trends.

Data are available from two programs that meet these criteria. The programs were developed and implemented by a county (New Jersey) community mental health center (Kalafat & Ryerson, 1999) and a county (Florida) public school Department of Crisis Management (Zenere & Lazarus, 1997). Each was systematically disseminated and had been sustained for ten (Kalafat & Ryerson, 1999) and six (Zenere & Lazarus, 1997) years at the time of the reports in all secondary schools in urban/suburban counties that had an average of approximately 130,000 school-age youth. Each aimed to prepare schools and communities to identify, respond to, and obtain help for at risk youth, as well as other health topics such as coping and self efficacy. The Florida program included additional health promotion programming for elementary and middle schools.

Follow up studies were done, comparing suicide rates in the New Jersey and Florida counties with state and national suicide rates for the time periods prior to and after program implementation. Both follow-up studies found a reduction in county youth suicide rates subsequent to the dissemination of the programs that did not occur in these states or nationally for the same time periods (Kalafat, 2000). While these data cannot be conclusively linked to the programs, taken together, they meet some of the epidemiological criteria for supporting the possibility of causal relationships. These include consistency of findings across studies, temporal sequence of exposure and outcome, and logical plausibility of the relationship (Potter, Powell, and Kachur, 1995); and, they provide encouraging initial support for comprehensive, community-oriented prevention approaches.

INDICATED PROGRAMS.   Eggert and her colleagues developed a conceptually grounded selective prevention program called *Reconnecting Youth* (Eggert, Thompson, Herting & Nicholas, 1995). Reconnecting Youth is a school-based prevention program for youth in grades nine through twelve (14–18 years old) who are at risk for school drop-out. Reconnecting Youth uses a partnership model involving peers, school personnel, and parents to deliver interventions that are organized into four components, including school bonding activities, parent involvement, school crisis response planning, and a Reconnecting Youth (RY) class offered for 50 minutes daily during regular school hours for one semester (80 sessions).

Subsequently, Eggert and her colleagues implemented and evaluated briefer versions of the RY class with potential drop out students who were identified as at risk for suicide through a subsequent screening. These interventions consisted of three conditions. One involved a structured assessment interview, a brief counseling protocol, and a referral to a school-based case manager and a parent or guardian (C-CARE). A second consisted of all of the above, plus a 12-session small group coping skills and securing support training program (CAST). The third condition was the standard school response to at-risk students, consisting of a brief assessment and referral to school and parental resources (control). Follow-up evaluations at four and ten weeks revealed reduction in suicidal ideation and less favorable attitudes toward suicide for all three groups. Most change occurred in the C-CARE and control conditions, while the CAST condition provided no additional benefits. These results indicate that a brief indicated intervention consisting of a risk assessment, crisis intervention, and enhanced connection with caring adults was sufficient for affecting short-term attitudes and ideation. A subsequent study involving a nine-month follow up of the same three conditions indicated that these suicidal attitudes and ideations declined faster and were more changed at the longer follow up period for the C-CARE and CAST conditions, as compared to the control condition (Thompson, Eggert, Randell & Pike (2001). This result, coupled with the findings of universal programs that promote identification of, and obtaining help for at risk youth, is encouraging in that schools may be able to effectively intervene with identified suicidal students with a relatively brief, focused intervention.

SCREENING PROGRAMS.   Universal screening programs are designed to identify and refer to treatment students at risk for suicidal behavior. Such programs focus specifically on identifying symptoms of psychopathology known to be related to adolescent suicidal behavior. Perhaps the most widely used screening program, the *Columbia TeenScreen Program* (CTSP), employs a multi-stage procedure. In the first stage, students complete a brief, self-report questionnaire. Those who screen positive on this measure are given a self-administered computerized instrument, the *Voice Diagnostic Interview for Children* (Voice DISC). In the next stage, youth who have been identified through Voice DISC as meeting specific diagnostic criteria for a psychiatric disorder are by a clinician, who determines whether the student needs to be referred for treatment or further evaluation. Ideally, the program also includes a case manager who contacts the parents of students who are referred and establishes links with a clinic to facilitate treatment compliance.

Columbia TeenScreen has been found to have good sensitivity and specificity (Shaffer, Fisher, Lucas, Dulcan & Schwab-Stone, 2000). The second stage of the screen that involves the Voice DISC is regarded as particularly important for avoiding over-assessment of students at reduced risk. Evaluation results reported to date indicate that most of the adolescents identified as high risk for suicide through the program were not previously recognized as such, and very few had received prior treatment. Slightly less than one-quarter of the students referred for treatment actually attended more than one treatment visit, however (Shaffer, 2003). In addition, the program's requirements of a clinician and a case manager may be a resource burden for many schools. In fact, school personnel have been less favorable toward screening programs than other school-based suicide prevention programs (Eckert et al., 2003; Hayden & Lauer, 2000). In addition to the low compliance rate with treatment referrals, which is likely a problem associated with all school-based programs, the often transient or episodic nature of suicidality among adolescents makes screening this population even more difficult. In most instances where school-based screening programs have been implemented, students are assessed at most only once a year, and in some cases, only once during their high school career.

In sum, school-based prevention programs that share the goal of promoting student awareness and help-seeking appear to be well received and sustainable, which are critical for effective prevention initiatives. Controlled studies have demonstrated knowledge gains, improved attitudes toward help seeking, increases in intent to seek help in analog situations, increases in actual help-seeking, and decreases in self-reported suicide attempts among program participants. Decreases in county youth suicide rates following county-wide implementation of programs have also been found. These universal programs are complemented by promising findings from controlled evaluations of indicated school programs for identified suicidal youth. All of these programs have a variety of components and findings are scattered among several similar programs. Large-scale dismantling studies are needed to identify the critical mediators or components of these programs associated with reductions in suicidal behavior. At present, universal school-based suicide prevention programs can be considered promising. Well-controlled evaluations with long-term follow-up provide strong support for indicated programs. Community gatekeeper programs and means restriction efforts are conceptually sound, but more controlled evaluations of gatekeeper programs are needed, and innovative strategies for implementing effective means restriction initiatives must be developed.

What Does Not Work

Based on research and field experience with school-based prevention programs aimed at a variety of problem behaviors, we also know what approaches do not work. One-time programs, such as assembly presentations, do not provide sufficient program dosage. Moreover, assembly presentations do not allow monitoring of students' reactions to the material. Programs should not include media depictions of suicidal behavior or presentations by youth who have made suicide attempts, as these might have modeling effects for vulnerable youth. Outsourcing programs rather than developing in-school expertise fails to enhance available local resources. Poorly implemented programs, regardless of content or intent, will not have positive effects. Also, there is no basis for promoting a single approach, such as indicated approaches or annual screenings, rather than emphasizing the complementary role of different empirically and conceptually grounded ones.

Recommendations

Suicide is not a medical condition that can be isolated and treated through traditional public health preventive "inoculations" or categorical clinical treatments. Rather, suicide is a multiply determined decision that arises out of complex biopsychosocial conditions. Initiating and evaluating interventions such as prevention and treatment in various contexts separately is not likely to affect youth suicide rates. Instead suicide, as with other youth dysfunctional behaviors, must be addressed through community or systemic efforts that combine complementary approaches in a coordinated continuum or system of care. Each of the approaches or programs reviewed in this chapter can be seen as components of an effective system. These approaches must take into account characteristics of systems: e.g., (a) systems take time to develop and require constant maintenance, (b) context is critical, and (c) everything in a system is connected and therefore a system is only as strong as its weakest component (Sanddal et al., 2003). For example, schools and communities may support a broad positive youth development program that focuses on resilience. There is longitudinal evidence that programs that promote generic protective factors such as social competence, decision-making, family connections, and school bonding moderate the appearance of a variety of risk behaviors, including substance abuse, delinquency, violent behavior, and problem sexual behavior and pregnancies (Hawkins et al., 1999; Lonczak et al., 2002). While these comprehensive programs have not included suicide in their outcome assessments, there is some evidence for an association between protective factors such as connection with school and prosocial norms and reduced suicidal thoughts and plans (Castle et al., 2002; Evans et al., 1996; McBride et al., 1995).

However, such programs alone will not be sufficient to prevent the emergence of suicidal behavior. They must be complemented by a comprehensive school-based suicide prevention program that prepares adults and students to respond to youths at risk for inter- and intrapersonal violence, as research indicates that both of these types of at-risk students often communicate their intent to others. If the program's lessons are to be *applied*, they must reside in a school climate that emphasizes competence, mutual support, and contributions of its members. In addition, the program must comply with the culture of the school and community as well as the school's primary education and protection mandates; and it must be implemented with a degree of fidelity and packaged in a way that promotes sustainability. However, even if a program proves to be effective in identifying youth at risk, it cannot succeed if effective school or community-based services are not available and accessible to students. These services can be group classes such as Orbach and Bar-Joseph's (1993) or those that have evolved from Reconnecting Youth (Thompson et al., 2001). Or, they may be evidence-based individual or family therapies. Moreover, if a student receives outpatient or inpatient services, there must be coordination between the mental health service sector, the family, and the school for the reintegration of the student to the community and school.

There is a model for such a comprehensive systemic approach to suicide prevention. The United States Air Force (USAF) specifically eschewed a strictly medical model in favor of a community approach under the rubric of the *competent community*. This initiative included a wide variety of components, including destigmatization of help-seeking, fostering mutual support, training for providers, screening, and service coordination. The program has resulted in a 33% reducion of suicide rates among USAF personnel, as well as reductions in homicide, accidental deaths, and moderate and severe family violence (Knox et al., 2003). It has been recognized as a model effective prevention program. Several states, including Maine, Maryland, and Washington have launched statewide multicomponent youth suicide prevention programs that are currently being evaluated.

Because of the interdependency of the components of these programs, they present challenges for evaluators. It will be necessary to carry out large-scale staged evaluations that first establish the efficacy or internal validity of each component, followed by evaluation using path analyses and structural equation modeling to assess the contributions of components to the reduction of suicidal behaviors.

Clearly, the evaluation of suicide treatment and prevention is still in its infancy. However, recent developments, such as the development of state plans (Hayden, 2003), the publication of The National Strategy for Suicide Prevention (2001), and the establishment of the Suicide Prevention Resource Center (SPRC, 2002), hold promise for concerted efforts to address this public health problem.

References

Adelman, H.S., & Taylor, L. (1999). Mental health in schools and system restructuring. *Clinical Psychology Review, 19,* 137–163.

American Academy of Pediatrics (2000). Firearm-related injuries affecting the pediatric population. *Pediatrics, 105,* 888–895.

American Foundation for Suicide Prevention (2001). *Reporting a Suicide: Recommendations for the Media.* Retrieved December 20, 2003, from *www.afsp.org.*

Aseltine, R.H. (2003). An evaluation of a school based suicide prevention program. *Adolescent & Family Health, 3*, 81–88.

Aseltine, R.H., & DeMartino, R. (2004). An outcome evaluation of the SOS suicide prevention program. *American Journal of Public Health, 94*, 446–452.

Bateman, A.W., & Fonagy, P. (1999). Effectiveness of partial hospitalization in the treatment of borderline personality disorder: A randomized controlled trial. *American Journal of Psychiatry, 156*, 1563–1569.

Berman, A.L., Jobes, D.A., & Silverman, M.M. (in press). *Adolescent Suicide: Assessment and Treatment.* Washington, DC: American Psychological Association.

Biglan, A., Mrazek, P.J., Carnine, D., & Flay, B.R. (2003). The integration of research and practice in the prevention of youth problem behaviors. *American Psychologist, 58*, 433–440.

Bongar, B. (2002). *The Suicidal Patient: Clinical and Legal Standards of Care.* Washington, DC: American Psychological Association.

Brent, D.A., & Bridge, J. (2003). Firearms availability and suicide: Evidence, interventions, and future directions. *American Behavioral Scientist, 46*, 1192–1210.

Brent, D.A., Perper, J., Moritz, G., Allman, C., Friend, A., Schweers, J., Roth, C., Balach, L., & Harrington, K. (1992). Psychiatric effects of exposure to suicide among friends and acquaintances of adolescent suicide victims. *Journal of the American Academy of Child & Adolescent Psychiatry, 31*, 629–640.

Brent, D.A., & Poling, D. (1997). *Cognitive Therapy Manual for Depressed and Suicidal Youth.* Pittsburgh: Western Psychiatric Institute and Clinic, University of Pittsburgh Medical Center.

Burns, B.J., Costello, E.J., Angold, A., Tweed, D., Stangle, D., Farmer, E.M.Z., & Erkaneli, A. (1995). Children's mental health service use across service sectors. *Health Affairs, 14*, 147–159.

Carlton, P.A., & Deane, F.P. (2000). Impact of attitudes and suicidal ideation on adolescents' intentions to seek professional psychological help. *Journal of Adolescence, 23*, 35–45.

Castle, K., Duberstein, P., Meldrum, S., Conner, K., & Fiscella, K., & Conwell, Y. (2002a, April). *Risk for black and white suicides.* Poster session presented at the annual conference of the American Association of Suicidology, Bethesda, MD.

Castle, K., Duberstein, P., Nelson, K., & Conwell, Y. (2002b, April). *Teen race differences in social connection, depression, and suicidal ideation.* Poster session presented at the annual conference of the American Association of Suicidology, Bethesda, MD.

Catalano, R.F., Berglund, L., Ryan, J.A.M., Lonczak, H.S., & Hawkins, J.D. (2002). Positive youth development in the United States: Research findings on evaluations of positive youth development programs. *Prevention & Treatment, 5*, Article 15. Retrieved December 10, 2003, from *http://journals.apa.org/prevention/volume5/pre0050015a.html*

Coyne-Beasley, T., Schoenbach, V.J., &. Johnson, R.M. (2001). Love Our Kids, Lock Your Guns: A Community-Based Firearm Safety Counseling and Gun Lock Distribution Program. *Archives of Pediatric Adolescent Medicine,155*, 659–664.

Dryfoos, J.G., Brindis, C., & Kaplan, D.W. (1996). Research and evaluation in school-baed health care. *Adolescent Medicine: State of the Art Reviews, 7*, 207–220.

Dubow, E.F., Kausch, D.F., Blum, M.C., Reed, J., & Bush, E. (1989). Correlates of suicidal ideation and attempts in a community sample of junior high and high school students. *Journal of Clinical Child Psychology, 18*, 158–166.

Durlak, J.A. (1998). Common risk and protective factors in successful prevention programs. *American Journal of Orthopsychiatry, 68*, 512–520.

Eastgard, S. (2000). *Youth suicide prevention program toolkit.* Seattle: Youth Suicide Prevention Program.

Eckert, T.L., Miller, D.N., DuPaul, G.J., & Riley-Tillman, T.C. (2003). Adolescent suicide prevention: School psychologists' acceptability of school-based programs. *School Psychology Review, 32*, 57–76.

Eggert, L.L., Thompson, E.A., Herting, J.R., & Nicholas, L.J. (1995). A prevention research program: Reconnecting at-risk youth. *Issues in Mental Health Nursing, 15*, 107–135.

Evans, W., Smith, M., Hill, G., Albers, E., & Nuefeld, J. (1996). Rural adolescent views of risk and protective factors associated with suicide. *Crisis Intervention, 3*, 1–12.

Fawcett, J., Busch, K.A., Jacobs D., Kravitz, H.M., & Fogg, L. (1997). Suicide: A four-pathway clinical-biochemical model. *Annals of the New York Academy of Sciences, 836*, 288–301.

Fawcett, J (2001). The anxiety disorders, anxiety symptoms and suicide. In D. Wasserman (Ed.), *Suicide—An Unnecessary Death* (pp. 59–63). London: Martin Duritz.

Felner, R.D., & Felner, T.Y. (1989). Primary prevention programs in the educational context: A transactional-ecological framework and analysis. In L.A. Bond & B.E. Compas (Eds.), *Primary Prevention and Promotion in the Schools* (pp. 13–49). Newbury Park, CA: Sage.

Goldsmith S.K., Pellmar T.C., Kleinman A.M., & Bunney W.E., (Eds.). (2002). *Reducing Suicide: A National Imperative*. Washington, DC: The National Academies Press.

Gould, M.S. (2001). Suicide and the media. In Hendin, H., & Mann, J.J. (Eds.), *Suicide Prevention: Clinical and Scientific Aspects. Annals of the New York Academy of Sciences*. New York: New York Academy of Sciences.

Gould, M.S., Greenberg T., Velting, D.M., & Shaffer, D. (2003). Youth suicide risk and preventive interventions: A review of the past 10 years. *Journal of the American Academy of Child Adolescent Psychiatry, 42*, 386–405.

Grossman, D.C., Cummings, P., Koepsell, T.D., Marshall, J., D'Ambrosio, L., Thompson, R.S., & Mack ,C. (2000). Firearm safety counseling in primary care pediatrics: a randomized, controlled trial. *Pediatrics, 106,* 22–26.

Grunbaum, I.A., Kann, L., Williams, B., Ross, I.G., et al. (2002). Youth risk behavior surveillance-United States, 2001. *MMWR Surveillance Summaries,* 51(SS-4):I-64.

Hawkins, J.D., Catalano, R.F., Kosterman, R., Abbott, R., & Hill, K.G. (1999). Preventing adolescent risk behaviors by strengthening protection during childhood. *Archives of Pediatric Adolescent Behavior, 153,* 226–234.

Hayden, D.C. (2003). *State plans for suicide prevention webpage*. Retrieved December 20, 2003 from http://www.ac.wwu.edu/~hayden/spsp/

Hayden, D.C., & Lauer, P. (2000). Prevalence of suicide programs in schools and roadblocks to implementation. *Suicide and Life-Threatening Behavior, 30,* 239–251.

Hazel, N., & McDonell, M.G. (2002, June). *QPR gatekeeper training results*. Retrieved December 20, 2003 from http://www.qprinstitute.com/

Hoagwood, K., & Erwin, H. (1997). Effectiveness of school-based mental health services for children: A 10-year research review. *Journal of Child and Family Studies, 6,* 435–461.

Illback, R.J., Cobb, C.T., & Joseph, H.M. (1997). *Integrated Services for Children and Families*. Washington, DC: American Psychological Association.

Iscoe, I. (1974). Community psychology and the competent community. *American Psychologist, 29,* 607–613.

Jessor, R., Van Den Bos, J., Vanderryn, J., Costa, F.M., & Turbin, M.S. (1995). Protective factors in adolescent problem behavior: Moderator effects and developmental change. *Developmental Psychology, 31,* 923–933.

Joiner, T.E., Pettit, J.W., Perez, M., Burns, A.B., Gencoz, T., Gencoz, F., et al. (2001). Can positive emotions influence problem-solving attitudes among adults? *Professional Psychology: Research & Practice, 32,* 507–512.

Joiner, T.E., Walker, R.L., Rudd, M.D., & Jobes, D.A. (1999). Scientizing and routinizing the assessment of suicidality in outpatient practice. *Professional Psychology: Research and Practice, 30,* 447–453.

Kalafat, J. (1997). The prevention of youth suicide. In R.P. Weissberg, T.P. Gullotta, B.A. Ryan, & G.R. Adams (Eds.), *Healthy Children 2010: Enhancing Children's Wellness* (pp. 175–213). Thousand Oaks, CA: Sage.

Kalafat, J. (2001). A systems approach to suicide prevention. In S.K. Goldsmith (Ed.), *Suicide prevention & Intervention: Summary of an Institute of Medicine Workshop* (pp. 4–7). Washington, DC: National Academy Press.

Kalafat, J. (2003). School approaches to youth suicide. *American Behavioral Scientist, 46,* 1211–1223.

Kalafat, J. & Ryerson, D.M. (1999). The implementation and institutionalization of a school-based youth suicide prevention program. *Journal of Primary Prevention, 19,* 157–175.

Kalafat, J. (2000). Issues in the evaluation of youth suicide prevention initiatives. In T. Joiner & M.D. Rudd (Eds.), *Suicide Science: Expanding the Boundaries* (pp. 241–249). Boston: Kluwer Academic Publishers.

Kalafat, J., & Mackey, K. (1994, April). *The school return of youths hospitalized for suicidal behavior*. Paper presented at the Annual Conference of the American Association of Suicidology, New York, NY.

Kalafat, J., & Underwood, M. (1989). *Lifelines: A School Based Adolescent Suicide Response Program*. Dubuque, IA: Kendall/Hunt Publishing Co.

Kazdin, A.E. (2003). Psychotherapy for children and adolescents. *Annual Review of Psychology, 54,* 253–276.

King, K.A., & Smith J. (2000). Project SOAR: A training program to increase school counselors' knowledge and confidence regarding suicide prevention and intervention. *Journal of School Health, 70,* 402–407.

Knox, K.L., Litts, D.A., Talcott, G.A., Feig, J.C., & Caine, E.D. (2003). Risk of suicide and related adverse outcomes after exposure to a suicide prevention programme in the US Air Force: Cohort study. *British Medical Journal, 237,* 1376–1378.

Konick, L.C., Brandt, L.A., & Gutierrez, P.M. (2002, April). *School-based suicide prevention programs: A meta-analysis*. Poster presentation at Annual Conference of the American Association of Suicidology, Bethesda, MD.

Linehan, M.M. Armstrong, H.E., Suarez, A., Allmon, D., & Heard, H.L. (1991). Cognitive-behavioral treatment of chronically parasuicidal borderline patients. *Archives of General Psychiatry, 48*, 1060–1064.

Lindsey, C.R., & Kalafat, J. (1998). Adolescents' views of preferred helper characteristics and barriers to seeking help. *Journal of Educational and Psychological Consultation, 9*, 171–193.

Links, P.S., Bergmans, Y., & Cook, M. (2003). Psychotherapeutic interventions to prevent repeated suicidal behavior. *Brief Treatment and Crisis Intervention, 3*, 445–464.

Lonczak, H.S., Abbott, R.D., Hawkins, J.D., Kosterman, R., & Catalano, R.F. (2002). Effects of the Seattle Social Development Project on sexual behavior, pregnancy, birth, and sexually transmitted disease outcomes by age 21 years. *Archives of Pediatric Adolescent Medicine, 156*, 438–447.

Mann, J.J., & Kapur, S. (1991). The emergence of suicidal ideation and behavior during antidepressant pharmacotherapy. *Archives of General Psychiatry, 48*, 1027–1033.

McBride, C.M., Curry, S.J. Cheadle, A., Anderman, C., Wagner, E.H., Diehr, P., & Psaty, B. (1995). School-level application of a social bonding model to adolescent risk-taking behavior. *Journal of School Health, 65*, 63–68.

McDaniel J.S., Purcell D., & D'Augelli A.R. (2001). The relationship between sexual orientation and risk for suicide: Research findings and future directions for research and prevention. *Suicide Life Threatening Behavior, 31*(suppl), 84–105.

Miller, M., Azrael, D., & Hemenway, D. (2001). Firearm availability and unintentional firearm deaths. *Accident Analysis and Prevention, 33*, 477–484.

Montgomery, S.A. (1997). Suicide and antidepressants. *Annals of New York Academy of Science, 836*, 329–338.

Montgomery, S.A., Dunner, D.L., & Dunbar, G.C. (1995). Reduction of suicidal thoughts with patoxetine in comparison with reference antidepressants and placebo. *European Neuropsychopharmacology, 5*, 5–13.

Morgan, H.G., Jones, E.M., Owen, J.H. (1993). Secondary prevention of non-fatal deliberate self-harm: The green card study. *British Journal of Psychiatry, 163*, 111–112.

Müller-Oerlinghausen, B. Müser-Causemann, B., & Volk, J. (1992). Suicides and parasuicides in a high risk patient group on and off lithium long-term medication. *Journal of Affective Disorders, 25*, 261–270.

National Center for Injury Prevention and Control (NCIPC), Center for Disease Control and Prevention, WISQARS, Available at: *http:llwww* .cdc.gov/nicip/wisqars/ .Accessed October, 2003.

The National Strategy for Suicide Prevention: Goals and Objectives for Action, 2001, U.S. Department of Health and Human Services.

Nabors, L.A., & Reynolds, M.W. (2000). Program evaluation activities: Outcomes related to treatment for adolescents receiving school-based mental health services. *Children's Services: Social Policy, Research, and Practice, 3*, 175–189.

O'Carroll, P.W., Berman, A., Maris, R.W., & Moscicki, E.K. (1996). Beyond the tower of Babel: A nomenclature for suicidology. *Suicide & Life-Threatening Behavior, 26*, 237–252.

Orbach, I., & Bar-Joseph, H. (1993). The impact of a suicide prevention program for adolescents on suicidal tendencies, hopelessness, ego identity, and coping. *Suicide and Life-Threatening Behavior, 23*, 120–129.

Oatis, P.J., Fenn-Buderer, N.M., Cummings, P., & Fleitz, R. (1999). Pediatric practice based evaluation of the Steps to Prevent Firearm Injury program. *Injury Prevention, 5*, 48–52.

Piacentini J., Rotherham-Borus, M.J., Gillis, J.R. et al., (1995). Demographic predictors of treatment attendance among adolescent suicide attempters. *Journal of Consulting and Clinical Psychology, 63*, 469–473.

Potter, L., Powell, K.E., & Kachur, P.S. (1995). Suicide prevention from a public health perspective. *Suicide & Life-Threatening Behavior, 25*, 82–91.

Quinnett, P.G. (1995). *QPR for Suicide Prevention.* Spokane, Washington: QPR Institute Inc.

Rathus, J.H., & Miller, A.L. (2002). Dialectical behavior therapy adapted for suicidal adolescents. *Suicidal and Life-Threatening Behavior, 32*, 146–157.

Rudd, M.D., & Joiner, T.E. (1998): The assessment, management, and treatment of suicidality: Towards clinically informed and balanced standards of care. *Clinical Psychology: Science and Practice, 5*, 135–150.

Rudd, M.D., Joiner, T.E., Jobes, D.A., & King, C.A. (1999). The outpatient treatment of suicidality. An integration of science and recognition of its limitations. *Professional Psychology:Research and Practice, 30*, 437–446.

Rudd, M.D., Joiner, T.E., & Rajab, M.H. (1995). Help negation after acute suicidal crisis. *Journal of Consulting and Clinical Psychology, 63*, 499–503.

Rudd, M.D., Joiner, T., & Rajab, H. (1996). Relationships among suicide ideators, attempters, and multiple attempters in a young adult sample. *Journal of Abnormal Psychology, 105*, 541–550.

Rudd, M.D., Joiner, T., & Rajab, M.H. (2001). *Treating Suicidal Behavior: An Effective Time-Limited Approach.* New York: Guilford Press.

Ryerson, D. (1990). Suicide awareness education in schools: The development of a core program and subsequent modifications for special populations or institutions. *Death Studies, 14,* 371–390.

Sanddal, N.D., Sanddal, T.L., Berman, A., & Silverman, M.M. (2003). A general systems approach to suicide prevention: Lessons from cardiac prevention and control. *Suicide and Life-Threatening Behavior, 33,* 341–352.

Saxe, L., Cross, T., & Silverman, T. (1988). Children's mental health services: The gap between what we know and what we do. *American Psychologist, 43,* 800–807.

Schou, M. (1999). Perspectives on lithium treatment of bipolar disorder: Action, efficacy, effect on suicidal behavior. *Bipolar Disorder, 9,* 5–10.

Shaffer, D., & Pfeffer, C.R. (2001). Practice parameter for the assessment and treatment of children and adolescents with suicidal behavior. *Journal of the American Academy of Child & Adolescent Psychiatry, 40* (7), Supplement: 24S–51S.

Shaffer, D. (2003, June). *Teen Screen program.* Presentation at Youth Suicide prevention workshop. New York, NY: American Foundation for Suicide Prevention.

Shaffer, D., Fisher, P., Lucas, C.P., Dulcan, M.K., & Schwab-Stone, M.E. (2000). NIMH Diagnostic Interview for Children Version IV: Description, differences from previous versions, and reliability of some common diagnoses. *Journal of the American Academy of Child and Adolescent Psychiatry, 39,* 28–38.

Shah, S., Hoffman, R.E., Wake, L., & Marine, W.M. (2000). Adolescent suicide and household access to firearms in Colorado: Results of a case-control study. *Journal of Adolescent Health, 26,* 157–163.

Silverman, M.M., & Felner, R.D. (1995). The place of suicide prevention in the spectrum of prevention: Definitions of critical terms and constructs. *Suicide and Life-Threatening Behavior, 25,* 70–81.

Sonneck, G., Etzersdorfer, E., & Nagel-Kuess, S. (1994). Imitative suicide on the Viennese subway. *Social Science Med,* (38), 453–457.

Suicide Prevention Resource Center (2002). http://www.sprc.org/index.asp

Thompson, E.A., Eggert, L.L., Randell, B.P., & Pike, K.C. (2001). Evaluation of indicated suicide risk prevention approaches for potential high school dropouts. *American Journal of Public Health, 91,* 742–752.

Tondo, L., Jamison, K.R., & Baldessarini, R.J. (1997). Effect of lithium maintenance on suicidal behavior in major mood disorders. *Annals of the New York Academy of Science, 836,* 340–351.

Trautman, P., Steart, N., & Morishima, A. (1993). Are adolescent suicide attempters non-compliant with outpatient care? *Journal of the American Academy of Child and Adolescent Psychiatry, 32,* 89–94.

Turley, C.B., & Tanney B.L. (1998). *Living Works Australian Field Trial Report.* Melbourne: Lifeline Australia. Report prepared for the Australian Commonwealth Government.

Van Heeringen, C., Jannes, S., Buylaert, W., Henderick, H., DeBacquer, D., & Van Remoortel, J. (1995). The management of non-compliance to referral to out-patient after-care among attempted suicide patients: A controlled intervention study. *Psychological Medicine, 25,* 963–970.

Wagner, B.M., Silverman, M.A.C., & Martin, C.E. (2003): Family factors in youth suicidal behaviors. *American Behavioral Scientist, 46,* 1171–1191.

Walker, P.V. (1996, August 2). Scientists decry lawmakers' decision to slash support for firearms research. Chronicle of Higher Education, Vol XLII (47), 19–21.

Zemetkin, A.J., Alter, M.R., & Yemini, T. (2001). Suicide in teenagers: Assessement, management, and prevention. *Journal of the American Medical Association, 286,* 3120–3125.

Zenere, F.J., III, & Lazarus, P.J. (1997). The decline of youth suicidal behavior in an urban, multicultural public school system following the introduction of a suicide prevention and intervention program. *Suicide and Life-Threatening Behavior, 4,* 387–403.

Chapter 12

Obsessive-Compulsive Disorder

Andre P. Bessette

Introduction

This chapter examines the construct of obsessive-compulsive disorder (OCD) in children and adolescents, and examines evidenced-based intervention and prevention strategies with this population.

Overview of Pediatric Obsessive-Compulsive Disorder (OCD)

Obsessive-compulsive disorder (OCD) is a debilitating, socially stigmatizing neurobehavioral condition that affects 1.8% to 2.5% of the general U.S. population (Weissman et al., 1994), and anywhere from 1% to 4% of the child and adolescent population in this country (Douglass, Moffitt, Dar, McGee & Silva, 1995; Flament et al., 1988; Valleni-Basile, Garrison & Jackson, 1994). It has been posited that of OCD cases recognized in adults, 80% experience symptom onset before the age of 18 (Pauls, Alsobrook, Goodman, Rasmussen & Leckman, 1995) and some may even demonstrate clear OC symptoms as early as age 3 years. Estimates as to the social and economic costs of treating OCD in 1990 hover around $8.4 billion (DuPont, Rice, Shiraki & Rowland, 1994). However, the true costs of pediatric OCD per se are most apparent in the formative social, academic, family, developmental opportunities, and related personal potential that a majority of these individuals never fully experience (Piacentini, Bergman, Keller & McCracken, 2003).

The Diagnostic and Statistical Manual of Mental Disorders, Fourth Edition, Treatment Revision (*DSM-IV-TR* [APA, 2000]) classifies obsessive-compulsive disorder (OCD) as an *anxiety disorder*. It is a largely chronic condition involving intrusive thoughts, impulses, or obsessions that an individual experiences as inappropriate and undesired, and which lead to intense anxiety and distress, and repetitive behaviors that a person feels driven to carry out (i.e., compulsions) in an effort to neutralize the obsessions and reduce the anxiety, distress, or sense of perceived threat. Essential features of these obsessions are that (1) they are recurrent, (2) are not merely unreasonable concerns about real-life problems, (3) the individual attempts to suppress the obsessions or otherwise distract themselves from the images or impulses, and (4) the individual recognizes that *they,* and not someone or something else, are producing these obsessions. Two core features of compulsions are that (1) they can be physical acts or *mental rituals* (e.g., counting, praying, prioritizing) meant to reduce distress, prevent a threatening event, or atone for a transgression, and (2) these acts are not logically or functionally related to the situation they are intended to address (e.g., touching a railing seven times to ward off possible intruders as opposed to repeatedly checking a stove to ensure that it has been turned off).

Criteria necessary to make the diagnosis of OCD are (1) at some point the individual demonstrates *some* insight in recognizing these obsessions and compulsions as excessive or unreasonable (however, this can vary for youngsters depending upon developmental level), (2) these behaviors are *ego-dystonic,* or experienced as unacceptable and distressing (this can vary somewhat with younger individuals); (3) they consume an inordinate amount of time and energy (sometimes several hours per day); and (4) these experiences impair social, occupational, family, and/or academic functioning.

Prevalence

In younger populations, epidemiologic studies have revealed a broad prevalence range of .25% to 4%. Specific to region, studies have revealed prevalence rates of 0.25% in the United Kingdom (Heyman et al., 2001), 0.5% in Germany (Grabe et al., 2000), 0.6% (adult sample) in Canada (Stein, Forde & Anderson, 1997), 1% (Flament et al., 1988) to 3% (Valleni-Basile et al., 1994) to 4% (Douglass, Moffitt, Dar, McGee & Silva, 1995) in the United States, 1.33% in Denmark (Thomsen & Mikkelsen, 1991), 3.6% in Israel (Zohar, et al., 1992; Zohar, 1999), and up to 5% in Japan (Honjo et al., 1989). Hypotheses for these differences are scarce at this time, and do not go much beyond implicating the different methods that researchers have used to gather these data.

Regarding gender, some studies have found a slight male predominance (Douglass, Moffitt, Dar, McGee & Silva,1995; Last & Strauss, 1989; Swedo et al., 1992). More commonly, the empirical evidence indicates that no significant gender difference exists with regard to prevalence (Karno, Golding, Sorenson & Burnam, 1988; Zohar, 1999), but that gender differences may be more apparent in symptom profiles (see Bogetto, Venturello, Albert, Maina & Ravizza, 2000).

Finally, a paucity of research exists that considers race and prevalence of OCD. However, in their epidemiologic study of OCD in five U.S. communities, Karno et al. (1988) discovered that obsessive-compulsive disorder is less common in African American individuals than it is in Caucasians.

Etiology and Theoretical Perspectives

No one cause or etiologic factor has been identified for obsessive-compulsive disorder. Rather, evidence supports physiologic and genetic contributions to this condition which combine biological, environmental, and learned determinants. Similarly, clinical research has given rise to models of how OCD symptoms are manifested, maintained, and remediated.

Beginning with Freud's seminal paper on the "Rat Man" and his subsequent theorizing about his patients' *compulsive neuroses* (Freud, 1966), and even up until the 1980s, psychodynamic theories of obsessive-compulsive disorder were widely accepted. According to this perspective, anxiety provoked by Oedipal conflicts led one to regress to anal phase defenses, characterized by doing and undoing, reaction formation, and affect isolation. Some contemporary theorists have even posited that anal fixations, arising from disturbances in early toilet training, as well as intrusive parenting styles are responsible for such regressions (Nemiah, 1988, as cited in Gabbard, 2001). However, Freud recognized the limitations of the psychoanalytic explanation for such a complex phenomenon and suggested that compulsive neuroses may best be understood from a medical or brain physiology perspective.

On this note, evidence has grown through neuroimaging, genetic, autoimmune, and pharmacotherapy studies that supports the notion that neurobiological abnormalities play a key role in the pathogenesis of OCD. Imaging studies (e.g., magnetic resonance imaging [MRI], computed tomography [CT], and positron emission tomography [PET]) have implicated a number of brain structures. One region of interest in such studies is the limbic system, including the cingulate and fronto-striatal areas (e.g., Jenike et al., 1996). These areas are considered responsible for regulating emotion, motivation, instinct, visceral processes, sexual and social relations, spontaneity, attention, and memory.

The dorsolateral prefrontal cortex (DLPFC) and its connection with the aforementioned limbic circuitry is another area of interest with regard to OCD symptomatology. Seen as being involved in governing purposeful behavior, evaluating external cues in order to self-adjust behavior, and exerting executive control over limbic function, abnormalities in the DLPFC may lead to OCD (Baxter et al., 1992).

Another line of inquiry has been the study of pediatric autoimmune neuropsychiatric disorders associated with streptococcal infection, or PANDAS (Allen Leonard & Swedo, 1995). Interestingly, PANDAS' relation to movement disorders (e.g., Sydenham's chorea) and comorbidity with tics has suggested the basal ganglia as a key structure underlying OC symptoms, where, in this case, anti-streptococcal antibodies that are produced in response to the infection end up attacking the neuronal cells of the basal ganglia rather than the infection itself. Studies have reported significantly increased basal ganglia volume in PANDAS individuals (Leonard & Swedo, 2001). However, aside from the neuroanatomical implications, the fact that such an infectious process can trigger the sudden onset and/or exacerbation of OC symptoms supports the contribution of biology to this phenomenon. Some researchers have investigated whether OCD may be altogether an autoimmune disorder (Arnold & Richter, 2001), but the presence of such symptoms in the absence of streptococcal infection contradicts this hypothesis.

Studies of regional cerebral blood flow (rCBF) and glucose metabolism under conditions of symptom stimulation and OCD treatment have been compelling in elucidating neural involvement in OCD.

Arising out of pharmacologic treatment studies, neurotransmitters have been identified as playing a major role in OCD. Specifically, the neurotransmitter serotonin has been studied, both as the target of the most effective OCD treatments and in terms of symptoms arising from dysfunctions in this system. The fact that both non-selective serotonin reuptake inhibitors (SRIs) and selective serotonin reuptake inhibitors (SSRIs) have received support as the pharmacologic treatments of choice for OCD is an indicator of this.

The genetic-based familial aggregation of OCD has received strong support. For example, Lougee, Perlmutter, Nicholson, Garvey, and Swedo (2000) found that of 54 PANDAS children, 26% had at least one first-degree relative with OCD, with 11% of parents qualifying for OC personality disorder. A subsequent meta-analytic study of family and twin studies confirmed significant family aggregation of OCD (Hettema, Neale & Kendler, 2001).

Complementary to the strong support of the biological underpinnings of OCD, researchers have examined the learned or behavioral aspects of this condition. It is axiomatic that early nurturing and socialization experiences are key in the shaping of behavior and personality. Behavioral learning work by Wolpe (1969) differed from the psychoanalytic views and suggested that neuroses (or unrealistic anxiety) are persistent maladaptive autonomic responses acquired through *classical conditioning*.

In OCD, obsessions are thought to arise from an inherently poor tolerance for uncertainty, difficulty discriminating real from imagined threat in a situation, and subsequent efforts to control or make predictable a world which is often seen as threatening and unpredictable (O'Leary & Wilson, 1975). The ambiguity and uncertainty become so intolerable that one feels compelled to bring certainty to the situation through either avoidance or through mental or physical rituals.

The current and most accepted *model* of OCD phenomenology integrates these aforementioned perspectives and is informed by a wealth of both theoretical and applied clinical work (e.g., Fitzgibbons & Pedrick, 2003; Barlow, 2000; Chansky, 2000; March & Mulle, 1998). This blueprint for how OCD "works" could best described as a *biopsychosocial* or *diathesis stress* model illustrated below.

Generalized biological (i.e., genetic), psychological, and specific *learned* vulnerabilities interact (Barlow, 2000) = vulnerability to emotional arousal/dysregulation, poor tolerance for uncertainty, diminished sense of control, and misinterpretation of cues/events.

⇓

Innocuous or *moderately* emotionally arousing events occur (e.g., dirty lunch table, counter, or toilet seat, or an interaction with a particular teacher)—they are catastrophically misinterpreted—"false alarm" is sounded—anxiety and dread are experienced in anticipation of catastrophic outcomes, and a perceived inability to control the situation.

⇓

What *might* be a problem is experienced as *definitely* a problem. For example, "I may get sick from these germs" experienced by most children is experienced as "I *will* get sick from these germs" by OCD youngsters. Or, in the case of aggressive obsessions, the unacceptable intrusive thought or image of hitting a teacher is experienced as if it is actually being acted upon—*thought–action fusion*.

⇓

These intrusive thoughts and images (i.e., obsessions) of negative outcomes and worst case scenarios persist. The urge to neutralize the threat and thus decrease the accompanying anxiety and "make things certain" grows.

Ú

> "I need to wash to make sure that this does not happen" or "I need to *avoid* such objects or situations so that I do not get sick," or "I need to block this out of my mind and distract myself or I will act on this unacceptable urge."

> So active compulsions or avoidance rituals ("safety behaviors") are carried out to "neutralize" the catastrophe and the accompanying distress: e.g., washing repeatedly to rid oneself of contamination, avoiding potentially contaminated objects, or distracting oneself, blocking out the aggressive thoughts/images (i.e., thought-blocking) or *purging* the images through prayer rituals.

Ú

> The averting of disaster is *misattributed* to the compulsion. Thus, the "safety" behavior is strengthened via negative reinforcement (i.e., the neutralization or removal of an aversive stimulus- in this case the anxiety and guilt experienced in relation to the contaminant or the unacceptable aggressive images respectively) (Wolpe, 1969).

> Distress is eased *but only temporarily*— The doubt- or uncertainty-laden intrusive thoughts and images eventually return, either spontaneously or in relation to relevant cues. Then the compulsion is repeated.

Ú

> Not unlike medicine tolerance and dependence, a more potent "dose" of the compulsion or "safety behavior" is necessary to produce "relief" from the increasing intensity of the thoughts, images, or urges.

Still, the challenge of teasing out the respective contributions of genetics versus environment persists. That is, persons with a biologic predisposition for OC symptoms and anxiety-related behaviors are likely to gravitate toward and/or create an environment and life-style that supports these symptoms. Subsequently, parents with such a predisposition are likely to have a parenting style that reinforces these behaviors in their children.

Comorbidity

OCD cases rarely exist alone. In fact, as many as 70% of OCD individuals present with *at least one* co-occurring, or comorbid, disorder such as a tic disorder (including Tourette's disorder), attention-deficit/hyperactivity disorder (ADHD) (see Geller et al., 2002), oppositional-defiant disorder (ODD), major depressive disorder, and other anxiety disorders such as phobias and generalized anxiety disorder (Swedo et al., 1989). These comorbidity findings have profound implications for diagnosis and treatment.

Symptom Presentation and Course of OCD

OCD is as diverse as the personalities of those who suffer from it. Thus, it can present in a variety of ways, particularly in light of the heterogeneity of symptom themes, symptom severity and impairment, and their differential manifestations over time. (Abramowitz et al., 2003; Leckman et al., 1997; Lin et al., 2002; Lochner & Stein, 2003; Rasmussen & Eisen, 1992). It is not uncommon to have two OCD youngsters present with completely different symptoms, and for these symptoms to shift themes over time. Common clinical cases involve, for example, the youngster who is fixated on the idea that she might become sick from the germs that she believes contaminate doorknobs and stair railings, and who thus avoids them at all costs and spends hours per day washing her hands in an effort to prevent infection. Another common scenario is that of the adolescent who is plagued with intrusive and undesired thoughts and images of incestuous situations, is obsessed with the idea that he is morally damned for allowing these images to persist, and who spends hours per day praying for absolution. And finally, there is the case of the child who is tormented by the thought that her parents will surely suffer a horrible accident should she not perform an elaborate bedtime ritual including ordering certain stuffed animals on her bureau, checking under her bed, and saying certain prayers three times each.

In their review of the literature to date on OCD in children and adolescents, Geller et al. (1998) found that the most common obsessions involved family catastrophes, hoarding, contamination, and sexual, somatic, and religious preoccupations. They also discovered that the most common compulsions were washing, repeating, checking, ordering, counting, hoarding, and touching. What was most compelling was the finding that compared to adults, children tended to present with a high frequency of compulsions *not* preceded by obsessions.

Regarding the predominance of certain symptoms by gender, Leckman et al. (1997) found two significant thematic differences: that symmetry and hoarding compulsions were more common in males. However, Lensi and her colleagues (Lensi, Cassano, Correddu, Ravagli & Kunovac, 1996) discovered that males demonstrated a higher frequency of sexual and symmetry obsessions and odd rituals, whereas females had a higher frequency of aggressive obsessions. Finally, Beckstein (2001) found that while there were no gender differences in subjective *experiences* of OCD, there emerged significant gender differences in terms of symptom *content*. Specifically, males more frequently reported violent or sexual obsessions and fear of contamination (animal-related), while females more frequently reported rereading or rewriting, and cleaning compulsions, in addition to the need to tell, ask, or confess.

Regarding gender and the *course* of OCD, Bogetto and colleagues (Bogetto et al., 2000) found an earlier age of onset of OCD symptoms and disorder in males (usually prepubertal), while females more commonly showed an acute onset and then episodic course of the condition. In addition, females more frequently reported the occurrence of a stressful event in the year preceding the onset of their OCD. Finally, in examining respective histories of their sample, these investigators discovered that males had a significantly more common experience of pre-OCD-onset anxiety disorders and hypomanic mood episodes *after* OCD onset, whereas females had a significantly more frequent history of eating disorders. This is consistent with other studies especially with regard to age-of-onset (Geller et al., 1998; Last & Strauss, 1989; Lensi et al., 1996; Zohar, 1999) and eating disorder profiles (Noshirvani, Kasvikis, Marks & Tsakiris, 1991).

Few studies have documented ethnicity differences in OCD symptom presentation. In his study of 27 Balinese OCD and comorbid OCD-tic individuals, Lemelson (2000) found that the most common obsessional themes centered on the need to gather information about a social network (e.g., the identity and status of passersby), somatic obsessions, and religious themes (e.g., witchcraft and spirits). This suggests a possible cultural-embeddedness of the symptom themes and makes a compelling case for further cross-cultural investigation.

Cognitive Processes in Pediatric OCD

It has been established that *how* one thinks about one's own condition can profoundly affect its impact. Particularly with OCD, which presupposes fundamental cognitive misinterpretations and distortions, there is no shortage of literature on the cognitive processes underlying this condition. In his examination of anxiety disorders from the perspective of emotion theory, David Barlow (2000) suggests that there is a sense of uncontrollability related to possible future threats, danger, or impending aversive events, that underlies anxiety. Consistent with current models of OCD phenomenology, he implicates the idea of individuals responding to "false alarms" or *perceived* threats as opposed to real threats. In this sense, he proposes that anxiety can be thought of as a state of helplessness due to a perceived inability to predict, control, or obtain desired outcomes in relation to anticipated events. In speaking to the third component of his tripartite vulnerability (or diathesis) model, Barlow describes a *learned* or *conditioned* vulnerability that predisposes a person to focus anxiety on certain objects or events. Regarding OCD in particular, he cites evidence that some individuals actually learn early on to equate dangerous thoughts with dangerous actions, thus leading to the notion of *thought-action fusion* (see also Zucker et al., 2002), where having an unwanted thought or intrusive image is experienced as synonymous with acting upon it.

Differential Diagnosis

The need to differentiate OCD from other conditions that share some of its characteristics is obvious. Whether it be distinguishing between clinical (i.e., pathological) and subclinical levels of these symptoms (i.e., typical of an OC personality style), elucidating developmentally or culturally normative forms, or teasing out bona fide OCD from OC-type symptoms secondary to *other* disorders, this process can be complicated simply due to how prevalent these behaviors are.

With regard to developmentally or culturally common obsessions and rituals, the simple distinction here is that such behaviors, however odd they may seem, tend to be volitional, manageable, temporary, innocuous, and do not cause excessive distress or functional impairment (e.g., Leonard, Goldberger, Rapoport, Cheslow & Swedo, 1990). Examples of such phenomena can include those childhood rituals, magical beliefs (see for example Evans, Milanak, Medeiros & Ross, 2002), and self-soothing compulsions, that may remit over time or become incorporated into a somewhat functional life-style.

However, a related issue to consider is whether such developmentally normative childhood obsessions and rituals are separate phenomena which children tend to manage over time or are a sign of premorbid OCD. While researchers may be apprehensive about formally stating that an obsessive-compulsive *style* is a risk factor in eventually developing OCD, evidence seems to be mounting in support of the notion, and that early and seemingly normative obsessive-compulsive/ritualistic behaviors may be precursors to OCD. In their examination of "normal" childhood rituals, Leonard et al. (1990) found that while OCD children and controls did not differ in frequency and type of superstitions, parents of the OCD children reported significantly more remarkable patterns of early ritualistic behaviors than did parents of the control group of children.

Thus, the possibility that such behavior reflects incipient OCD remains a serious question and one, for obvious early intervention purposes, demands study.

PANDAS

Within the past decade or so, the notion of an autoimmune-based OCD subtype has taken hold. Susan Swedo and her National Institute of Mental Health (NIMH) colleagues (see Allen, Leonard & Swedo, 1995) noticed the intriguing pattern of sudden-onset or marked exacerbation of OC and tic symptoms in youngsters who had developed strep infections (commonly, strep throat). Specifically, these researchers had recognized that in Sydenham's chorea, which is a neurological variant of rheumatic fever and involves involuntary and awkward (i.e., choreoform) writhing movement of the extremities, OC symptoms were quite common. In then recognizing that Sydenham's chorea involves anti streptococcal antibodies that attack the brain's basal ganglia tissue instead of the strep infection itself, these researchers reasoned that the emergence of the OC and tic symptoms might involve the same process.

Subsequent and careful investigations of this phenomenon indeed revealed a distinct subtype of OCD in which youngsters presented with sudden onset of OC and/or tic symptoms following a positive finding for group A beta-hemolytic streptococci (GABHS) infection. Originally labeled with the acronym PITANDS (pediatric infection-triggered autoimmune neuropsychiatric disorder), this condition is now referred to as pediatric autoimmune neuropsychiatric disorder associated with streptococcal infection or *PANDAS*. The most recent examinations of this syndrome using increasingly larger sample sizes have arrived at a solid understanding of the pathophysiology of this condition and criteria for it. Leonard and Swedo (2001) have established five inclusionary criteria for this disorder: (1) presence of OCD and/or a tic disorder, (2) prepubertal symptom onset, (3) sudden onset or episodic course of symptoms, (4) a temporal association between streptococcal infections and neuropsychiatric symptom exacerbations, and (5) neurological abnormalities. Recent investigations have found evidence for family aggregation of OCD in relatives of PANDAS children. For example, Lougee et al. (2000) found that of 54 PANDAS children, 26% had at least one first-degree relative with OCD, with 11% of parents qualifying for OC personality disorder.

Risk and Resiliency in Pediatric Obsessive-Compulsive Disorder

The notion of risk refers to "those characteristics, variables, or hazards that, if present for a given individual, make it more likely that this individual, rather than someone selected from the general population, will develop a disorder" (Mrazek & Haggerty, 1994, p. 6). On the other hand, the characteristic of *resiliency* refers to an individual's ability to adapt to and thrive in their environment in spite of the presence of such risk factors. Factors that promote such resiliency are often referred to as *protective factors* or those "positive behaviors or features of the environment that lessen the likelihood of negative outcomes or increase the possibility [i.e., probability] of positive outcomes" (Mrazek & Haggerty, 1994, p. 6).

Individual Factors

With regard to *individual* risk factors in pediatric OCD, personality, cognitive vulnerability and deficits, a preexisting pattern of ritualistic or perfectionistic behaviors, comorbid conditions, and neuropsychological deficits are potential influences. In light of PANDAS, a history of strep infection and a positive strep titer are risk factors and should be considered regardless of whether tics and OC symptoms are apparent.

Personality characteristics such as temperament (e.g., behavioral inhibition), poor insight, defensiveness, oppositionality, low self-esteem, social and emotional immaturity, and avoidant coping style pose problems for youngsters with or without OCD. The temperament quality of *behavioral inhibition* has been well-studied in developmental research (e.g., Kagan, 1997) and found to be relatively common. It manifests as excessive crying and irritability in infants, fearfulness and clinginess in toddlers, and cautiousness, shyness, and social withdrawal in older children (see Hudson, Flannery-Schroeder & Kendall, 2004).

Even though insight can vary developmentally, limited awareness of one's deficits and a tenuous desire to deal with them, which is common in younger individuals, poses a serious impediment to addressing early OC symptoms, and thus is a risk factor. Attitude-wise, and within OCD youngsters per se, defensiveness and oppositionality have been identified as treatment barriers (Swedo et al., 1989) and have been posited to contribute to symptom maintenance and exacerbation, developing an ego-syntonic perception of one's OC behaviors, and perhaps to the development of OCD (e.g., Baer & Jenike, 1992). Apathy has also been identified as a psychopathology risk factor, as have low self-esteem and social and emotional immaturity (Greenberg et al., 2001).

Cognitive vulnerabilities to "over-perceiving" threat, underestimating one's control over a situation, and possessing poor "uncertainty tolerance" have been theorized as core aspects of most anxiety disorders (e.g., Barlow, 2000). Moreover, the autonomic or emotional arousal dysregulation that often interacts with these thoughts and thus completes the vicious "cognitive-affective cycle" is a factor. Thus, a youngster evidencing such a cognitive-affective style could be considered at risk for developing anxiety disorders such as OCD, or for experiencing further symptom complication. With regard to early ritualistic and perfectionistic behaviors, it may be a predisposing factor for OCD (e.g., Evans et al., 2002; Frost & Steketee, 1997).

Comorbid conditions have long been considered risk factors in developing pediatric OCD (Geller et al., 2002) and have been observed to predict poorer outcomes. The presence of tic disorders, externalizing behaviors, and comorbid schizotypy have been found to be concerning risk factors as they can exacerbate cognitive and affective distortions and pose significant impediments to treatment. Interestingly, though, initial OCD severity and types of symptoms have received mixed support as risk factors for poor outcomes (Keijsers, Hoogduin & Schapp, 1994; March et al., 2001). Finally, neuropsychological deficits such as organizational strategy problems, difficulty recalling unstructured information (Greisberg & McKay, 2003), impaired learning strategies (Savage & Rauch, 2000), and impairment in inhibiting and filtering out visual-perceptual interference (Hartston, 2000), may be risk factors. Even though this research is in its infancy, results so far are consistent with the processing, learning, coping, and threat discrimination deficits commonly observed in OCD individuals.

Individual factors promoting resiliency, or protective factors, have received little attention in the literature, and so we are left to extrapolate from what we know of the promotion of stress resilience in general and from the study of the aforementioned risks. Thus, personality characteristics such as agreeableness, extroversion, a flexible coping style, balanced attributional style, ego strength (i.e., stable and positive self-concept), openness to treatment, and insightfulness, are logical protective factors. Having the intellectual capacity to benefit from prescribed therapies is important. A longitudinal study of pediatric OCD found that premorbid social functioning predicted treatment response and course of illness, thus suggesting that nurturing strong interpersonal skills early on may be beneficial (Ayres, 2000). Clearly, there needs to be further study of individual resiliency in pediatric OCD, and might best be accomplished in comparing OCD youngsters having experienced positive treatment response and improved quality of life (QOL) to those who have evidenced little or no functional benefits.

Very few studies have examined gender and ethnicity issues with regard to individual risk and resiliency factors in pediatric OCD. Those that have done so have reported largely qualitative functional impairment differences by gender (e.g., Piacentini et al., 2003), no significant ethnicity (or religious) differences at all (Raphael et al., 1996), or some race differences, suggesting higher incidence in whites as compared to blacks. However, in their review of the current state of the prevention field, Greenberg et al. (2001) have identified racial injustice as a psychopathology risk factor.

Family Factors Affecting Risk and Resilience

While this area is still tenuously studied, family factors affecting risk and resiliency in pediatric OCD have received the most attention to date. Genetic vulnerability (including parental and familial psychopathology), attachment quality, family dynamic (including parenting style), and effective parental involvement (or lack thereof) in treatment are among the most notable risk factors related to OCD.

As noted earlier, the genetic vulnerability and family aggregation of OCD has been well-established (Nestadt et al., 2000; Pauls et al., 1995; Black et al., 2003; Ayres, 2000.)

Attachment style has been well researched as a predictor of later-life adjustment and well-being (e.g., Bartholomew, 1993; Bowlby, 1979, 1986; Ainsworth, Blehar, Waters & Wall, 1978;) and as such, has received much attention in the anxiety literature. Warren and colleagues (Warren, Huston, Egeland & Stroufe, 1997) found that an anxious-resistant attachment style in the first year of life was predicative of anxiety disorders at age 18. Insofar as the notions of threat perception, predictability, uncertainty, and emotional dyscontrol have been established as core factors in OCD symptomatology, it stands to reason that attachment styles predisposing children to these challenges (and perhaps contributing to behavioral inhibition) need to be considered as risk factors.

Related to this, family dynamic plays a key role as either a risk or resiliency factor in pediatric OCD. In contrast to adults, children with OCD tend to be "embedded" in their families and very dependent upon them. In fact, especially with younger children, family influences play a larger role than do peer and social factors. Thus, this dependence can render them vulnerable to many familial influences over which they have little if any control (Freeman et al., 2003). Marital discord, family disorganization (Black et al., 2003), family coping style, parent–child enmeshment and involvement in rituals (Freeman et al., 2003), and parenting style have all been cited as risk factors in increasing the likelihood of developing of pediatric OCD, or in further impairment. In addition, family circumstances such as low SES, large family size, and stressful life events have been found to place children at risk for developing psychopathology in general (Greenberg, Dimitrovich & Bumbarger, 2001). Given that compromised stress resilience is a characteristic of OCD, such factors maintaining symptoms, or increasing stress within the family and thus taxing a youngster's coping resources are of concern.

With regard to parenting style, Yoshida, Taga & Fukui (2001) examined differences in perceptions parental rearing style in OCD persons compared with "normal" controls. The results indicated that perceptions of paternal protectiveness and interference were significantly higher in OCD individuals than in controls. Turgeon and colleagues (Turgeon, O'Connor, Marchand & Freeston, 2002) likewise found parental protectiveness to be more common in pediatric OCD when compared with control families. One study looking at whether families of OCD youngsters could be distinguished from those of control families based upon parent–child behaviors, found that this was indeed so (Barrett, Shortt & Healy, 2002).

Unfortunately, no studies are available that examine family-related resiliency factors with respect to pediatric OCD. However, looking at family involvement in the treatment of OCD has provided valuable information regarding the possible *positive* family contributions to the improvement of their affected member. Grunes (1999) examined the effectiveness of inclusion a family member in the Exposure/Response Prevention (E/RP) treatment protocol. They found that compared to control groups where there was no family participation, the family treatment group demonstrated greater reduction in OCD symptoms. Interestingly, they also found that anxiety and depression in treatment *family members* (not patients) diminished significantly more than in control group family members.

Apart from this, it is clear that adaptive variants of the aforementioned risk factors, as well as awareness of these risk factors and efforts to address them and promote well-being, can be considered protective. For instance, an awareness of a familial vulnerability to OCD or other anxiety disorders, and how best to address their emergence could be considered a resiliency factor. A secure attachment characterized by parental emotional attunement, availability, warmth, and a healthy balance between gratification and frustration can be protective. In this vein, a parenting style balancing protectiveness with support of autonomy and reasonable risk-taking (including failure and recovery from failure), parental modeling of flexible coping and emotional resilience, access to extra-familial support, and maintaining healthy boundaries and communication within the family could be considered core factors affecting resiliency.

Social and Community Factors

As children grow older, early parent and family influences become eclipsed by social and community influences. Peer relations become crucial in helping children develop self-advocacy skills, a sense of identity in a variety of social contexts, social competence, and a sense of what is socially acceptable. Peer groups, as well as school and community adult figures, serve as valuable reinforcers and punishers of behaviors, thus shaping behaviors that are culturally accepted (Hudson et al., 2004). It stands to reason that dysfunction in these relationships, where acceptance is so highly valued, can be stressful and can pose a risk for developing behavior problems. In fact, social withdrawal has been well-supported as a correlate of anxiety in youngsters (Strauss et al., 1986), just as peer rejection, alienation, and isolation have been identified as risk factors for developing psychopathology (Greenberg et al., 2001). Furthermore, a cycle has been posited wherein "social reservedness has been found to be associated with anxiety, vulnerability, submissiveness, lack of adventuresomeness, and negative self-perceptions of social, cognitive, physical, and general attributes" and "these negative self-perceptions may generalize to the social realm, resulting in impaired peer interactions" (Hartup, 1983, as cited in Hudson et al., 2004, p. 106).

Insofar as OC symptoms in part mediated by a youngster's tenuous ability to manage stress and perceived threat, any social or community event, characteristic, or interaction that may tax a child in this way could be considered a risk factor. Such factors include an insensitive school or neighborhood culture, hostile peer interactions, unsympathetic treatment by school staff or community elders, related school failure, extreme poverty, and a resulting lack of support resources (Greenberg et al., 2001).

Again, little attention has been paid to ethnicity and gender issues with regard to social and community factors affecting risk and resiliency. However, Guerrero et al. (2003) studied over 600 adolescents in Hawaii to examine if OCD is more prevalent amongst native Hawaiians as opposed to other ethnicities, suspecting that this was so since Hawaiian and Polynesian youth are at particular risk for developing rheumatic fever (which is associated with PANDAS). The authors found indeed, that native Hawaiians had a twofold higher risk of developing OCD relative to other ethnicities. In terms of race, Greenberg et al. (2001) have identified racial injustice as a phenomenon that may place children at increased risk for psychopathology.

Social and community factors promoting resiliency have received no formal study in the pediatric OCD literature per se. However, drawing upon the anxiety and resilience work in general, and looking at the adaptive alternatives to these risk factors is a logical approach to identifying those factors that my decrease the likelihood of OCD, or at least lessen its impact. In this sense, a supportive peer group; school personnel educated in and sympathetic to OCD and other internalizing disorders;

availability of school counseling and problem-solving resources; a cohesive and peaceful neighborhood community; availability of habilitative and therapeutic community resources; stable and supportive community role models; opportunities to be challenged, to fall short, and to recover within a "safe" context; and sufficient economic means to access key resources are factors that could be considered protective or promoting of resiliency.

Evidence-Based Treatment Interventions in Community Settings

What Works

With both phobia treatment protocols (Emmelkamp, 1994) and adult OCD intervention models (Foa et al., 1980) as a logical springboard, the study of psychosocial treatments for pediatric OCD has burgeoned within the past 10 years (e.g., Piacentini et al., 2002; March, Franklin, Nelson & Foa, 2001; Franklin et al., 1998; March, Frances, Kahn & Carpenter, 1997). Specifically, cognitive-behavioral therapy (CBT) has emerged as the most efficacious psychosocial treatment to date for pediatric OCD. Emerging out of the behavioral, cognitive, and psychodynamic traditions (see Hollon & Beck, 1994; Meichenbaum, 1992), CBT approaches are based on the premise that one's beliefs, perceptions (e.g., *schemas*), and affect, and not just reinforcement or punishment, are key determinants of behavior, and vice versa (Bandura, 1978). In particular, exposure and response prevention strategies (E/RP) have proven helpful in bringing about lasting behavioral change and symptom relief. This approach is based on the belief that since threat misperception, autonomic dysregulation (i.e., the erroneous sounding of the anxiety "false alarm"), and obsessions emerge for OCD-vulnerable youngsters in response to innocuous cues or situations, sufficient exposure to this stimuli (Foa, Steketee & Millby, 1980) and to the reality that no real threat exists, facilitates the "resetting" of the "anxiety thermostat" to normal. Additionally, the preventing of the compulsion or response that a child has ritualistically engaged in order to diminish the threat and accompanying anxiety and obsessions, serves to break the maladaptive cycle of negative reinforcement wherein the temporary relief from the obsessions and fear had reinforced the "safety behavior" that had been superstitiously used.

Based upon the effectiveness of CBT approaches in treating adults with obsessive-compulsive disorder (e.g., Foa, Steketee, Grayson, Turner & Latimer, 1984; Foa et al., 1980), researchers began to adapt a protocol for treating youngsters (March & Mulle, 1998; March, Mulle & Herbel, 1994). While still considered cognitive-behavioral in orientation, this approach is a hybrid in that it integrates the most effective and appropriate techniques from several accepted therapeutic orientations, thereby ensuring that it can be applied as flexibly and efficaciously as possible (March et al., 2001). For instance, this approach integrates cognitive therapy techniques (CT) such as cognitive restructuring, self-talk or self-coaching, and attribution retraining; psychoeducation for children and parents around OCD and its neurobehavioral and chemical aspects; narrative techniques like *externalizing* the problem (Chansky, 2000; White & Epston, 1990) and addressing *unique outcomes;* family systems concepts focusing on integrating family; work and addressing the reciprocal influences of OCD between a child and his or her family; more active-directive behavioral strategies such as limit-setting, modeling, homework, and contingency management (e.g., positive reinforcement contingent upon progress); and even psychodynamic approaches involving nurturing the therapeutic alliance, insight, and internalization of behavior and perceptions.

Within the past decade, March and his colleagues (e.g., March & Mulle, 1998; March et al., 1994) have streamlined this approach into a *manualized* treatment protocol that has served as a template for numerous subsequent treatment studies of pediatric OCD. It was explicitly designed to enhance (a) patient and parental compliance, (b) exportability to other populations and settings, and (c) empirical evaluation. This involves five phases of treatment over the course of 12–20 sessions. The protocol, adapted and expanded upon from March and Mulle (1998) and March et al. (2001) is summarized in Table 1.

Table 1. 12-week OCD Treatment Protocol

Visit/step	Goals	Components	Considerations
Weeks 1 and 2	Psychoeducation and cognitive training	Establish rapport; present neurobehavioral model; externalize OCD as an "unwelcome visitor"; use appropriate metaphors: "brain hiccups," "brain lock," "false alarms," etc.	Assess treatment factors (e.g., age, developmental issues, OC features, medical profile, family psychopathology, etc); assess OC content, severity, and impairment (CY-BOCS, OCS, CGS/CHI)
Week 2	Mapping OCD, cognitive training	"Bossing back" OCD, self-talk, flexible coping strategies, positive reinforcement of accurate perceptions; determine specific obsessions, compulsions, triggers, avoidance behaviors; "easy trial" E/RP to gauge child's tolerance and compliance	Increasing sense of self-efficacy, predictability, and controllability; "map out" where child has success, where OCD has control, and where they both "win"; determine "work zone" and stimulus hierarchy: what can safely be addressed first, and so on
Weeks 3, 12	Exposure and response-prevention	Address therapy variables (e.g., comorbidity, symptom severity, family psychopathology, etc.); address situation at school via behavioral consultation model (Adams et al., 1995)	Graded (gradual) vs. flooding exposure? maximize child's control of the pace within reason; imaginal and in vivo work; in-session practice and review; homework monitored by clinician
Weeks 11, 12	Relapse prevention and generalization training	Greater use of imaginal exposure (as opposed to in vivo) and RP along with CT	Discuss relapse prevention; address termination issues and booster sessions; focus on internalization and generalization
Visits 1, 7, and 9	Parent Sessions	*Graded* involvement. Parents as collaborators/coaches.	Address family pathology, motivation, and involvement in/impact from OCD; collaboration

Beginning with this protocol's pilot use (March et al., 1994) and extending to the present (e.g., Benazon, Ager & Rosenberg, 2002; Piacentini et al., 2002;), this CBT approach has demonstrated efficacy.

In providing an overarching assessment of the pediatric OCD field and specifically, the value of various treatment protocols, periodic reviews of the literature (March et al., 2001; Riddle, 1998; March et al., 1997; March & Leonard, 1996; Thomsen, 1996; March, 1995) have consistently supported the CBT and E/RP approaches. Moreover, they have provided a valuable summary of *moderator* variables (i.e., pre-existing individual or systemic characteristics, such as demographics, comorbidity, and family functioning that may affect treatment response), *mediator* variables (i.e., characteristics or conditions within the treatment, such as compliance, that can affect treatment response) (Kazdin, 2001), and best-match characteristics. While consensus is still tenuous regarding this "which treatment, for whom, and under what circumstances?" question, some basic positive and negative predictors have emerged. More severe obsessions and OCD-related academic impairment (Piacentini et al., 2003), comorbid schizotypy (Geller et al., 2002), oppositionality (Wever & Rey, 1997), tics, family dysfunction, intellectual immaturity, poor insight, and noncompliance with treatment have all been found to be *likely* impediments to positive outcomes. Conversely, strong motivation to get well, insight into symptoms, lack of comorbidity, and the presence of clear rituals have been cited as predictors of successful OCD treatment response (March et al., 2001). However, these findings are not conclusive and thus demand further study, especially with pediatric populations.

The Expert Consensus Treatment Guidelines for Obsessive-Compulsive Disorder (March et al., 1997) surveyed 69 experts on OCD and provided an assessment of the above-mentioned factors. Specifically, selecting the components, pacing, and structure of treatment (e.g., CBT, CT, medication, combined) based on age, patient response, symptoms, time constraints, medication side effects, and comorbidity was a major focus. Additionally, treatment decision flow charts based upon these factors and interim treatment response are provided. An in-depth summary of this seminal work is beyond the purview of this chapter. However, the common findings of these experts further support CBT or combined CBT and medication as the treatment of choice for pediatric OCD and for those with milder symptoms. Specifically, the CBT and E/RP tacks are cited as best suited to clearly circumscribed symptoms such as contamination fears, symmetry, and hoarding, while less concrete symptoms such as scrupulosity, pathological doubt, and obsessive slowness are most amenable to cognitive approaches. Still, as these authors have concluded, challenges remain regarding generalizability to various populations, exportability to other settings, exactly what works in treatment (and how), how psychosocial interventions compare to placebo, and how to address relapse.

What Might Work

Considering the question of which psychosocial treatment interventions might work is an exciting prospect. This is so because several treatment directions have been explored lately which appear to hold promise for these youngsters' long-term prognoses and for the further study of pediatric OCD. One such intervention is the use of the Behavioral Avoidance Test (BAT) as a means of both achieving patient-controlled exposure to feared stimuli in the home, and assessing avoidance and related distress (Barrett, Healy & March, 2003).

Looking at treatment in the group milieu, Thienemann and colleagues (Thienemann et al., 2001) adapted March and Mulle's (1998) manualized pediatric OCD treatment protocol for use in the group format. After a 14-week CBT treatment process including E/RP, with weekly two-hour groups, 9 of the 18 participants experienced 25% or greater symptom improvement and 5 showed between 13% and 18% improvement. While the magnitude of these treatment gains are not on par with those seen in previous individual-format studies, this was likely due to several treatment adherence issues, including difficulty ensuring conscientious E/RP practice, early withdrawal from exposure trials, and limited opportunity for in vivo exposure. However, the authors of this study support the group context it promotes normalizing or "universalizing" youngsters' experiences, provides support and modeling, and may help with treatment adherence.

Gold-Steinberg & Logan (1999) investigated the possibility of integrating psychodynamically oriented *play therapy* with OCD children. While conducted in a more descriptive case study format, and admittedly a *component* of the overall treatment protocol (and not the sole approach) these authors offer a rationale for the use of play therapy based upon its recognized effectiveness in addressing treatment resistance, OCD-related feelings of shame, negative self-concept, and issues of psychosocial adjustment. In a similar adjunctive component/case-study fashion, Tolin (2001) looked at bibliotherapy in addition to the accepted CBT protocol for a 5-year-old boy with severe reassurance-seeking OCD. While no control was available, this boy's OCD symptoms remained significantly improved at one- and three-month follow-up assessments.

In the same vein, integrating psychodynamic work with established CBT protocols, and especially in later and more adjustment- and maintenance-oriented phases, could be effective with pediatric individuals. Especially as functional impairment attenuates, and identity/self-concept, family adjustment, and future issues become more conscious and developmentally salient, focused, insight-oriented work may prove to be an adjunctive treatment of choice. Psychodynamic techniques have been widely criticized as inaccessible to younger individuals, those with tenuous insight, or those with limited intellectual capacities. However, further maturation of this orientation and cross-pollination with other therapies has changed this (Marmor, 1992; Meichenbaum, 1992). Gabbard (2001) and Leib (2001) both laud the effectiveness of CBT approaches but recognize that no single treatment approach, not even CBT, will suffice for everyone. They make a case for the judicious inclusion of psychodynamic formulations to aid in working through possible developmental disruptions and disturbances in one's sense of self. Focused, time-limited dynamic psychotherapy (TLDP) techniques such as those discussed by Levenson (1995) may be best suited to this task, especially with more introspective youngsters, in later sessions, and as a child attempts to rebuild their social connections and reconcile who they were with who they have become.

Although conducted with adults, Danger Ideation Reduction Therapy (DIRT) has been investigated as a very focused "imaginal exposure" CBT variant with a cognitive "collaborative empiricism" component (Jones & Menzies, 1998). In this study, the DIRT approach was tailored specifically for compulsive washers. Components included attentional focusing, filmed interviews, corrective information, cognitive restructuring, expert testimony, microbiological experiments, and a probability of catastrophe assessment task. The objective of this protocol was to decrease danger-related expectancies, as cognitions focusing on danger and disastrous outcomes are a common characteristic of OCD individuals. In one of the few studies not using specific E/RP techniques, Jones and Menzies reported significant symptom decrease at post-treatment relative to the non-treatment comparison group. These authors argue that one advantage of DIRT over E/RP is that DIRT does not involve direct exposure to anxiety-provoking stimuli, and that the prospect of such direct interaction can lead to treatment resistance and attrition. However, comparisons to other active treatments would need to be made in order to examine DIRT's relative effectiveness.

Finally, in what may represent the cutting edge of exposure-based CBT interventions, the use of computer-generated (virtual reality) exposure continues to be explored as a useful approach with anxiety disorders, and phobias in particular. While to this writer's knowledge, no studies of these techniques have been conducted with regard to treating OCD, Robillard and colleagues (Robillard, Bouchard, Fournier & Renaud, 2003) discuss evidence of past studies (e.g., Emmelkamp et al., 2001, cited in Robillard et al., 2003) for the continued use and refinement of this methodology. In their study of anxiety arousal in therapeutic virtual environments derived from computer games (TVEDG), these investigators found that consistent with their objectives, these environments were moderately *phobogenic* and produced therapeutically useful levels of anxiety. Moreover, this milieu was demonstrated to be safe, and thus may have broad implications for therapeutically and cost-effective alternatives to in vivo techniques. What may indeed prove helpful in the treatment of pediatric OCD is that TVEDG (1) may be a logical alternative to in vivo procedures which are often logistically difficult to carry out consistently; (2) may be seen by youngsters as safer and more controllable, easier to manipulate the exposure gradient, and thus promote greater investment in the therapy; (3) may be seen by youngsters as a more contemporary, novel, and thus attractive intervention thereby maximizing investment and adherence potential; (4) may be customizable to specific and perhaps less common symptom profiles; and (5) may be well-suited to homework activities and in-home interventions.

What Does Not Work

The question of which treatments do *not* work is a difficult one to answer for two reasons: (1) the OCD literature tends not to review studies of ineffective treatments, and (2) an approach "not working" is largely a function of certain *aspects* of the treatment that are not well-suited to a particular population (e.g., or that are in need of further examination and refinement). This being said, several investigators have suggested that more insight-oriented psychodynamic psychotherapy (e.g., Gabbard, 2001; Esman, 1989; Hollingsworth, Tanguay & Grossman, 1980), particularly for younger persons with OCD, is not well-suited (March et al., 2001; March & Mulle, 1998) and has demonstrated disappointing outcomes. However, it may be that psychodynamic therapy in its purest form (which has been used effectively to treat OC personality disorder) is ineffective, while integrating aspects of it in established treatment protocols in response to certain symptom profiles, at certain phases of treatment, and framed in a developmentally appropriate fashion may be helpful (e.g., Gabbard, 2001; Leib, 2001).

Evidence-Based Treatment Interventions in Residential Settings

To this writer's knowledge, no outcome studies have been published looking at treatment of pediatric OCD in residential settings.

Psychopharmacology

In addition to the aforementioned psychosocial interventions for pediatric OCD, the pharmacological treatment of this condition has become common practice and has received significant research attention within the past 15 years. In particular, serotonin reuptake inhibitors (SRIs) and more recently, *selective* serotonin reuptake inhibitors (SSRIs) have demonstrated encouraging effectiveness in addressing pediatric OCD symptoms. An early investigation of this (Leonard et al., 1989) established the effectiveness of clomipramine (a tricyclic antidepressant and SRI under the trade name Anafranil) compared to both placebo and desipramine in 48 youngsters. A subsequent study (DeVeaugh-Geiss et al., 1992) noted a 37% CY-BOCS symptom improvement in young participants compared to 8% placebo improvement, and facilitated FDA approval of clomipramine for youngsters of aged ten years and older. Widespread study and administration of this agent (e.g., Geller et al., 2003; Haan, Hoogduin & Buttelaar, 1998; Scahill & Lynch, 1995) has since burgeoned, as has the recommendation for its judicious use, especially in combination with cognitive-behavioral interventions (March et al., 1994; 1997). Typical side effects of clomipramine, such as dry mouth, urinary retention, sexual side effects, weight gain, hepatic problems, and increased heart rate, have been noted to be similar to those found in adults (e.g., Scahill & Lynch, 1995). However, these reactions have largely been determined to be moderate relative to therapeutic gains, and have been reliably noted in pediatric studies (e.g., DeVeaugh-Geiss et al., 1992; Pigott et al., 1990). A 12-week trial of clomipramine versus behavior therapy in treating pediatric OCD (Haan et al., 1998) found significant improvement with both treatments, but interestingly, determined that stronger therapeutic changes emerged in the behavior therapy group.

The recent advent of SSRIs such as fluoxetine (trade name Prozac), paroxetine (trade name Paxil), sertraline (trade name Zoloft), and fluvoxamine (trade name Luvox) as first-line somatic treatments for adult OCD have led to their consideration for use with pediatric OCD populations. An early study of fluoxetine treatment of OCD children (Riddle et al., 1992) found a 44% symptom severity improvement with this medicine compared to 27% placebo effect after eight weeks. A later chart review investigation of fluoxetine and its relative effectiveness in children and adolescents (Geller, Biederman, Reed, Spencer & Wilens, 1995) indicated moderate to marked improvement in OCD symptoms over the 19-month follow-up period. In a subsequent study of the efficacy and tolerability of this agent (Geller, Hoog & Heiligenstein, 2001), fluoxetine (of 20–60 mg per day) was found to be associated with significantly greater improvement in OCD symptoms as compared with placebo. Moreover, it was well tolerated and with no significant difference in discontinuation of the treatment compared to placebo. Similar findings have since been demonstrated by Liebowitz et al. (2002), but again most notably after eight weeks of treatment, with a 57% symptom severity decrease at 16 weeks compared with 27% in the placebo group.

Pediatric OCD studies of other SSRIs such as sertraline have demonstrated similar efficacy. In their randomized double-blind, placebo-controlled investigation, March et al. (1998) noted significant symptom improvement in their sample of 187 youngsters on the CY-BOCS after three weeks. Using similarly rigorous methodology, a long-term study of sertraline treatment of 135 pediatric OCD individuals (Cook, Wagner & March, 2001) revealed a 25% CY-BOCS symptom severity decrease over one year. The most recent investigation of this somatic agent (Wagner, Cook, Chung & Messig, 2003) looking specifically at remission found that of those with severe OCD at baseline (i.e., CY-BOCS of 26 or greater), 55% achieved full remission (i.e., CY-BOCS of 8 or less) and 31% achieved partial remission (i.e., CY-BOCS of 15 or less).

While currently receiving less attention compared to other SSRIs in treating pediatric OCD, fluvoxamine has likewise been found to be safe and efficacious and perhaps more fast-acting. Riddle et al. (2001) found that 42% of fluvoxamine subjects achieved 25% or greater symptom reduction as compared to 26% of placebo youngsters. A review of fluvoxamine treatment in pediatric anxiety disorders (Cheer & Figgitt, 2002) supports its tolerability and efficacy not only in addressing OCD, but also in a positively affecting conditions such as generalized anxiety disorder (GAD), social phobia, and separation anxiety, with relatively moderate adverse effects. The most notable study to date on another SSRI, paroxetine, has examined its efficacy with regard to disorders comorbid with pediatric OCD (Geller et al., 2003). As has been posited previously, these investigators found that despite an encouraging 71% paroxetine response rate, these effects were significantly less in youngsters with comorbid disorders. They also noted that greater relapse rate was associated with comorbidity.

The newest of the SSRIs, citalopram (trade name Celexa), has just begun to be systematically investigated as an efficacious pharmacologic treatment for pediatric OCD. A recent long-term examination of citalopram (Thomsen, Ebbesen & Persson, 2001) observed mean CY-BOCS scores drop from 28.7 to 17.9 over the course of two years, suggesting a similar response profile to it fellow medicines in this class. Finally, in an attempt to answer the question of which SRI treatment is best for pediatric OCD, Geller et al. (2003) conducted a meta-analysis of 12 randomized, controlled, double-blind studies, including 1,044 children. These investigators found that clomipramine had the greatest effect compared with placebo, and that there were no efficacy differences among the SSRIs. However, they clarified that despite clomipramine's stronger efficacy, it is still not considered first-line therapy for pediatric OCD largely because of side effects and the need for cardiac monitoring. They concluded that medication selection should be based upon the pharmacokinetics and possible adverse effects of each agent considered.

As many youngsters may simply not respond to monotherapy, pharmacological *augmentation* may be warranted. Complementing SSRIs with an SRI such as clomipramine, and vice versa, is common and has demonstrated some efficacy. The use of typical neuroleptics (e.g., haloperidol), atypical neuroleptics (e.g., risperidone), and anti-anxiety agents such as benzodiazepines (e.g., clonazepam) to address a range of symptom and drug-response profiles has been reviewed (Grados & Riddle, 2001). Regardless of the first-line drug therapy or augmentation strategy, issues such as comorbid psychopathology (particularly depression), possible drug–drug interactions, diet, comorbid medical involvement, side effects, ethnicity, and compliance are essential considerations and demand a high level of interdisciplinary treatment coordination.

As with the management of many medical conditions such as asthma and diabetes, pharmacological effectiveness is maximized when combined with psychosocial strategies, thus equipping youngsters with the necessary behavioral "tool kit" or resources to manage their condition and help protect against loss of treatment progress (March et al, 1997; Thomsen, 1996; March & Mulle, 1998).

PANDAS

Due to the biological etiology of PANDAS, and the medical nature of the current treatments for this condition, these treatments will be discussed briefly here. The proposed model of PANDAS has opened the door for several possible and unique treatment approaches: antibiotic prophylaxis, intravenous immunoglobulin (IVIG), and plasmapheresis or plasma exchange (PEX). In short, PEX is a six- to ten-procedure protocol wherein the antibody-rich plasma of the blood is separated by a cell separator and discarded, while the cells are returned to the individual. IVIG involves intravenously administering a sterile solution of concentrated antibodies. In an early small-scale study of these treatments, Allen, Leonard, and Swedo (1995) found that in the two youngsters treated with PEX, one with IVIG, and one with prednisone, all demonstrated clinically significant responses immediately following treatment. A later double-blind, balanced, cross-over study of penicillin prophylaxis in 37 strep-positive children (Garvey et al., 1999) however, failed to produce significant symptom relief with this treatment. A recent study of this approach (Murphy & Pichichero, 2002), focused more on the *timing* of antibiotic prophylaxis, found that in children treated with antibiotics effective in eradicating GABHS infection at the sentinel episode, OCD symptoms disappeared quickly. Of those individuals who later experienced recurrence of OCD symptoms, each case was clearly associated with subsequent GABHS infection and responded once again to antibiotics.

Immunomodulatory approaches such as PEX and IVIG, which are more invasive than simple antibiotic treatment, have also been effectively applied (Snider & Swedo, 2003; Leonard & Swedo, 2001).

The Prevention of Obsessive-Compulsive Disorder in Adolescence

What Works

Unfortunately, there are no available studies on the prevention of OCD.

What Might Work

Obviously, early identification of youngsters at possible risk for developing OCD is important. This would involve coordination between parents, school counselors and staff, and possibly community mental health professionals. As of yet, no reliable risk factors for OCD have been convincingly identified. However, individual characteristics such as behavioral inhibition, anxiety, OC and ritualistic tendencies, tic symptoms, the tendency to catastrophize and personalize relatively innocuous stressors, coping fragility, and the inordinate need to maintain a semblance of predictability and controllability may be important to note. In addition, parental over- protectiveness and intrusiveness, a parental OC style, family accommodation of a child's rituals, and parental "rescuing" of their child when facing a conflict or other stressful situation are important factors. Finally, identifying social and community risk factors such as insensitive or poorly trained school staff, peer rejection or bullying, self-isolation, academic struggle, and a generally hostile and/or competitive school environment is important. The challenge here is that compared to classic "high-risk" behaviors such as drug abuse, sexual acting out, and antisocial behavior, pediatric OCD and other anxiety disorders are less visible, may be seen as less problematic, and thus fall low on a priority list when it comes to mobilizing school resources.

Minimizing these identified risk factors while enhancing internal resiliency resources would be important in any prevention efforts. This could be accomplished in a variety of ways. With regard to minimizing risk factors, educating parents (especially in relation to family aggregation issues), school and community leaders, and students about anxiety disorders and OCD in particular, and the very visible functional impairment implications, is a logical first step. This could aid early identification as well as help create more tolerant environments for those with the condition. With regard to enhancing resiliency, and as socially mediated stress can play a significant role in symptom exacerbation and functional impairment, efforts to help youngsters cope more flexibly with such challenges is crucial. This should involve supportive exposure to moderately stressful situations, and a systematic titration of external supports, such that these children can eventually manage increasing demands without perceiving them as threatening or overwhelming.

In their comprehensive examination of the state of the prevention field, Greenberg et al. (2001) reviewed a number of notable internalizing and stress-related programs that address these notions. Specifically, the Stress Inoculation Training (SIT) I and SIT II programs (Hains & Ellman, 1994; Hains, 1992) aimed at reducing negative emotional arousal and increasing coping and assertiveness skills in youngsters, demonstrated significant changes in anxiety and depressive symptomatology. While aimed at preventing depression, the Coping with Stress Program (Clarke et al., 1995, as cited in Greenberg et al., 2001) and the Penn Prevention Program (Gilham, Reivich, Jaycox & Seligman, 1994, as cited in Greenberg et al., 2001; Jaycox, Reivich, Gilham & Seligman, 1994) seemed to demonstrate initial promise and perhaps could be modified to address anxiety disorders. The only anxiety-specific prevention program reviewed was the Queensland Early Intervention and Prevention of Anxiety Project (Dadds et al., 1999; Dadds, Spence, Holland, Barrett & Laurens, 1997). This project was designed to teach youngsters cognitive, behavioral, and physiological coping strategies while exposing them to increasingly fearful situations. Encouragingly, anxious individuals developed significantly less internalizing disorders than the placebo group at six months post-intervention.

Finally, in one study aimed at addressing anxiety associated with intrusive thoughts and thought-action fusion, Zucker, Craske, Barrios, and Holguin (2002) demonstrated the efficacy of listening to a brief psychoeducational audiotape about the fallacy of thought–action fusion. Furthermore, Zucker and Craske (cited in Story, Zucker & Craske, 2004) are currently investigating a three-hour group CBT intervention for college students with subclinical OC symptoms, based on the premise that this condition may be a precursor to bona fide OCD.

What Does Not Work

Data does not exist to identify preventive practices that would not work.

Recommendations

While pediatric OCD is a heterogeneous condition in terms of symptom breadth and severity, the current literature and clinical wisdom are clear in their recommendations for best practice. Cognitive-behavioral therapy (CBT) centered on systematic exposure and response prevention (E/RP), and combined with a selective serotonin reuptake inhibitor (SSRI) regimen, remains the current treatment of choice for children and adolescents (e.g., Franklin et al., 2003; Geller et al., 2003; March et al., 1997; March & Mulle, 1998). Tailoring this protocol with respect to a child's symptom severity, developmental, familial, and comorbidity issues is crucial. This may involve, for example, taking a more cognitive and less directive approach, adjusting the pacing or patient control of the process, modifying or excluding family involvement, an extended rapport-building phase, and first addressing more emergent conditions behaviorally and/or pharmacologically before addressing a child's OCD challenges. This may also involve imbuing later stages of the therapy with more insight-oriented work to address the meanings that a child ascribes to having (or having struggled with OCD), as well as addressing changes in a youngster's sense of self, their interpersonal relatedness, and future strivings in relation to treatment gains they may have made. Interventions should be conducted by qualified clinicians specifically trained in these approaches, and should include multisystemic involvement and support (i.e., key individuals from school, clinic, family, community) whenever feasible.

As school and related developmental experiences play such a significant role in youngsters' lives, coordinating intervention and support with trained and sensitive school counselors is an important component of treatment (Adams, Waas, March & Smith (1995). In addition, and just as a child's obsessions and rituals can entangle a family system, these behaviors can also negatively impact a child's school *system*. Thus, effective collaboration is likely to aid in preventing this dynamic, as well as in maintaining treatment gains, minimizing peer alienation, making appropriate referrals, improving social and coping skills, and enhancing key stress- and anxiety-management skills. Most importantly, however, it can serve as a valuable vehicle for preventing further functional impairment, which can be devastating in the school environment and beyond.

Finally, ever-improving computer technology means that we are closer than ever to developing effective computer-aided exposure interventions specific to treating pediatric patients. While to this writer's knowledge there are no such known applications in current use with pediatric OCD, recommendations for best practice should include a call to develop such technologies. This would be crucial in providing a reasonable alternative or preliminary step toward in vivo exposure; may be experienced as easier to manipulate the exposure gradient, and thus promote greater investment in the therapy; may be seen by youngsters as a more contemporary, novel, and thus attractive intervention, thereby maximizing investment and adherence potential; may help make treatment protocols easier to follow, more consistent, and thus more replicable both for research and clinical purposes; may be customizable to specific and perhaps less common symptom profiles; and may be well suited to homework activities and in-home interventions.

References

Abramowitz, J.S., Franklin, M.E., Schwartz, S.A., & Furr, J.M. (2003). Symptom presentation and outcome of cognitive-behavioral therapy for obsessive-compulsive disorder. *Journal of Consulting and Clinical Psychology, 71(6)*, 1049–1057.

Adams, G.B., Waas, G.A., March, J.S., & Smith, M.C. (1995). Obsessive-compulsive disorder in children and adolescents: The role of the school psychologist in identification, assessment, and treatment. School Psychology Quarterly, 91(4), 274–294.

Ainsworth, M.D.S., Blehar, M., Waters, E., & Wall, S. (1978). *Patterns of attachment: a psychological study of the strange situation.* Hillsdale, NJ: Erlbaum.

Allen, A.J., Leonard, H.L., & Swedo, S.E. (1995). Case study: A new infection-triggered autoimmune subtype of pediatric obsessive-compulsive disorder and tourette's syndrome. *Journal of the American Academy of Child and Adolescent Psychiatry, 34*, 307–311.

American Psychiatric Association. (2000). *Diagnostic and Statistical Manual of Mental Disorders* (4th ed.), treatment revision. Washington, DC: Author.

Arnold, P.D., & Richter, M.A. (2001). Is obsessive-compulsive disorder an autoimmune disease? *Canadian Medical Association Journal, 165*(10), 1353–1358.

Ayres, J.L. (2000). Obsessive-compulsive disorder in children and adolescents: A longitudinal study. *Dissertation Abstracts International, 61*(6–B), 3269. University Microfilms International.

Baer, L., & Jenike, M.A. (1992). Personality disorders in obsessive-compulsive disorder. *The Psychiatric Clinics of North America, 15*(4), 803–812.

Bandura, A. (1978). The self-system in reciprocal determinism. *American Psychologist, 33*, 344–358.

Barlow, D.H. (2000). Unraveling the mysteries of anxiety and its disorders from thee perspective of emotion theory. *American Psychologist, 55*(11), 1247–1263.

Barrett, P., Healy, L., & March, J.S. (2003). Behavioral avoidance test for childhood obsessive-compulsive disorder. *American Journal of Psychotherapy, 57*(1), 80–100.

Barrett, P., Shortt, A., & Healy, L. (2002). Do parents and child behaviours differentiate families whose children have obsessive-compulsive disorder from other clinic and non-clinic families? *Journal of Child Psychology & Psychiatry & Allied Disciplines, 43*(5), 597–607.

Bartholomew, K. (1993). From childhood to adult relationships: Attachment theory and research. In S. Duck (Ed.), *Understanding Relationship Process Series: Vol. 2. Learning About Relationships* (pp. 30–62). Newbury Park: Sage Publications.

Baxter, L.R.J., Schwartz, J.M., Bergman, K.S., Szuba, M.P., Guze, B.H., Mazziotta, J.C., Alazraki, A., Selin, C.E., Ferng, H.K., & Munford, P. (1992). Caudate glucose metabolic rate changes with both drug and behavioral therapy for obsessive-compulsive disorder. *Archives of General Psychiatry, 49*, 681–689.

Beckstein, C.L. (2001). Gender differences in obsessive-compulsive disorder symptomatology. *Dissertation Abstracts International, 62*(6B), 2950. University Microfilms International.

Benazon, N.R., Ager, J., & Rosenberg, D.R. (2002). Cognitive behavior therapy with treatment-naïve children and adolescents with obsessive-compulsive disorder: An open trial. *Behaviour Research and Therapy, 40*, 529–539.

Black, D.W., Gaffney, G.R., Schlosser, S., & Gabel, J. (2003). Children of parents with obsessive-compulsive disorder: A 2-year follow-up study. *Acta Psychiatrica Scandinavica, 107*(4)., 305–313.

Bogetto, F., Venturello, S., Albert, U., Maina, G., & Ravizza, L. (2000). Gender-related clinical differences in obsessive-compulsive disorder. *European Psychiatry, 14*(8), 434–441.

Bowlby, J. (1979). The Making and Breaking of Affectional Bonds. London: Tavistock.

Bowlby, J. (1986). The nature of the child's tie to his mother. In P. Buckley (Ed.), *Essential Papers on Object Relations* (pp. 153–199). New York: New York University Press.

Chansky, T.E. (2000). *Freeing Your Child from Obsessive-Compulsive Disorder.* New York: Three Rivers Press.

Cheer, S.M., & Figgitt, D.P. (2002). Spotlight on fluvoxamine in anxiety disorders in children and adolescence. *CNS Drugs, 16*(2), 139–144.

Cook, E.H., Wagner, K.D., & March, J.S. (2001). Long-term sertraline treatment of children and adolescents with obsessive-compulsive disorder. *Journal of the American Academy of Child and Adolescent Psychiatry, 40*(10), 1175–1181.

Dadds, M.R., Holland, D.E., Laurens, K.R., Mullins, M., Barrett, P.M., Spence, S.H. (1999). Early intervention and prevention of anxiety disorders in children: Results at 2-year follow-up. *Journal of Consulting
and Clinical Psychology, 67*, 145–150.

Dadds, M.R., Spence, S.H., Holland, D.E., Barrett, P.M., Laurens, K.R. (1997). Prevention and early intervention of anxiety disorders: A controlled trial. *Journal of Consulting and Clinical Psychology, 65*,
627–635.

DeVeaugh-Geiss, J., Moroz, G., Biederman, J., Cantwell, D., Fontaine, R., Greist, J.H., Reichler, R., Katz, R.,
& Landau, P. (1992). Clomipramine hydrochloride in childhood and adolescent obsessive-compulsive
disorder- a multicenter trial. *Journal of the American Academy of Child and Adolescent Psychiatry, 31*, 45–59.

Douglass, H.M., Moffitt, T.E., Dar, R., McGee, R., & Silva, P. (1995). Obsessive-compulsive disorder in a
birth cohort of 18-year olds: Prevalence and predictors. *Journal of the American Academy of Child and
Adolescent Psychiatry, 34*(11), 1424–1431.

DuPont, R.L., Rice, D.P., Shiraki, S. & Rowland, C. (1994). *Economic Costs of Obsessive-Compulsive Disorder.*
Unpublished manuscript.

Emmelkamp, P.M.G. (1994). Behavior therapy with adults. In A.E. Bergin & S.L. Garfield (Eds.), *Handbook
of Psychotherapy and Behavior Change* (4th ed., pp. 379–427). New York: Wiley.

Esman, A. (1989). Psychoanalysis in general psychiatry: Obsessive-compulsive disorder as a paradigm.
Journal of the American Psychoanalytical Association, 37, 319–336.

Evans, D.W., Milanak, M.E., Medeiros, B., & Ross, J.L. (2002). Magical beliefs and rituals in young children.
Child Psychiatry and Human Development. 33(1), 43–58.

Fitzgibbons, L. & Pedrick, C. (2003). *Helping Your Child with OCD: A Workbook for Parents of Children with
Obsessive-Compulsive Disorder.* Oakland, CA: New Harbinger Publications.

Flament, M.F., Whitaker, A., Rapoport, J.L., Davies, M., Berg, C.Z., Kalikow, K., Sceery, W., & Shaffer, D.
(1988). Obsessive-compulsive disorder in adolescence: An epidemiological study. *Journal of the American
Academy of Child and Adolescent Psychiatry, 27*(6), 764–771.

Foa, E.B., Steketee, G., Grayson, B., Turner, M., & Latimer, P. (1984). Deliberate exposure and blocking of
obsessive-compulsive rituals: Immediate and long-term effects. *Behavior Therapy, 15*, 450–472.

Foa, E.B., Steketee, G., & Millby, J.B. (1980). Differential effects of exposure and response prevention in
obsessive-compulsive washers. *Journal of Consulting and Clinical Psychology, 48*(1), 71–79.

Franklin, M., Foa, E., & March, J.S. (2003). The pediatric obsessive-compulsive disorder treatment study:
Rationale, design, and methods. *Journal of Child and Adolescent Psychopharmacology, 13*(Suppl. 1), 39–51.

Franklin, M.E., Kozak, M.J., Cashman, L.A., Coles, M.E., Rheingold, A.A., & Foa, E.B. (1998). Cognitive
behavior treatment of pediatric obsessive-compulsive disorder: An open clinical trial. *Journal of the
American Academy of Child and Adolescent Psychiatry, 37*(4), 412–419.

Freeman, J.B., Garcia, A.M., Fucci, C., Karitani, M., Miller, L., & Leonard, H.L. (2003). Family-based treatment of early-onset obsessive-compulsive disorder. *Journal of Child and Adolescent Psychopharmacology,
13*(1), 71–80.

Freud, S. (1966). *Introductory Lectures on Psychoanalysis.* New York: Norton.

Frost, R.O., & Steketee, G. (1997). Perfectionism in obsessive-compulsive disorder. *Behaviour Research and
Therapy, 35*, 291–296.

Gabbard, G.O. (2001). Psychoanalytically informed approaches to the treatment of obsessive-compulsive
disorder. *Psychoanalytic Inquiry, 21*(2), 208–221.

Garvey, M.A., Perlmutter, S.J., Allen, A.J., Hamburger, S., Lougee, L., Leonard, H.L., Witowski, M.E., Dub-
bert, B., & Swedo, S.E. (1999). A pilot study of penicillin prophylaxis for neuropsychiatric exacerbations triggered by streptococcal infections. *Biological Psychiatry, 45*(12), 1564–1571.

Geller, D.A., Biederman, J., Faraone, S.V., Cradock, K., Hagermoser, L., Zaman, N., Frazier, J.A., Coffey,
B.J., Spencer, T.J. (2002). Attention-deficit/hyperactivity disorder in children and adolescents with
obsessive-compulsive disorder: Fact or artifact? *Journal of the American Academy of Child and Adolescent
Psychiatry, 41*(1), 52–58.

Geller, D.A., Biederman, J., Jones, J., Park, K., Schwartz, S., Shapiro, S., & Coffey, B. (1998). Is juvenile
obsessive-compulsive disorder a developmental subtype of the disorder? A review of the pediatric literature. *Journal of the American Academy of Child and Adolescent Psychiatry, 37*(4), 420–427.

Geller, D.A., Biederman, J., Reed, E.D., Spencer, T., & Wilens, T.E. (1995). Similarities in response to fluoxetine treatment of children and adolescents with obsessive-compulsive disorder. *Journal of the American
Academy of Child and Adolescent Psychiatry, 34*(1), 36–44.

Geller, D.A., Biederman, J., Stewart, E., Mullin, B., Farrell, C., Wagner, K.D., Emslie, G., & Carpenter, D.
(2003). A meta-analysis of pharmacotherapy trials in pediatric obsessive-compulsive disorder. *American
Journal of Psychiatry, 160*, 1919–1928.

Geller, D.A., Hoog, S.L., & Heiligenstein, J.H. (2001). Fluoxetine treatment for obsessive-compulsive disorder in children and adolescents: A placebo-controlled clinical trial. *Journal of the American Academy of Child and Adolescent Psychiatry, 40*(7), 773–779.

Geller, D.A., Wagner, K.D., Emslie, G.J., Murphy, T.K., Gallagher, D., Gardiner, C., & Carpenter, D.J. (2002). Efficacy of paroxetine in pediatric OCD: Results of a multicenter study. *Annual Meeting New Research Program and Abstracts* (No. 349). Washington DC: American Psychiatric Association.

Gold-Steinberg, S., & Logan, D. (1999). Integrating play therapy in the treatment of children with obsessive-compulsive disorder. *American Journal of Orthopsychiatry, 69*(4), 495–503.

Grabe, H.J., Meyer, C., Hapke, U., Rumpf, H.J., Freyberger, H.J., Dilling, H., & John, U. (2000). Prevalence, quality of life and psychosocial function in obsessive-compulsive disorder and subclinical obsessive-compulsive disorder in northern Germany. *European Archives of Psychiatry & Clinical Neurosciences, 250*(5), 262–268.

Grados, M.A., & Riddle, M.A. (2001). Pharmacological treatment of childhood obsessive-compulsive disorder: From theory to practice. *Journal of Clinical Child Psychology, 30*(1), 67–79.

Greenberg, M.T., Dimitrovich, C., & Bumbarger, B. (2001). The prevention of mental disorders in school-aged children: Current state of the field. *Prevention & Treatment, 4,* Article 1. Retrieved from http://journals.apa.org/prevention/volume4/pre0040001a.html

Greisberg, S., & McKay, D. (2003). Neuropsychology of obsessive-compulsive disorder: A review and treatment implications. *Clinical Psychology Review, 23*(1), 95–117.

Grunes, M.S. (1999). Family involvement in the behavioral treatment of obsessive-compulsive disorder. *Dissertation Abstracts International, 59*(9–B), 5083. University Microfilms International.

Guerrero, A.P., Hishinuma, E.S., Andrade, N.N., Bell, C.K., Kurahara, D.K., Lee, T.G., Turner, H., Andrus, J., Yuen, N.Y., & Stokes, A.J. (2003). Demographic and clinical characteristics of adolescents in Hawaii with obsessive-compulsive disorder. *Archives of Pediatrics and Adolescent Medicine, 157*(7), 665–670.

Haan, E.de, Hoogduin, K.A., & Buttelaar, J.K. (1998). Behavior therapy versus clomipramine for the treatment of obsessive-compulsive disorder in children and adolescents. *Journal of the American Academy of Child and Adolescent Psychiatry, 37*(10), 1022–1029.

Hains, A.A. (1992). Comparison of cognitive-behavioral stress management techniques with adolescent boys. *Journal of Counseling & Development, 70,* 600–605.

Hains, A.A., & Ellman, S.W. (1994). Stress inoculation training as a preventative intervention for high school youths. *Journal of Cognitive Psychotherapy, 8,* 219–232.

Hartston, H.J. (2000). Inhibitory deficits in obsessive-compulsive disorder. *Dissertation Abstracts International, 60*(11B). University Microfilms International.

Hettema, J.M., Neale, M.C., & Kendler, K.S. (2001). A review and meta-analysis of the genetic epidemiology of anxiety disorders. *American Journal of Psychiatry, 158*(10), 1568–1578.

Heyman, I., Fombonne, E., Simmons, H., Ford, T., Meltzer, H. & Goodman, R. (2001). Prevalence of obsessive-compulsive disorder in the British nationwide survey of child mental health. *The British Journal of Psychiatry: The Journal of Mental Science, 179,* 324–329.

Hollingsworth, C., Tanguay, P., & Grossman, L. (1980). Long-term outcome of obsessive-compulsive disorder in childhood. *Journal of the American Academy of Child Psychiatry, 19,* 134–144.

Hollon, S.D. & Beck, A.T. (1994) Cognitive and cognitive behavioral therapies. In A.E. Bergin & S.L. Garfield (Eds.), *Handbook of Psychotherapy and Behavior Change* (4th ed., pp. 428–466). New York: Wiley.

Honjo, S., Hirano, C., Murase, S., Kaneko, T., Sugiyama, T., Ohtaka, K., Aoyama, T., Takei, Y., Inoko, K., & Wakabayashi, S. (1989). Obsessive-compulsive symptoms in childhood and adolescence. *Acta Psychiatrica Scandinavica, 80,* 83–91.

Hudson, J.L., Flannery-Schroeder, E., & Kendall, P.C. (2004). Primary prevention of anxiety disorders. In D.J.A. Dozois & K.S. Dobson (Eds.), *The Prevention of Anxiety and Depression: Research, Theory, and Practice* (pp. 101–130). Washington, DC: American Psychological Association.

Jaycox, L.H., Reivich, K.J., Gilham, J.E., & Seligman, M.E.P. (1994). Prevention of depression symptoms in school children. *Behavior Research & Therapy, 32,* 801–816.

Jenike, M.A., Breiter, H.C., Baer, L., Kennedy, D.N., Savage, C.R., Olivares, M.J., O'Sullivan, R.L., Shera, D.M., Rauch, S.L., Keuthen, N., Rosen, B.R., Caviness, V.S., & Filipek, P.A. (1996). Cerebral structural abnormalities in obsessive-compulsive disorder. A quantitative morphometric magnetic resonance imaging study. *Archives of General Psychiatry, 53,* 625–632.

Jones, M.K., & Menzies, R.G. (1998). Danger ideation reduction therapy (DIRT) for obsessive-compulsive disorder. *Behaviour Research & Therapy, 36,* 959–970.

Kagan, J. (1997). Temperament and the reactions to unfamiliarity. *Child Development, 68,* 139–143.

Kazdin, A. (2001). Bridging the enormous gaps of theory with therapy research and practice. *Journal of Clinical Child Psychology, 30*(1), 59–66.

Karno, M., Golding, J.M., Sorenson, S.B., & Burnam, M.A. (1988). The epidemiology of obsessive-compulsive disorder in five US communities. *Archives of General Psychiatry, 45*, 1094–1099.

Keijsers, G.P., Hoogduin, C.A., & Schaap, C.P. (1994). Predictors of treatment outcome in the behavioral treatment of obsessive-compulsive disorder. *The British Journal of Psychiatry: The Journal of Mental Science, 165*(6), 781–786.

Last, C.G., & Strauss, C.C. (1989). Obsessive–compulsive disorders in childhood. *Journal of Anxiety Disorders, 3*(4), 295–302.

Leckman, J.F., Grice, D.E., Boardman, J., Zhang, H., Vitale, A., Bondi, C., Alsobrook, J., Peterson, B.S., Cohen, D.J., Rasmussen, S.S., Goodman, W.K., McDougle, C.J. & Pauls, D.L. (1997). Symptoms of obsessive-compulsive disorder. *American Journal of Psychiatry, 152*, 76–84.

Leib, P.T. (2001). Integrating behavior modification and pharmacotherapy with the psychoanalytic treatment of obsessive-compulsive disorder: A case study. *Psychoanalytic Inquiry, 21*(2), 222–241.

Lemelson, R.B. (2000). Re-checking the color of chickens: Indigenous, ethnographic, and clinical perspectives on obsessive-compulsive disorder and tourette's syndrome in Bali. *Dissertation Abstracts International, 60*(9-A), 3419. University Microfilms International.

Lensi, P., Cassano, G.B., Correddu, G., Ravagli, S., & Kunovac, J.L. (1996). Obsessive-compulsive disorder. Familial developmental history, symptomatology, comorbidity and course with special reference to gender-related differences. *British Journal of Psychiatry, 169*(1), 101–107.

Leonard, H.L., Goldberger, E.L., Rapoport, J.L., Cheslow, D.L., & Swedo, S.E. (1990). Childhood rituals: Normal development or obsessive-compulsive symptoms? *Journal of the American Academy of Child and Adolescent Psychiatry, 29*(1), 17–23.

Leonard, H.L., & Swedo, S.E. (2001). Paediatric autoimmune neuropsychiatric disorders associated with streptococcal infection (PANDAS). *International Journal of Neuropsychopharmacology, 4*(2), 1919–198.

Leonard, H.L., Swedo, S.E., Rapoport, J.L., Koby, E.V., Lenane, M., Cheslow, D.L., & Hamburger, S.D. (1989). Treatment of obsessive-compulsive disorder with clomipramine and desipramine in children and adolescents. A double-blind cross-over comparison. *Archives of General Psychiatry, 46*, 1088–1092.

Levenson, H. (1995). *Time-Limited Dynamic Psychotherapy: A Guide to Clinical Practice*. New York: Basic Books.

Liebowitz, M.R., Turner, S.M., Piacentini, J., Beidel, D.C., Clarvit, S.R., Davies, S.O., Graae, F., Jaffer, M., Lin, S.H., Sallee, F.R., Schmidt, A.B., & Simposon, H.B. (2002). Fluoxetine in children and adolescents with OCD: A placebo-controlled trial. *Journal of the American Academy of Child and Adolescent Psychiatry, 41*(12), 1431–1438.

Lin, H., Yeh, C.B., Peterson, B.S., Scahill, L., Grantz, H., Findley, D.B., Katsovich, L., Otka, J., Lombroso, P.J., King, R.A., Leckman, J.F. (2002). Assessment of symptom exacerbations in a longitudinal study of children with Tourette's syndrome or obsessive-compulsive disorder. *Journal of the American Academy of Child and Adolescent Psychiatry, 41*(9), 1070–1077.

Lochner, C. & Stein, D.J. (2003). Heterogeneity of obsessive-compulsive disorder: A literature review. *Harvard Review of Psychiatry, 11*(3), 113–132.

Lougee, L., Perlmutter, S.J., Nicholson, R., Garvey, M.A., & Swedo, S.E. (2000). Psychiatric disorders in first-degree relatives of children with pediatric autoimmune neuropsychiatric disorders associated with streptococcal infections (PANDAS). *Journal of the American Academy of Child and Adolescent Psychiatry, 39*(9), 1120–1126.

March, J.S. (1995). Cognitive-behavioral psychotherapy for children and adolescents with OCD: A review and recommendations for treatment. *Journal of the American Academy of Child and Adolescent Psychiatry, 34*(1), 7–18.

March, J.S., Biederman, J., Wolkow, R., Safferman, A., Mardekian, J., Cook, E.H., Cutler, N.R., Dominguez, R., Ferguson, J., Muller, B., Riesenberg, R., Rosenthal, M., Sallee, F.R., & Wagner, K.D. (1998). Sertraline in children and adolescents with obsessive-compulsive disorder: A multicenter randomized controlled trial. *Journal of the American Medical Association, 280*, 1752–1756.

March, J.S., Frances, A, Kahn, D., & Carpenter, D. (1997). Expert consensus guidelines: Treatment of obsessive-compulsive disorder. *Journal of Clinical Psychiatry, 58*(Suppl. 4), 1–72.

March, J.S., Franklin, M., Nelson, A., & Foa, E. (2001). Cognitive-behavioral psychotherapy for pediatric obsessive-compulsive disorder. *Journal of Clinical Child Psychology, 30*(1), 8–18.

March, J.S., & Leonard, H.L. (1996). Obsessive-compulsive disorder in children and adolescents: A review of the past 10 years. *Journal of the American Academy of Child and Adolescent Psychiatry, 35*(10), 1265–1273.

March, J.S. & Mulle, K. (1998). *OCD in Children and Adolescents: A Cognitive-Behavioral Manual*. New York: Guilford.

March, J.S., Mulle, K., & Herbel, B. (1994). Behavioral psychotherapy for children and adolescents with obsessive-compulsive disorder: An open trial of a new protocol-driven treatment package. *Journal of the American Academy of Child and Adolescent Psychiatry, 33*, 333–341.

Marmor, J. (1992). The essence of dynamic psychotherapy. In J.K. Zeig (Ed.), *The Evolution of Psychotherapy: The Second Conference* (pp. 189–200). New York: Brunner Mazel.

Meichenbaum, D. (1992). Evolution of cognitive behavior therapy: Origins, tenets, and clinical examples. In J.K. Zeig (Ed.), *The Evolution of Psychotherapy: The Second Conference* (pp. 114–128). New York: Brunner Mazel.

Mrazek, P.J., & Haggerty, R.J. (Eds.). (1994). *Reducing Risks for Mental Disorders: Frontiers for Preventive Intervention Research*. Washington, DC: National Academy Press.

Murphy, M.L., & Pichichero, M.E. (2002). Prospective identification and treatment of children with pediatric autoimmune neuropsychiatric disorder associated with group A streptococcal infection (PANDAS). *Archives of Pediatric Adolescent Medicine, 156*(4), 356–361.

Nestadt, G., Samuels, J., Riddle, M., Bienvenu, O.J., Liang, K.Y., LaBuda, M., Walkup, J., Grados, M., & Hoehn-Saric, R. (2000). A family study of obsessive-compulsive disorder. *Archives of General Psychiatry, 57*(4), 358–363.

Noshirvani, H.F., Kasvikis, Y., Marks, I.M., Tsakiris, F., et al. (1991). Gender-divergent aetiological factors in obsessive-compulsive disorder. *British Journal of Psychiatry, 158*, 260–263.

O'Leary, K.D. & Wilson, T.G. (1975). *Behavior therapy: Application and outcome*. New Jersey: Prentice Hall.

Pauls, D.L., Alsobrook, J.P., Goodman, W., Rasmussen, S., & Leckman, J.F. (1995). A family study of obsessive-compulsive disorder. *American Journal of Psychiatry, 152*, 76–84.

Piacentini, J., Bergman, R.L., Jacobs, C., McCracken, J.T., & Kretchman, J. (2002). Open trial of cognitive behavior therapy for childhood obsessive-compulsive disorder. *Journal of Anxiety Disorders, 16*(2), 207–219.

Piacentini, J., Bergman, L., Keller, M., & McCracken, J. (2003). Functional impairment in children and adolescents with obsessive-compulsive disorder. *Journal of Child and Adolescent Psychopharmacology, 13*(Suppl. 1), 61–69.

Pigott, T.A., Pato, M.T., Bernstein, S.E., Grover, G.N., Hill, J.L., Tolliver, T.J., & Murphy, D.L. (1990). Controlled comparisons of clomipramine and fluoxetine in the treatment of obsessive-compulsive disorder. Behavioral and biological results. *Archives of General Psychiatry, 47*, 926–932.

Raphael, F.J., Rani, S., Bale, R., & Drummond, L.M. (1996). Religion, ethnicity, and obsessive-compulsive disorder. *International Journal of Social Psychiatry, 42*(1), 38–44.

Rasmussen, S., & Eisen, J. (1992). The epidemiology and clinical features of obsessive-compulsive disorder. *Psychiatric Clinics of North America, 15*, 743–758.

Riddle, M. (1998). Obsessive-compulsive disorder in children and adolescents. *The British Journal of Psychiatry, 35*(Suppl.), 91–96.

Riddle, M.A., Reeve, E.A., Yaryura-Tobias, J.A., Yang, H.M., Claghorn, J.L., Gaffney, G., Greist, J.H., Holland, D., McConville, B.J., Pigott, T., & Walkup, J.T. (2001). Fluvoxamine for children and adolescents with obsessive-compulsive disorder: A randomized, controlled, multicenter trial. *Journal of the American Academy of Child and Adolescent Psychiatry, 40*(2), 222–229.

Riddle, M.A., Scahill, L., King, R.A., Hardin, M.T., Anderson, G.M., Ort, S.I., Smith, J.C., Leckman, J.F., & Cohen, D.J. (1992). Double-blind, crossover trial of fluoxetine and placebo in children and adolescents with obsessive-compulsive disorder. *Journal of the American Academy of Child and Adolescent Psychiatry, 31*, 1062–1069.

Robillard, G., Bouchard, S., Fournier, T., & Renaud, P. (2003). Anxiety and presence during VR immersion: A comparative study of the reactions of phobic and non-phobic participants in therapeutic virtual environments derived from computer games. *CyberPsychology & Behavior, 6*(5), 467–476.

Savage, C.R., & Rauch, S.L. (2000). Cognitive deficits in obsessive-compulsive disorder. *American Journal of Psychiatry, 157*(7), 1182.

Scahill, L., & Lynch, K.A. (1995). *Clomipramine and obsessive-compulsive disorder*. *Journal of Child and Adolescent Psychiatric Nursing, 8*(2), 42–45.

Snider, L.A., & Swedo, S. E. (2003). Childhood-onset obsessive-compulsive disorder and tic disorders: Case report and literature review. *Journal of Child and Adolescent Psychopharmacology, 13*(Suppl. 1), 81–88.

Stein, M.B., Forde, D.R., & Anderson, G. (1997). Obsessive-compulsive disorder in the community: An epidemiological survey with clinical reappraisal. *The American Journal of Psychiatry, 54*, 1120–1126.

Story, T.J., Zucker, B.G., & Craske, M.G. (2004). Secondary prevention of anxiety disorders. In D.J.A. Dozois & K.S. Dobson (Eds.), *The Prevention of Anxiety and Depression: Theory, Research & Practice*. Washington, DC: American Psychological Association.

Strauss, C.C., Forehand, R., Smith, K., & Frame, C.L. (1986). The association between social withdrawal and internalizing problems of children. *Journal of Abnormal Psychology, 14,* 525–535.

Swedo, S.E., Leonard, H.L., & Rapoport, J.L. (1992). Childhood onset obsessive-compulsive disorder. *Psychiatric Clinics of North America, 15*(4), 767–775.

Swedo, S.E., Rapoport, J.L., Leonard, H., Lenane, M.C., & Cheslow, D.L. (1989). Obsessive-compulsive disorder in children and adolescents: Clinical phenomenology of 70 consecutive cases. *Archives of General Psychiatry, 46,* 335–341.

Swedo, S. E., Schapiro, M.B., Grady, C.L., Cheslow, D.L., et al. (1989). Cerebral glucose metabolism in childhood onset obsessive-compulsive disorder. *Archives of General Psychiatry, 46*(6), 518–523.

Thienemann, M., Martin, J., Cregger, B., Thompson, H.B., & Dyer-Friedman, J.J. (2001). Manual-driven group cognitive-behavioral therapy for adolescents with obsessive-compulsive disorder: A pilot study. *Journal of the American Academy of Child and Adolescent Psychiatry, 40*(11), 1254–1260.

Thomsen, P.F. (1996). Treatment of obsessive-compulsive disorder in children and adolescents: A review of the literature. *European Child and Adolescent Psychiatry, 5*(2), 55–66.

Thomsen, P.H., Ebbesen, C., & Persson, C. (2001). Long-term experience with citalopram in the treatment of adolescent OCD. *Journal of the American Academy of Child and Adolescent Psychiatry, 40*(8), 895–902.

Thomsen, P.H., & Mikkelsen, H.U. (1991). Children and adolescents with obsessive-compulsive disorder: The demographic and diagnostic characteristics of 61 Danish patients. *Acta Psychiatrica Scandinavica, 83*(4), 262–266.

Tolin, D.F. (2001). Case study: Bibliotherapy and extinction in the treatment of obsessive-compulsive-disorder in a 5-year-old boy. *Journal of the American Academy of Child and Adolescent Psychiatry, 40*(9), 1111–1114.

Turgeon, L., O'Connor, K.P., Marchand, A., & Freeston, M.H. (2002). Recollections of parent-child relationships in patients with obsessive-compulsive disorder and panic disorder with agoraphobia. *Acta Psychiatrica Scandinavica, 105*(4), 310–316.

Valleni-Basile, L.A., Garrison, C.Z., & Jackson, K.L. (1994). Frequency of obsessive-compulsive disorder in a community sample of young adolescents. *Journal of the American Academy of Child and Adolescent Psychiatry. 33,* 782–791.

Wagner, K.D., Cook, E.H., Chung, H., & Messig, M. (2003). Remission status after long-term sertraline treatment of pediatric obsessive-compulsive disorder. *Journal of Child and Adolescent Psychopharmacology, 13*(Suppl. 1), 53–60.

Warren, S.L., Huston, L., Egeland, B., & Stroufe, L.A. (1997). Child and adolescent anxiety disorders and early attachment. *Journal of the American Academy of Child and Adolescent Psychiatry, 36,* 637–644.

Weissman, M.M., Bland, R.C., Canino, G.J., Greenwald, S., Hwu, H.G., Lee, C.K., Newman, S.C., Oakley-Brown, M.A., Rubio-Stipec, M., Wickramaratne, P.J., Wittchen, H-U., & Yeh, E-K. (1994). The cross national epidemiology of obsessive-compulsive disorder. The Cross National Collaborative Group. *Journal of Clinical Psychiatry, 55*(Suppl.), 5–10.

Wever, C., & Rey, J.M. (1997). Juvenile obsessive-compulsive disorder. *The Australian and New Zealand Journal of Psychiatry, 31*(1), 105–113.

White, M., & Epston, D. (1990). *Narrative Means to Therapeutic Ends.* New York: Norton.

Wolpe, J. (1969). *The Practice of Behavior Therapy.* New York: Pergamon Press.

Yoshida, T., Taga, C., & Fukui, K. (2001). Gender difference of parental rearing style of obsessive-compulsive disorder patients: A study using the parental bonding instrument. *Seishin Igaku (Clinical Psychiatry), 43*(9), 951–956.

Zohar, A.H. (1999). The epidemiology of obsessive-compulsive disorder in children and adolescents. *Child and Adolescent Psychiatric Clinics of North America, 8*(3), 445–460.

Zohar, A.H., Ratzoni, G., Pauls, D.L., et al. (1992). An epidemiological study of obsessive-compulsive disorder and related disorders in Israeli adolescents. *Journal of the American Academy of Child and Adolescent Psychiatry, 31:* 1057–1061.

Zucker, B.G., Craske, M.G., Barrios, V., & Holguin, M. (2002). Thought-action fusion: Can it be corrected? *Behaviour Research and Therapy, 40,* 653–664.

Chapter 13

Oppositional Defiant Disorder and Conduct Disorder

Deborah M. Capaldi and J. Mark Eddy

Introduction

Young children who display temper tantrums, poor self-control, noncompliance with parent and teacher requests, and unskilled or aggressive behaviors with peers cause problems for themselves and those around them at home, at school, and in the neighborhood. During adolescence, such conduct problem behaviors have more serious consequences than during early childhood and often bring the youth to the attention of authorities in the school and juvenile justice systems. Conduct problems are the most common reason for referrals to child mental health clinics in the western hemisphere (Frick, 1998) and have the poorest prognosis for adult adjustment of any childhood disorder (Kohlberg, Ricks & Snarey, 1984). Conduct problems are associated not only with pervasive developmental failures (Capaldi & Stoolmiller, 1999) in various key domains, such as academics, but also with serious and maladaptive behaviors during adulthood, such as substance abuse (Wiesner, Kim & Capaldi, in press) and violence toward romantic partners (Capaldi & Clark, 1998). Conduct problems thus have been the target of nationwide efforts in a variety of countries to understand causes and consequences, to prevent emergence, and to treat symptoms.

There are two main diagnoses given for conduct problems, with the primary being *conduct disorder* (CD). In the *DSM-IV* (American Psychological Association, 1994) classification system, the essential feature of CD is a repetitive and persistent pattern of behavior in which either the basic rights of others and/or major age-appropriate societal norms are violated in a way that significantly impairs functioning in social, academic, and/or work settings. The major behavioral domains of importance in CD are aggression toward people and/or animals, destruction of property, stealing or lying, and serious rule violations. To receive a diagnosis of CD, children must exhibit at least three conduct problem behaviors during the past year. The behaviors that are most prognostic of CD tend to be illegal throughout the United States and include both criminal and status offenses–the latter being offenses for juveniles only (e.g., minor in possession of alcohol). Diagnostic criteria for CD in the

ICD-10 Classification of Mental and Behavior Disorders (World Health Organization, 1997) are similar.

In the *DSM-IV* only, *oppositional defiant disorder* (ODD) is a secondary diagnosis that is given to children and adolescents who exhibit hostile, defiant, and antisocial behavior at a higher rate than their peers for at least six months, but who do not meet criteria for CD. At least four behaviors indicative of hostility and defiance must be present, including temper tantrums, arguments with adults, and blaming others for mistakes; and the symptoms must be associated with impairment in at least one area of functioning. Occurrence of such behaviors during the course of a psychotic or mood disorder precludes this diagnosis. The behaviors that lead to a diagnosis of ODD do not involve illegal acts per se, but can lead to serious consequences in certain settings, such as at school. CD tends to develop at later ages than ODD, and ODD is thought to develop into CD frequently (Hinshaw, Lahey & Hart, 1993). CD and ODD are typically diagnosed through clinician-administered interviews with the parent or child. However, structured interviews (e.g., DISC; Shaffer, Fisher, Dulcan & Davies 1996) can be administered by a nonclinician.

The diagnostic systems used to classify conduct problems as CD or ODD are based on a disease model and are intended to help guide decisions regarding treatment at any particular point in time. While this type of present/absent model fits well for certain childhood problems, conduct problem behaviors show a continuous distribution among both boys and girls at any given point in time, and these behaviors change in prevalence, frequency, and severity with age. The peak age for conduct problems (as indexed by self-reports) is between ages 14 and 17 years (Blumstein, Cohen, Roth & Visher, 1986).

For the purposes of understanding the development, causes, and outcomes of CD and ODD, conduct problems are usually studied as they occur within a particular population of adolescents, rather than by using diagnostic criteria. A variety of checklists and rating scales are available for such assessment. The most widely used is the *Child Behavior Checklist* (CBC-L; Achenbach, 1993) with parent, teacher and youth self-report versions, and it includes queries on aggression, delinquency, and hyperactivity symptoms. Together, these symptoms are thought to form the broader category of externalizing behaviors. Also frequently used is the *Elliott Delinquency Scale* (Elliott, 1983), which queries on a wide variety of behaviors for which an adolescent could be arrested, including both criminal and status offenses.

Conduct disorders frequently are comorbid with other child and adolescent psychiatric disorders, including disorders involving anxiety, depression, attention deficit hyperactivity, and substance use. Similarly, co-occurrence of these problem behaviors has been found in youth below diagnostic thresholds (e.g., Capaldi, 1991). It is beyond the scope of the current chapter to address issues of co-occurrence in depth. However, there are developmental associations between some of these domains of psychopathology and conduct problems that are addressed to some degree. For a recent review of issues of comorbidity, see Angold, Costello, and Erkanli (1999).

Prevalence

In order to estimate the prevalence of conduct problem diagnoses, Lahey, Miller, Gordon, and Riley (1999) examined 39 general population studies, and they calculated the median prevalence estimate for CD as 2.0% and the equivalent estimate for ODD as 3.2%. Angold and Costello (2001) concluded that the prevalence of CD and ODD is rather higher, at between 5% and 10%. Of significance is that the range in prevalence estimates across the population of studies is quite wide, 1–20%. These higher estimates may not be unreasonable. General population studies may tend to underestimate the prevalence of youth that meet diagnostic criteria due to the difficulty of recruiting families that are highly likely to have youth with conduct problems. For example, in the Oregon Youth Study (Capaldi & Patterson, 1987), a longitudinal study of boys who were recruited by inviting the participation of the families of all fourth-grade boys from selected schools with a higher than usual incidence of delinquency in their neighborhoods, boys from the most difficult-to-recruit families later showed the highest incidence of delinquency. Specifically, 13% of the families had no phone at the time of recruitment and, therefore, had to be recruited by personal visits, with several visits often being required to find the family at home. Of these boys, 62% had three or more police referrals prior to age 18 years, compared with 19% of boys from families with a phone. Further, 23% of these boys had between three and five referrals for violence, compared with 1% of the rest of the sample.

Boys are more likely than girls to be diagnosed with a CD (Cohen et al., 1993; Zoccolillo, 1993), although some studies have found a scant difference in prevalence during mid to late adolescence (Cohen et al., 1993). A common conception is that the prevalence of CD is approximately 6–16% of adolescent boys and 2–9% of adolescent girls (Mandel, 1997). A further indicator of gender differences in CD is juvenile arrest rates. Uniform Crime Reports for 1990 indicate that girls accounted for only 20% of juvenile arrests (Steffensmeier, 1993). Although various factors affect the likelihood of arrest, this indicates a potentially substantial difference in conduct problem rates during adolescence for boys and girls. However, there may be an increasing number of girls becoming involved in antisocial and delinquent behaviors (American Bar Association & the National Bar Association, 2001), and the long-term consequences for girls persistently engaging in such behaviors are quite serious (Lewis, Yeager, Cobham–Portorreal, Klein, Showalter, & Anthony, 1991).

Theoretical Approaches

Gottfredson and Hirschi (1990) have argued that individual dispositions are the cause of youth conduct and closely related problems, such as serious failures in school, social relationships, and heavy substance use (i.e., behaviors related in nature to crime in that they break fundamental societal norms or rules). They posit that a *lack of self-control* is the underlying propensity factor driving such behavior throughout the life course, and that this parsimonious explanation is all that is required to explain the occurrence of antisocial behavior. This propensity could be genetic or could be due to other factors, such as physiological conditions in utero (e.g., exposure to nicotine). Their theory further implies that all relationships between conduct problems and associated analogous behaviors or possible cumulative consequences are spurious (see also Evans, Cullen, Burton, Dunaway & Benson, 1997).

Genetic theories of antisocial behavior also posit that individual dispositions, in this case caused by familial genetic factors, place some individuals at higher risk for such behavior due to temperamental tendencies such as a relatively high activity level, or a greater vulnerability to feelings of negative affect and anger, or a higher tolerance for risk taking. The most common studies of genetic contributions to date have been via behavior genetic designs, and through such studies there is some evidence of a genetic basis for conduct problems (Simonoff, 2001). A popular hypothesis is that genes relevant to the display of ADHD symptoms are probably also related to the display of CD symptoms (e.g., Comings, 2000). Regardless, the strength of this finding depends on the type of measures that are used as well as on other methodological factors (Leve, Winebarger, Fagot, Reid & Goldsmith, 1998). Whereas there are not yet clear answers regarding the relationship of genetics to conduct problems, rapid advances in molecular approaches have spawned an increased interest in using such approaches for the study of antisocial behavior and, hopefully, much will be learned in the next several decades.

Cognitive researchers have proposed a theory regarding individual differences in interpreting social environmental cues that attempts to identify proximal mechanisms involving biases in social information processing that may trigger aggressive behavior (Dodge, 1993). Adolescents who show higher levels of conduct problems are found both to be more likely to interpret the ambiguous behaviors of others as being aggressive and to show a more limited repertoire of responses, particularly positive solutions to specific interpersonal problems (Dodge, 1993). Such biases may be partly due to having learned to negotiate more hostile environments. Adolescents showing such hostile attribution biases in their social information processing tend to be higher in conduct problem behaviors. However, such biases explain only a small proportion of the variance in longer-term antisocial behavior (Dodge, Pettit, Bates & Valente, 1995).

Beyond theories such as these that focus on the casual importance of one or relatively few factors, there is a general consensus that the development of antisocial behavior involves a prolonged process of interplay between the characteristics of the individual youth and their key social environments (e.g., Baltes, 1983; Cairns & Cairns, 1995; Elder, 1985). These environments include those created by family, by school personnel and students, by peer groups, and by pertinent community members. The social interactions that occur within each environment may affect antisocial behavior across the life span. Figure 1 illustrates the interaction of the individual

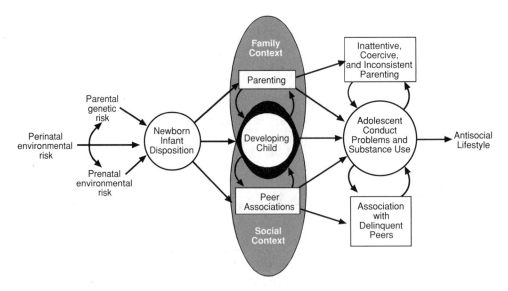

Figure 1. Interactional developmental model.

characteristics of the developing child with the social environment (for simplicity only parent and peer associations are illustrated). These social transactions occur within and are affected by larger contextual factors. Bronfenbrenner (1986) conceptualized such settings and processes as a hierarchy of four nested systems involving intrapersonal factors (e.g., temperament), microsystems of face-to-face interactions, behavioral settings (e.g., neighborhood), and finally macrocontextual factors involving cultural and community practices. Social interactions begin to affect behavior significantly in infancy, and thus it is difficult to assess the relative contribution of temperament or propensity and socialization even from very early in life using conventional assessment approaches.

Interactions between the individual child and their social environment may be characterized or typed according to the direction of influence and degree of active involvement (Scarr & McCartney, 1983). The first type is *passive*, whereby the individual has no choice in the selection of the environment and only limited ability to affect the environment, and thus may be very vulnerable to environmental effects. This pertains particularly to environments provided by caregivers in early childhood, but also to institutional environments, including detention centers, schools to some degree, and to cultural and community practices such as portrayals of violence in the media. The second type is *evocative* (i.e., through responses elicited from others). Thus, explosive temper tantrums and aggression by a child may partially predict both harsh parental discipline (Ge et al., 1996) and peer rejection (Coie & Dodge, 1988). Such rejection by prosocial peers deprives the aggressive child of positive developmental influences in the peer group. An individual also can affect their social environment through more active attempts at change or *manipulation* (Buss, 1987) that may be either positive (e.g., working hard to make a good impression on a new teacher) or negative (e.g., lying to parents to avoid punishment). Individuals may also *react* to environmental events or evocative triggers (e.g., an aggressive response to an insult). Adolescents who are proactively aggressive (e.g., attacking another person without a reason) versus reactively aggressive (i.e., self-defense) are found to be lower in self-control, constructive behavior, and in adult adjustment than those showing reactive patterns (Pulkkinen, 1996). Further, proactively aggressive boys were found to be prone to externalizing problems and criminality in adulthood, whereas girls were more prone to internalizing problems, including depressive symptoms. The final type of interactive effect described by Scarr and McCartney is through the *active* selection of environments. Youth have some latitude in selecting social environments that suit them, particularly in relation to their friends who may vary from very prosocial to highly antisocial. Friendships play a critical role in conduct problem behavior during adolescence, and involvement with delinquent peers per se is a major contributor to the continuance of conduct problems (Dishion, Spracklen, Andrews & Patterson, 1996).

A key individual–environment interaction effect with long-term consequences for conduct problem youth is *restriction of environmental options*. Such restriction may start in early childhood through family contextual factors, including low income and residence in a deprived neighborhood. Critically for development, individual characteristics may expand or contract the range of environmental options. Developmental success may lead to expansion of options, whereas developmental failures and conduct problems lead to restriction (e.g., rejection by socially skilled peers due to unskilled or aggressive behavior may occur early in development). In adolescence, restriction may continue through such pathways as academic failure and high school drop-out, which limit future education and employment opportunities. Such restrictions are an unintended and pervasive consequence of conduct problem behaviors affecting future developmental trajectories in a variety of ways. Such failures and restrictions, along with overlapping family risk factors, may account at least partially for the association of conduct problems with depressive symptoms in adolescence (Capaldi, 1991).

Remaining in or entering higher risk and antisocial environments is more likely when these prior failures in development have occurred (Capaldi & Stoolmiller, 1999). Such environments may provide a variety of supports for continued conduct problem behaviors, as well as provide fewer interpersonal sanctions against such behaviors. The net effect is to either maintain the stability of conduct problem behaviors or to increase engagement in such behaviors. Co-occurring and problematic levels of substance use may be a key factor in these processes. Wiesner et al. (in press) found that drug use was strongly associated with remaining in a high-crime trajectory through early adulthood. Substance use may impact conduct problems through multiple means, including relationships (i.e., peers and dating partners who do not use substances may reject individuals who do use) and detrimental financial impacts (i.e., substance use can be costly and significantly interfere with performance on the job).

Dishion and colleagues (e.g., Dishion et al., 1996) examined the processes by which conduct problems can form the basis for adolescent friendships and labeled the reinforcement of rule-breaking talk that was observed to occur in some dyads as delinquency training. Rule-breaking talk was more frequent for dyads high in anti-social behavior and was associated with positive affective exchanges and laughter. In contrast, prosocial boys tended to laugh mostly in normative discussions. This process of delinquency training in adolescence predicted escalations in serious delin-quent behavior (Dishion, Andrews, Kavanagh & Soberman, 1996). Interviews with delinquent adolescent girls indicate that they are also involved in friendship networks that encourage their delinquent behavior (Giordano & Cernkovich, 1997). What appears to be particularly salient in these networks is the perception of peer approval for law violations. In short, adolescence is a critical period for the influence of peers, with respect to establishing norms, values, and behaviors that account for subsequent individual differences in conduct problem behaviors.

Individual Factors

The earliest manifestations of individual factors that may affect social interactions are temperamental differences in infancy. Temperament is the response tendencies an infant displays early in life in the areas of attention, activity level, emotionality (positive and negative), approach, risk-taking, and inhibitory control (see Rothbart, Posner & Hershey, 1995). These tendencies not only affect the way that the infant interacts with his or her environment but also how caregivers and others interact with the infant.

Children who exhibit more difficult temperamental characteristics may be at particularly high risk for the development of externalizing behavior problems (Campbell & Ewing, 1990). Lahey and Waldman (2003) identified three dimensions of temperament that they considered to place the child at high risk for conduct problems: negative emotionality, daring or risk-taking behavior, and lack of prosocial behaviors (e.g., sharing, empathy, and kindness). The latter dimension, although associated with positive emotionality, is strongly associated with socialization and thus is not usually considered an indicator of underlying temperament. Children who are highly active, persistent in attempting to reach goals (versus more easily distracted from an undesirable activity), angry in mood, irritable, and difficult to soothe are particularly at risk. Gilliom, Shaw, Beck, Schonberg, and Lukon (2002) found that anger at age 3 ½ years was significantly predictive of externalizing behaviors and lack of cooperation at age 6 years, as rated by teachers. Several longitudinal studies have followed children from preschool or first grade through a major portion of adolescence, and all provide at least some confirmation that early childhood risks for conduct problems include poor impulse control, serious disobedience, and aggressive behavior both at school and at home (e.g., Caspi, Moffitt, Newman & Silva, 1996).

Intergenerational associations have been found for conduct problems and difficult temperament. Capaldi, Pears, Patterson, and Owen (2003) found that father's conduct problems, assessed in adolescence, were predictive of their offspring's more difficult temperament (anger and activity level) at age 2 years. Temperament is presumed to be associated with biological factors and especially with genetic predispositions. Adoption studies have found that both antisocial behaviors in the biological parent and in the adoptive parent are influence on antisocial behavior in the offspring (Bohman, 1996). Cadoret, Yates, Troughton, Woodworth, and Stewart (1995) found interactions between the presence of antisocial personality in the biological parent and psychiatric disorder in the adoptive parents that predicted childhood and adolescent aggression and CD. Behavior-genetic approaches to the study of the transmission of conduct problems are common, in particular, twin and adoption designs. Such studies indicate strong effects of genetics and unshared environment on conduct problems and less of a role for shared environmental factors (e.g., familial factors). Such studies suggest that there may be a difference between the relative importance of genetic and environmental influences on different dimensions of CD, with shared environmental factors being more influential for delinquency than for aggression (Edelbrock, Rende, Plomin & Thompson, 1995). In general, behavior genetic studies do not find gender differences in the degree of genetic and environmental effects (Simonoff, 2001). Behavior genetic designs suffer from some problems that may affect the estimates of heritability and shared versus unshared environmental effects, including the failure to control for the effects of assortative partnering of the parents (i.e., nonrandom mating), the reliance on parental reports of child behavior, the limited measures of environmental contributions, and in the case of adoption studies, the tendency for higher-risk families to be screened out as adoptive parents, thus limiting the possible range of environmental contributions (Stoolmiller, 1999).

Simonoff (2001) reviewed genetic influences on CD and noted that to date there are no molecular genetic studies using CD per se as the phenotype of interest. However, there have been studies using such approaches to examine the contributions to related risk factors and aspects of CD, such as sensation seeking, impulsivity, and physical aggression. Genetic loading may be associated particularly with dimensions of temperament that relate to brain activity and, thus, to neural pathways (Hill, 2002). Two behavioral systems, the *Behavioral Activation System* (BAS) and the *Behavioral Inhibition System* (BIS), are hypothesized to be critical to the way an individual responds to environmental stimuli that offer reward or punishment (Gray, 1987). The BAS is posited to activate behaviors in response to likely rewards, and the BIS to inhibit behaviors when punishment cues are present. During behavioral activation, the dopaminergic system in the brain is believed to be facilitating approach responses. The noradrenergic and serotonergic systems are believed to be associated with behavioral inhibition (Rogeness & McClure, 1996).

There are promising findings of associations of several candidate genes and implicated brain metabolic pathways. Associations with neurotransmitters hypothesized to be associated with low behavioral inhibition have been found, including lower noradrenaline (Rogeness et al., 1984) and serotonin (Kruesi et al., 1990; Moffitt et al., 1997) levels in the brain. Genes affecting dopamine function have been found to be associated with hyperactivity (Thapar, Holmes, Poulton & Harrington, 1999). Caspi et al. (2002) examined the association of child maltreatment and a genetic variant that results in brain monoamine oxidase levels being too low to break down some neurotransmitters (e.g., norepinephrine, serotonin, and dopamine) that may become overactive due to maltreatment. Findings indicated an interaction effect between this polymorphism and maltreatment in predicting antisocial behavior.

Of note, however, is that findings regarding the associations of candidate genes and neurotransmitter levels and activity often do not replicate consistently, and effects may differ by age (Hill, 2002). The current picture is that most psychiatric disorders, including CD, are considered genetically complex, with evidence that multiple genes are involved that confer some degree of vulnerability, but with no single gene being sufficient to produce the disorder. Several genes may affect an individual neural pathway in ways that interact; and further, there are interactions among neurotransmitters. It is currently assumed that conduct problems have complex or multifactorial inheritance—involving both multiple genetic susceptibilities and multiple environmental risk factors for disease or behavioral expression (Simonoff, 2001).

In addition to genetics, the prenatal environment may also relate to individual differences in temperament and risk for conduct problems. This is usually considered in terms of the intra-uterine environment, and smoking during pregnancy has been found predictive of conduct problems in boys, controlling for related factors (Fergusson, Woodward & Horwood, 1998). However, it is also the case that there may be environmental effects on the eggs and sperm prior to fertilization. For example, marijuana has been found to affect male fertility by affecting sperm (Schuel et al., 2002). Thus, it is likely that environmental factors prior to birth affect brain functioning.

Family Factors

In contrast to genetic approaches, social learning theories focus on contributions of the social environment to the development of conduct problems. Only the highly unusual parent would purposely socialize their child toward conduct problems and criminal behavior. However, Patterson and colleagues (Patterson, 1982; Reid, Patterson & Snyder, 2002) have detailed the mechanisms by which parents may *inadvertently* contribute to their child's development in these directions. Central to Patterson's *coercion model* is the role of poor discipline practices, including patterns of alternating inattention to children's behavior and ineffective nattering (i.e., verbal negatives, such as yelling, complaining, and lecturing) that are punctuated periodically by angry explosions and overly harsh discipline. In particular, parents may positively reinforce aggression by initially refusing a child's request (e.g., for a treat or money), but then submit if the child becomes negative or aggressive. Parents also may negatively reinforce noncompliance and aggression by making a request (e.g., that the child switch off the television and go to bed), but then failing to follow through on the request if the child responds in an aversive manner. Thus, children may learn to get their way through persistent noncompliance and aggression. At the extreme of the continuum of poor parental discipline is physically abusive behavior, which is also associated with conduct problems, and patterns of physically abusive behavior have been shown to occur across generations within families (Pears & Capaldi, 2001).

One critical set of parenting behaviors that underlie positive parental discipline practices come under the rubric of *parental monitoring*. We have posited that the foundation of parental monitoring is parental awareness of all aspects of their child's life and development, including activities in and outside the home, friendships and other relationships, progress in school, and health-related behaviors (Capaldi, 2003). This awareness is based on the parents' placing a high priority on the welfare of the youth and involves regular and positive communication. Parents must track the indicators of normal development, watch for signals of potential problems, and adjust their parenting behaviors accordingly. Dishion and McMahon (1998) argue that parental monitoring plays an important role from infancy into young adulthood and should be developmentally as well as contextually appropriate. They propose a broad definition, including both *structuring* the child or adolescent's home, school, and community environments and *tracking* the child's behavior in these environments. Monitoring is associated both with conduct problems and with associated outcomes of conduct problems, such as health-risking sexual behavior (Capaldi, Stoolmiller, Clark & Owen, 2002) and substance use (Friedman, Lichtenstein & Biglan, 1985). The association of poor discipline and monitoring practices with conduct problems has been found in many studies (e.g., Forgatch, 1991; Lipsey & Derzon, 1998). A recent study (Galambos, Barker & Almeida, 2003) found that parents' firm control seemed to halt the upward trajectory in externalizing problems among adolescents who associated with deviant peers.

Monitoring, however, is just one of several behaviors that are required for effective parenting. As discussed in Capaldi, Chamberlain, and Patterson (1997), *effective parenting* involves (a) accurately tracking and classifying problem behaviors; (b) ignoring trivial coercive events, yet intervening before a problem escalates; (c) structuring situations and redirecting toward positive behaviors; (d) consistent use of a mild to moderate consequence when punishment is necessary (e.g., time out, privilege loss); (e) following up on behavioral change; and (f) encouraging positive behaviors. Parents of children with higher levels of conduct problems tend to have difficulty with each of these skills (see also Reid et al., 2002).

Social and Community Factors

There is a considerable body of evidence indicating associations between community factors and child well-being and problem behaviors (see Leventhal & Brooks-Gunn, 2000). For example, Wichstrom, Skogen, and Oia (1996) examined the association of urbanization and conduct problems and found that rates of conduct problems were higher only at high levels of urbanization, and this finding was not explainable by a variety of control or neighborhood factors. However, the finding was associated with involvement with delinquent peers and with drug use.

Delinquency tends to be a social activity, with adolescents most typically being arrested along with peers (Aultman, 1980). However, the relationship between peers and delinquency is qualified by family factors. Pettit, Bates, Dodge, and Meece (1999) found that unsupervised peer contact predicted worsening conduct problems among adolescents who were monitored less by their parents and who lived in neighborhoods perceived by their parents to be unsafe. Beyers, Bates, Pettit, and Dodge (2003) examined whether census-based measures of neighborhood factors, including structural disadvantage, residential instability, and concentrated affluence, moderated the effects of parenting processes, particularly parental monitoring, on conduct problems. Low supervision and less positive parental involvement were associated with increases in externalizing behavior across time. The decreases in externalizing levels associated with more parental monitoring was significantly more pronounced when the family lives in a neighborhood with higher residential instability.

A well-documented phenomenon associated with conduct problems at adolescence is that such adolescents take a more precocious or accelerated pathway to adulthood, taking on certain adult-like roles at an earlier age than usual. Engagement with delinquent peers is a key factor in such acceleration (Dishion, Poulin & Medici-Skaggs, 2000). Newcomb (1987) has described the process whereby risk or problem behaviors are associated with more rapid movement into adult roles as pseudomaturity, indicating that the taking on of such roles does not necessarily indicate the capacity to succeed in them. Similarly, Burton, Obeidallah, and Allison (1996) have described the accelerated life courses of inner-city African American adolescents. Thus, both conduct problems and higher-risk communities may be associated with such developmental acceleration. High school drop-out may be a key factor in such acceleration, because drop-outs are likely to enter employment earlier and leave the family-of-origin home prior to age 18 years (Capaldi & Stoolmiller, 1999). Dropping out of high school is strongly associated with conduct problems (Elliott & Voss, 1974).

A second major factor in acceleration into adult roles is initiation of sexual intercourse at an early age. Early initiation of intercourse is predicted by childhood and adolescent conduct problems (Capaldi, Crosby & Stoolmiller, 1996) and shows a particularly strong association with arrests. Youth who initiate intercourse early are also likely to become parents at a young age. Although conduct problem youth may take on some adult roles, including employment and parenthood, at an earlier age than their peers, they may not become fully autonomous, but are often financially reliant on their parents. This may be especially true in the case of teenage girls who have had a child.

Peers are not the only social and community factor related to conduct problems. Wikstrom and Loeber (2000) examined the association of neighborhood socioeconomic context and offending. They found that adolescents with high scores on risk characteristics commit serious criminal offenses at a similar rate regardless of the socioeconomic context of their neighborhood, but youth with higher levels of protective factors were directly and negatively impacted by neighborhood context. In a study that included white, black, and Latino populations in two major cities, Elliott et al. (1996) found that higher levels of neighborhood disadvantage were associated with lower levels of informal control, including neighbor involvement. Informal control was related to lower levels of conduct problems for the African American population in Chicago. Informal networks of friends and family members within neighborhoods were related to lower conduct problems in the more diverse ethnic populations in Denver.

In terms of more extreme conduct problems, although youth violence occurs in all communities, the prevalence varies, and the concentration is highest in inner cities (Tolan & Gorman-Smith, 2002). Black youth are five times more likely to be murdered than white youth (Snyder, 1998), and because ethnicity is related to inner-city residence, these differences may be due to community differences. The social ecology of inner city neighborhoods is such that they may present a qualitatively different context for families and youth, whereby parental behaviors that promote positive youth adjustment in lower risk communities may not work (Tolan et al., 2003). There is a higher density of delinquent peers in high-crime neighborhoods and fewer school and community resources. Tolan et al. (2003) found that there was a perceived lack of support, a lower sense of belonging to the neighborhood, and a lower involvement in the community. Violence in the peer group, particularly delinquent gang memberships, were high-risk factors, and the most effective parents worked to prevent gang membership.

Overall, it appears that neighborhood risk factors are more highly associated with conduct problems in boys than girls. This may be because boys are more likely to participate in neighborhood activities and especially to spend more time in unsupervised activities with peers or join gangs. Thus, in neighborhoods with poor resources and higher densities of delinquent peers, they may be at particular risk (Ensminger, Lamkin & Jacobson, 1996).

Evidence-Based Interventions for CD/ODD

There are two interventions that are recommended for the treatment and prevention of CD and ODD according to the evidence based criterion of three or more successful trials; namely, *parent management training* (PMT) and *child social skills training* (CSST) (see Eddy, 2001; Taylor & Biglan, 1998). The basic tenets and techniques of PMT were developed by behavior therapists during the 1960s and refined during the 1970s (e.g., Patterson, Reid, Jones & Conger, 1975). Via group or individual formats, PMT coaches parents in discouraging child problem behaviors and encouraging child prosocial behaviors. Most PMT programs teach parents skills in the area of positive reinforcement, nonviolent and consistent discipline, effective monitoring and supervision, and constructive family problem-solving. Interactive exercises, role plays, and skills practice homework are commonly used. In a meta-analysis of the 26 studies that have compared a PMT condition to a comparison group condition, the average effect size for child antisocial outcomes immediately post intervention was $d = 0.80$ (Serketich & Dumas, 1996). Only a few studies that include PMT have been published since that time, and most are studies of the impact of multimodal interventions (e.g., PMT, CSST, and the Good Behavior Game playground intervention; Reid, Eddy, Fetrow & Stoolmiller, 1999) and thus would not be utilized in a PMT meta-analysis. Insufficient data are available to calculate effect sizes for the long-term impact of PMT.

CSST was developed during the 1970s (Shure, Spivack & Gordon, 1972). Youth are taught cognitive and behavioral techniques and strategies that are useful in solving interpersonal problems. Most programs teach some combination of problem-solving skills, anger-control skills, social skills, coping skills, and assertive skills. CSST can be delivered via group or individual formats, although most programs require group settings. Like PMT, CSST utilizes a variety of interactive exercises, such as skills practice within small and large groups and dyadic role plays. In a meta-analysis of 84 studies that compared a child social skills training condition to a comparison group condition, the average effect size for antisocial outcomes immediately post intervention was $d = 0.38$ and at follow-up was $d = 0.28$ (Losel & Beelmann, 2003). Only 20% of studies included a follow-up, and 90% of these studies followed children for less than one year post-intervention.

Evidence-Based Treatment Interventions in Community Settings

Treatment or clinical interventions are targeted to youth who are already exhibiting antisocial behavior at problematic levels. The parents may seek help for their child, or the youth may be identified at school, by police, or by service agencies as in need of intervention to improve their behavior and increase their chance of future successful adjustment.

What Works

The most extensively researched intervention for community settings, and one of only two programs to be classified as well established for the treatment of conduct problems by the American Psychological Association Division 30 (Brestan & Eyberg, 1998) is the video-based PMT program designed by Carolyn Webster-Stratton (Webster-Stratton, 1990). The other well-established program is the closely related PMT program developed by Patterson et al. (1975).

Over the years, the Webster-Stratton program has expanded to encompass a variety of parent and child-based modules and is now known as *The Incredible Years Series*. This series is designed to treat and/or reduce conduct problems in young children ages 2–8 years and includes separate but linked programs for PMT, child social skills training, and teacher behavior management training. The Basic Program teaches parents interactive play and reinforcement skills, nonviolent discipline techniques, logical and natural consequences, and problem-solving strategies. The Advanced Curriculum addresses family risk factors, including depression, marital discord, poor coping skills, poor anger management, and lack of support. A School Curriculum assists parents to further their young child's social and academic competence. The Teacher Curriculum is designed to strengthen teacher's classroom management skills, and includes encouragement and motivational techniques, promotion of social skills and cooperation with peers and teachers, anger management and problem-solving, and reducing classroom aggression. The Children's Curriculum includes developing recognition of emotions, empathy with others, peer relations, problem-solving and anger management, following school rules, and school success.

The Webster–Stratton interventions have been shown to reduce conduct problems and improve parenting interactions for approximately two-thirds of families whose children have conduct disorders and who have been treated in clinics, and improvements have been sustained for up to three years (e.g., Webster-Stratton, 1990). The teacher program has also been shown to improve children's classroom behavior and the teacher's classroom management skills (e.g., Webster-Stratton, Reid & Hammond, 2000). The child training component was shown to improve social and peer group skills, as well as to reduce child behavior problems (e.g., Webster-Stratton & Hammond, 1997).

A more intensive community based program is *multisystemic therapy* (MST; Henggeler, 1990), an individualized case management program that often incorporates many aspects of PMT and CSST. MST is designed for youth with serious behavior disorders who are at risk for out-of-home placement. MST targets the multiple factors that can contribute to antisocial behavior at the individual, family, and broader social levels, including peer, school, and neighborhood factors. MST identifies strengths in each youth's social network and capitalizes on these to promote positive change. By helping both parents and youth to manage their lives more effectively, the need for out-of-home placement may be eliminated. Treatment is designed in collaboration with the family, and therapists have low caseloads and are available around the clock. The average duration of treatment is four months; during this time, therapists work very closely (e.g., multiple times per week in the home and community) with youth and families. In a variety of studies, reductions of 25–70% in long-term re-arrest rates and of 47–64% in out-of-home placements have been achieved, and positive improvements in youth and family functioning have been observed for several years following intervention (e.g., Borduin, Henggeler, Blaske, & Stein, 1990; Henggeler, Cunningham, Pickrel, Schoenwald & Brondino, 1996; Henggeler, Melton & Smith, 1992; Henggeler, Melton, Smith, Schoenwald & Hanley, 1993). Further and importantly, the costs associated with MST are less than those for institutional placement (Henggeler, Mihalic, Rone, Thomas & Timmons-Mitchell, 1998).

What Might Work

Functional family therapy (FFT; Alexander & Parsons, 1982) focuses on improving communication within the family. Whereas FFT includes instruction for parents in PMT skills in the area of discipline and positive reinforcement, it focuses primarily on teaching parents and children problem-solving skills, including how to describe thoughts and feelings clearly and how to negotiate solutions to family problems effectively. Functional family therapy involves three phases: engagement and motivation, behavior change, and generalization. The generalization phase is particularly important and involves helping families to apply positive change to other areas in order to create support for maintaining change and preventing relapse. To assist in long-term maintenance, FFT therapists attempt to link families with available and on-going community resources. Although less researched than the Webster-Stratton program, FFT is widely acknowledged as a best practice (e.g., see Blueprints for Violence Prevention *www.colorado.edu/cspv/blueprints/*). In several studies, high participation and completion rates have been demonstrated for FFT. Impacts have been found on recidivism rates for targeted youth for up to 18 months following treatment (Alexander & Parsons, 1973), as well as on the subsequent delinquency of the siblings of the youth who were the original targets of the program (Klein, Alexander & Parsons, 1977).

Evidence-Based Treatment Interventions in Residential Settings

What Works

Whereas residential treatment is commonly mandated for delinquent youth, only a few interventions either have been studied sufficiently or incorporate components that have been studied sufficiently to be considered evidence based. Like community based interventions, these also incorporate elements of PMT and CSST. There are no interventions of this type with three or more successful trials.

What Might Work

In *multidimensional treatment foster care* (MTFC; Chamberlain & Reid, 1998), youth are placed with foster parents who have received extensive training in PMT skills and who receive ongoing and intensive support. An individual treatment plan is created for each youth and his or her family. A typical plan includes PMT for the natural parents, an individual therapist for the youth, academic goals, and plans to minimize contact between the youth and any delinquent or otherwise deviant peers.

Removing the youth from the contexts that supported conduct problem behaviors, placing them in a specialized setting designed to reduce such behaviors, and providing the natural parents respite and training in how to better manage the youth once he or she is home can produce the leverage needed to change very serious behavior patterns. Study outcomes indicate that MTFC youth had about 50% fewer criminal referrals than a control group of youth placed in residential group care programs, were less likely to be incarcerated, and returned to live with relatives more often than youth placed in more traditional care (Chamberlain & Reid, 1998). Longer-term outcomes include significant reductions in violent behavior (Eddy, Whaley, & Chamberlain, 2004). Eddy and Chamberlain (2000) found that reductions in arrest rates for the treatment group were mediated by contextual changes related to lower conduct problems; namely, increases in structured discipline and supervision, relationships with a prosocial adult mentor, and less engagement with antisocial peers.

PMT and CSST have been adapted specifically for use in the *inpatient hospital setting* by Kazdin and colleagues (Kazdin, Siegel & Bass, 1992). In this iteration, CSST is delivered during individual therapy sessions. Between sessions, youth are assigned specific tasks that help them apply the interpersonal skills that they learn and practice during sessions. PMT is also delivered during individual family therapy sessions. In a series of studies examining various combinations of these versions of PMT and CSST, positive effects on child antisocial behavior have been found both immediately following treatment and at 1-year follow-up (e.g., Kazdin, Bass, Siegel & Thomas, 1989; Kazdin, Esveldt-Dawson, French & Unis, 1987a, b; Kazdin et el., 1992).

Psychopharmacology

A variety of medications have been examined as *adjuncts* to treatment for CD and ODD. In cases of severe aggressive behavior, for example, lithium or one of the neuroleptics (e.g., haloperidol) may be prescribed (Campbell, Gonzalez & Silva, 1992). However, even in extreme cases, medication is not recommended as either the sole or the primary treatment for these disorders. The most common medication that a youth with CD or ODD may receive is one of the stimulants, such as methylphenidate or dextroamphetamine (Wilens & Biederman, 1992). These medications are prescribed to address symptoms of attention-deficit/hyperactivity disorder (ADHD), which commonly co-occurs with CD or ODD (e.g., Barkley, 1990), but they may impact certain conduct problem behaviors such as noncompliance and aggression.

There is some evidence that lithium can be beneficial for the short-term treatment of severe aggression (Campbell et al., 1984). The neuroleptics can be effective in this way as well, but have more numerous and serious side effects (Whitaker & Rao, 1992). Approximately 50–75% of patients accurately diagnosed with ADHD respond in at least some positive ways (e.g., increases in attention, decreases in impulsivity, decreases in verbal and/or physical aggression) to one of the stimulants (Greenhill, 1992). These effects are only seen for a limited period of time after ingestion (i.e., usually for several hours). Common side effects of stimulant treatment include insomnia, decreased appetite, stomachaches, headaches, and irritability (see Eddy, 2001).

The Prevention of CD/ODD

What Works

Programs to prevent conduct problems are designed either to prevent the onset of clinical levels of conduct problems or to lower the current level of conduct problems. Prevention programs fall into three general categories: universal interventions, which target the general population of children; selected interventions, which target individuals who belong to a subgroup of the population that is considered at risk for the development of ODD and/or CD; and indicated interventions, which target children who have a risk factor or condition that indicates that they are at high risk for the development of ODD and/or CD (see Mrazek & Haggerty, 1994). Most preventive intervention programs that have received at least some empirical support include elements of PMT and/or CSST, and many are multimodal in design, targeting multiple risk factors through multiple interventions. Few of these programs have been rigorously studied more than once, at least in reference to outcomes on antisocial behavior, and thus all can be considered programs that might work.

What Might Work

UNIVERSAL INTERVENTIONS.   To date, most research on universal interventions for ODD and CD has focused on elementary public schools as the medium for program delivery. Three types of programs appear most promising: classroom behavior management programs; CSST programs; and multimodal programs, which often combine various aspects of CSST and PMT with environmental interventions. Classroom behavior management programs provide encouragement for desired behaviors and discouragement for undesired behaviors, usually through a combination of individual and group contingencies. In a randomized trial, first-graders who received the classroom-based *Good Behavior Game* (GBG) were rated as less aggressive by teachers and peers post-intervention (Dolan et al., 1993); by middle school, however, only the most aggressive first-grade boys were impacted by the program (Kellam, Rebok, Mayer, Ialongo & Kalodner, 1994). CSST prevention programs are similar to those discussed earlier and are delivered in a group format. The CSST program, *Promoting Alternative Thinking Strategies* (PATHS), has been shown to decrease conduct problem behavior for up to several years following intervention (Greenberg & Kusché, 1998; Greenberg, Kusché, Cook & Quamma, 1995). Multimodal programs have also been shown to impact conduct problems. In a randomized controlled study, the *Linking the Interests of Families and Teachers* (LIFT) program, which combined PMT, CSST, and the GBG, decreased child aggressive behavior in multiple settings immediately following the intervention, particularly for the most aggressive children, and decreased overall rates of juvenile crime for at least the next 3 years (Eddy, Reid, Stoolmiller & Fetrow, 2003; Reid et al., 1999; Stoolmiller, Eddy & Reid, 2000).

SELECTED INTERVENTIONS.   Two promising selected interventions for CD and ODD that have frequently appeared on best practices lists are the *Nurse Family Partnership* (NFP) and the *Adolescent Transitions Program* (ATP). The NFP was designed to reduce very early risk factors by targeting mother's health-risking behavior during pregnancy, problematic maternal adjustment, and child abuse and neglect. Nurse home visitors work to develop a supportive relationship with low-income, first-time mothers. The program emphasizes education, mutual goal setting, and the development of the mother's problem-solving skills and self-efficacy, as well as preventing future unintended pregnancies and employment for the mother. Adolescents whose mothers received nurse home visits were 60% less likely to have run away, 55% less likely to have been arrested, and 80% less likely to have been convicted of a crime than adolescents whose mothers did not receive visits (Olds, Hill, Mihalic & O'Brien 1998). In contrast, the ATP targets at-risk early adolescents through community-based PMT groups. In a controlled study, youth whose parents received PMT were rated by teachers as displaying fewer conduct problems (Dishion & Andrews, 1995).

INDICATED INTERVENTIONS.   Promising indicated interventions, like universal interventions, have focused on the public elementary school as the base for program delivery. Two examples are the *Montreal Prevention Project* (MPP) and *Fast Track*. In the MPP, children were identified in kindergarten as at risk for ODD and CD. PMT and CSST programs were provided during first and second grade. In a controlled study, children in the intervention group were less likely to report delinquent behavior during middle school than children in the control group (Tremblay, Pagani-Kurtz, Masse, Vitaro & Pihl, 1995). Fast Track targets at-risk kindergarten children and combines universal, selected, and indicated components. In contrast to all of the other programs mentioned in this chapter, intervention continues throughout the school years. The program includes CSST, PMT, academic tutoring, mentoring, and a variety of other components. After the first three years of intervention in a controlled trial of Fast Track, children in the intervention group displayed fewer conduct problems than children in the control group (Conduct Problems Prevention Research Group, 2002).

What Does Not Work

Defining harm in reference to interventions for antisocial behavior is somewhat different than with other emotional or behavioral disorders. If youth are displaying antisocial behaviors, by definition they are harming those around them through acts against person and/or property. Thus, delivering an intervention to such individuals that is ineffective, particularly when an intervention with evidence of effectiveness exists that could be used, could be considered contributing to harm. There are a variety of interventions that are used with antisocial youth that fall into this category of harm in the sense that they do not seem to make much difference in subsequent youth behavior.

In a meta-analysis of treatments for delinquency, Lipsey (1992) found that among programs delivered by juvenile justice sponsors, *deterrence programs* (including shock incarceration and "Scared Straight" programs) and *vocational programs* showed negative outcomes compared to control groups. For example, in Scared Straight programs, at-risk or delinquent youth are brought into prisons and given frank talks by inmates about the realities of prison life in the hope that the youth will avoid a life of crime. A second meta-analysis of randomized controlled studies on these types of programs also found that, on average, the interventions were associated with an increase in the criminal behavior of youth (Petrosino, Turpin-Petrosino & Buehler, 2003). Among programs administered by non-juvenile justice sponsors, Lipsey (1992) found that individual counseling and employment/vocational programs also had negative effects, but of a very small magnitude.

There is recent controversy regarding the possible negative effects of interventions involving groups of youth (Arnold & Hughes, 1999; Dishion, McCord & Poulin, 1999). Group approaches to prevention and treatment are popular in both community and residential settings, in part, because they seem to capitalize on the economy of scale and, in part, because youth usually prefer to be with their age-mates. *Group approaches* are used with youth with conduct problems both in community (e.g., in the schools) and residential settings, including group homes and incarceration facilities. However, CD and ODD are fostered within social relationships, particularly within groups of same-age peers. Thus, a potential side effect of group treatments, particularly with adolescent youth who have CD, is that youth are introduced to other youth with antisocial behavior problems, thereby enlarging their friendship networks and providing them with new opportunities for delinquent peer influences and delinquency training.

Lipsey (1992) reported positive, albeit small to moderate, intervention effects from group counseling. However, Dishion, McCord, and Poulin (1999) summarized evidence that group interventions can result in iatrogenic effects, with youth who received group-based interventions showing *poorer* outcomes than youth who received no intervention at all. They argued that it is hard to tell how frequently such negative effects may occur, as studies with negative effects may not be submitted for publication as frequently as those with positive effects. Probably the best-known example of this is the randomized controlled *Cambridge Somerville Study*, which examined the impact of a mentoring program during adolescence on participant outcomes during middle age. At-risk youth in the intervention met regularly with a mentor and also participated in a variety of activities, including group-based programs such as summer camps. Initially, the program had no impact on youth, but over the long run, participants in the intervention group had more adverse outcomes than participants in the control group (McCord, 1978, 1981). Enough evidence has accumulated around this issue that in a summary of research on child and adolescent violence, staff at the National Institute of Mental Health (NIMH) concluded that "current policies and approaches grouping or housing troubled adolescents together may be the wrong approach, and it is clear that there are no quick, inexpensive answers . . . Some proposed interventions have been found to actually increase the negative behavior and so due care must be taken" (p. 1, <*http://www.nimh.nih.gov/publicat/violenceresfact.cfm*>). Dishion et al. (1999) posited that young high-risk adolescents may be most at risk in homogeneous group treatments, whereas older and younger children may be less at risk, and heterogeneous groups including prosocial youth may be more efficacious (Feldman & Caplinger, 1983). At a minimum it seems that in practice, group approaches should be approached cautiously, and in future research, group approaches should be compared to alternative approaches, and that data should be collected regarding potential harmful effects, such as contacts between the antisocial youth outside of the group setting and participation in rule-breaking activities together.

Recommendations

In the past 20 years, much has been learned about the development of conduct problems and related behaviors, particularly from long-term longitudinal studies that began in childhood and traced social environmental factors related to such development. The field has moved from relatively simplistic measurement of risk factors to the development of explanatory lifespan models that involve multiple levels of influence and the individual child's transactions with the overlapping social influences that make up their world. More recent work that also examines the contribution of parental genetic risk using molecular genetic approaches and perinatal as well as prenatal environmental risk will lead to more comprehensive etiological models of biological and social processes in the development of problem behaviors in the next 20 years. Findings in all these areas suggest that there are probably multiple routes to elevated levels of conduct problem behaviors. Findings also suggest that although the prevalence of conduct problem behaviors is lower among girls than boys, the developmental factors related to the emergence of such problems may be relatively similar across genders, although girls appear to have a later onset of more serious conduct problem behaviors (Keenan, Loeber & Green, 1999). Once underway, however, these behaviors can be reduced through leveraging the social environments through interpersonal relationships.

A key feature of effective prevention and treatment is inclusion of the adults who are involved in the child's socialization from day-to-day, particularly parent figures (e.g., stepparents, foster parents) and teachers. Improving the social-interactional and child-management skills of such adults has been shown to improve children's conduct problem behavior. Early intervention with higher-risk parents, such as through nurse home visitors, is particularly helpful in preventing destructive cycles of coercive interactions from developing between parents and children and in improving other risk factors such as prenatal environment. Early intervention has the benefits of preventing the development of negative behaviors in childhood before they have detrimental consequences, such as rejection by prosocial peers. Further, it is much more difficult for a parent to change the behavior of an older child who is noncompliant and out of control, especially as the parent may have lost hope that improvement is possible. Treatments for conduct problems that *only* focus on the child are generally less useful, as they do nothing to manipulate environmental factors that have powerful effects in evoking and reacting to the child's problem behavior. Because such children generally have low social skills and are more impulsive, they need adult coaching in order to make substantive changes in behavior. For school-aged children, universal interventions that affect the school environment, including peer behavior, are also very beneficial in reducing problem behaviors by reducing support for such behaviors in the school social system, including programs that reduce bullying in school (Olweus, 1993).

Despite encouraging findings regarding prevention and treatment of conduct problems through interventions affecting the social environment, there are relatively few U.S. programs that have outcome data in multiple randomized trials, or trials conducted by more than one research group. This leads to the concern that more replications of efficacy are needed for these programs. On a positive note, enough studies have now been conducted with relatively similar approaches that we can be relatively confident of the efficacy of various basic components, such as participation in parenting groups. However, as discussed by Eddy (in press), effectiveness trials for such programs generally have yet to be conducted. Efficacy trials are generally conducted under controlled conditions with a high degree of supervision and monitoring of the fidelity of the intervention, whereas effectiveness trials for such programs are on a larger scale and usually in less ideal delivery settings with less supervision and tracking. Effectiveness studies are urgently needed so that interventions that have been shown to be helpful may be made more widely available.

A major concern is that interventions and treatment for different populations, including girls and particularly ethnic groups, need further development and testing. Although many studies have included girls and ethnically diverse samples, differential effectiveness across groups needs further testing, and further adaptation of programs to account for potentially important cultural factors is required.

It is encouraging that much progress has been made on both developmental models of conduct problems that reflect the true complexity of the world of the developing child and also in testing interventions spanning universal to indicated levels and from prenatal to adolescent developmental stages. We have learned much about components of interventions that can improve conduct problem behaviors and about features of programs that may actually make them worse. Future work on examining the interactional effects of biological and social risk in development, on interventions for diverse groups, and on tests of effectiveness should further advance our ability to prevent these domain of behaviors that can have long-term destructive effects for affected youth.

Author Note. The Antisocial and Other Personality Disorders Program, NIMH, U.S. PHS provided support for the Oregon Youth Study (grant MH 37940). The Cognitive, Social, and Affective Development, NICHD, and Division of Epidemiology, Services and Prevention Branch, NIDA, NIH, U.S. PHS provided support for the Couples Study (HD 46364). Additional support was provided by grant DA 051485 from the Division of Epidemiology, Services and Prevention Branch, NIDA, and Cognitive, Social, and Affective Development, NICHD, NIH, U.S. PHS; and grant MH 46690 from the Prevention, Early Intervention, and Epidemiology Branch, NIMH, and Office of Research on Minority Health, U.S. PHS.

References

Achenbach, T.M. (1993). Taxonomy and comorbidity of conduct problems: Evidence from empirically based approaches. *Development and Psychopathology, 5,* 51–64.

Alexander, J.F., & Parsons, B. (1973). Short-term behavioral intervention with delinquent families: Impact on family process and recidivism. *Journal of Abnormal Psychology, 81,* 219–225.

Alexander, J.F., & Parsons, B. (1982). *Functional family therapy.* Monterey, CA: Brooks/Cole.

American Bar Association & National Bar Association. (2001). *Justice by gender: The lack of appropriate prevention, diversion, and treatment alternatives for girls in the justice system* (Report): American Bar Association and National Bar Association.

American Psychological Association. (1994). *Diagnostic and Statistical Manual of Mental Disorders* (4th ed.). Washington, DC: Author.

Angold, A., & Costello, E.J. (2001). The epidemiology of disorders of conduct. Nosological issues and comorbidity. In J. Hill & B. Maughan (Eds.), *Conduct Disorders in Childhood and Adolescence.* Cambridge: Cambridge University Press.

Angold, A., Costello, E.J., & Erkanli, A. (1999). Comorbidity. *Journal of Child Psychology and Psychiatry, 40,* 57–87.

Arnold, M.E., & Hughes, J.N. (1999). First do no harm: Adverse effects of grouping deviant youth for skills training. *Journal of School Psychology, 37,* 99–115.

Aultman, M. (1980). Group involvement in delinquent acts: A study of offense type and male-female participation. *Criminal Justice and Behavior, 7,* 185–192.

Baltes, P.B. (1983). Life-span developmental psychology: Observations on history and theory revisited. In R.M. Lerner (Ed.), *Developmental Psychology: Historical and Philosophical Perspectives* (pp. 79–11). Hillsdale, NJ: Lawrence Erlbaum.

Barkley, R.A. (1990). A critique of current diagnostic criteria for attention deficit hyperactivity disorder: Clinical and research implications. *Journal of Developmental and Behavioral Pediatrics, 11,* 343–352.

Beyers, J.M., Bates, J.E., Pettit, G.S., & Dodge, K.A. (2003). Neighborhood structure, parenting processes, and the development of youths' externalizing behaviors: A multilevel analysis. *American Journal of Community Psychology, 31,* 35–53.

Blumstein, A., Cohen, J., Roth, J.A., & Visher, C.A. (Eds.). (1986). *Criminal Careers and "Career Criminals."* Washington, DC: National Academy Press.

Bohman, M. (1996). Predispositions to criminality: Swedish adoption studies in retrospect. In G.R. Bock & J.A. Goode (Eds.), *Genetics of Criminal and Antisocial Behavior: Ciba Foundation Symposium 194* (pp. 179–197). New York: Wiley.

Borduin, C.M., Henggeler, S.W., Blaske, D.M., & Stein, R. (1990). Multisystemtic treatment of adolescent sexual offenders. *International Journal of Offender Therapy and Comparative Criminology, 34,* 105–113.

Brestan, E.V., & Eyberg, S.M. (1998). Effective psychosocial treatments of conduct-disordered children and adolescents: 29 years, 82 studies, and 5,272 kids. *Journal of Clinical Child Psychology, 27,* 180–189.

Bronfenbrenner, U. (1986). Ecology of the family as a context for human development: Research perspectives. *Developmental Psychology, 22,* 723–742.

Burton, L.M., Obeidallah, D.A., & Allison, K. (1996). Ethnographic insights on social context and adolescent development among inner-city African-American teens. In R. Jessor & A. Colby (Eds.), *Ethnography and Human Development: Context and Meaning in Social Inquiry* (pp. 395–418). The John D. And Catherine T. MacArthur Foundation Series on Mental Health and Development. Chicago, IL: University of Chicago Press.

Buss, D.M. (1987). Selection, evocation, and manipulation. *Journal of Personality and Social Psychology, 53,* 1214–1221.

Cadoret, R.J., Yates, W.R., Troughton, E., Woodworth, G., & Stewart, M.A. (1995). Adoption study demonstrating two genetic pathways to drug abuse. *Archives of General Psychiatry, 52,* 42–52.

Cairns, R.B., & Cairns, B.D. (1995). Social ecology over time and space. In P. Moen, G.H. Elder Jr., & K. Luscher (Eds.), *Examining Lives in Context* (pp. 397–421). Washington, DC: American Psychological Association.

Campbell, S.B., & Ewing, L.J. (1990). Follow-up of hard-to-manage preschoolers: Adjustment at age 9 and predictors of continuing symptoms. *Journal of Child Psychology and Psychiatry, 31,* 871–889.

Campbell, M., Gonzalez, N.M., & Silva, R.R. (1992). The pharmacologic treatment of conduct disorders and rage outbursts. *Pediatric Psychopharmacology, 15,* 69–85.

Campbell, M., Small, A.M., Green, W.H., Jennings, S.J., Perry, R., Bennett, W.G., & Anderson. L. (1984). Behavioral efficacy of haloperidoal and lithium carbonate: A comparison in hospitalized aggressive children with conduct disorder. *Archives of General Psychiatry, 41,* 650–656.

Capaldi, D.M. (1991). The co-occurrence of conduct problems and depressive symptoms in early adolescent boys: I. Familial factors and general adjustment at Grade 6. *Development and Psychopathology, 3,* 277–300.

Capaldi, D.M. (2003). Parental monitoring: A person-environment interaction perspective on this key parenting skill. In A.C. Crouter & A. Booth (Eds.), *Children's Influence on Family Dynamics: The Neglected Side of Family Relations* (pp. 171–179). Mahwah, NJ: Lawrence Erlbaum.

Capaldi, D.M., Chamberlain, P., & Patterson, G.R. (1997). Ineffective discipline and conduct problems in males: Association, late adolescent outcomes, and prevention. *Aggression and Violent Behavior, 2,* 343–353.

Capaldi, D.M., & Clark, S. (1998). Prospective family predictors of aggression toward female partners for at-risk young men. *Developmental Psychology, 34,* 1175–1188.

Capaldi, D.M., Crosby, L., & Stoolmiller, M. (1996). Predicting the timing of first sexual intercourse for at-risk adolescent males. *Child Development, 67,* 344–359.

Capaldi, D.M., & Patterson, G.R. (1987). An approach to the problem of recruitment and retention rates for longitudinal research. *Behavioral Assessment, 9,* 169–177.

Capaldi, D.M., Pears, K.C., Patterson, G.R., & Owen, L.D. (2003). Continuity of parenting practices across generations in an at-risk sample: A prospective comparison of direct and mediated associations. *Journal of Abnormal Child Psychology, 31,* 127–142.

Capaldi, D.M., & Stoolmiller, M. (1999). Co-occurrence of conduct problems and depressive symptoms in early adolescent boys: III. Prediction to young-adult adjustment. *Development and Psychopathology, 11,* 59–84.

Capaldi, D.M., Stoolmiller, M., Clark, S., & Owen, L.D. (2002). Heterosexual risk behaviors in at-risk young men from early adolescence to young adulthood: Prevalence, prediction, and STD contraction. *Developmental Psychology, 38,* 394–406.

Caspi, A., McClay, J., Moffitt, T.E., Mill, J., Martin, J., Craig, I.W., Taylor, A., & Poulton, R. (2002). Role of genotype in the cycle of violence in maltreated children. *Science, 297,* 851–854.

Caspi, A., Moffitt, T.E., Newman, D.L., & Silva, P.A. (1996). Behavioral observations at age 3 years predict adult psychiatric disorders. *Archives of General Psychiatry, 53,* 1033–1039.

Chamberlain, P., & Reid, J. (1998). Comparison of two community alternatives to incarceration for chronic juvenile offenders. *Journal of Consulting and Clinical Psychology, 6,* 624–633.

Cohen, P., Cohen, J., Kasen, S., Velez, C.N., Hartmark, C., Johnson, J., Rojas, M., Brook, J.S., & Struening, E.L. (1993). An epidemiological study of disorders in late childhood and adolescence: I. Age- and gender-specific prevalence. *Journal of Child Psychology and Psychiatry and Allied Disciplines, 34,* 851–867

Coie, J.D., & Dodge, K. (1988). Multiple sources of data on social behavior and social status in the school: A cross-age comparison. *Child Development, 59,* 815–829.

Comings, D.E. (2000). The role of genetics in ADHD and Conduct Disorder-Relevance to the treatment of recidivistic antisocial behavior. In D.H. Fishbein (Ed.), *The Science, Treatment, and Prevention of Antisocial Behaviors: Application to the Criminal Justice System* (pp. 16-11–16-25). Kingston, NJ: Civic Research Institute.

Conduct Problems Prevention Research Group. (2002). The implementation of the Fast Track program: An example of a large-scale prevention science efficacy trial. *Journal of Abnormal and Child Psychology, 30,* 1–17.

Dishion, T.J., & Andrews, D.W. (1995). Preventing escalation in problem behaviors with high risk young adolescents: Immediate and 1-year outcomes. *Journal of Consulting and Clinical Psychology, 63,* 538–548.

Dishion, T.J., Andrews, D.W., Kavanagh, K., & Soberman, L.H. (1996). Preventive interventions for high-risk youth: The Adolescent Transitions Program. In R.D. Peters & R.J. McMahon (Eds.), *Preventing Childhood Disorders, Substance Abuse, and Delinquency* (pp. 184–214). Thousand Oaks, CA: Sage.

Dishion, T.J., McCord, J., & Poulin, F. (1999). When interventions harm: Peer groups and problem behavior. *American Psychologist, 54,* 1–10.

Dishion, T.J., & McMahon, R.J. (1998). Parental monitoring and the prevention of child and adolescent problem behavior: A conceptual and empirical formulation. *Clinical Child and Family Psychology Review, 1,* 61–75.

Dishion, T.J., Poulin, F., & Medici Skaggs, N. (2000). The ecology of premature autonomy in adolescence: Biological and social influences. In K.A. Kerns, J. Contreras, & A.M. Neal-Barnett (Eds.), *Family and Peers: Linking Two Social Worlds* (pp. 27–45). Westport, CT: Praeger.

Dishion, T.J., Spracklen, K.M., Andrews, D.W., & Patterson, G.R. (1996). Deviancy training in male adolescent friendships. *Behavior Therapy, 27*, 373–390.

Dodge, K.A. (1993). Social-cognitive mechanisms in the development of conduct disorder and depression. *Annual Review of Psychology, 44*, 559–584.

Dodge, K.A., Pettit, G.S., Bates, J.E., & Valente, E. (1995). Social-information-processing patterns partially mediate the effect of early physical abuse on later conduct problems. *Journal of Abnormal Psychology, 104*, 632–643.

Dolan, L.J., Kellam, S.G., Brown, C.H., Werthamer-Larsson, L., Rebok, G.W., Mayer, L.S., et al. (1993). The short-term impact of two classroom-based preventive interventions on aggressive and shy behaviors and poor achievement. *Journal of Applied Developmental Psychology, 14*, 317–345.

Eddy, J.M. (in press). Prevention of aggression and conduct disorders in childhood. In C.M.H. Hosman, E. Jane-Lopis, & S. Saxena (Eds.), *Prevention of Mental Disorders: An Overview on Evidence-Based Strategies and Programs*.

Eddy, M. (2001). *Aggressive and defiant behavior: The Latest Assessment and Treatment Strategies for the Conduct Disorders*. Kansas City, MO: Compact Clinicals.

Eddy, J.M., & Chamberlain, P. (2000). Family management and deviant peer association as mediators of the impact of treatment condition on youth antisocial behavior. *Journal of Consulting and Clinical Psychology, 5*, 857–863.

Eddy, J.M., Reid, J.B., Stoolmiller, M., & Fetrow, R.A. (2003). Outcomes during middle school for an elementary school-based preventive intervention for conduct problems: Follow-up results from a randomized trial. *Behavior Therapy, 34*, 535–552.

Eddy, J.M., Whaley, R.B., & Chamberlain, P. (2004). The prevention of violent behavior by chronic and serious male juvenile offenders: A 2-year follow-up of a randomized clinical trial. *Journal of Emotional and Behavioral Disorders, 12*, 2–8.

Edelbrock, C., Rende, R., Plomin, R., & Thompson, L.A. (1995). A twin study of competence and problem behavior in childhood and early adolescence. *Journal of Child Psychology and Psychiatry, 36*, 775–785.

Elder G.H. Jr. (1985). Perspectives on the life course. In G.H. Elder, Jr. (Ed.), *Life Course Dynamics: Trajectories and Transitions* (pp. 23–49). Ithaca, NY: Cornell University Press.

Elliott, D.S. (1983). *Interview schedule, National Youth Survey*. Behavioral Research Institute, Boulder, Colorado.

Elliott, D.S., & Voss, H.L. (1974). *Delinquency and Dropout*. Lexington, MA: Lexington Books.

Elliott, D.S., Wilson, W.J., Huizinga, D., Sampson, R.J., Elliott, A., & Rankin, B. (1996). The effects of neighborhood disadvantage on adolescent development. *Journal of Research in Crime and Delinquency, 33*, 389–426.

Ensminger, M.E., Lamkin, R.P., & Jacobson, N.S. (1996). School leaving: A longitudinal perspective including neighborhood effects. *Child Development, 67*, 2400–2416.

Evans, D.T., Cullen, F.T., Burton, V., Dunaway, R. & Benson, M.L. (1997). The social consequences of self-control: Testing the general theory of crime. *Criminology 35*, 475–504.

Feldman, R.A., & Caplinger, T.E. (1983). The St. Louis experiment: Treatment of antisocial youths in prosocial peer groups. In J.R. Kluegel (Ed.), *Evaluating Juvenile Justice* (pp. 121–148). Beverly Hills, CA: Sage.

Fergusson, D.M., Woodward, L.J., & Horwood, L.J. (1998). Maternal smoking during pregnancy and psychiatric adjustment in late adolescence. *Archives of General Psychiatry, 55*, 721–727.

Forgatch, M.S. (1991). The clinical science vortex: Developing a theory for antisocial behavior. In D.J. Pepler & K.H. Rubin (Eds.), *The Development and Treatment of Childhood Aggression* (pp. 291–315). Hillsdale, NJ: Lawrence Erlbaum Associates.

Frick, P.J. (1998). *Conduct Disorders and Severe Antisocial Behaviour*. New York: Plenum.

Friedman, L.S., Lichtenstein, E., & Biglan, A. (1985). Smoking onset among teens: An empirical analysis of initial situations. *Addictive Behaviors, 10*, 1–13.

Galambos, N.L., Barker, E.T., & Almeida, D.M. (2003). Parents do matter: Trajectories of change in externalizing and internalizing problems in early adolescence. *Child Development, 74*, 578–594.

Ge, X., Conger, R.D., Cadoret, R.J., Neiderhiser, J.M., Yates, W., Troughton, E., et al. (1996). The developmental interface between nature and nurture: A mutual influence model of child antisocial behavior and parent behaviors. *Developmental Psychology, 32*, 574–589.

Gilliom, M., Shaw, D.S., Beck, J.E., Schonberg, M.A., & Lukon, J.L. (2002). Anger regulation in disadvantaged preschool boys: Strategies, antecedents, and the development of self-control. *Developmental Psychology, 38*, 222–235.

Giordano, P.C., & Cernkovich, S.A. (1997). Gender and antisocial behavior. In D.M. Stoff, J. Breiling, & J.D. Maser (Eds.), *Handbook of Antisocial Behavior* (pp. 496–510). New York: Wiley.

Gottfredson, M.R., & Hirschi, T. (1990). *A General Theory of Crime*. Stanford, CA: Stanford University Press.

Gray, J.A. (1987). Anxiety and depression. In J.A. Gray (Ed.), *The Psychology of Fear and Stress* (2nd ed., pp. 356–365). New York: Cambridge University Press.

Greenberg, M.T. & Kusché, C.A. (1998) *Promoting Alternative Thinking Strategies*. Institute of Behavioral Sciences, University of Colorado.

Greenberg, M.T., Kusché, C.A., Cook, E.T., & Quamma, J.P. (1995). Promoting emotional competence in school-aged children: The effects of the PATHS curriculum. *Development and Psychopathology, 7*, 117–136.

Greenhill, L.L. (1992). Pharmacologic treatment of attention deficit hyperactivity disorder. *Pediatric Psychopharmacology, 15*, 1–26.

Henggeler, S.W. (1990). *Family Therapy and Beyond: A Multisystemic Approach to Treating the Behavior Problems of Children and Adolescents*. Pacific Grove, CA: Brooks/Cole.

Henggeler, S.W., Cunningham, P.B., Pickrel, S.G., Schoenwald, S.K. & Brondino, M.J. (1996). Multisystemic therapy: An effective violence prevention approach for serious juvenile offenders. *Journal of Adolescence, 19*, 47–61.

Henggeler, S.W., Melton, G.B., & Smith, L.A. (1992). Family preservation using multisystemic therapy: An effective alternative to incarcerating to incarcerating serious juvenile offenders. *Journal of Consulting & Clinical Psychology, 60*, 953–961.

Henggeler, S.W., Melton, G.B., Smith, L.A., Schoenwald, S.K., & Hanley, J.H. (1993). Family preservation using multisystemic treatment: Long-term follow up to a clinical trial with serious juvenile offenders. *Journal of Child and Family Studies, 2*, 283–293.

Henggeler, S.W., Mihalic, S.F., Rone, L., Thomas, C., & Timmons-Mitchell, J. (Eds.). (1998). *Blueprints for Violence Prevention; Book 6: Multisystemic Therapy*. Boulder, CO: Center for the Study and Prevention of Violence.

Hill, J. (2002). Biological, psychological and social processes in the conduct disorders. *Journal of Child Psychology and Psychiatry, 43*, 133–164.

Hinshaw, S.P., Lahey, B.B., & Hart, E.L. (1993). Issues of taxonomy and comorbidity in the development of conduct disorder. *Development and Psychopathology, 5*, 31–49.

Kazdin, A.E., Bass, D., Siegel, T., & Thomas, C.C. (1989). Cognitive-behavioral treatment and relationship therapy in the treatment of children referred for antisocial behavior. *Journal of Consulting and Clinical Psychology, 57*, 522–535.

Kazdin, A.E., Esveldt-Dawson, K., French, N.H., & Unis, A.S. (1987a). Effects of parent management training and problem-solving skills training combined in the treatment of antisocial child behavior. *Journal of the American Academy of Child and Adolescent Psychiatry. 26*, 416–424.

Kazdin, A.E., Esveldt-Dawson, K., French, N.H., & Unis, A.S. (1987b). Problem-solving skills training and relationship therapy in the treatment of antisocial child behavior. *Journal of Consulting and Clinical Psychology, 55*, 76–85.

Kazdin, A.E., Siegel, T.C., & Bass, D. (1992). Cognitive problem-solving skills training and parent management training in the treatment of antisocial behavior in children. *Journal of Consulting and Clinical Psychology, 60*, 733–747.

Keenan, K., Loeber, R., & Green, S. (1999). Conduct disorder in girls: A review of the literature. *Clinical Child and Family Psychology Review, 2*, 3–19.

Kellam, S.G., Rebok, G.W., Mayer, L.S., Ialongo, N., & Kalodner, C.R. (1994). Depressive symptoms over first grade and their response to a developmental epidemiologically based preventive trial aimed at improving achievement. *Developmental Psychopathology, 6*, 463–481.

Klein, N.C., Alexander, J.F., & Parsons, B.V. (1977). Impact of family systems intervention on recidivism and sibling delinquency: A model of primary prevention and program evaluation. *Journal of Consulting and Clinical Psychology, 45*, 469–474.

Kohlberg, L., Ricks, D., & Snarey, J. (1984). Childhood development as a predictor of adaptation in adulthood. *Genetic Psychology Monographs, 110*, 91–172.

Kruesi, M.J.P., Rapoport, J.L., Hamburger, S., Hibbs, E.D., Potter, W.Z., Lenane, M., & Brown, G.L. (1990). Cerebrospinal fluid monoamine metabolites, aggression, and impulsivity in disruptive behavior disorders of children and adolescents. *Archives of General Psychiatry, 47*, 419–426.

Lahey, B.B., Miller, T.L., Gordon, R.A., & Riley, A. (1999). Developmental epidemiology of the disruptive behavior disorders. In H.C. Quay & A. Hogan (Eds.), *Handbook of the Disruptive Behavior Disorders*. San Antonia, TX: Academic Press.

Lahey, B.B., & Waldman, I.D. (2003). The developmental propensity model of the origins of conduct problems during childhood and adolescence. In B.B. Lahey, T.E. Moffitt, & A. Caspi (Eds.), *Causes of Conduct Disorder and Juvenile Delinquency* (pp. 76–117). New York: Guilford Press.

Leve, L.D., Winebarger, A.A., Fagot, B.I., Reid, J.B., & Goldsmith, H.H. (1998). Environment and genetic variance in children's observed and reported maladaptive behavior. *Child Development, 69*, 1286–1298.

Leventhal, T., & Brooks-Gunn, J. (2000). The neighborhoods they live in: The effects of neighborhood residence on child and adolescent outcomes. *Psychological Bulletin, 126*, 309–337.

Lewis, D.O., Yeager, C.A., Cobham-Portorreal, C.S., Klein, N., Showalter, C., & Anthony, A. (1991). A follow-up of female delinquents: Maternal contributions to the perpetuation of deviance. *Journal of the American Academy of Child and Adolescent Psychiatry, 30*, 197–201.

Lipsey, M.W. (1992). Juvenile delinquency treatment: A meta-analytic inquiry into the variability of effects. In T.D. Cook, H. Cooper, D.S. Cordray, H. Hartmann, L.V. Hedges, R.J. Light, T.A. Louis, & F. Mosteller (Eds.), *Meta-Analysis for Explanation: A Casebook* (pp. 83–127). New York: Russell Sage Foundation.

Lipsey, M.W., & Derzon, J.H. (1998). Predictors of violent or serious delinquency in adolescence and early adulthood: A synthesis of longitudinal research. In R. Loeber & D.P. Farrington (Eds.), *Serious and Violent Juvenile Offenders: Risk Factors and Successful Interventions* (pp. 86–105). Thousand Oaks, CA: Sage.

Losel, F, & Beelmann, A. (2003). Effects of child skills training in preventing antisocial behavior: A systematic review of randomized evaluations. *Annals of the American Academy of Political and Social Science, 587*, 84–109.

Mandel, H.P. (1997). *Conduct disorder and underachievement*. New York: Wiley.

McCord, J. (1978). A thirty-year follow-up of treatment effects. *American Psychologist, 33*, 284–289.

McCord, J. (1981). Consideration of some effects of a counseling program. In S.E. Martin, L.B. Sechrest, & R. Redner (Eds.), *New Directions in the Rehabilitation of Criminal Offenders* (pp. 394–405). Washington, DC: The National Academy of Sciences.

Moffitt, T., Caspi, A., Fawcett, P., Brammer, G.L., Raleigh, M., Yuwiler, A., et al. (1997). Whole blood serotonin and family background relate to male violence. In A. Raine, P.A. Brennan, D.P. Farrington, & S.A. Mednick (Eds.), *Biosocial Bases of Violence. NATO ASI Series: Series A: Life Sciences* (vol. 292, pp. 231–249). New York: Plenum.

Mrazek, P.G., & Haggerty, R.J. (Eds.). (1994). *Reducing Risks for Mental Disorders: Frontiers for Preventive Intervention Research*. Washington, DC: National Academy Press.

Newcomb, M.D. (1987). Consequences of teenage drug use: The transition from adolescence to young adulthood. *Drugs and Society, 1*, 25–60.

Olds, D., Hill, P., Mihalic, S., & O'Brien, R. (Eds.). (1998). *Blueprints for Violence Prevention; Book 7: Prenatal and Infancy Home Visitation by Nurses*. Boulder, CO: Center for the Study and Prevention of Violence.

Olweus, D. (1993). *Bullying at School: What We Know and What We Can Do*. Cambridge, United Kingdom: Blackwell.

Patterson, G.R. (1982). *Coercive Family Process*. Eugene, OR: Castalia.

Patterson, G.R., Reid, J.B., Jones, R.R., & Conger, R.E. (1975). *A Social Learning Approach to Family Intervention: Families with Aggressive Children* (Vol. 1). Eugene, OR: Castalia Publishing.

Pears, K.C., & Capaldi, D.M. (2001). Intergenerational transmission of abuse: A two-generation, prospective study of an at-risk sample. *Child Abuse & Neglect: The International Journal, 25*, 1439–1461.

Petrosino, A., Turpin-Petrosino, C., & Buehler, J. (2003). Scared Straight and other juvenile awareness programs for preventing juvenile delinquency. *The ANNALS of the American Academy of Political and Social Science, 589*, 41–62.

Pettit, G.S., Bates, J.E., Dodge, K.A., & Meece, D.W. (1999). The impact of after-school peer contact on early adolescent externalizing problems is moderated by parental monitoring, perceived neighborhood safety, and prior adjustment. *Child Development, 70*, 768–778.

Pulkkinen, L. (1996). Proactive and reactive aggression in early adolescence as precursors to anti- and prosocial behavior in young adults. *Aggressive Behavior, 22*, 241–257.

Reid, J.B., Eddy, J.M., Fetrow, R.A., & Stoolmiller, M. (1999). Description and immediate impacts of a preventative intervention for conduct problems. *American Journal of Community Psychology, 27*, 483–517.

Reid, J.B., Patterson, G.R., & Snyder, J. (Eds.). (2002). *Antisocial Behavior in Children and Adolescents: A Developmental Analysis and Model for Intervention*. Washington, DC: American Psychological Association.

Rogeness, G.A., Hernadez, J.M., Macedo, C.A., Mitchell, E.L., Amrung, S.A., & Harris, W.R. (1984). Clinical characteristics of emotionally disturbed boys with very low activities of dopaminemetahydroxylase. *Journal of the American Academy of Child and Adolescent Psychiatry, 23,* 203–208.

Rogeness, G.A., & McClure, E.B. (1996). Development and neurotransmitter-environmental interactions. *Development and Psychopathology, 8,* 183–199.

Rothbart, M.K., Posner, M.I., & Hershey, K.L. (1995). Temperament, attention, and developmental psychopathology. In D. Cicchetti & D.J. Cohen (Eds.), *Developmental Psychopathology: Vol. 1. Theory and Methods* (pp. 315–341). New York: Wiley.

Scarr, S., & McCartney, K. (1983). How people make their own environments: A theory of genotype leading to environment effects. *Child Development, 54,* 424–435.

Schuel, H., Burkman, L.J., Lippes, J., Crickard, K., Mahony, M.C., Giuffrida, A., Picone, R.P., & Makriyannis, A. (2002). Evidence that anandamide-signaling regulates human sperm functions required for fertilization. *Molecular Reproduction and Development, 63,* 376–387.

Serketich, W.J., & Dumas, J.E. (1996). The effectiveness of behavioral parent training to modify antisocial behavior in children: A meta-analysis. *Behavior Therapy, 27,* 171–186.

Shaffer, D., Fisher, P., Dulcan, M.K., & Davies, M. (1996). The NIMH Diagnostic Interview Schedule for Children Version 2.3 (DISC-2.3): Description, acceptability, prevalence rates, and performance in the MECA study. *Journal of the American Academy of Child and Adolescent Psychiatry, 35,* 865–877.

Shure, M.D., Spivack, G., & Gordon, R. (1972). Problem-solving thinking: A preventative mental health program for preschool children. *Reading World, 11,* 259–273.

Simonoff, E. (2001). Genetic influences on conduct disorder. In J. Hill & B. Maughan (Eds.), *Conduct Disorders in Childhood and Adolescence* (pp. 202–234). New York: Cambridge University Press.

Snyder, H.N. (1998). *Juvenile Arrests 1997,* Washington, DC: U.S. Department of Justice, Office of Justice Programs, Office of Juvenile Justice and Delinquency Prevention.

Steffensmeier, D. (1993). National trends in female arrests, 1960–1990: Assessment and recommendations for research. *Journal of Quantitative Criminology, 9,* 411–441.

Stoolmiller, M. (1999). Implications of the restricted range of family environments for estimates of heritability and nonshared environment in behavior-genetic adoption studies. *Psychological Bulletin, 125,* 392–407.

Stoolmiller, M., Eddy, J.M., & Reid, J.B. (2000). Detecting and describing preventative intervention effects in a universal school-based randomized trail targeting delinquent and violent behavior. *Journal of Consulting and Clinical Psychology, 68,* 296–306.

Taylor, T.K., & Biglan, A. (1998). Behavioral family interventions for improving child-rearing: A review of the literature for clinicians and policy makers. *Clinical Child and Family Psychology Review, 1,* 41–60.

Thapar, A., Holmes, J., Poulton, K., & Harrington, R. (1999). Genetic basis of attention deficit and hyperactivity. *British Journal of Psychiatry, 174,* 105–111.

Tolan, P.H., & Gorman-Smith, D. (2002). What violence prevention research can tell us about developmental psychopathology. *Development and Psychopathology, 14,* 713–729.

Tolan, P.H., Gorman-Smith, D., & Henry, D.B. (2003). The development ecology of urban males' youth violence. *Developmental Psychology, 29,* 274–291.

Tremblay, R.E., Pagani-Kurtz, L., Masse, L.C., Vitaro, F., & Pihl, R.O. (1995). A bimodal preventive intervention for disruptive kindergarten boys: Its impact through mid-adolescence. *Journal of Consulting and Clinical Psychology, 63,* 560–568.

Webster-Stratton, C. (1990). Long-term follow-up of families with young conduct-problem children: From preschool to grade school. *Journal of Clinical Child Psychology, 19,* 144–149.

Webster-Stratton, C., & Hammond, M. (1997). Treating children with early-onset conduct problems: A comparison of child and parent training interventions. *Journal of Consulting and Clinical Psychology, 65,* 93–109.

Webster-Stratton, C., Reid, J., & Hammond, M. (2000). *Preventing conduct problems, promoting social competence: A parent and teacher training partnership for a multi-ethic, Head Start population.* Unpublished. Seattle: University of Washington, School of Nursing, Department of Family and Child Nursing, Parenting Clinic.

Whitaker, A., & Rao, U. (1992). Neuroleptics in pediatric psychiatry. *Pediatric Psychopharmacology, 15,* 243–275.

Wichstrom, L., Skogen, K., & Oia, T. (1996). Increased rate of conduct problems in urban areas: What is the mechanism? *Journal of the American Academy of Child and Adolescent Psychiatry, 35,* 471–479.

Wiesner, M., Kim, H.K., & Capaldi, D.M. (in press). Developmental trajectories of offending: Validation and prediction to young adult alcohol use, drug use, and depressive symptoms. *Development and Psychopathology*.

Wikstrom, P.H., & Loeber, R. (2000). Do disadvantaged neighborhoods cause well-adjusted children to become adolescent delinquents? A study of male juvenile serious offending, individual risk and protective factors, and neighborhood context. *Criminology, 38,* 1109–1142.

Wilens, T.E., & Biederman, J. (1992). The stimulants. *Pediatric Psychopharmacology, 15,* 191–222.

World Health Organization. (1997). *Composite International Diagnostic Interview (CIDI). Core Version 2.1.* Geneva, Switzerland: World Health Organization.

Zoccolillo, M. (1993). Gender and the development of conduct disorder. *Development and Psychopathology, 5,* 65–78.

Chapter 14

Pervasive Developmental Delay

Raymond W. DuCharme and Kathleen A. McGrady

Introduction

This chapter examines pervasive developmental delay and in particular Asperger syndrome. Interventions for these disorders and the question of prevention are examined.

What is a pervasive developmental delay (PDD)? Is a diagnostic description of pervasive development delay, not otherwise specified (PDD, NOS) helpful to the individual, his family, and those responsible to provide treatment?

The purpose of a diagnosis is to describe a condition in need of correction and to determine a regimen of treatment. The diagnosis should state that if a treatment is provided, then a prediction of prognosis can be made. The correctness of the diagnosis is critical to the identification of the proper interventions that should be present in order to treat the individual.

In recent years the diagnosis of pervasive developmental delay or pervasive developmental delay, not otherwise specified (*DSM-IV* PDD, NOS) has increased dramatically in referrals of individuals to residential schools and special education classrooms. Individuals with a pervasive developmental delay, not otherwise specified diagnosis are those persons who do not fit all of the criteria for a cluster of diagnoses that are part of a spectrum of disorders that involve developmental delays (see Table 1).

There is a strong case to be made that autism, high-functioning autism, and Asperger syndrome are aspects of a continuum that reflect a spectrum of developmental delay (Volkmar et al., 1998; Rourke, 1995). There is a concern, however, that differences between the current *DSM-IV* and ICD-10 of the World Health Organization criteria for the diagnosis of Asperger syndrome threaten the external validity of a correct diagnosis (DuCharme & McGrady, 2004) (See Table 2).

These differences in diagnostic criteria can result in error and misdiagnosis. Misdiagnosis can result in errors in the selection and duration of treatment which can yield poor prognosis and little evidence of efficacy.

The prevalence data of Asperger syndrome (AS) are limited by the validity measures associated with basic research. Ehlers and Gillberg (1993) report the prevalence

Table 1. Pervasive Developmental Delay

Diagnosis	Onset of Symptoms	Gender	Social Skills	Head Circumference	Language Skills	Cognitive Functioning	Motor Skills
Autism	Prior to age 3 years; symptoms in infancy are subtle	Males (8 times greater than females)	Social skill deficits		Delay, or lack of development	75% have mental retardation	Repetitive and Stereotyped
Rett's disorder	Five months normal development; diagnosed at 5–48 months	Females	Loss of social interaction early; may develop later	Decelerates at 5–48 months	Expressive and receptive language problems	Severe to profound mental retardation	"Hand-wringing"; gait and truck coordination problems
Childhood disintegrative disorder	Two years normal development; diagnosed before age 10	Males—more common	Loss of social skills (after age 2 years)		Expressive or receptive (after age 2 years)	Severe mental retardation (usually)	Loss of motor skills after age 2 years
Asperger syndrome	Recognition and diagnosis later (e.g., school age, ages 7–11 years)	Males (8 times greater than females)	Social skill deficits		No general delay in language; but pragmatic language deficits; theory of mind—subvocal speech	Normal IQ, verbal performance deviation	Motor delays and clumsiness: absence of research
PDD, NOS	Does not meet criteria for any of the above, but has some of the behaviors	Does not meet criteria for any of the above, but has some of the behaviors	Does not meet criteria for any of the above, but has some of the behaviors	Does not meet criteria for any of the above, but has some of the behaviors	Does not meet criteria for any of the above, but has some of the behaviors	Does not meet criteria for any of the above, but has some of the behaviors	Does not meet criteria for any of the above, but has some of the behaviors

The Learning Clinic, Inc., January 16, 2004.

Table 2. Asperger Syndrome Criteria

	DSM-IV	ICD-10
Qualitative impairment in social interaction	X	X
Restricted repetitive and stereotyped patterns of behavior, interests, and activities	X	X
No general language delay	X	X
No delay in cognitive development	X	X
Normal general intelligence (most)		X
Markedly clumsy (common)		X
No delay in development of—	X	
Age-appropriate self-help skills		
Adaptive behavior (excluding social interaction)		
Curiosity about environment		

of Asperger syndrome to be 26–36 per 10,000 school-age individuals. Paul Shattuck detailed prevalence data of autism in public schools. He reported an increase of 24% between 1994 and 2000 (cited in Blacher, 2002). Other researchers report similiar data (Blacher, 2002).

Klin et al. (1995) conclude that AS appears to be a "very mild" form of pervasive developmental disorder. The authors question the value of creating the Asperger syndrome grouping apart from the pervasive developmental disorder, not otherwise specified category. This idea of a broadband diagnostic grouping creates the need for answering what constitutes a "significant" delay and what combination of delayed performances suggests pervasiveness. Further, the status of a developmental delay does not imply that there will be continued future development toward the maturation of that measured delay.

A search of the literature using the keyword "Asperger" produced 385 studies, articles, and other references. One hundred sixty-six studies pertained to diagnosis. These articles examine autism, Asperger syndrome, high-functioning autism, pervasive developmental delay, not otherwise specified, and non-verbal learning disability.

Raja and Anzzoni (2001) discuss the autistic condition described almost simultaneously by Dr. Asperger in Vienna (1944) and Dr. Kanner (1943) in Baltimore. Both men were medically trained in Vienna at about the same time. Dr. Kanner (1943) described the children that he diagnosed as having "infantile autism." Dr. Asperger (1944) observed children in his hospital unit in Vienna that he characterized as "autistic psychopathy" (Frith, 1991). Kanner's diagnosis of infantile autism is more severe than Asperger's label. Their work has inspired decades of research that has attempted to clarify the differences and similarities between the two clinical descriptions.

In recent years Asperger syndrome (AS) was considered to be a pervasive developmental disorder and was included as a new diagnosis in the World Health Organization (1992) International Classification of Diseases (ICD-10) and the United States (1994) Diagnostic and Statistical Manual of Mental Disorders (DSM-IV) (APA, 1994) (see Table 2).

Eisenmajer et al. (1996) point out that the DSM-IV criteria for Asperger's disorder (now called Asperger syndrome) is the same as that for autism disorder (AD) with three exceptions: communication and imagination impairment criteria for Autism Disorder are not listed for AS; the child with an AS diagnosis does not suffer from a clinically significant general delay in language (single words by age 2 years and phrases by age 3); and the child with AS does not have a clinically significant delay in cognitive development, age appropriate self-help skills, adaptive behavior, or curiosity about the environment.

Raja and Anzzoni (2001, pp. 285–293) note that ". . . the syndrome Hans Asperger originally described may not be captured by the present DSM-IV or ICD-10 criteria." There are differences between the diagnostic criteria provided by the *DSM-IV* and the ICD-10. While the ICD-10 endorses the traits of normal intelligence and clumsy behavior, the *DSM-IV* does not. Further, the *DSM-IV* lists that there is no delay in the development of age appropriate self-help skills, adaptive behavior (excluding social interaction), and curiosity about the environment, while the ICD-10 does not list these criteria.

Behavior Patterns

Fundamental differences in criteria produce a serious threat to the external validity of the diagnosis of Asperger syndrome. The similarity between an autistic disorder diagnosis and a pervasive developmental disorder, not otherwise specified (PDD, NOS) diagnosis adds to the difficulty in interpreting diagnostic categories.

Leekham et al. (2000) developed algorithms for a Diagnostic Interview for Social and Communication Disorders (DISCO). The interview models were used to compare the ICD-10 for AS with those developed by Gillberg in 1993. Two hundred children and adults were studied who met the ICD-10 criteria for childhood autism or atypical autism. Of these only 1% met the ICD-10 criteria for Asperger syndrome. Forty-five percent of the sample met the Asperger syndrome criteria defined by Gillberg. This study revealed that the discrepancy in diagnoses was due to the ICD-10 requirement for "normal" development of cognitive skills. The authors question the benefit of defining a separate AS subgroup. They suggest, as do Klin et al. (1995), Volkmar et al. (1998), and Schopler et al. (1998), that a dimensional view of the autistic spectrum is more appropriate than a categorical one. The definition of a "syndrome" or pattern of symptoms along a continuum is more useful than the term "disorder."

Gillberg's six criteria (Ehlers and Gillberg, 1993) comprise social impairments, narrow interests, repetitive routines, speech and language peculiarities, non-verbal communication problems, and motor clumsiness. The ICD-10 and *DSM-IV* note an absence of any clinical delay in language and cognitive development in the first 3 years of life. The *DSM-IV* adds no delay in the development of self-help skills, adaptive behavior, and curiosity about the environment. Gillberg's (Ehlers and Gillberg, 1993) broader criteria appears to differentiate between groups more reliably than do either the *DSM-IV* or ICD-10.

It is also important to note that the developmental signpost of 3 years of age for evidence of delays may be too limiting, as critical functions may become deficient over time, through subsequent developmental stages. Also, the criterion of an IQ of 70 or above may place the lower level too low, given the normal range of IQ that other researchers use as the standard for an Asperger syndrome characteristic. Other research (DuCharme, 2003) suggest that patterns of pragmatic skill deficits persist across ages for Asperger syndrome individuals.

Research suggests that a dimensional view of the autism spectrum is more appropriate than the categorical approach represented by the ICD-10 and *DSM-IV*. A dimensional view considers patterns of symptoms, or characteristics, and degrees of severity. For example, Ozonoff et al. (2000) compared 23 children with high-functioning autism with 12 children who were diagnosed with Asperger syndrome. Both groups were matched for chronological age, gender, and intellectual ability. The sources of difference between the groups are categorized as cognitive functions, current symptoms, and early history. The authors conclude that high-functioning Autism and Asperger syndrome involve the same symptomatology and differ only in degree of severity.

Klin et al. (1995) report on the validity of neuropsychological characterization of Asperger syndrome and the convergence of Asperger syndrome with non-verbal learning disability. Their research used the ICD-10 diagnostic criteria. The authors compared neuropsychological profiles of Asperger syndrome (AS) and high-functioning autism (HFA) and the assets and deficits described by the term "non-verbal learning disability" (NLD) reported by Rourke (1995). The groups were described to differ significantly in 11 neuropsychological areas.

The aspects of non-verbal learning disorder, typical of child functioning, include deficits in tactile perception, psycho-motor coordination, visual-spatial organization, non-verbal problem solving, appreciation of incongruity, and humor. The non-verbal learning disability child demonstrates poor pragmatic language skill and impaired prosody in speech, along with deficits in social perception, social judgment, and social interaction skills. These examples of child functioning for non-verbal Learning Disability are also typical of the Asperger syndrome child. Both groups, Asperger syndrome and non-verbal learning disability, share the tendency toward social withdrawal and mood disorder (Klin et al., 1995). Non-verbal learning disability is not part of the diagnostic nosology of either the ICD-10 or *DSM-IV*.

Characteristics of Asperger Syndrome

MOTOR DEVELOPMENT.   It is reported that delayed motor milestones and the presence of motor clumsiness are Asperger syndrome characteristics. But there is a paucity of research to corroborate a clear association between motor delay and other Asperger syndrome characteristics (Ghaziuddin and Butler, 1998).

Motor development and "clumsiness" were investigated by Ghaziuddin and Butler (1998) and Ghaziuddin et al. (1994). The authors found no significant relationship between coordination scores and diagnostic category after adjusting scores for intelligence.

Weimer et al. (2001) suggest that the motor clumsiness reported by Green et al. (2002) and Miyahara et al. (1997) may be the result of the proprioceptive deficits that underlie the cases of uncoordination observed in some Asperger syndrome cases. Motor delay and early language delay prior to age 3 are not predictive of other Asperger syndrome characteristics or of later developmental problems. The definition of "language delay" may be too limited, as this usually pertains to the child's saying single words or simple phases.

SPEECH AND PROSODY.   Shriberg et al. (2001) investigated the speech and prosody characteristics of adolescents and adults with high-functioning autism and AS. Prosody includes phrasing, variability in speech production, same word duration in sentences, and grammatical placement of stressed and unstressed syllables and words. Voice loudness, pitch, and quality were also compared.

There were minor differences between Asperger syndrome and high-functioning autism subjects in volubility differences and articulation errors. Asperger syndrome subjects used higher volume, and there was a high prevalence of speech-sound distortion in both groups.

Findings associated with prosody and voice analyses identified significant differences between clinical and control groups in the areas of phrasing, stress, and nasal resonance. Two-thirds of the Asperger syndrome speakers were coded as having non-fluent phrasing on more than 20% of their utterances. It is speculated that Asperger syndrome individuals use repetition and revision to compensate for formulation difficulties. There is also a suggestion that increasing length of utterance is associated with increased phrasing errors. Higher levels of grammatical complexity were also associated with increased phrasing errors and length of utterance.

LANGUAGE AND MEANING.   Jolliffe and Baron-Cohen (2000) examined linguistic processing in high-functioning adults with autism or Asperger syndrome. The ability to establish causal connections and to interrelate "local chunks[1]" into higher-order "chunks" so that most linguistic elements are linked together thematically is defined as "global coherence." The authors hypothesized that adults on the autism spectrum, including those with Asperger syndrome, would have difficulty integrating information so as to derive meaning. Results showed that the clinical groups were less able to arrange sentences coherently and to use context to make a global inference.

The findings of the study on the abilities called "global coherence" are inconsistent with the classroom experience of adolescent high-functioning autism and Asperger syndrome student performance at The Learning Clinic (DuCharme & McGrady, 2003). Thirty students were assigned a task with directions for writing a news story. They were given seven statements of instruction and ten individual descriptive informational statements, six of which were relevant to a theme; and four, irrelevant. The assignment was to create a news story that had a main point by selecting relevant information from the sentences provided. All students successfully completed the task set, but demonstrated an inability to select information less relevant or irrelevant to the main theme.

Jolliffe and Baron-Cohen (2000) required an inference and use of connotative meaning to demonstrate comprehension. Global coherence may be different from inference. The Learning Clinic student behavior demonstrated the ability to identify a main theme and related, supporting data that were "coherent." No inference was required. But students were not able to differentiate the relative importance of information provided.

The "global coherence" requirement of the Jolliffe & Baron-Cohen (2000) study to interpret and infer within the context of a story is different from combining facts into a coherent statement or conclusion. The definition of their task has connotative implications. Connotative and denotative meaning derive from linguistic processes that may differ from the processes used to infer meaning from factual content.

For example, Channon et al. (2001) presented videotaped real-life problems to 30 pre-teen and adolescent youth. Fifteen were diagnosed with AS and 15 were placed in a control group. The AS group differed in their ability to provide socially appropriate

---

[1]Chunking. The process of reorganizing materials in working memory to increase the number of items successfully recalled.

solutions to the problems as compared to the control group responses. The inability to draw inferences and to assign appropriate attribution to key factors present in social situations are also discussed by Barnhill (2001) and Barnhill and Myles (2001).

COGNITIVE PROCESSES.   Cognitive flexibility required to solve a novel problem, or a familiar problem in a novel situation, is absent for AS persons to a degree beyond what their normal to superior IQ scores should predict. Shulman et al. (1995) report that individuals on the autism spectrum have difficulties with tasks that necessitate internal manipulation of information.

Theory of mind (TOM) is defined as the ability to infer mental states, including beliefs, intentions, and thoughts (Perner & Wimmer, 1985). Happe (1995) describes these internalized manipulations of information as mentalizing. How "mentalizing" is related to "global coherence" and theory of mind is unclear. But these processes suggest an interface among auditory processing, language, cognition, and the "load" of factors present in any situation.

Dunn et al. (2002) support the view that clear differences exist in the sensory processing patterns of children with AS when compared with non-clinical peers. Asperger syndrome students are reported to have difficulty with auditory processing. They demonstrate poor ability to modulate their responses from one situation to another. The authors advocate for a student to receive a sensory measurement that will yield a profile that reflects the assessment of sensory processing, modulation of behavioral-emotional responses, and level of response to "sensory events." Sensory processing deficits may alter the ability to cognitively manipulate data accurately.

Observations by Frith (1991) and Frith and Happe (1994) that AS children are limited in their ability to demonstrate pretend play, imagination, and creativity has some support in the research literature (Craig and Cohen, 1999). This apparent restricted ability to predict future events by manipulating past experience, as part of problem-solving, may be related to measures of limited creativity and theory of mind factors identified early in Asperger syndrome child development (Baron-Cohen et al., 1999; Jolliffe & Baron-Cohen, 2000).

Asperger Syndrome Profile

Barnhill (2001) provides a synthesis of research conducted by the "Asperger Syndrome Project." The Asperger Syndrome Project was designed to provide an "empirically valid profile of individuals with Asperger Syndrome" (p. 300). A series of studies were summarized to provide a description of Asperger syndrome children and youth. The following characteristics were reported:

1. IQs similar to the general population, ranging from deficient to very superior.
2. Significantly less capable written than oral language skills.
3. Limited ability to problem-solve in contrast to verbal fluency skill.
4. Measured emotional difficulties not endorsed by the Asperger syndrome students themselves.
5. Problems with inferential comprehension.
6. Attributions that parallel a learned helplessness approach.
7. Sensory problems similar to a cognitively deficient person.

Barnhill (2000) omits other characteristics such as eye gaze, pragmatic language deficiencies, poor speech characteristics of prosody, volume, phrasing, grammatical structure, and word stress.

The cluster of factors associated with socialization, social skill development, and social reality testing are important discriminate variables associated with Asperger syndrome. The tendency to prefer aloneness, to avoid peers in preference to adult interaction, other avoidant behaviors, and marginal independent living skills are related to diagnosis and prognosis for Asperger syndrome persons (Dewey, 1991; Dyer et al., 1996; Matthews, 1996; Mawhood & Howlin, 1999; Nesbitt, 2000; Tantam, 2000).

The inability to draw inferences, to interpret connotative meaning, and to apprehend relationships between factual knowledge and higher-order thinking also need to be included as Asperger syndrome characteristics worthy of investigation. Evidence of over- and under-reactivity to ordinary stimuli, and attentional shift problems are important characteristics (Courchesne et al., 1994). Level of cognitive rigidity in the presence of anxiety-producing stimuli reported anecdotally has important heurestic value in future researches.

Asperger syndrome is a complex continuum of symptoms, and these problematic symptoms of communication and language, cognition, adaptability, lack of generalization of skill, socialization, and sensory processing are more evident in the interactions that are part of the daily activities in the natural environment than the testing room. The clarity of the diagnostic nosology that fits the child's environment is important. And the need to assess Asperger syndrome persons as part of the natural daily routine is also important in order to obtain a valid assessment of their competencies.

Associated Comorbid Conditions

The method to obtain an accurate diagnosis and treatment for an Asperger child is not straightforward. Asperger syndrome is a multifaceted disorder with subtle manifestation of deficits (Mesibov et al., 2001). The diagnostic process is further complicated by comorbid conditions or other secondary problematic behaviors. These may include difficulties with attention and concentration, anxious behaviors, depression, motor or vocal tics, obsessive-compulsive behaviors, noncompliant or aggressive behaviors, or learning disabilities (Klin, Volkmar & Sparrow, 2000). Behaviors associated with these conditions tend to be disruptive, and therefore become the focus of treatment and diagnosis. Before it is recognized that a youngster has Asperger syndrome, the child may be given one or more of the following diagnostic labels: attention-deficit/hyperactivity disorder (ADHD), depression, anxiety disorder, obsessive-compulsive disorder (OCD), oppositional-defiant disorder, or schizophrenia. In some cases the child may have a comorbid condition, which warrants the diagnosis. In other cases, the behaviors are a manifestation of one of the many features of Asperger syndrome, and do not meet the criteria for a second diagnosis.

Attention-Deficit/Hyperactivity Disorder

Difficulties with attention and concentration are not uncommon with Asperger syndrome children, especially in younger children (Klin, Volkmar & Sparrow, 2000).

According to Klin and Volkmar (1997) 28% of Asperger Syndrome children have a comorbid diagnosis of attention-deficit/hyperactivity disorder. However, the Asperger syndrome child can present with impaired attention without having attention-deficit/hyperactivity disorder. Some features of Asperger syndrome that interfere with attention include sensory overload and fixated attention. With sensory overload, the Asperger syndrome child has difficulty filtering out irrelevant stimuli, and can become overloaded with sensory input. Instead of focusing attention on what is relevant, s/he is "distracted" by too much sensory input, failing to attend to what is important. With fixated attention the Asperger syndrome child becomes intensely preoccupied and selectively focused on an object or activity. Because of this fixated attention, they fail to attend to other stimuli (verbal information or interactions) in their environment.

Anxiety Disorders and Depression

Anxiety and depression are more common among older Asperger syndrome children and adults (Klin, Volkmar & Sparrow, 2000). As Asperger syndrome children mature, they become increasingly aware of how they differ from their peers, and the difficulty they have in social relationships. They are aware of "standards" of behavior and achievement which are difficult for them to attain. As a result of these differences, the AS child becomes the victim of peer teasing or ostracizing. In response to these very real differences, taunting, and social consequences, the AS child may become depressed. Adolescent depression tends to manifest differently than in adults. Instead of expressed sadness or withdrawn behaviors, it is manifested through acting-out or an irritable demeanor.

If the AS child responds with anxious behaviors, it could manifest as nail-biting, tugging at clothing, hair pulling, avoidance of school or other social situations, etc. In some cases, the anxious behaviors may meet the criteria of an anxiety disorder such as social anxiety, or school phobia. Similarly, if the depression becomes chronic and significantly interferes with daily life, it may meet the criteria for a mood disorder. In a study by Klin et al. (2000), 15% of Asperger Syndrome children had a co-existing mood disorder.

Obsessive-Compulsive Disorder

Although obsessive-compulsive disorder does occur in some individuals with Asperger syndrome (19% according to Klin et al., 2000), some features of AS can be mistaken for obsessive-compulsive disorder: cognitive rigidity, rigid adherence to routines and schedules, and a restricted range of interests. For example, it is common for Asperger syndrome children and adults to have a consuming interest in a specific limited topic (trains, elevators, dinosaurs, etc.) They typically develop extensive knowledge about their specific area of interest. What distinguishes behaviors associated with these interests from obsessive-compulsive disorder is that the Asperger syndrome individual does not feel compelled to read about "trains" or "ride a train" as a means of reducing feelings of anxiety—they simply find pleasure in pursuing their area of interest.

Another feature of the Asperger syndrome child's restricted range of interests is that they are ego-syntonic (the AS youngster does not see anything wrong with engaging in the absorbing interest). An obsessive-compulsive disorder youngster is generally bothered by the obsessive thoughts and compulsive behaviors, and experiences them as intrusive and disruptive to his/her life, and is a source of anxiety. Not so for the Asperger syndrome child.

Oppositional Defiant Disorder

Asperger syndrome children can be difficult to manage and exhibit noncompliant behaviors. However, the reasons for the apparent noncompliance are different. An important difference between an AS child and an oppositional defiant child is volition. While the oppositional defiant child will planfully disobey the "rules," the AS child will generally make an effort to follow the rules as he understands them. However, his understanding of the rule may be impaired either because of a miscommunication (comprehension or language pragmatics), sensory overload, misreading of contextual (nonverbal) cues, inattention, or because he acted impulsively. Additionally, when an AS child learns a rule in one environment, the behavior will not generalize to a new setting. In the new setting the contextual cues are different, and the AS child will perceive the similar setting/situation as entirely different.

Schizophrenia

Many aspects of Asperger syndrome can be confused with psychotic behavior. An untreated AS child can present as a solitary individual, uninterested in social interaction and intensely preoccupied with internal thoughts. Poor language pragmatic skills can contribute to a child verbalizing tangential thoughts that are loosely related to ongoing discussions.

Individual Factors

Youth who demonstrate significant and pervasive developmental delays are at risk of school failure, unemployment, and psychological and psychiatric symptoms of a debilitating nature over time.

Asperger syndrome individuals' college drop-out and failed-employment rates are high. These high rates are due not to lack of intellectual capability or the inability to understand job performance and competency requirements. Failures are associated with a lack of social skill, pragmatic language skill, failed attendance, and poor self-advocacy skills. Psychological and psychiatric symptoms increase over time and the corresponding medication therapy of increased levels of neuroleptic and other psychological medications tends to interfere with alertness, responsiveness, and other cognitive functions.

Asperger syndrome individuals are observed to incorporate symptoms of dysfunctional behavior into their performance and these dysfunctional behaviors become ego-syntonic. The Asperger syndrome individual perceives his behavior as "normal" and not in need of change. Increased attention, focus, and treatment attempts at intervention often result in increasing the level of rigidity and resistance on the part of the AS individual.

Importantly, preschool and elementary-age children are more malleable and responsive to treatment. This contrasts with adolescent individuals, who demonstrate behavior patterns and preferences that are more resistant to modification. Adolescents are less able and willing to perceive their own patterns of behavior and specific symptoms as problematic and in need of change.

Family Factors

There is little research specific to risk and resiliency in families of Asperger syndrome individuals. There is anecdotal evidence that Asperger syndrome is linked to male family members. The evidence suggests that male Asperger syndrome characteristics are genetically linked to male children and their fathers or paternal grandfathers. There are more male than female individuals identified with Asperger syndrome (ratio 8:1). And, if one child is born with characteristics of autistic symptoms, then there is a higher probability of siblings being diagnosed as demonstrating symptoms on the autism spectrum.

The family setting is the most influential factor in socializing and educating a child. Therefore, the composition and "health" of the family exerts significant influence on the degree of success of these efforts at intervention.

Family factors which provide a child with resiliency include family history of mental health, effective behavior management skills, parental support of treatment interventions, and ability to advocate for needed services. The degree to which any of these factors are diminished or absent increases the risk of failure to successfully socialize and educate a child.

Social and Community Factors

A "syndrome" is defined as a group of signs and symptoms that occur together (Merriam-Webster, 1990). The term Asperger's "disorder" was changed to Asperger "syndrome" to reflect more accurately the fact that it is characterized by a group of symptoms on a continuum. Many of these symptoms require specific interventions. The resiliency of children is enhanced when these resources are readily available through social networks and community services and preplanned transition services are provided after high school graduation.

Peer Groups

Social skill training is essential for Asperger syndrome and pervasive developmental disorder children. However, the skills that are learned in a therapeutic setting must also be put into practice in daily life. The goal is for them to be able to self-initiate age-appropriate social skills in non-therapeutic settings. Asperger and pervasive developmental disorder youth learn best when there is the opportunity for repeated practice in multiple settings. The concept of exposure to environmental social interaction as necessary for the development of social skills is well understood (Bandura, 1969; Tharpe & Wetzel, 1969). Therefore, the availability of a peer group who can encourage, support, and role-model appropriate social skills—and provide the opportunity for social interaction—facilitates the development of these skills.

Social "Clubs"

One of the defining traits of Asperger and pervasive developmental disorder children is their restricted areas of interest, topics in which they have an intense interest, and about which they tend to accumulate extensive knowledge. Teachers have learned that these children will become very attentive and motivated to learn when their area of special interest is incorporated into the concept being taught. Similarly, their area of special interest can be used to compete with the tendency to isolate: social clubs/activities in their area of special interest.

Community Resources

Children in general, and developmentally disabled children in particular, thrive and are resilient when their communities are able to provide the services they need. The community-based services that may be needed include special education, occupational therapy, physical therapy, speech and language therapy, psychiatric and psychological interventions, neurological and neuropsychological assessments, and social skill training, apprenticeship and employment opportunities, and independent living skills and transition plans for post-high school years.

Special Education

In our experience, special education schools and contained classrooms are better able to provide for the educational needs of developmentally handicapped children. Academic modifications which enhance learning for Asperger syndrome and other pervasive developmental disorder students include multi-sensory learning, adaptations for dysgraphia and visual-motor processing problems, required extra processing time, self-paced program, frequent repetitions and cues, hands-on learning experiences for the concrete learner, distraction-free environments, structured and self-contained classrooms that minimize transitions, and modifications for sensory hypersensitivities, receptive-expressive language deficits, and other learning disabilities.

Because of impaired nonverbal skills and receptive/expressive language deficits, Asperger syndrome and other pervasive developmental disorder children learn better through multisensory approaches to learning. Special education teachers are skilled at using teaching techniques that involve use of multiple senses. One manifestation of visual-motor integration difficulties faced by AS/PPD children is poor handwriting (dysgraphia), necessitating a way of expressing themselves by means other than paper and pencil, such as computer keyboarding or video and audio recording. These are common teaching modifications available at special education schools. Other teaching modifications available at special education schools include providing one-on-one instruction that incorporates the need for extra processing time, simplified (one or two steps at a time) instruction, repetitive hands-on practice for the concrete learner, backwards chaining to address global coherence deficits, and self-contained classrooms to minimize distractions and transitions.

The degree to which these special education services are provided for Asperger syndrome and pervasive developmental disorder youngsters contributes to or detracts from their resiliency. It is important to note that the class composition is critical. In our experience, youth with the diagnosis of PDD/AS do not do well with conduct-disordered youth, nor should they be placed with youth who are mentally challenged.

Professionals Knowledgeable in Diagnosing and Treating Asperger Syndrome and Pervasive Developmental Disorder, NOS

Some students may require occupational or physical therapy to improve visual-motor integration skills, and to minimize sensory hypo/hypersensitivities and self-stimulating behaviors. Speech and language therapists may be needed to remediate expressive and receptive language deficits. Psychologists, neuropsychologists, and psychiatrists are essential to diagnose and treat psychiatric and behavioral difficulties. This requires an understanding of the neurobiology of the Asperger/pervasive developmental disorder brain, and the resulting individual patterns of strengths and weaknesses, to develop effective treatment interventions.

Comorbidity is common in Asperger syndrome and pervasive developmental delay children, and often interferes with accurate diagnosis. Children are accurately diagnosed at an earlier age when they are seen by medical and psychiatric professionals who are familiar with pervasive developmental disorders. The resiliency of these children is enhanced when they receive an early, accurate diagnosis because they begin to receive needed services at an earlier age.

Employment

In general, Asperger syndrome and pervasive developmental disorder children have average to high-average intelligence and develop employable skills. However, because of their social skill deficits, they often "fail" the employment interview. Employers who are unfamiliar with the developmentally disabled sometimes interpret their poor social skills as lack of interest in the job, low intelligence, or rudeness.

Educating employers about the deficits—and strengths—of the developmentally disabled helps to overcome interview misunderstandings, and to provide an appropriate fit between employment opportunities and employee skills. Increasing employment opportunities for Asperger syndrome and pervasive developmental disorder youth increases the probability that they will be able to enter the job market and work towards financial independence. Sufficient planning of transition programs that include in vivo rehearsal, training, and monitoring of employment skills is critically important to the Asperger syndrome or PDD, NOS client.

Evidenced-Based Treatment Interventions in Community Settings

What Works

A review of the literature did not reveal an intervention that met the criteria of three successful research trials for what works.

What Might Work

There is little difference in treatment approaches between the community and residential setting. Both require a comprehensive integrated approach that marshals the family and professional resources around the youth to maximize his potential. This includes family interventions, learning modifications, and social support.

SOCIAL SKILLS TRAINING.   Social skills training is accepted as an appropriate treatment for AS children (Mesibov et al., 2001; Klin et al., 2000; DuCharme & McGrady, 2003). For students enrolled in our program at The Learning Clinic (a private residential school in northeastern Connecticut), a treatment intervention plan begins with an analysis of pragmatic skills strengths and weaknesses, and an Adult Mentor is used to facilitate these skills with peers. An example of a treatment plan for integrating pragmatic language and social skills is shown below:

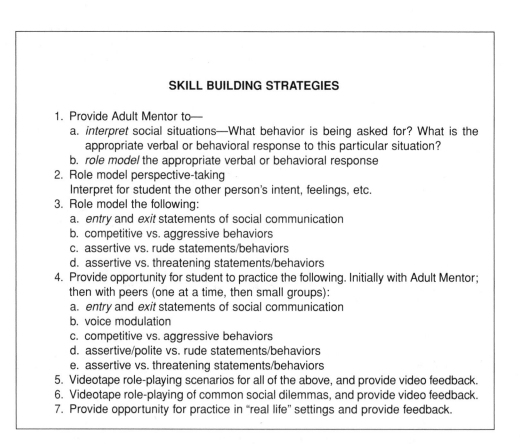

SKILL BUILDING STRATEGIES

1. Provide Adult Mentor to—
   a. *interpret* social situations—What behavior is being asked for? What is the appropriate verbal or behavioral response to this particular situation?
   b. *role model* the appropriate verbal or behavioral response
2. Role model perspective-taking
   Interpret for student the other person's intent, feelings, etc.
3. Role model the following:
   a. *entry* and *exit* statements of social communication
   b. competitive vs. aggressive behaviors
   c. assertive vs. rude statements/behaviors
   d. assertive vs. threatening statements/behaviors
4. Provide opportunity for student to practice the following. Initially with Adult Mentor; then with peers (one at a time, then small groups):
   a. *entry* and *exit* statements of social communication
   b. voice modulation
   c. competitive vs. aggressive behaviors
   d. assertive/polite vs. rude statements/behaviors
   e. assertive vs. threatening statements/behaviors
5. Videotape role-playing scenarios for all of the above, and provide video feedback.
6. Videotape role-playing of common social dilemmas, and provide video feedback.
7. Provide opportunity for practice in "real life" settings and provide feedback.

The importance of practicing social skills in real life situations is understood as necessary for the development of social skills (Bandura, 1969; Tharpe and Wetzel, 1969). Exposure to environmental social interaction enhances the learning of these skills.

TRANSITION AND INDEPENDENT LIVING SKILLS TRAINING. Twenty-four years of experience with children at The Learning Clinic revealed that students required a graduated, planned withdrawal of structure and supervision to facilitate maintenance of skills after transition to post-secondary education, employment, or home. Asperger syndrome students, in particular, require a period of training in transitional skills and independent living skills. As structure and supervision are gradually reduced, students are increasingly involved in the community through employment, community college classes, driving, use of community resources, and establishing community social contacts.

What Does Not Work

There is no evidence that a change in diet will prevent the onset of AS/PDD. While our personal experience suggests that psychodynamic interventions are not useful with this population, the published literature does not identify at the present time interventions that do not work.

Evidence-Based Treatment Interventions in Residential Settings

What Works

A review of the literature did not uncover an intervention that met the criteria for what works.

What Might Work

The psychological, social, psychiatric, and educational issues associated with an Asperger syndrome diagnosis require a cohesive, multimodal intervention.

Cohesiveness is determined by the degree of cooperation and collaboration between those professionals involved in the treatment objectives and the integration of treatment strategies across the primary treatment settings, home, school or work, and community.

Multimodal intervention requires that the treatment components include medication therapy, cognitive-behavioral therapy, and psycho-educational interventions. Quality residential treatment settings that demonstrate an identified cognitive behavioral theoretical treatment model within a well-defined set of admissions and treatment development processes have the potential to generate a cohesive, multimodal implementation of research-based treatment.

Evidence-based treatment requires the use of data collection systems that are integrated into the treatment setting and its practices. The residential treatment milieu offers the opportunity to provide an engineered environment for the purpose of creating specific treatment outcomes. Student-clients with an Asperger syndrome diagnosis require a prescribed environment that will teach pragmatic, social, psychological, educational, and community living skills. The way in which the treatment environment is described by its schedules, activities, and priorities for self-reliant behavior will influence the competencies to be elicited and practiced.

The design of residential milieu using a cognitive behavioral theoretical treatment model may create reliable performance standards and authentic community application. The use of well-designed, small-scale, multiple treatment settings provides the opportunity to measure skills, define individual treatments, establish self-paced programs with performance standards and prescribe steps toward independent living, work, or advanced education.

The use of technology is a necessary part of the treatment environment. Computers for education, training, self-assessment, and performance records is critical. Video-monitoring for behavior assessment and self-modeling is an effective application of computer-video integration. Also, the use of video monitoring of classrooms, residential, and work setting enable treatment settings to provide mentoring and coaching to the Asperger syndrome person from a distance. Video-monitoring also provides a method for less intrusive immediate feedback and performance cueing.

The quality residential milieu offers a closed environment in which to provide safe, well-structured opportunities to elicit, practice, and apply key competencies required for independent living.

What Does Not Work

There is no evidence that a change in diet will prevent the onset of AS/PDD. While our personal experience suggests that integrating this population with conduct disordered youth is very ill-advised, the current published literature does not identify specific ineffective interventions.

However, experience with 150 Asperger students over a ten-year period at The Learning Clinic reveals treatment and school factors that are contraindicated:

1. "Open" environment that requires self-regulation of transitions, interactions with others, and movement in space.
2. Multiple transitions between classes and activities.
3. Large class size: over 10 students.
4. Unguided instruction without cues, prompts, and structure (daily plan, checklists, assigned work station; use of icons and ideograms, etc.).
5. Discipline that is lacking, inconsistent, or not clearly defined.
6. Mixed diagnostic groups, particularly students diagnosed with conduct disorder, peers who have disruptive or aggressive behaviors, and those with below-average IQ.
7. Traditional classroom setting where teacher instructs the class as a whole (as opposed to one-to-one tutorial).
8. Instructional methods
   - lack of multisensory methods of instruction
   - inconsistent format, mode, and pace of presentation of tasks
   - increases in task complexity that are not based on evidence of performance
   - delayed and noncontingent response feedback
   - uncontrolled pace of learning
   - focus on what was done "wrong" other than what to do now
   - presentation or assessment that is judgmental
   - motivation contingencies that are not based on interests of the Asperger student

- inconsistent pace for reading text to the Asperger student
- lack of computer-assisted instruction
- indirect, ambiguous instruction.

Psychopharmacology

There is limited research on the efficacy of psychotropic medications for children with Asperger syndrome, pervasive developmental disorder, not otherwise specified, or autistic spectrum disorders.

There are no medications designed specifically to treat autistic spectrum disorders. There is no medication that is going to "cure" or eliminate the disorder. However, there are medications that can treat some of the symptoms associated with these disorders. These behaviors include irritability, aggression, stereotypy, hyperactivity, inattention, anxiousness, and mood lability. Comorbid conditions are not unusual with pervasive developmental disorders (PDD). As the number of comorbid diagnoses increase, the number of prescribed medications generally increase. Typical classes of drugs used include the atypical antipsychotics, mood stabilizers, SSRIs, and anti-anxiety medications.

Two studies published in 2003 reported on the effectiveness of the atypical antipsychotics with pervasive developmental disorder youngsters. A three-year study of preschool children with severe behavior problems, and diagnosed with autism or pervasive developmental disorder, not otherwise specified, found that risperidone was effective in improving affect and behavior control (Masi et al., 2003).

Hollander et al. (2003) also evaluated the use of risperidone with preschoolers who had severe behavior problems. This study concluded that risperidone was effective in reducing irritability, repetitive movements, and hyperactivity. They noted there were no significant improvements in social withdrawal or inappropriate speech. Another atypical antipsychotic, olanzapine (Zyprexa), produced a modest decrease in disruptive behaviors (Hollander et al., 2003). The main side effect reported for these atypical antipsychotics was weight gain.

Hollander et al. (2003) also reported the effectiveness of other categories of prescription medications for autism: mood stabilizers and SSRIs. The mood stabilizers valproate (Depakene) and levetiracetam (Keppra) were found to decrease aggression, labile mood, and impulsive behaviors. In patients diagnosed with mild autism and a family history of manic depression, lithium was reported to be beneficial.

In non-controlled and retrospective studies, some of the SSRIs were associated with a reduction in symptoms (Hollander et al., 2003). For example, in adult autistic patients, fluvoxamine (Luvox) and sertraline (Zoloft) were associated with improvement in repetitive thoughts and behavior, aggression, social skills, and language. Decreased inattention, hyperactive and repetitive behaviors, and social skill deficit, and improved communication skills, were associated with low doses of venlafaxine (Effexor). Overall, the SSRIs were found to be more effective in reducing symptoms associated with the mood disorders and obsessive-compulsive disorder.

In summary, although there are no medications designed specifically to treat pervasive developmental disorders, there are medications used to treat many of the symptoms associated with these disorders. The following table summarizes the typical categories of medications for behavioral and psychiatric problems:

**Table 3. Categories of Medications for
Behavioral and Psychiatric Problems**

Hyperactivity, inattention, and impulsivity
Psychostimulants
Alpha-adrenergics
Atypical antipsychotics

Aggression & irritability
SRIs
Alpha-adrenergics
Beta-blockers
Mood stablizers
Atypical antipsychotics

Anxiety
SRIs
Alpha-adrenergics
Minor tranquilizers
Busprione

Preoccupations, rituals, compulsions
SRIs
TCAs
Atypical antipsychotics
Alpha-adrenergics

Depression
SRIs
TCAs

The Prevention of PDD

What Works

A review of the literature did not identify a preventive intervention for PDD.

What Might Work

In the section on obsessive-compulsive disorder (see Chapter 12), there is a discussion of the role the streptococcus bacteria plays in the onset of OCD in some individuals. Is it possible that a similar environmental agent, whether bacterial, viral, or chemical, could trigger PDD in some vulnerable individuals? If, indeed, this is the case, then the possibility arises that in some cases PDD could be avoided, or symptoms mitigated through timely medical intervention for the "environmental" agent.

While we have discussed the importance of social support elsewhere in this chapter, its importance as a health-promotion activity for parents and youth with AS should be noted. Here, the interest is in enabling the family to understand and assist their adolescent as well as find support for themselves. Likewise, for the adolescent, the planned provision of social support can help to counteract the depression that frequently accompanies AS.

What Does Not Work

There is no evidence that a change in diet will prevent the onset of AS/PDD.

Recommendations

Asperger syndrome is a life-long condition. The effects of specific symptom manifestation at different developmental stages are important to identify because early identification of developmental difficulties facilitates early diagnosis and treatment. The corresponding treatment, environmental modification, education, and medication adjustment to changing symptom profiles are important because Asperger syndrome is not a static condition. As changes occur in the performance and abilities of the Asperger syndrome individual, appropriate service and treatment options need to be available to the (Asperger syndrome) individual and family.

Our current approaches to Asperger syndrome lack a comprehensive lifespan view of treatment. The day-to-day, developmental stage, or academic year focus is too limited and tends to be reactive rather than proactive. There is enough current research to inform us that if we do not provide a comprehensive, long-view approach, then the needed resources will most probably not be available to individuals, because over time Asperger syndrome individual's incorporate their symptoms into their pattern of behavior; i.e., symptoms become ego-syntonic.

The challenges associated with evidence-based treatment of Asperger syndrome over the affected individual's lifespan are formidable. However, the evidence of effective intervention outcomes for Asperger syndrome and other individuals with pervasive developmental delays makes it worthwhile to put forth the effort to meet these challenges.

References

American Psychiatric Association. (1994). *Diagnostic and Statistical Manual of Mental Disorders* (4th ed.) (DSM-IV). Washington, DC.

Asperger, H. (1944). Die 'autistischen Psychopathen' im Kindesalter, *Archiv fur Psychiatric und Nervenkrankheiten, 117*, 76–136. Translated by U. Frith (Ed.), *Autism and Asperger syndrome* (1991, pp. 37–92). Cambridge: Cambridge University Press.

Bandura, A. (1969). *Principles of Behavior Modification.* Holt, Rinehart and Winston, Inc.

Baron-Cohen, S., O'Riordan, M., Stone, V., Jones, R., & Plaisted, K. (1999). Recognition of Faux Pas by Normally Developing Children and Children with Asperger Syndrome or High-Functioning Autism, *Journal of Autism and Developmental Disorders, 29,* 5.

Barnhill, G.P. (2001). What's New in AS Research: A Synthesis of Research Conducted by the Apserger Syndrome Project. *Intervention in School and Clinic, 36*(5), 300–305.

Barnhill, G.P., & Myles, B.S. (2001). Attributional style and depression in adolescents with Asperger syndrome. *Journal of Positive Behavior Interventions,* Sum 3(3), 175–182.

Blacher, J. (2002). Autism Rising: Delivering Services without draining parents and school systems. *Exceptional Parent Magazine,* Oct. 32, 10, 94–97.

Channon, S., Charman, T., Heap, J., Crawford, C., & Rios, P. (2001). Real-life-type problem-solving in Asperger's syndrome. *Journal of Autism & Developmental Disorders, 3*(5), 461–469.

Courchesne, E., Townsend, J., Akshoomoff, N.A., Saitoh, O., Yeung Courchesne, R., Lincoln, A., Hector, E.J., Haas, R.H., Schreibman, L., & Lau, L. (1994) Impairment in shifting attention in autistic and cerebellar patients. *Behavioral Neuroscience, 108,* 5, 848–865.

Craig, J., Baron-Cohen, S. (1999) Creativity and imagination in autism and Asperger syndrome. *Journal of Autism & Developmental Disorders,* Aug 29, 4, 314–326.

Dewey, M. (1991). Living with Asperger's syndrome. In U. Frith (Ed.), *Autism and Asperger Syndrome,* (pp. 184–206). New York: Cambridge University Press.

DuCharme, R.W. (2003). *Promoting the Healthy Development of Children with Asperger Syndrome: Education & Life Skills Issues.* New London, CT: Connecticut College.

DuCharme, R.W., & McGrady, K. (2003). *Promoting the Healthy Development of Children with Asperger Syndrome: Education & Life Skills Issues.* New London, CT: Connecticut College.

DuCharme, R.W. & McGrady, K (2004). What is Asperger Syndrome? In *Asperger Syndrome: A Guide for Professionals and Families.* (pp. 1–20). New York: Kluwer Academic/Plenum Publishers.

Dunn, W., Myles, B.S., & Orr, S. (2002). Sensory processing issues associated with Asperger Syndrome: A preliminary investigation. *The American Journal of Occupational Therapy, 56*(1), 97–102.

Dyer, K., Kneringer, M.J., & Luce, S.C. (1996). An efficient method of ensuring program quality for adults with developmental disabilities in community-based apartments. *Consulting Psychology Journal: Practice & Research,* Sum *48*(3), 171.

Ehlers, S., & Gillberg, C. (1993). The epidemiology of Asperger syndrome: A total population study. *Journal of Child Psychology & Psychiatry & Allied Disciplines,* Nov *34*(8), 1327–1350.

Eisenmajer, R., Prior, M., Leekham, S., Wing, L., et al. (1996). Comparison of clinical symptoms in autism and Asperger's disorder. *Journal of the Academy of Child & Adolescent Psychiatry,* Nov *35*(11), 1523–1531.

Frith, U. (1991). *Autism and Asperger syndrome.* New York: Cambridge University Press.

Frith, U., & Happe, F. (1994). Autism: Beyond "theory of mind." *Cognition, 50,* 115–132.

Ghaziuddin, M., & Butler, E. (1998). Clumsiness in autism and Asperger syndrome: A further report. *Journal of Intellectual Disability Research,* Feb *42*(1), 43–48.

Ghaziuddin, M., Butler, E., Tsai, L., & Ghaziuddin, N. (1994). Is clumsiness a marker for Asperger syndrome? *Journal of Intellectual Disability Research,* Oct, *38*(5), 519–527.

Gillberg, C. (1993). Asperger syndrome and clumsiness. *Journal of Autism & Develomental Disorders,* Dec *23*(4), 686–687.

Green, D., Baird, G., Barnett, A.L., Henderson, L., Huber, J., & Henderson, S.E. (2002). The severity and nature of motor impairment in Asperger's syndrome: A comparison with Specific Developmental Disorders of Motor Function. *Journal of Child Psychology & Psychiatry & Allied Disciplines,* Jun *43*(5), 655–668.

Happe, F.G.E. (1995). The role of age and verbal ability in the theory of mind task performance of subjects with autism. *Child Development, 66,* 843–855.

Hollander, E., Phillips, A., & Yeh, C. (2003). Targeted treatments for symptom domains in child and adolescent autism. *Lancet, 362* (August 30): 732–734. Mount Sinai School of Medicine, New York, NY.

Joliffe, T., & Baron-Cohen, S. (2000). Linguistic processing in high-functioning adults with autism or Asperger's syndrome. Is global coherence impaired? *Psychological Medicine, 30,* 1169–1187.

Kanner, L. (1943). Autistic disturbance of affective contact. *Nervous Child, 2,* 217–250.

Klin, A., & Volkmar, F.R. (1997). Asperger's syndrome. In D.J. Cohen & F.R. Volkmar (Eds.), *Handbook of Autism and Pervasive Developmental Disorders* (2nd ed., pp. 94–112). New York: Wiley.

Klin, A., Volkmar, F., & Sparrow, S. (2000). *Asperger Syndrome.* New York: The Guilford Press.

Klin, A., Volkmar, F.R., Sparrow, S.S., & Cicchetti, D.V. (1995). Validity and *neuropsychological characterization of Asperger Syndrome: Convergence with Nonverbal Learning Disabilities syndrome. Journal of Child Psychology & Psychiatry & Applied Disciplines,* 1127–1140.

Leekham, S., Libby, S., Wing, L., Gould, J., & Gillberg, C. (2000). Comparison of ICD-10 and Gillberg's Criteria for Asperger Syndrome. *Autism: The International Journal of Research and Practice, 4(1),* 85–100.

Masi, G., Cosenza, A., Mucci, M., & Brovedani, P. (2003). A 3-year naturalistic study of 53 preschool children with pervasive developmental disorders treated with resperidone. *Journal of Clinical Psychiatry,* 64 (September):1039–1047. From the Scientific Institute of Child Neurology and Psychiatry, Calambrone, Italy.

Matthews, A. (1996). Employment training and the development of a support model within employment for adults who experience Asperger syndrome and autism: The Gloucestershire Group Homes Model. In Morgan, H. (Ed.), *Adults with Autism: A Guide to Theory and Practice* (pp. 163–184). New York: Cambridge University Press.

Mawhood, L., & Howlin, P. (1999). The outcome of a supported employment scheme for high-functioning adults with autism or Asperger syndrome. *Autism,* Sep *3*(3), 229–254.

Merriam-Webster (1990). *Webster's Ninth New Collegiate Dictionary.* Springfield, MA: Merriam-Webster, Inc.

Mesibov, G.B., Shea, V., & Adams, L.W. (2001). *Understanding Asperger Syndrome and High Functioning Autism.* New York: Kluwer Academic/Plenum Publishers.

Miyahara, M., Tsujii, M., Hori, M., Nakanishi, K., Kageyama, H., & Sugiyama, T. (1997). Motor incoordination in children with Asperger syndrome and learning disabilities. *Journal of Autism & Developmental Disorders*, Oct, 27(5), 595–603.

Nesbitt, S. (2000). Why and why not? Factors influencing employment for individuals with Asperger syndrome. *Austim*, Dec 4(4), 357–369.

Ozonoff, S., South, M., & Miller, J. (2000). DSM-IV defined Asperger syndrome: cognitive, behavioral and early history differentiation from high-functioning autism. *Autism: The International Journal of Research and Practice, 4*, 29–46.

Perner, J., & Wimmer, H. (1985). "John thinks that Mary thinks that . . ." Attribution of second-order beliefs by 5–10 year old children. *Journal of Experimental Child Psychology, 39*, 437–471.

Raja, M., & Azzoni, A. (2001). Asperger's disorder in the emergency psychiatric setting. *General Hospital Psychiatry, 23*, 285–293.

Rourke, B.P. (1995). *Syndrome of Nonverbal Learning Disabilities.* New York: Guilford Press.

Schopler, E. Mesibov, G.B., & Kunce, L.J. (1998). *Asperger Syndrome or High-functioning Autism?* New York: Plenum Press.

Shriberg, L.D., Paul, R., McSweeny, J.L., Klin, A., & Cohen, D.J. (2001) Speech and prosody characteristics of adolescents and adults with high-functioning autism and Aspeger syndrome. *Journal of Speech, Language, & Hearing Research*, Oct 44(5), 1097–1115.

Shulman, C., Yirmiya, N., & Greenbaum, C.W. (1995) From categorization to classification: A comparison among individuals with a retardation, and normal development. *Journal of Abnormal Psychology*, Nov 104(4), 601–609.

Tantam, D. (2000). Adolescence and adulthood of Individuals with Asperger Syndrome. *Asperger Syndrome*, 367–399.

Tharpe, R.G., & Wetzel, R.J. (1969) *Behavior Modification in the Natural Environment.* New York: Academic Press, Inc.

Volkmar, F.R., Klin, A., & Pauls, D. (1998). Nosological and Genetic Aspects of Asperger Syndrome. *Journal of Autism and Developmental Disorders*, 28(5), 457–463.

Weimer, A.K., Schatz, A.M., Lincoln, A., Ballantyne, A.O., & Trauner, D.A. (2001). "Motor" impairment in Asperger Syndrome: Evidence for a deficit in proprioception. *Journal of Developmental & Behavioral Pediatrics*, Apr 22(2), 92–101.

World Health Organization. (1992). *International Classification of Diseases* (10th ed.). Geneva, Switzerland: Author.

Chapter 15

Prevention and Treatment of Post-Traumatic Stress Disorder in Adolescents

Theresa Kruczek, Jill R. Salsman, and Stephanie Vitanza

Introduction

The idea that traumatic life events can lead to the development of reactive psychopathology is one of the earliest in psychology (e.g., Breuer & Freud, 1955). However, only recently have we begun to investigate the impact of traumatic life events on the development of post-traumatic reactions in children and adolescents (Davis & Siegel, 2000). At the same time, we have developed an increased awareness of the extent to which children and adolescents experience traumatic life events (Klingman, 2001). Even though post-traumatic stress disorder (PTSD) first emerged as a diagnostic category in the third version of the *Diagnostic and Statistical Manual of Mental Disorders (DSM-III;* American Psychiatric Association, 1980), the diagnosis was not specifically applied to children and adolescents until the next revision *(DSM-III-R;* American Psychiatric Association, 1987). PTSD has a significant negative impact on the biological, psychological, and social development of those youth who develop the disorder following exposure to a traumatic event (Pynoos, 1994). Given the frequency with which young people today experience traumatic events it is important that we develop a model for primary prevention and health promotion in those youth who have experienced trauma.

DSM IV-TR (American Psychiatric Association, 2000) estimates suggest that one-third to one-half of those exposed to a traumatic life event will go on to develop PTSD. The prevalence of PTSD in the general population of adolescents is estimated at 6.3% (Reinherz, Giaconia, Lefkowitz, Pakiz & Frost, 1993). PTSD symptoms generally fall within three categories: (1) re-experiencing the trauma, which includes flashbacks, intrusive thoughts, nightmares, and an exaggerated startle response; (2) avoiding stimuli related to the trauma and numbing, which includes feeling detached or estranged from others and deriving significantly less pleasure from previously enjoyed activities; and (3) hyper-arousal, which includes irritability, hypervigilance, and sleep and concentration disturbance. The symptoms of PTSD in adolescents are fairly consistent with adult symptomatology (Amaya-Jackson & March, 1995), although there is some suggestion that children and adolescents may alternate between periods of re-experiencing and avoidance/numbing symptoms (Cohen, 1998). When adolescents use avoidance and numbing to cope they may appear asymptomatic or their symptoms of PTSD may be masked (Cohen, 1998).

Theoretical models for the development of PTSD are grounded in *stress reaction theory* or as it is more popularly known the "fight or flight" response. Hans Selye (1952) first developed the *general adaptation syndrome* to describe the human response to chronic stressors. More recently, Miller and Veltkamp (1988, 1993, as described in Clark & Miller, 1998) have elaborated a specific *Trauma Accommodation Syndrome* for children and adolescents to describe their stages of adaptation to traumatic stressors. Stage I involves the adolescent's actual experience of the traumatic event. At stage II the adolescent may have to deal with the aftermath of physical injuries sustained in the trauma and often experiences psychological fear, horror, and helplessness. The initial two stages, the actual trauma and the acute reaction to the trauma, are followed by a third stage characterized by a period of intrusive thoughts and feelings related to the trauma. This third stage often includes reenacting the trauma, having frightening dreams, avoiding activities related to the trauma, re-experiencing thoughts and feelings from the trauma, and displaying disorganized and/or agitated behavior. Stage IV heralds the beginning of successful accommodation. In this stage the adolescent uses cognitive reasoning to reevaluate both the original trauma and their subsequent re-experiences of the trauma. It is at this stage that the adolescent may begin to mourn losses associated with the trauma and work to find meaning from the experience. The final stage (V) involves successful accommodation or resolution of the traumatic issues. By this stage the adolescent is using coping strategies to deal with the aftermath of the trauma and has integrated the traumatic experience within his or her overall life experience and identity.

A five-phase *Child Sexual Abuse Accommodation Syndrome* has been proposed to describe trauma adaptation specific to child sexual abuse (O'Donahue, Fanetti & Elliott, 1998; Summit, 1983) These phases include, secrecy, helplessness, accommodation, delayed disclosure, and retraction. During the accommodation phase the adolescent is most likely to suffer dissociative experiences and repress memories about the abuse, particularly if her/his disclosure is met with disbelief, rejection, continued abuse or threats of violence by the perpetrator. These adolescents are at significant risk for developing PTSD, and even personality changes, in reaction to the trauma of child sexual abuse (Briere, 1997).

The stress reaction of a given adolescent is moderated by many variables, including the nature of the stressor and whether the stressor occurs as a single, acute event or as chronic, repeated events. Adolescents can be exposed to a wide variety of traumatic events, including natural and technological disasters (e.g., earthquakes, hurricanes, ferry boat accidents), exposure to war, sexual and physical abuse or interpersonal violence, community violence, life-threatening illnesses, and medical procedures (Pynoos, 1994). Additionally, Terr (1991) distinguishes between two types of traumatic events. Type I events are often a single traumatic experience that is short-term, unexpected, and more likely to result in a quick recovery. Type II events are either exposure to a series of traumatic events (e.g., a series of earthquakes) or are chronic and repetitive traumatic experiences (e.g., repeated sexual molestation). Type II trauma is more likely to result in more severe stress reactions and difficulty with adjustment. Certain type I stressors can result in more severe stress reactions, particularly those resulting in loss of a significant other (e.g., death of a parent) or loss of function (e.g., loss of a limb or paralysis). There are also risk and protective factors, specifically age or developmental factors and gender, that contribute to an adolescent's stress reaction and that will be discussed later in this chapter.

Exposure to any traumatic event can result in adverse stress reactions. Most adolescents can cope with these experiences provided they receive appropriate prevention and intervention. Primary prevention can be used to promote healthy functioning and prevent the development of PTSD in those youth experiencing traumatic life events. Most models of prevention typically consist of a multilevel approach to prevention. Gullotta and Bloom's (2003) definition of primary prevention will be used as a conceptual framework for the discussion of prevention programming in this chapter. When adapted to PTSD, this model emphasizes programming to help youth, their families, and communities to prevent the predictable outcomes of trauma exposure. The main goal of primary prevention in this context is to preserve existing health and functioning in trauma survivors and to promote psychological and social well being in these youth. Further, this approach distinguishes between universal prevention that targets whole populations, selective prevention programming with those youth at risk for developing PTSD, and indicated prevention programming with very high risk groups. This latter level of programming may include elements of prevention and treatment.

This model is consistent with Klingman's (2001) suggestion that a five-level model is relevant for PTSD prevention, particularly with traumatic exposure to natural and technological disasters. The first level of Klingman's model is a universal effort that involves working with youth, their families and communities to develop disaster plans and to foster development of life skills to deal with traumatic events. His second two levels are selective efforts that occur after a collective traumatic event. The second level consists of traditional primary prevention programs provided to the general population following trauma exposure. These primary prevention efforts occur with youth (and their caregivers) who are not yet displaying coping difficulties and typically consist of psychoeducational programs, social support, and crisis coping skill development. The next level of selective effort follows mass screening of the general population designed to identify those adolescents with early signs of PTSD. Those adolescents identified as "at risk" receive proactive interventions to minimize development of "full-blown" PTSD symptoms. The final two levels of intervention occur with these indicated groups. The fourth level involves providing more intensive and follow-up services to those identified as having gone on to develop PTSD. The purpose of this level is rapid intervention to contain and manage the PTSD symptoms as well as to provide support to these youth and their families. The fifth and final level of intervention occurs once the adolescent's PTSD symptoms have stabilized, in an attempt to prevent relapse and to promote healthy development in these youth.

Individual Factors

Childhood trauma is a risk factor for the development of PTSD in both children and adolescents. Individual factors contributing to risk for PTSD include the child's age (chronological and developmental at both the onset of the trauma and at the time of disclosure), gender, cognitive maturity, coping skills, attributional style, existing psychopathology, and social connectedness (O'Donohue, Fanetti & Elliott, 1998). Courtois (2003) also stresses the importance of the child's attachment history, personality functioning, defenses, beliefs, values, and abilities. Prior and subsequent life events, including repeated victimization, affect response to the trauma and the likelihood of the development of PTSD (Courtois, 2003).

Age and Developmental Factors

Research investigating the relationship between age at the time of trauma exposure and development of PTSD is mixed. Some investigations have found that for children who experienced trauma before age 11 there was an up to three times increased risk for the development of PTSD (Davidson & Smith, 1990). Others, however, report no empirical support for age as a factor in predicting the development of PTSD (Foa, Keane & Friedman, 2000; Garrison et al., 1995; Silverman & La Greca, 2002; Yule, Perrin & Smith, 1999). In fact, some argue that age may be a protective factor in younger children as they may not have a depth of cognitive understanding and therefore may not be as impacted by a trauma as an older teen or adult, who can fully appreciate the danger of the circumstances (Davis & Siegel, 2000).

Most agree that a youth's response to trauma and subsequent risk for development of PTSD is broadly related to how the youth perceives the trauma (Yule et al., 1999; Pandit & Shah, 2000). Yule et al. (1999, p. 37) specifically identify that the experience of "subjective threat is determined by the developmental stage the child [adolescent] has reached." This perception of threat not only applies to the child, but also to his/her perception of possible danger or fear for a parent's safety (Silverman & La Greca, 2002). Wraith (2000) and DiNicola (1996) describe how a child's developmental level can affect not only their reaction to the trauma, but the method of recovery and the subsequent adjustment or distress of the adolescent or child. Thus, each age group of children is susceptible to particular vulnerabilities. For example, preverbal children may exhibit regressive behaviors, fears, or increased attachment and the need to "play out" their anxiety, while verbal children may need to tell their story repeatedly, behave aggressively, or exhibit psychosomatic complaints. Teens, on the other hand, mimic more adult responses and are likely to turn to peers, feign pseudomaturity, or to "pretend it didn't happen" (DiNicola, 1996; Tyler, Hoyt & Whitbeck, 2000; Wraith, 2000). Empirical evidence further supports that a child or adolescent's cognitive appraisal of an event leads to either a maladaptive or an adjusted response to the traumatic event (Pandit & Shah, 2000; Silverman & La Greca, 2002; Stallard, 2000; Tolin & Foa, 2002; Udwin, Boyle, Yule, Bolton & O'Ryan, 2000). Not only does the child's developmental level affect how PTSD symptoms may be shown, but PTSD symptomatology may affect or disrupt a child's subsequent development (Davis & Siegel, 2000; DiNicola, 1996). The most common long-term effects of PTSD include impairment in the areas of trust, intimacy, healthy relationships, self-esteem, and impulse control.

Gender

Research consistently demonstrates that girls display greater symptoms of anxiety, depression, and distress after experiencing a trauma (Elklit, 2002; Davis & Siegel, 2000; Foa et al., 2000; Pandit & Shah, 2000; Silverman & La Greca, 2002; Yule et al., 1999). These gender differences hold whether the experience is a natural disaster (Garrison et al., 1995) or repeated, personal trauma. Horowitz, Weine & Jekel (1995) found rates of PTSD symptomatology as high as 67% in their sample of urban females. However, it is not yet clear whether these differences are due to cultural factors and the type of traumatic experience, or whether represent "true" gender differences (Clark & Miller, 1998; Foa et al., 2000; Silverman & La Greca, 2002).

Norris, Foster, and Weisshar (2002) found that female's greater risk for the development of PTSD begins in childhood and continues through middle age. Tolin and Foa (2002) believe these gender differences may arise from several factors, including the type of trauma typically experienced by males and females (females are more likely to experience sexual assault, males physical assault) and gender differences in cognitive appraisal following the trauma. Female victims seem more likely than males to assign self-blame following trauma exposure and to subsequently evaluate the world as a more negative or dangerous place. Overall, most authors agree that continued research is needed to delineate further the specific nature of gender differences in the development of PTSD.

Research also provides some evidence that higher levels of cognitive ability provide a protective buffer against the development of PTSD (Yule et al.,1999). Related research suggests that children with preexisting academic difficulties, behavior problems, and attentional difficulties may be at greater risk for the development of PTSD symptomatology (Silverman & La Greca, 2002). Additional protective factors include a high level of self-esteem, good problem-solving and communication skills, an internal locus of control, a history of adaptive coping, and family support and/or a connection with a positive adult (Clark & Miller, 1998; Silverman & La Greca, 2002).

Family Factors

Violence within the family is often one source of trauma for children. Children growing up in homes where there is domestic violence and even high parental conflict are at greater risk for developing PTSD symptoms following subsequent trauma exposure (McCloskey & Walker 2000; Wasserstein & La Greca, 1998). The effects of family violence on the development of PTSD are moderated by whether the violence is witnessed versus experienced, involves a loss, or is based on single vs. multiple trauma exposure (Wasserstein & La Greca, 1998). Other family factors such as the parent's marital status, psychological functioning, stability, and level of education have been associated with the development of PTSD in children and adolescents (Davis & Siegel, 2000; Elklit, 2002; Silverman & La Greca, 2002). Not surprisingly, children are less likely to develop PTSD following a trauma exposure when their family environment is characterized as being stable, having a higher socioeconomic level, and having parents who themselves demonstrate healthy psychological functioning. Divorce and remarriage are considered specific risk factors for the development of sexual abuse as many adult perpetrators are stepfathers (Davis & Siegel, 2000).

Perhaps the most important familial mediating factor is the parent's reaction to the traumatic event or disclosure (Davis & Siegel, 2000; Silverman & La Greca, 2002). Research has long demonstrated that positive family support serves as a protective factor, while a lack of family or caregiver support often results in an increased risk for serious mental illnesses. Parental support is considered one of the most important buffers for traumatic events (Wasserstein & La Greca, 1998). Broader familial support is also important and can come from the youth's immediate family or a wider network of caregivers or supportive individuals, such as extended family or even foster parents (de Silva, 1999). Research has further demonstrated that a strong relationship with grandparents can serve as a mediator with regard to the development of PTSD symptomatology (Pandit & Shah, 2000).

Social and Community Factors

For over 200 years PTSD symptoms have been seen across cultures in those exposed to war, terrorism, or natural disasters. Thus, it is evident that the development of PTSD is not culturally limited (de Silva, 1999). Community-based violence is known to have a negative effect on children and adolescents and can be considered a risk factor for the development of PTSD. In fact, recent studies have shown rates of PTSD ranging from 34.5% to 67% in urban youth exposed to community violence (Horowitz et al., 1995). Horowitz and her colleagues (1995) introduced the notion of *compounded community trauma* for some high-risk youth. These predominantly urban adolescents (and those living in war zones) experience multiple types of trauma exposure within their homes and communities. These youth have an increased risk for developing PTSD following specific traumatic events, given the overall pattern of violence exposure in their lives. Their risk is exacerbated by issues related to culture and poverty.

Ethnicity

Rabalais, Ruggerio, and Scotti (2002) reviewed the literature investigating ethnicity as a risk and protective factor in children exposed to trauma. Their review revealed mixed results with regard to differences in PTSD symptomatology. However, they concluded that Hispanic American and African American youth were at higher risk for developing PTSD after experiencing a traumatic life event and that these groups might be less likely to demonstrate a decrease in PTSD symptoms over time as compared to their Caucasian counterparts. It is likely socioeconomic status and available social support interact with cultural customs and beliefs to influence the development of PTSD. Culture may be a specific risk factor when traumatized youth belong to an ethnic group that has been historically oppressed. As poverty is considered to be an even greater risk factor for child abuse than race, members of oppressed minority groups (e.g., African Americans, Hispanic Americans, Native Americans) may be at a higher risk for the development of PTSD. Certainly prejudice and prior discrimination are risk factors. If the youth and their families experienced pre-disaster discrimination they may be less likely to seek support from "outsiders," particularly when those outsiders are from the majority culture (Rabalais et al., 2002). On the other hand, culture may serve as a protective factor in groups that emphasize extended kin networks, spirituality, and positive family relationships (Gonzales & Kim, 1997). There is some evidence that religion serves as a positive moderating variable (de Silva, 1999).

Media

Finally, media exposure can have a negative influence on a child's adjustment to a natural disaster or traumatic life event. Repetitive media exposure can evoke powerful images for adolescents and children who may not have the skills to cope with or dismiss these images from their mind (Pandit & Shah, 2000). Investigations of media exposure to a variety of traumatic events ranging from natural disasters (Kiser, Heston, Hickerson & Millsap, 1993) to terrorist attacks (e.g., Pfefferbaum, 2001; Saylor, Coward, Lipovsky, Jackson & Finch, 2003) have demonstrated the potential for PTSD symptoms to develop from this indirect mechanism of trauma exposure. Most startling is the finding that mere predictions of impending disaster can result in the development of mild, but prevalent symptoms of PTSD (Kiser et. al., 1993). Contrary to popular thought, exposure to heroic images and positive role models did not moderate the adverse impact of media exposure (Saylor et al., 2003). Further, older youth and boys are likely to experience greater media exposure and concurrent PTSD symptoms related to this exposure (Saylor et al., 2003), making adolescent males the most vulnerable to this effect.

Evidence-Based Treatment Interventions in Community Settings

Few empirical studies exist that specifically examine the treatment of PTSD in the adolescent population (Cohen, Berliner & March, 2000). This represents a drawback of the literature in this area as treatment approaches and guidelines for PTSD in adolescents are often adapted from research studying adults (Yule, 2001) and children with PTSD (Cohen, 1998). General guidelines and practice parameters for the treatment of PTSD in adolescents have been proposed (i.e., Cohen, 1998; Cohen, Berliner & March, 2000) based on a combination of theory and empirical investigation. However, research evidence involving the treatment of PTSD in children and adolescents varies considerably in terms of methodological rigor. Therefore, when discussing treatment interventions for PTSD in adolescents, the authors of this chapter suggest treatment interventions that "work" based on empirical evidence; "may work," as they have inadequate empirical support or can be substantiated by theory; and "do not work."

What Works

Research examining the efficacy of individual therapy versus group therapy in the treatment of PTSD in children and adolescents is sparse (Cohen, 1998). However, group interventions, as compared to individual treatment, seem to be preferred in community-based settings as they afford an opportunity to reach large adolescent populations (Yule, 2001). Further, group interventions help combat the sense of isolation that often accompanies PTSD, especially in cases of abuse (Kruczek & Vitanza, 1999). The efficacy of group therapy interventions in alleviating post-traumatic stress symptoms in response to crisis among adolescents has been demonstrated in earlier studies (Cohen, 1998) and in a more recent pilot study (Salloum, Avery & McClain, 2001). However, definitive conclusions about the efficacy of group therapy based on these studies is limited due to lack of comparison control groups.

Effective primary prevention for adolescents with PTSD in community-based settings often emphasizes acute crisis intervention via psychoeducational groups (Cohen, 1998). These psychoeducational groups educate adolescents about normal emotional reactions to trauma, effective coping strategies for re-exposure (Cohen, Berliner & March, 2000) and ways to reduce re-enactment and risk-taking behaviors related to the traumatic experience (Nader, 2001). Glodich (1999) as cited in Nader (2001) found that adolescents exposed to violence were less likely to re-enact the trauma and engage in risk-taking behaviors after participation in a psychoeducational group. Psychoeducational groups that provide information to teachers and parents about how to support traumatized children and teens also reduce the psychological effects of trauma and have been used in both hospital (i.e., Butler, Rizzi & Handwerger, 1996) and school settings. (i.e., Blom, 1986; La Greca, Silverman, Vernberg & Prinstein, 1996; Rigamer, 1986). *Psychological debriefing* is another primary prevention tool that is similar to, but slightly different from, psychoeducation. During psychological debriefing, a group facilitator reconstructs the traumatic event, encourages adolescents to discuss their thoughts and feelings related to the event, fosters a sense of universality and normalizes their reactions to the event, and provides information about how they can cope with their reactions (Stallard, 2000). The facilitator also discusses the expected course of their symptoms and provides additional resources if symptoms persist. A form of psychological debriefing called *"psychological first aid"* has been proposed by Pynoos and Nader (1988) and is provided in an individual, family, or group context near or on the site that trauma occurred. Psychological first aid involves screening children at risk for PTSD, establishing teacher and parental support systems through psychoeducation, and referring children with severe symptoms for more extensive treatment. Literature in the area of psychological debriefing is less extensive in adolescents than in adults; however, several investigations of debriefing with adolescents (i.e., Stallard & Law, 1993; Yule, 1992; Yule & Udwin, 1991) suggest the technique effectively reduces fear reactions, intrusive thoughts, and psychological distress in teens.

Cognitive-behavioral therapy (CBT) is the most frequently researched treatment modality for PTSD in youth and is typically recommended as the treatment of choice when used alone or in combination with other approaches (Cohen, Berliner & March, 2000; Perrin, Smith & Yule, 2000). Research in community-based settings has consistently demonstrated a reduction of post-traumatic stress symptoms in children when using CBT (Cohen, Berliner & March, 2000). Two studies have specifically investigated the efficacy of CBT implemented with adolescents in a school-based setting (Goenjian et al. 1997; March, Amaya-Jackson, Murray & Schulte, 1998). Both studies demonstrated a reduction of PTSD symptoms in adolescents with trauma exposure, following participation in CBT groups. Case studies of adolescents with PTSD (i.e., Saigh, 1989) also offer support for the use of a multifaceted behavioral intervention in reducing the cognitive, affective, and behavioral symptoms that accompany PTSD.

Trauma-focused CBT commonly utilizes a combination of exposure to trauma-related stimuli, anxiety management, relaxation techniques, and cognitive restructuring related to the traumatic event (Cohen, Berliner & March, 2000; Perrin, Smith & Yule, 2000). While treatment outcome studies of trauma-focused CBT have demonstrated general effectiveness, it remains unclear which specific elements of CBT are most strongly related to its efficacy. Therefore, no established guidelines currently exist with regards to the "dosage" and "frequency" of each technique needed or for what degree a traumatic event should be recapitulated in therapy in order to achieve the desired treatment effect (Cohen, Berliner & March, 2000).

What Might Work

In contrast to CBT, other treatments are not as frequently investigated using empirical methods. Consequently, there is not clear empirical evidence to support the use of these interventions. Therefore, the following interventions "might" be effective. Adequate support for the use of *psychodynamic psychotherapy* in treating PTSD in adolescents is not available (Cohen, Berliner & March, 2000; Cohen, 1998). However, case studies of children of abuse (i.e., McElroy & McElroy, 1989; Seinfeld, 1989; Van Leeuwen, 1988) do offer some support for the use of psychoanalytic therapy with traumatized children. Nevertheless, it is unknown whether this finding can be replicated in the adolescent population.

Eye Movement Desensitization and Reprocessing (EMDR) consists of a combination of cognitive therapy techniques and exposure techniques (Shapiro, 1996). This treatment approach involves having adolescents generate an image or memory associated with a traumatic event and simultaneously follow a therapist's hand with their eyes, with or without interpretations or verbal interventions being made by the therapist (Yule, 2001). Although controversial, EMDR has been frequently cited as a treatment approach used in childhood PTSD (Perrin, Smith & Yule, 2000). While empirical support exists for the use of EMDR in adults with PTSD (Cohen, 1998), currently there are no published controlled trials studying the efficacy of EMDR with adolescents. Chemtob, Nakashima, Hamada, and Carlson (2002) used a randomized, lagged-group design to investigate the effect of EMDR with traumatized children. These authors reported therapeutic gains, but their investigation did not provide comparison data with other treatment approaches such as CBT. Chemtob et al.'s (2002) study, along with EMDR case studies treating PTSD in children (i.e., Coco & Sharpe, 1993; Greenwald, 1994; Muris & de Jonghe, 1996, Tinker & Wilson, 1999) suggest that EMDR "might" work when treating the adolescent population.

Family therapy treatment models have been proposed, but not empirically validated, when working with adolescents and their families in community settings. Figley (1988) formulated a systematic therapy approach to treating traumatized families. A similar family crisis intervention model for addressing symptoms of post-traumatic stress was later developed by Harris (1991). Both treatment models share the following treatment objectives: building trust and rapport with the family, examining symptoms related to maladaptive family coping styles in response to the trauma, increasing familial communication and support, and formulating more adaptive coping strategies. However, the efficacy of these therapeutic approaches has not been investigated (Riggs, 2000).

Creative therapies that utilize art, drama, dance, music, or poetry have also been recommended for use with children who have difficulty talking abstractly about their traumatic experiences (Read Johnson, 2000). Support for the efficacy of creative therapies is derived from case studies and clinical reports, and further research is needed that confirm the efficacy of these treatments.

What Does Not Work

Sufficient evidence does not currently exist to delineate which treatment interventions are not effective in community-based settings.

Evidence-Based Treatment Interventions in Residential Settings

To date there has been very little research specifically assessing interventions for PTSD in residential treatment settings. Consequently, treatment recommendations for these settings are based primarily on theoretical models. The few available studies involving adolescents in residential treatment settings are included in this review, as are interventions with incarcerated adolescents who have a history of trauma exposure.

What Works

As the majority of studies examining the efficacy of interventions for PTSD in children and adolescents have been conducted in community settings, there is not sufficient empirical support for any particular intervention specifically applied within residential settings.

What Might Work

A limited research base exists for PTSD interventions with adolescents in residential settings. Nevertheless, traumatized children and adolescents are frequently admitted to residential and inpatient psychiatric treatment settings (Lawson, 1998). Literature examining treatment approaches for PTSD in these settings with adolescent survivors of sexual abuse consists of two studies. Kruczek and Vitanza (1999) used a combination of CBT and creative arts therapies with adolescent female sexual abuse survivors. Their brief therapy group in an inpatient psychiatric setting emphasized the development of adaptive skills for coping with the trauma. Their intervention targeted skill development in the following areas: normalizing the PTSD experience, increasing safety, managing internalizing and externalizing emotions, developing healthy self-esteem, fostering healthy relationships, and developing positive self-assertion skills. Group participants demonstrated improved adaptive functioning on completion of the brief therapy group. In a similar study, survivors made significant positive changes in coping skill mastery on completion of the group and showed an increase in functional behaviors at three-month follow-up (Kruczek & Watson, 1995).

Suggestions regarding what might work with this population can also be derived from theoretical literature and research findings with incarcerated youth with a history of trauma exposure. *Multimodal interventions* involving a combination of individual, group, and family therapy and psychopharmacology are often recommended when treating incarcerated youth (Arroyo, 2001). Individual treatment with this population may incorporate a combination of treatment interventions (i.e., CBT and psychodynamic therapy). A controlled study by Soberman, Greenwald, and Rule (2002) has also demonstrated the efficacy of EMDR in reducing PTSD symptoms in boys and adolescents in residential or day treatment for conduct problems. *Group treatments* may also be appropriate for this population, especially in cases where many adolescents are exposed to a similar traumatic event (Arroyo, 2001). A preliminary investigation of a trauma-focused therapy group with incarcerated juvenile offenders resulted in the following therapeutic gains: increased awareness of the connection between trauma and aggression, better anger management, and a regulation of sleep disturbance. This intervention consisted of psychoeducation, verbal processing of the trauma, creative art expressions, and coping skill development (McMackin, Leisen, Sattler, Krinsley & Riggs, 2002).

Although empirical literature investigating treatment interventions in residential settings for adolescents with PTSD is sparse, trauma-focused treatment models have been outlined that may prove useful with this population. The *Sanctuary Model* (Bloom, 1997) was originally developed for adult survivors of child abuse in hospital settings (Bills & Bloom, 1998; Bloom et al., 2003) and adapted for use with traumatized children and adolescents in residential settings (Abramovitz & Bloom, 2003; Rivard et al., 2003). This model conceptualizes PTSD symptomatology in terms of normal reactions and coping mechanisms to deal with an abnormal stressor. The core concept of this model is providing a safe, therapeutic environment for teens that is free from physical and verbal violence (Bills & Bloom, 1998). Proponents of this approach report that adolescents with a history of trauma (i.e., physical abuse, sexual abuse, substantiated neglect, family or community violence) demonstrate a decrease in maladaptive behaviors and an increase in social, psychological, and physical safety within the context of this treatment environment (Bloom et al., 2003; Rivard et al., 2003). Similarly, a *milieu therapy approach* (Gunderson, 1978) to residential treatment with these adolescents involves providing a sense of security through physical containment, applying structure to emotional and arousal patterns (Burgess, 1993, as cited in Lawson, 1998), validating feelings, promoting differentiation and balance between interpersonal distance and intimacy, and raising self-esteem (Lawson, 1998). Doyle & Bauer's (1989) *recovery model* provides a third and similar approach to residential treatment. This model emphasizes the following treatment objectives: building a therapeutic relationship, normalizing the stress response, labeling emotions, encouraging the expression of emotions, recapitulating the traumatic event, cognitive reframing, and formulating an integrated perspective of the trauma. The similarity of treatment objectives in these three models suggests a conceptual consensus for residential treatment of adolescents with PTSD. However, controlled trials are needed to substantiate their treatment efficacy.

What Does Not Work

The limited research available in this area does not yet indicate any specific intervention that is ineffective in residential treatment settings.

Psychopharmacology

There is limited empirical data to guide medication decisions with adolescent trauma survivors. To date, only one investigation has used a control comparison group and randomized assignment to the medication or control group. There have been several promising open trial studies. In open trial studies everyone (adolescent, physician, and family) involved is aware of the medication being used. The problem with open trial studies is that there is no way to distinguish between improvement due to the medication and improvement due to positive expectations because the adolescents are being treated with a psychoactive medication (the placebo effect). At present, the medication recommendations for treating PTSD in children and adolescents are guided primarily by *rational* pharmacotherapy (Friedman, 1990). That is, the recommendations are derived logically based on the known physiology of the disorder and the medication action of the drug. In order to understand these recommendations it is first necessary to briefly review the neurobiology of PTSD.

Understanding the normal stress response provides a basis for understanding the biological underpinnings of the stress response in traumatized adolescents. The limbic system, particularly the amygdala, seems to play a primary role in the normal stress response via a "fear conditioning" response (LeDoux, 1996). The limbic system is primarily responsible for modulating and expressing emotions. It is the amygdala that integrates input from our sensory organs so that information the brain receives about particular life experiences can be encoded in and retrieved from memory. The amygdala is also involved in assigning emotional valence to the experience. Further, when an experience is perceived as stressful, it is action in the amygdala that triggers the physiological and psychological stress response. The PTSD symptoms of hyperarousal, intrusive memories, and nightmares are thought to result from hyperresponsive action in the amygdala (Cohen, 2001). Stress, particularly when it is uncontrollable and unpredictable, also increases responsiveness in the locus ceruleus (Chronister & DeFrance, 1981). Increased activity in the locus ceruleus increases adrenergic activity in those brain areas impacting memory, emotion, arousal, and attention and this increased activity is thought to underlie the "fight or flight" response (Donnelly, Amaya-Jackson, & March, 1999). Further, the neurobiological systems regulating this stress response are probably not as adaptive and well developed in children (Perry, 1994).

Several neurotransmitters have been implicated in PTSD symptoms. The catecholamines [norepinephrine (NE), epinephrine (EPI), and dopamine DA)] show the most evidence of involvement in PTSD symptoms. Both adults and children with a trauma history have demonstrated elevations in DA and the severity of PTSD symptoms has been correlated positively with DA elevations (DeBellis, et al., 1999). As described above the adrenergic system, NE and EPI, seems to play a key role in PTSD. Seratonin (5-HT) influences several mood regulation symptoms associated with PTSD, including, anxiety, aggression, impulsivity, obsessive-compulsive symptoms, and suicidality (Friedman, 1990).

Those medications affecting the catecholamine system have been most investigated as treatments for PTSD in adolescents. Specifically, the antihypertensive medications (adrenergic agents), which were originally developed to treat high blood pressure, are often used to remediate the physical symptoms of anxiety that are commonly part of PTSD. These medications include clonidine (Catapres), guanfacine

(Tenex), and propranolol (Inderal) and several open trial studies have demonstrated their efficacy with children and adolescents (i.e., Famularo, Kinscherff & Fenton, 1988; Harmon & Riggs, 1996; Perry, 1994). Antipsychotics (DA agents) also affect the catecholamine system and have been regularly used in the treatment of adult PTSD (Donnelly et al., 1999). The atypical antipsychotics [i.e., risperidone (Risperdal), olanzapine (Zyprexa), and quetiapine (Seroquel)] are more often used currently because they seem to have a lower risk of adverse side effects (Friedman, 1998). To date there has been only one published study suggesting a positive response to res-peridone in male children with severe PTSD symptoms (Horrigan & Barnhill, 1999). Cohen and her colleagues (2002) urge caution when using this class of medication because of the risk of adverse side effects, including increased risk in adolescents of developing diabetes (Koller, Malozowski & Doraiswamy, 2001).

In spite of the fact that there has been only one open trial investigation of the efficacy of serotonergic agents, specifically the selective serotonin reuptake inhibitors (SSRIs), they have recently been the medication treatment of choice for this population (Cohen, Mannarino & Rogal, 2001). The SSRIs include fluoxetine (Prosac), ser-traline (Zoloft), paroxetine (Paxil), fluvoxamine (Luvox), and citaloram (Celexa). Seedat et al. (2002) found that PTSD symptoms were decreased in children and adolescents treated with citalopram at a level comparable to adults. Until recently this class of medications was seen as having a low risk of adverse side effects in the child and adolescent population and this perception likely accounts for their recent popularity in treating PTSD. However, the possibility of an increased risk of suicide attempts and completed suicides in adolescents treated with SSRIs is currently under investigation. The FDA (2003) has issued a public health advisory urging caution when using these medications with at risk adolescents. Similarly, the United Kingdom MHRA (2003) has issued a precautionary statement about this class of medications and specifically banned the use of paroxetine with youth because of the greater risk for self-harm and potentially suicidal behavior.

Two classes of medication, monoamine oxidase inhibitor (MAOI) and tricyclic antidepressants (TCAs), act on both the adrenergic and seratonergic systems. Both these medications have been used successfully to treat PTSD in adults (Cohen, 2001). The only double-blind randomized investigation of the efficacy of medication in treating stress disorders has been with one of the TCAs, imipramine (Tofranil). Robert et al. (1999) investigated the development of PTSD symptoms in acutely burned children who were treated with imipramine versus chloral hydrate. Those children treated with imipramine were significantly less likely to develop PTSD symptoms. It is unclear how generalizable these findings are to adolescents who have experienced other types of trauma. Further, the side effects of these two classes of medication can be life-threatening and so they are not typically recommended as a first-line medication when treating PTSD in children and adolescents (Cohen, 2001).

The Prevention of PTSD

The best way to prevent PTSD is to prevent adolescents' exposure to traumatic life events. However, research suggests many children and adolescents are likely to experience trauma (Yule, 2001). When adolescents are exposed to trauma, Klingman's (2001) five-level approach provides a useful conceptual framework to guide our work with these youth. The first three levels (the universal and selective efforts) typically occur as community-based interventions. The fourth level of intervention, with indicated groups, may be provided at community or residential treatment facilities, depending on the level of symptom severity displayed by the adolescent. The fifth level, again with an indicated group, is most likely to be provided in the community. It is important to note that progression through these levels of prevention and intervention does not always occur in a linear fashion. Adolescents with more severe PTSD may progress up and down through the levels as they encounter developmental and life experiences that precipitate a relapse of PTSD symptoms.

What Works

There is very little empirical data to identify what works across all levels of prevention and intervention. However, there exists an emerging credible body of evidence to guide our selective efforts with the general population of adolescents exposed to trauma and those youth displaying early signs of PTSD. There is empirical support for the efficacy of psychological debriefing and psychoeducational interventions in response to natural and technological disasters. More intensive indicated interventions and follow-up services can be provided to those adolescents identified as displaying early symptoms of PTSD following exposure to a traumatic event. Cognitive behavioral interventions seem to help these youth contain and manage the PTSD symptoms. Group therapies to provide support to these adolescents and their families are also effective.

What Might Work

The majority of the literature about prevention of PTSD in adolescents falls within the category of "what might work ." The universal level of anticipatory prevention programming exists primarily as a conceptual recommendation at this time and has yet to be empirically investigated. Selective primary prevention provides proactive interventions to youth who have been identified as being "at risk" for developing PTSD. Thorough assessment for PTSD in adolescents involves gathering information from both the teen and their parents. Semi-structured interviews are often recommended to assess PTSD in youth (e.g., Lipovsky, 1992; O'Donahue, Fanetti & Elliott, 1998; Perrin, Smith & Yule, 2000), but are costly and time-consuming. Self-report measures afford greater opportunity to screen large numbers of adolescents and several authors provide a comprehensive review of self-report instruments to assess PTSD (e.g., March, 1998; Nader, 1997). The instruments most often used to assess broad symptoms of PTSD include the Children's Post-Traumatic Stress Reactions Index (CPTS-RI; Frederick, 1985), the Children's Post-Traumatic Stress Disorder Inventory (Saigh, 1989), and an adaptation (Perrin, Smith & Yule, 2000) of the adult Impact of Events Scale (IES; Horowitz, Wilner & Alvarez, 1979). The Trauma Symptom Checklist for Children (TSCC; Briere, 1996) and The Children's Impact of Traumatic Events Scale-Revised (CITES-R; Wolfe, Gentile, Michienzi, Sas & Wolfe, 1991) are often used with abuse survivors. These instruments can help identify those adolescents displaying an adverse reaction to the traumatic event.

There are several recommendations at the level of interventions with indicated populations that might work. EMDR has been recommended and might be an effective indicated intervention method; however, there is limited empirical support for this method as the majority of investigations with adolescents have used case study methodologies. Similarly, case studies, but not empirical investigations, have supported the psychodynamic and creative therapies. Until recently, the SSRIs have been the most frequently used medications with adolescents demonstrating PTSD symptoms. However, there have been recent concerns about use of this class of medications and there has only been one open trial study of their efficacy. The antihypertensives have been supported by open trial studies but are less commonly used because of their negative side-effect profiles. Atypical antipsychotics, MAOIs, and TCAs have been investigated and shown to reduce PTSD symptoms. However, they are not considered first-line medications because they have potentially dangerous side effects.

The final level of intervention is provided to those adolescents who have developed symptoms of and been treated for PTSD. The goal of this level is to prevent relapse and promote healthy development in these youth. Intervention at this level is important as the neurobiological changes that accompany PTSD predispose adolescents with trauma exposure to chronic stress reactions (DeBellis, et al., 1999). Further, adolescents with a history of victimization have an increased likelihood for runaway and re-victimization (Tyler, Hoyt & Whitbeck, 2000). To date, programs for this level of programming have been recommended conceptually, but there have been no specific programs developed and investigated.

What Does Not Work

At present, there have been no specific investigations at any level that indicate interventions that clearly do not work.

Recommendations

Even though continued research is needed to validate further specific methods of prevention programming and intervention for PTSD in adolescents, the current review does suggest recommendations for best practice. In community settings, group interventions are recommended, as they allow clinicians to intervene with large number of adolescents both at risk for development of PTSD and with emerging or existing symptoms of PTSD. Psychological debriefing (provided in a group format) with the traumatized adolescents is also recommended as an effective tool for preventing psychological distress. *Cognitive-behavioral therapy* is the most extensively researched treatment for adolescents who have developed PTSD and is most often recommended as the treatment of choice for containing and managing symptoms of post-traumatic stress (Cohen, Berliner & March, 2000). However, current evidence does not allow the authors to make suggestions regarding the "dosage" or "frequency" of individual CBT techniques, such as exposure, relaxation, or cognitive restructuring. Again, there seems to be most support for providing CBT in a group format. Group therapy can also help combat the sense of isolation that often accompanies trauma recovery. Psychoeducational and support groups designed to help parents and teachers provide support to these adolescents can also help prevent these youth from developing post-traumatic stress symptoms.

Further empirical evidence is needed to support the application of specific interventions in residential settings. Therefore, it is difficult to derive conclusions for best
practice in these settings. However, there is a theoretical consensus that interventions
for these youth should combine cognitive behavioral, group, and family therapies,
within the context of a safe and supportive milieu. Finally, some adolescents with
more severe PTSD symptoms may need medication intervention. SSRIs are most frequently used to treat adolescents with PTSD (Cohen, Mannarino & Rogal, 2001).
Antihypertensives have also been used to reduce the physiological symptoms of
anxiety that accompany PTSD, and this class of medications has been studied most
frequently in children and teens. However, given the risk factors associated with
each, caution should be exercised with any medication intervention, particularly
when the risk of suicide is high.

References

Abramovitz, R., & Bloom, S. L. (2003). Creating sanctuary in residential treatment for youth: From the
    "well ordered asylum" to a "living learning environment." *Psychiatric Quarterly, 74*(2), 119–133.
Amaya-Jackson, L., & March, J. (1995). Posttraumatic stress disorder in adolescents: Risk factors, diagnosis,
    and intervention. *Adolescent Medicine, 6*, 251–269.
American Psychiatric Association. (1980). *Diagnostic and Statistical Manual of Mental Disorders* (3rd ed.).
    Washington, DC: Author.
American Psychiatric Association. (1987). *Diagnostic and Statistical Manual of Mental Disorders* (3rd ed.,
    revised). Washington, DC: Author.
American Psychiatric Association. (2000). *Diagnostic and Statistical Manual of Mental Disorders* (4th ed., text
    revisions). Washington, DC: Author.
Arroyo, W. (2001). PTSD in children and adolescents in the juvenile justice system. In S. Eth (Ed.), *PTSD
    in Children and Adolescents* (pp. 59–85). Washington, DC: American Psychiatric Publishing.
Bills, L.J., & Bloom, S.L. (1998). From chaos to sanctuary: Trauma-based treatment for women in a state
    hospital system. In B. Lubotsky Levin, A.K. Blanch, & A. Jennings (Eds.), *Women's Mental Health Ser-
    vices: A Public Health Perspective* (pp. 348–367). Thousand Oaks, CA: Sage.
Blom, G.E. (1986). A school disaster: Intervention and research aspects. *Journal of the American Academy of
    Child Psychiatry, 25*, 336–345.
Bloom, S.L. (1997). *Creating Sanctuary: Toward the Evolution of Sane Societies.* New York: Routledge.
Bloom, S.L., Bennington-Davis, M., Farragher, B., McCorkle, D., Nice-Martini, K., & Wellbank, K. (2003).
    Multiple opportunities for creating sanctuary. *Psychiatric Quarterly, 74*(2), 173–190.
Breuer, J., & Freud, S. (1955). Studies on hysteria. In *The Standard Edition* (Vol.2). London: Hogarth Press
    (original work published 1895).
Briere, J. (1996). *Trauma Symptoms Checklist for Children (TSCC): Professional Manual.* Odessa, FL: Psycho-
    logical Assessment Resources.
Briere, J. (1997). *Psychological Assessment of Adult Posttraumatic States.* Washington, DC: American Psycho-
    logical Association.
Butler, R.W., Rizzi, L.P., & Handwerger, B.A. (1996). Brief report: The assessment of posttraumatic stress
    disorder in pediatric cancer patients and survivors. *Journal of Pediatric Psychology, 21*(4), 499–504.
Chemtob, C.M., Nakashima, J., & Carlson, J.G. (2002). Brief treatment for elementary school children with
    disaster-related post-traumatic stress disorder: A field study. *Journal of Clinical Psychology, 58*, 99–112.
Clark, D.B., & Miller, T.W. (1998). Stress response and adaptation in children: Theoretical Models. In T.W.
    Miller (Ed.), *Children of Trauma: Stressful Life Events and Their Effects on Children and Adolescents* (pp.
    3–29). Madison, CT: International Universities Press, Inc.
Chronister, R.B., & DeFrance, J.F. (1981). Functional organization of monoamines. In G.C. Palmer (Ed.), *Neu-
    ropharmacology of Central Nervous System and Behavior Disorders* (pp. 435–462). New York: Academic Press.
Coco, N., & Sharpe, L. (1993). An auditory variant of eye movement desensitization in a case of childhood
    post-traumatic stress disorder. *Journal of Behavior Therapy and Experimental Psychiatry, 24*, 373–377.

Cohen, J.A. (1998). Practice parameters for the assessment and treatment of children and adolescents with posttraumatic stress disorder. *Journal of the American Academy of Child and Adolescent Psychiatry, 37,* 4S–26S.

Cohen, J.A. (2001). Pharmacologic treatment of traumatized children. *Trauma, Violence, and Abuse, 2(2),* 155–171.

Cohen, J.A., Berliner, L., & March, J.S. (2000). Treatment of children and adolescents. In. E.B. Foa, T.M. Keane, & M.J. Friedman (Eds.), *Effective Treatments for PTSD: Practice Guidelines from the International Society for Traumatic Stress Studies* (pp. 106–138). New York: Guilford Press.

Cohen, J.A., Mannarino, A.P., & Rogal, S.S. (2001). Treatment practices for childhood posttraumatic stress disorder, *Child Abuse and Neglect, 25,* 123–136.

Cohen, J.A., Perel, J.M., DeBellis, M.D., Friedman, M.J., & Putnam, F.W. (2002). Treating traumatized children: Clinical implications of the psychobiology of posttraumatic stress disorder. *Trauma, Violence, & Abuse, 3(2),* 91–108.

Courtois, C. (2003). *Advances in trauma treatment.* Paper presented at the 26th Annual Networker Symposium, Washington, D.C.

Davidson, S., & Smith, R. (1990). Traumatic experiences in psychiatric outpatients. *Journal of Traumatic Stress Studies, 3,* 459–475.

Davis, L., & Siegel, L.J. (2000). Posttraumatic stress disorder in children and adolescents: A review and analysis. *Clinical Child and Family Psychology Review, 3(3),* 135–154.

DeBellis, M.D., Baum, A.S., Birmaher, B., Keshavan, M.S., Eccard, C.H., Boring, A.M., Jenkins, F.J., & Ryan, N.D. (1999). Developmental traumatology, part I: Biological stress systems. *Biological Psychiatry, 45,* 1259–1270.

de Silva, P. (1999). Cultural aspects of posttraumatic stress disorder. In W. Yule (Ed.), *Post Traumatic Stress Disorders: Concepts and Therapy* (pp. 116–137). New York: John Wiley & Sons.

DiNicola, V.F. (1996). Ethnocultural aspects of PTSD and related disorders among children and adolescents. In A.J. Marsella, M.J. Friedman, E.T. Gerrity, & R.M Scurfield (Eds.), *Ethnocultural Aspects of Posttraumatic Stress Disorder* (pp. 389–414). Washington, DC: American Psychological Association.

Donnelly, C.I., Amaya-Jackson, L., & March, J.S. (1999). Psychopharmacology of pediatric posttraumatic stress disorder. *Journal of Child and Adolescent Psychopharmacology, 9(3),* 203–220.

Doyle, J.S., & Bauer, S.K. (1989). Post-traumatic stress disorder in children: Its identification and treatment in a residential setting for emotionally disturbed youth. *Journal of Traumatic Stress, 2,* 275–288.

Elklit, A. (2002). Victimization and PTSD in a Danish national youth probability sample. *Journal of the American Academy of Child and Adolescent Psychiatry, 41(2),* 174–181.

Famularo, R., Kinscherff, R., & Fenton, T. (1988). Propranolol treatment for childhood PTSD acute type. *American Journal of Diseases of Childhood, 142,* 1244–1247.

Figley, C.R. (1988). A five-phase treatment of post-traumatic stress disorder in families. *Journal of Traumatic Stress, 1,* 127–141.

Foa, E.B., Keane, T.M., & Friedman, M.J. (2000). Introduction. In. E.B. Foa, T.M. Keane, & M.J. Friedman (Eds.), *Effective Treatments for PTSD: Practice Guidelines from the International Society for Traumatic Stress Studies* (pp. 106–138). New York: Guilford Press.

Food and Drug Administration. (2003). *Reports of suicidality in pediatric patients being treated with antidepressant medications for major depressive disorder.* Retrieved January 13, 2004, from http://www.fda.gov/cder/drug/advisory/mdd.htm

Frederick, C.H. (1985). Children traumatized by catastrophic situations. In S. Eth & R.S. Pynoos (Eds.), *Posttraumatic Stress Disorder in Children* (pp. 71–100). Washington, DC: American Psychiatric Press.

Friedman, M.J. (1990). Interrelationships between biological mechanisms and pharmacotherapy of posttraumatic stress disorder. In M.E. Wolfe & A.D. Mosnian (Eds.), *Posttraumatic Stress Disorder: Etiology, Phenomenology, and Treatment* (pp. 204–225). Washington, DC: American Psychiatric Press.

Friedman, M.J. (1998). Current and future drug treatment for posttraumatic stress disorder patients. *Psychiatric Annals, 28,* 461–468.

Garrison, C.Z., Bryant, E.S., Addy, C.L., Spurrier, P.G., Freedy, J.R., & Kilpatrick, D.G. (1995). Posttraumatic stress disorder in adolescents after Hurricane Andrew. *Journal of the American Academy of Child and Adolescent Psychiatry, 34(9),* 1193–1201.

Goenjian, A.K., Karayan, I., Pynoos, R.S., Minassian, D., Najarian, L.M., Steinberg, A.M., & Fairbanks, L.A. (1997). Outcome of psychotherapy among early adolescents after trauma. *American Journal of Psychiatry, 154,* 536–542.

Gonzales, N., & Kim, L. (1997). Stress and coping in an ethnic minority context. In S.A. Wlochik & I.N. Sandler (Eds.), *Handbook of Children's Coping: Linking Theory and Intervention* (pp. 481–511). New York: Plenum Press.

Greenwald, R. (1994). Applying eye movement desensitization and reprocessing (EMDR) to the treatment of traumatized children: Five case studies. *Anxiety Disorders Practice Journal, 1*, 83–97.

Gunderson, J.G. (1978). Defining the therapeutic processes in psychiatric milieus. *Psychiatry, 41*, 327–355.

Gullotta, T.P., & Bloom, M. (2003) (eds.). *The Encyclopedia of Primary Prevention and Health Promotion*. New York: Kluwer/Academic.

Harmon R.J. & Riggs, P.D. (1996). Clinical perspectives: Clonidine for PTSD in preschool children. *Journal of the American Academy of Child and Adolescent Psychiatry, 35*, 1247–1249.

Harris, C.J. (1991). A family crisis-intervention model for the treatment of posttraumatic stress reaction. *Journal of Traumatic Stress, 4*, 195–207.

Horowitz, K., Weine, S., & Jekel, J. (1995). PTSD symptoms in urban adolescent girls. *Journal of the American Academy of Child and Adolescent Psychiatry, 34*(10), 1353–1361.

Horowitz, M., Wilner, N., & Alvarez, W. (1979). Impact of Event Scale: A measure of subjective stress. *Psychosomatic Medicine, 41*, 209–218.

Horrigan, J.P., & Barnhill, L.J. (1999). Risperidone and PTSD in boys. *Journal of Neuropsychiatry and Clinical Neuroscience, 11*, 126–127.

Kiser, L., Heston, J., Hickerson, S., & Millsap, P. (1993). Anticipatory stress in children and adolescents. *American Journal of Psychiatry, 150*(1), 87–92.

Koller, E., Malozowski, S., & Doraiswamy, M.P. (2001). Atypical antipsychotic drugs in adolescents. *Journal of the American Medical Association, 286*, 2547–2548.

Klingman, A. (2001). Prevention of anxiety disorders: The case of posttraumatic stress disorder. In W.K. Silverman & P.D.A. Treffers (Eds.), *Anxiety Disorders in Children and Adolescents: Research, Assessment and Intervention* (pp. 368–391). Cambridge, UK: Cambridge University Press.

Kruczek, T., & Vitanza, S. (1999). Treatment effects with an adolescent abuse survivor's group. *Child Abuse & Neglect, 23*(5), 477–485.

Kruczek, T., & Watson, W. (1995). *The efficacy of group therapy with sexually abused adolescent females*. Unpublished manuscript.

La Greca, A.M., Silverman, W.K., Vernberg, E.M., & Prinstein, M.J. (1996). Symptoms of posttraumatic stress in children after Hurricane Andrew: A prospective study. *Journal of Consulting and Clinical Psychology, 64*, 712–723.

Lawson, L. (1998). Milieu management of traumatized youngsters. *Journal of Child and Adolescent Psychiatric Nursing, 11*(3), 99–106.

LeDoux, J.E. (1996). *The Emotional Brain: The Mysterious Underpinnings of Emotional Life*. New York: Simon & Schuster.

Lipovsky, J.A. (1992). Assessment and treatment of posttraumatic stress disorder in child survivors of sexual assault. In D.W. Foy (Ed.), *Treating PTSD: Cognitive-Behavioral Strategies* (pp. 127–165). New York: Guilford Press.

March, J.S. (1998). Assessment of pediatric posttraumatic stress disorder. In P.A. Saigh & J.D. Bremner (Eds.), *Posttraumatic Stress Disorder: A Comprehensive Text* (pp. 199–218). Needham Heights, MA: Allyn & Bacon.

March, J.S., Amaya-Jackson, L., Murray, M.C., & Schulte, A. (1998). Cognitive-behavioral psychotherapy for children and adolescents with postraumatic stress disorder after a single incident stressor. *Journal of the American Academy of Child and Adolescent Psychiatry, 37*, 585–593.

McCloskey, L.A., & Walker, M. (2000). Posttraumatic stress in children exposed to family violence and single-event trauma. *Journal of the American Academy of Child and Adolescent Psychiatry, 39*(1), 108–115.

McElroy, L.P., & McElroy, R. A. (1989). Psychoanalytically oriented psychotherapy with sexually abused children. *Journal of Mental Health Counseling, 11*(3), 244–258.

McMackin, R.A., Leisen, M.B., Sattler, L., Krinsley, K., & Riggs, D.S. (2002). Preliminary development of trauma-focused treatment groups for incarcerated juvenile offenders. In R. Greenwald (Ed.), *Trauma and Juvenile Delinquency: Theory, Research, and Interventions* (pp.175–199). Binghampton, NY: Hayworth Press.

Medicines and HealthCare Products Regulatory Agency (MHRA). (2003). *Use of Selective Serotonin Reuptake Inhibitors (SSRIs) in children and adolescents with major depressive disorder (MDD)*. Retrieved January 13, 2004, from http://www.mhra.gov.uk/news/2003.htm#ssri.

Muris, P., & deJongh, A. (1996). Eye movement desensitization and reprocessing: A new treatment method for trauma-related anxiety complaints (in Dutch). *Kind en Adolescent, 17*, 190–199.

Nader, K. (1997). Assessing traumatic experiences in children. In J.P. Wilson and T.M. Keane (Eds.), *Assessing Psychological Trauma and PTSD* (pp. 291–348). New York: Guilford Press.

Nader, K. (2001). Treatment methods for childhood trauma. In J.P. Wilson, M.J. Friedman, & J.D. Lindy (Eds.), *Treating Psychological Trauma and PTSD* (pp. 278–334). NewYork: Guilford Press.

Norris, F.H., Foster, J.D., Weisshar, D.L. (2002). The epidemiology of sex differences in PTSD across developmental, social, and research contexts. In R. Kimmerling, P. Ouimette, and J. Wolfe (Eds.), *Gender and PTSD* (pp. 3–42). New York: Guilford Press.

O'Donahue, W., Fanetti, M., & Elliott, A. (1998). Trauma in children. In Follette, V.M., Ruzek, J.I., & Abueg, F.R. (Eds.), *Cognitive-Behavioral Therapies for Trauma* (pp. 355–382). NewYork: Guilford Press.

Pandit, S., & Shah, L. (2000). Post-traumatic stress disorder: causes and aetiological factors. In K.N. Dwivedi (Ed.), *Post-Traumatic Stress Disorder in Children and Adolescents* (pp. 25–38). London, England: Whurr Publishers, Ltd.

Pfefferbaum, B. (2001). The impact of the Oklahoma City bombing on children in the community. *Military Medicine, 166(12),* 49–50.

Perrin, S., Smith, P., & Yule, W. (2000). Practitioner review: The assessment and treatment of post-traumatic stress disorder in children and adolescents. *Journal of Child Psychology and Psychiatry, 41*(3), 277–289.

Perry, B.D. (1994). Neurobiological sequelae of childhood trauma: PTSD in children. In M.M. Murburg (Ed.), *Catecholamine Function in Posttraumatic Stress Disorder: Emerging Concepts* (pp. 223–255). Washington, DC: American Psychiatric Press.

Pynoos, R.S. (1994). Traumatic stress and developmental psychopathology in children and adolescents. In R.S. Pynoos (Ed.), *Posttraumatic Stress Disorder: A Clinical Review* (pp. 64–98). Lutherville, MD: The Sidran Press.

Pynoos, R.S., & Nader, K. (1988). Psychological first aid and treatment approach to children exposed to community violence: Research implications. *Journal of Traumatic Stress, 1,* 445–473.

Rabalais, A.E., Ruggerio, K.J., & Scotti, J.R. (2002). Multicultural issues in the response of children to disasters. In A.M. LaGreca, W.K. Silverman, E.M. Vernberg, and MC. Roberts (Eds.), *Helping Children Cope with Disasters and Terrorism* (pp. 73–100). Washington, DC: American Psychological Association.

Read Johnson, D. (2000). Creative Therapies. In. E.B. Foa, T.M. Keane, & M.J. Friedman (Eds.), *Effective Treatments for PTSD: Practice Guidelines from the International Society for Traumatic Stress Studies* (pp. 302–314). New York: Guilford Press.

Reinherz, H.Z., Giaconia, R.M., Lefkowitz, E.S., Pakiz, B., & Frost, A.K. (1993). Prevalence of psychiatric disorders in a community population of older adolescents. *Journal of the American Academy of Child and Adolescent Psychiatry, 32,* 369–377.

Riggs, D. (2000). Marital and family therapy. In. E.B. Foa, T.M. Keane, & M.J. Friedman (Eds.), *Effective Treatments for PTSD: Practice Guidelines from the International Society for Traumatic Stress Studies* (pp. 280–301). New York: Guilford Press .

Rivard, J.C., Bloom, S.L., Abramovitz, R., Pasquale, L.E., Duncan, M., McCorkle, D, & Gelman, A. (2003). Assessing the implementation and effects of a trauma-focused intervention for youths in residential treatment. *Psychiatric Quarterly, 74*(2), 137–154.

Rigamer, E.F. (1986). Psychological management of children in a national crisis. *Journal of the American Academy of Child Psychiatry, 25,* 364–369.

Robert, R., Blackeney, P.E., Villareal, C., Rosenbert, L., & Meyer, W.J. (1999). Imipramine treatment in pediatric burn patients with symptoms of adult stress disorder. *Journal of the American Academy of Child Psychiatry, 38,* 873–882.

Saigh, P.A. (1989). The use of an in vitro flooding package in the treatment of traumatized adolescents. *Journal of Developmental and Behavioral Pediatrics, 10*(1), 17–21.

Salloum, A., Avery, L., & McClain, R.P. (2001). Group psychotherapy for adolescent survivors of homicide victims: A pilot study. *Journal of the American Academy of Child and Adolescent Psychiatry, 40,* 1261–1267.

Saylor, C.F., Coward, B.L., Lipovsky, J.A., Jackson, C., & Finch A.J. (2003). Media exposure to September 11: Elementary school students' experiences and posttraumatic symptoms, *American Behavioral Scientist, 46,* 1622–1642.

Seedat, S., Stein, D.J., Ziervogel, C., Middleton, T., Kaminer, D., Emsley, R.A., & Rossouw, W. (2002). Comparison of response to a selective serotonin reuptake inhibitor in children, adolescents and adults with PTSD. *Journal of Child and Adolescent Psychopharmacology, 12,* 37–46.

Seinfeld, J. (1989). Therapy with a severely abused child: An object relations perspective. *Clinical Social Work Journal, 17*(1), 40–49.

Selye, H. (1952). *The Story of the Adaptation Syndrome.* Montreal, Canada: Acta, Inc.

Shapiro, F. (1996). Eye movement desensitization and reprocessing (EMDR): Evaluation of controlled PTSD research. *Journal of Behavior Therapy and Experimental Psychiatry, 27*(3), 209–218.

Silverman, W.K., & La Greca, A.K. (2002). Children experiencing disasters: Definitions, reactions, and predictors of outcomes. In A.M. LaGreca, W.K. Silverman, E.M. Vernberg, and MC. Roberts (Eds.), *Helping Children Cope with Disasters and Terrorism* (pp. 11–34). Washington, DC: American Psychological Association.

Soberman, G.B., Greenwald, R., & Rule, D.L. (2002). A controlled study of eye movement desensitization and reprocessing (EMDR) for boys with conduct problems. In R. Greenwald (Ed.), *Trauma and Juvenile Delinquency: Theory, Research, and Interventions* (pp. 217–236). Binghampton, NY: Hayworth Press.

Stallard, P. (2000). Debriefing adolescents after critical life events. In B. Raphael & J.P. Wilson (Eds.), *Psychological Debriefing: Theory, Practice, and Evidence* (pp. 213–224). New York: Cambridge University Press.

Stallard, P., & Law, F.D. (1993). Screening and psychological debriefing of adolescent survivors of life-threatening events. *British Journal of Psychiatry, 163,* 660–665.

Summit, R.C. (1983). The child sexual abuse accommodation syndrome. *Child Abuse and Neglect, 7,* 177–193.

Terr, L.C. (1991). Childhood traumas: An outline and overview. *American Journal of Psychiatry, 148,* 10–19.

Tinker, R.H., & Wilson, S.A. (1999). *Through the Eyes of a Child: EMDR with Children.* New York: Norton and Company.

Tolin, D.E., & Foa, E.B. (2002). Gender and PTSD: A cognitive model. In R. Kimmerling, P. Ouimette, and J. Wolfe (Eds.), *Gender and PTSD* (pp. 76–97). NewYork: Guilford Press.

Tyler, K.A., Hoyt, D.R., & Whitbeck, L.B. (2000). The effects of early sexual abuse on later sexual victimization among female homeless and runaway adolescents. *Journal of Interpersonal Violence, 15,* 235–250.

Udwin, O., Boyle, S., Yule, W., Bolton, D., & O'Ryan, D. (2000). Risk factors for long-term psychological effects of a disaster experienced in adolescence: Predictors of post traumatic stress disorder. *Journal of Child Psychology and Psychiatry, 41*(8), 969–979.

Van Leeuwen, K. (1988). Resistances in the treatment of a sexually molested 6-year-old girl. *International Review of Psycho-Analysis, 15*(2), 149–156.

Wasserstein, S.B., & La Greca, A.M. (1998). Hurricane Andrew: Parent conflict as a moderator of children's adjustment. *Hispanic Journal of Behavioral Sciences, 20*(2), 212–224.

Wolfe, V.V. Gentile, C., Michienzi, T., Sas, L., & Wolfe, D.A. (1991). The Children's Impact of Traumatic Events Scales: A measure of post-sexual-abuse PTSD symptoms. *Behavioral Assessment, 13,* 359–383.

Wraith, R. (2000). Children and debriefing: theory, interventions and outcomes. In B. Raphael & J.P. Wilson (Eds.), *Psychological Debriefing: Theory, Practice, and Evidence* (pp. 195–212). New York: Cambridge University Press.

Yule, W. (1992). Post-traumatic stress disorder in child survivors of shipping disasters: The sinking of the "Jupiter." *Psychotherapy and Psychosomatics, 57,* 200–205.

Yule, W. (2001). Post-traumatic stress disorder in children and adolescents. *International Review of Psychiatry, 13,* 194–200.

Yule, W., Perrin, S., & Smith, P. (1999). Post-traumatic stress reactions in children and Adolescents. In W. Yule (Ed.), *Post-Traumatic Stress Disorders* (pp. 25–50). New York: John Wiley & Sons.

Yule, W., & Udwin, O. (1991). Screening child survivors for post-traumatic stress disorders: Experiences from the "Jupiter" sinking. *British Journal of Clinical Psychology, 30*(2), 131–138.

Chapter 16

Schizophrenia

Judy A. McCown

Introduction

Schizophrenia is a complex, serious psychiatric illness that is characterized by disruptions in cognitive, affective, and social functioning. The term *schizophrenia* comes from the Greek words meaning "split mind" and many people mistakenly believe that this disorder refers to individuals who have multiple personalities. In fact, the term was intended to refer to the disconnection among thinking, feeling, and behavior (Bleuler, 1911/1950). In the general population, about 1% of the population develops schizophrenia. Onset of symptoms typically occurs in late adolescence or early adulthood. Very early onset before age 13 is extremely rare, with incidence rates increasing throughout adolescence. Because it is uncommon, few epidemiological studies have been conducted for children and adolescents. However, Remschmidt, Schulz, Martin, Warnke, and Trott (1994) have estimated that 1 child in 10,000 is likely to develop schizophrenia.

The diagnostic criteria for both early-onset and adult-onset schizophrenia are the same. Persons with schizophrenia typically demonstrate a combination of symptoms categorized broadly as positive and negative symptoms. Positive symptoms are more active behaviors and include hallucinations, delusions, disorganized speech and thought, and disorganized or catatonic or bizarre behaviors. Negative symptoms reflect deficits in functioning and include dampening of emotions, decrease in verbal productivity, and inability to initiate or sustain goal-directed activity.

A diagnosis of schizophrenia requires the presence of two or more of these characteristic symptoms for six months accompanied by problems in social and/or occupational functioning (American Psychiatric Association, 2000). Because many of these symptoms may be found in other disorders and because the presentation of symptoms varies among people and over time, diagnosing schizophrenia is particularly challenging. With early-onset presentation, it is imperative to rule out disorders such as depression, bipolar disorder, developmental disorders, or substance abuse before deciding on a diagnosis of schizophrenia. Asarnow and Asarnow (1996) recommend conducting longitudinal diagnostic evaluations since studies indicate a high rate of misdiagnosis of early-onset schizophrenia.

Over time, the development of schizophrenic symptoms may occur acutely or follow a slower progression. For children and adolescents, the development tends to be gradual and insidious and often results in deterioration in social and academic functioning. This pattern tends to be associated with poorer prognosis.

Although the specific causes of schizophrenia are not known, theories regarding etiology focus on the biological and environmental domains. Contemporary thinking suggests a vulnerability-stress model that describes schizophrenia as a disease of the brain that is likely caused by an inherited genetic vulnerability that interacts with certain environmental and psychosocial stressors to produce the symptoms of schizophrenia.

Individual Factors

How schizophrenia develops is uncertain but research suggests that brain abnormalities, birth complications, and neurotransmitter dysfunction may be important risk factors. Studies examining neurological anomalies in persons with schizophrenia indicate that ventricular enlargement, gross reduction of cerebral gray matter, and reduced metabolism in the frontal lobes may be related to the development of positive and negative symptoms (Gur & Pearlson, 1993; Schlaepfer et al., 1994; Andreasen et al., 1992; Bogerts et al., 1993). Prenatal stressors during the second trimester of pregnancy have also been implicated (Weinberger, 1987). These stressors may include exposure to a viral infection during a critical period of brain development, delivery complications, and poor maternal nutrition (Pallast, Jongbloet, Straatman & Zielhuis, 1994; Dalman, Allebeck, Cullberg, Grunewald & Koster, 1999). In adults, inadequate levels of dopamine have been associated with the development of psychosis (Carlsson, 1987). Other neurotransmitters such as the seratonin, noradrenergic and glutamate systems (Inayama et al., 1996; Harrison, 1999) are also being considered. However, few brain imaging or neurochemical studies have been done with children and adolescents so these theories must be considered conservatively.

While lifetime prevalence rates are equivalent for men and women, gender differences are seen in age of onset. In both adult-onset and childhood-onset schizophrenia, men show higher prevalence rates at a ratio of 2:1. However, gender differences decrease for incidence rates in adolescence (Remschmidt et al., 1994; Howard, Castle, Wessley & Murray, 1993).

Early-onset patients often display a number of abnormalities before psychotic symptoms are noted. These difficulties include social withdrawal and isolation, speech and language problems, developmental delays, disruptive behaviors, and general academic difficulties (Alaghband-Rad, McKenna & Gordon, 1995; Hollis, 1995; McClellan & McCurry, 1998). Retrospective interviews with families of very early-onset patients reported most problematic behaviors were noticed when the children first entered school although most problems began two to three years before that time (Schaeffer & Ross, 2002).

Individually, intelligence and social competence may be protective factors for early-onset schizophrenia (Arsarnow & Goldstein, 1986). Adolescents who function at a higher level intellectually may have greater resources for problem-solving and may be able to develop better insight into managing the symptoms of their disorder.

Stronger social skills may serve as a buffer against social isolation. Together these factors may reduce the risk of schizophrenic exacerbations.

Family Factors

Another aspect of the vulnerability-stress model is consideration of an inherited genetic predisposition to schizophrenia. Research studies examining the concordance rates of schizophrenia in families provide compelling evidence that genetics play an important role in the development of this disease. First-degree relatives of schizophrenic patients are ten times more likely to develop schizophrenia than the rate in the general population (Kety, 1987). Additionally, the risk of developing schizophrenic spectrum disorders including schizoaffective disorder, nonaffective psychoses, and schizotypal and paranoid personality disorder is much higher in families of persons with schizophrenia than in unaffected families (Kendler et al., 1993).

Twin studies allow researchers to explore the roles of genetic and environmental factors in the development of schizophrenia. Monozygotic twins share 100% of their genetic material. If genetic factors are solely responsible for the development of schizophrenia, both twins should always develop the disease. However, studies have demonstrated that concordance rates for monozygotic twins vary from 33% to 78%. Furthermore, concordance rates for same-sex dizygotic twins range from 8% to 28% (Gottesman, 1991). These findings suggest that while vulnerability for schizophrenia is indeed inherited, environmental factors are also important, if not the controlling influence in some cases.

Social and Community Factors

Since environment seems significantly to influence the risk of developing schizophrenia, several studies have explored social and community factors that may be related with this disorder. Again, few studies of early-onset cases are available but some longitudinal research provides important data on the impact of environmental stress on schizophrenic expression. A recent prospective study by Ventura, Nuechterlein, Lukoff, and Hardesty (1989) tracked the occurrence of stressful life events of subjects who developed schizophrenia for one year after the onset of schizophrenic symptoms. Results revealed that 37% of the participants experienced a significant relapse following stressful life events.

What constitutes life stress may vary considerably from person to person, but one area that seems to be important is the family environment.

Early psychoanalytic theories (Fromm-Reichmann, 1948) presented the concept of the schizophrenogenic mother and suggested that maladaptive mother–child relationships caused the onset of schizophrenic symptoms. However, empirical studies have demonstrated that there is no support for these ideas and this theory is no longer accepted today.

Although no evidence exists that family environment directly leads to the development of schizophrenia, several studies have noted the correlation between conflicted home environments and relapse. One particular area of interest looks at a family communication style known as expressed emotion and how it might contribute to environmental stress. Expressed emotion is defined as a familial interaction style characterized by criticism, hostility, emotional overinvolvment, and controlling behaviors (Leff & Vaughn, 1985). Ratings of high expressed emotion in families of schizophrenic patients are strongly correlated with higher rates of relapse and rehospitalization (Kavanaugh, 1992); high expressed emotion ratings in adolescence were also associated with later development of schizophrenic spectrum disorders (Goldstein, 1987). Although these findings may be interpreted as supporting the hypothesis that communication deviance in families leads to relapse, we must also consider the possible impact an adolescent's schizophrenic symptoms may have on family functioning. Concurrently, healthy family communication styles characterized by flexibility, acceptance, and support are associated with decreased risk of psychotic episodes (Mueser, Bellack, Wade, Sayers, Tierney, & Haas, 1993). If the family system is adaptable, greater social support will be available for all family members.

Although the presentation of schizophrenia is universal across cultures, rate of diagnosis varies considerably. Research in the United States and England has revealed that minority groups receive a diagnosis of schizophrenia significantly more often than majority ethic groups. In the United States, African Americans and Puerto Ricans are more likely to be diagnosed with schizophrenia than whites, suggesting that misdiagnosis may be a factor (Lewis, Croft-Jeffreys & Anthony, 1990).

Evidence-Based Treatment Interventions in Community Settings

What Works

Many studies have been conducted looking at the efficacy of various treatment interventions with adult schizophrenic patients. However, very few studies have focused on treatment interventions for early-onset schizophrenia. Since the presentation of the disorder is identical for both adolescents and adults, the evidence gained from the adult literature is very likely applicable to the younger population. Only psychopharmacological treatment has been deemed to be effective in the treatment of early-onset schizophrenia and is considered to be the most appropriate first-line treatment for schizophrenia. Those interventions will be discussed in the section below (Psychopharmacology and Schizophrenia).

In general, adolescents with schizophrenia need a multimodal approach, including medication, psychotherapy, psychoeducation, stress management, and social skills training as well as any treatment for comorbid conditions such as substance abuse. Ideally, a range of services can be provided which will address both the specific symptoms of schizophrenia as well as other needs of the adolescent and the family (McClellan, et al., 2001).

In community settings, adolescents with schizophrenia and their families can benefit from psychotherapy, social support services, and, in a more limited way, specialized educational and vocational training programs. These interventions can be delivered in a variety of settings—outpatient clinics, community centers, or schools.

Individual or group psychotherapy should focus on the practical aspects of coping with schizophrenia. Learning about the nature of schizophrenia, developing strategies and skills to monitor and manage medications, and identifying the warning signs of relapse can help adolescents regain a feeling of control and predictability at a time when they may be particularly distressed. Behavioral therapy can be effective in increasing skills necessary for day-to-day functioning in such areas as time and money management, household chores, and personal hygiene. Cognitive therapy helps patients cope with the stigma of having a chronic mental illness and learn alternative, adaptive ways of responding to everyday demands and situations (Kingdon, Turkington & John, 1994). Group therapy can be particularly helpful in decreasing social isolation and increasing social support (Scott & Dixon, 1995).

Psychoeducational family interventions can help family members understand what schizophrenia is and how it affects their own family. People with schizophrenia must often rely on family members to assist them in finding appropriate treatment and in accessing support services. Family members often feel overwhelmed and isolated and may need supportive therapy themselves. Family support groups in the community are often very helpful in these circumstances (Bustillo, Lauriella, Horan & Keith, 2001).

Families with high levels of expressed emotion may benefit from cognitive-behavioral family therapy that can help them learn to communicate and problem-solve more effectively. In turn, improved communication can help to prevent relapse and lead to improved relationships for all involved (Tarrier, Barrowclough, Porceddu & Fitzpatrick, 1994). Therapy groups consisting of several families may be helpful in developing a support network for both patients and family members.

Community-based social services may also be helpful for adolescents with schizophrenia. Some of the more common systems of care include partial hospitalization, day treatment aftercare, case management, assertive community treatment (ACT), and rehabilitation programs.

Partial hospitalization is typically conducted on an outpatient basis in a community clinic and includes intensive treatment several days per week with medication management and individual and group therapy. Day treatment is usually less structured but also serves as a transitional program between acute phase care and maintenance.

What Might Work

Beyond formal therapeutic interventions, some adolescents with schizophrenia may benefit from self-help groups. After symptoms have stabilized, participation in a peer support group may provide opportunities for discussion, sharing, and socialization that are especially important in order to maintain adaptive functioning.

In school, adolescent patients may need to take advantage of special education services. Smaller classrooms with teachers experienced in working with mentally ill children are necessary. Academic curricula can be modified to take into consideration the individual adolescent's cognitive limitations and need for a less stimulating environment.

Case management and assertive community treatment both involve in-home follow-up. Individual case managers or multidisciplinary teams work directly with schizophrenic individuals to offer intensive support services. Patients who have had a severe and unstable course of illness often need extensive support to maintain adequate functioning and these types of interventions allow them to avoid hospitalization and have a higher quality of life than would otherwise be possible.

Specialized rehabilitation programs generally focus on helping an individual acquire the skills needed to assume an active role in the community. A review of the literature by Mueser, Drake, and Bond (1997) outlined components of rehabilitation programs that were deemed essential for effective intervention. These included developing specific behavioral goals, focusing on long-term strategies, and providing interventions in naturalistic settings whenever possible. Rehabilitation programs usually provide training in several areas, including personal goal setting, development of job, independent living and social skills, assistance with housing arrangements, and development of social support networks (World Health Organization, 1997).

What Does Not Work

While certain insight-oriented approaches to psychotherapy, including psychoanalytic, humanistic, existential, and gestalt techniques may be helpful to some individuals, there is insufficient empirical evidence to support recommending these interventions for the treatment of schizophrenia in adolescents (McClellan et al., 2001).

Evidence-Based Treatment Interventions in Residential Settings

What Works

Many of the interventions described above are also employed in residential settings such as inpatient hospitals, group homes, and residential schools. However, at times of acute exacerbations of psychotic symptoms, adolescents with schizophrenia may require inpatient hospitalization. This becomes particularly important if individuals are experiencing severe hallucinations or delusions and may be suicidal or in danger of harming others. Since approximately 10% of people with schizophrenia commit suicide, appropriate response to acute episodes is vital.

What Might Work

Residential settings for adolescents often provide the same interventions used in community settings. As noted previously, the literature provides strong support for the effectiveness of individual and group psychotherapy, peer-support groups, and special education services for adolescents with schizophrenia. However, more research is needed to provide solid evidence for their efficacy with this population.

What Does Not Work

The American Academy of Child and Adolescent Psychiatry (McClellan et al., 2001) reports that electroconvulsive therapy (ECT) has been used on rare occasions to address treatment-resistant schizophrenic symptoms in adolescents. However, it does not appear to be very effective and is not recommended except in extreme cases in which all other interventions have failed.

Psychopharmacology

The recent report of the Surgeon General of the United States on mental health (U.S. Department of Health and Human Services, 1999) recommends that the first-line of treatment for schizophrenia should be the use of antipsychotic medications.

One of the strongest predictors for long-term remission of psychotic symptoms and for prevention of relapse is the consistent use of antipsychotic medication (Lehman & Steinwachs, 1998). However, as with psychotherapy, there are few well-designed studies examining the use of antipsychotic medications with adolescents and children. The studies that have been done suggest that the pattern of response in early-onset patients is similar to that of adult patients.

Two classifications of antipsychotic medications are considered: traditional and atypical neuroleptics. Traditional neuroleptic medications such as chlorpromazine and haloperidol have demonstrated effectiveness in reducing positive symptoms by blocking dopamine D2 receptors (Dixon, Lehman & Levine, 1995). They are less effective at addressing negative symptoms, however. Furthermore, adolescents have demonstrated the same unpleasant side effects from these medications as adults, including sedation, tremors, muscle rigidity, spasms, and tardive dyskinesia (Campbell, Rapoport & Simpson, 1999; Ernst, Malone, Rowan, George, Gonzalez & Silva, 1998). Approximately 40% of patients experience these side effects and compliance with the medication regimen is problematic (U.S. Department of Health and Human Services, 1999).

More recently, another classification of antipsychotic medications has been introduced which target a number of neurotransmitter systems, including both the dopamine D2 and seratonin 5-HT2 systems. Research indicates that these medications are as effective as traditional neuroleptics for positive symptoms and may be more effective in treating negative symptoms (Meltzer, 1997). Clozapine has been shown to be effective with treatment-resistant patients but is not used as a first-line treatment because of significant side effects. Although potentially very effective, the use of atypical neuroleptics is associated with weight gain and, more seriously, agranulocytosis, neutropenia, and seizures. Use of atypical antipsychotic medications requires close monitoring. Also, since these medications are relatively new, the long-term effectiveness and safety is unknown. Continued research in this area is imperative.

The Prevention of Schizophrenia

What Works

In a review of the literature on primary prevention of schizophrenia, Larson et al. (2001) found no studies that proved that schizophrenia could be prevented. Identifying potential schizophrenia victims in the prodromal phase is fraught with ethical problems as efforts result in a preponderance of false positives. They indicated that research aimed at reducing the duration of untreated psychosis seems more promising for the immediate future.

What Might Work

For decades, schizophrenia was regarded as an unfortunate but inevitable legacy for those predisposed to the disease. Recently, however, researchers have begun to explore whether early identification and intervention can slow down the development of schizophrenia or, perhaps, prevent it entirely.

McGlashan (1998) suggests that effective prevention must include accurate identification of those at risk for schizophrenia followed by effective intervention. The current literature strongly suggests that persons who later develop schizophrenia present with marker behaviors long before the disorder manifests itself. Adolescents who have one or more first- or second-degree relatives with schizophrenia should be assessed for declines in social, academic, and occupational functioning, particularly if they demonstrate deterioration in school performance, social withdrawal, or odd and unusual thinking or behavior. Two recent studies indicate that interventions prior to the onset of such symptoms may be able to interrupt the progression of the disease and thereby lessen its severity.

McGorry and Jackson (1999) completed a study in which subjects with prodromal symptoms were randomly assigned to a control group receiving "supportive following" or a treatment group receiving low-dose resperidone, cognitive behavioral therapy, and antianxiety or antidepressant medication (as needed). The results indicated that 36% of the control group converted to schizophrenia, while only 13% of the treatment group met diagnostic criteria. These results strongly suggest that early intervention can be beneficial to the prevention of schizophrenia.

The Recognition and Prevention (RAP) program at Hillside Hospital and Schneider's Children's Hospital in New York state is examining the impact of community-based interventions in the prevention of schizophrenia. By identifying which symptoms are most predictive for the development of schizophrenia, researchers hope to provide services strategically to those at risk (Cornblatt, Obuchowski, Schnur & O'Brien, 1998). Thus far, results indicated that prodromal symptoms of social withdrawal/isolation, decline in academic functioning, and odd behaviors or magical beliefs were the best predictors of later conversion to schizophrenia for the adolescent participants in this study. Treatment protocols were developed based on the individual patient's needs and could include medication, psychoeducation, and individual, group, and/or family therapy. Findings suggest that medication significantly reduced the likelihood of developing full-blown schizophrenia and should be considered crucial to first-line intervention for adolescents.

Some very promising research has examined the efficacy of psychosocial interventions as primary and secondary interventions. Two areas in particular—problem-solving and family relationships—have been investigated at the secondary intervention level and are now being explored as applicable as primary interventions.

Ian Falloon (2000) has proposed a training program for at-risk individuals, schizophrenic patients and their families that focuses on combining education about mental illness with the development of effective personal problem solving skills. With proficient problem-solving skills, more efficient management of life stress is possible. Looking at the development of schizophrenia from a vulnerability/stress perspective, decreased stress is associated with prevention or delay of symptom onset. Falloon suggests that training in stress management, goal setting, and identification and activation of social support networks can significantly decrease the rate of recurrence of psychotic episodes.

A second domain for prevention strategies for family relationships—specifically with respect to expressed emotion (EE). As mentioned previously, family communication patterns characterized by criticism and emotional over-involvement are associated with increased rates of relapse and rehospitalization of individuals with schizophrenia. Some researchers suggest that high EE may be included as a source of significant stress that may adversely affect vulnerable persons. Patterson, Birchwood, and Cochrane (2000) propose that identifying the early precipitants of EE in families can help in the development of more effective interventions.

What Does Not Work

Research on the prevention of early-onset schizophrenia is in its infancy. Clear evidence of any effective or ineffective prevention methods is not yet available.

Recommendations

Schizophrenia is a devastating disease. The development of symptoms in adolescence often deprives its victims of normal experiences. Fortunately, great strides have been made in the prevention and treatment of this disorder and continuing progress in these areas looks promising.

Best practice parameters should begin with identification of risk factors and accurate diagnosis. Any child with a family history of schizophrenia should be considered "at risk." Particular attention should be paid to individual behaviors such as social withdrawal, decline in academic functioning, bizarre preoccupations, academic problems, and odd beliefs or magical thinking. Clinicians should follow up with a thorough assessment of psychiatric, physical, and psychological functioning using interviews with the adolescent and the family and a review available past records (McClellan et al., 2001) noting any history of birth complications, developmental delay, mood disorder, or substance abuse.

Current research suggests that, even before criteria for schizophrenia is met, early intervention may be helpful. Although prophylactic medication is not yet recommended, psychosocial interventions show promise. Since environmental stress has been implicated in the development of schizophrenia, the adolescent's family functioning needs to be assessed. Psychoeducational interventions including stress management, communication skills training, and problem-solving may be particularly helpful.

The most effective protocol for prevention and treatment of schizophrenia in adolescents will have an individualized, multimodal approach. If psychotic symptoms are present, antipsychotic medication is recommended. The American Academy of Child and Adolescent Psychiatry (McClellan et al., 2001) suggests that first-line agents may include traditional or atypical antipsychotic medications based on the prescribing physicians recommendation. In addition to the previously mentioned psychosocial interventions, social skills training, social support services, and specialized educational programs should be accessed. Whenever possible, adolescents should receive treatment in the least restrictive settings; however, if the symptoms become severe, residential placement needs to be considered.

As research continues to refine our understanding of the precipitants and causes of schizophrenia, our interventions are likely to become more strategic and more effective. For at-risk adolescents and their families, these efforts provide hope for a brighter future.

References

Alaghband-Rad, J., McKenna, K., & Gordon, C. (1995). Childhood-onset schizophrenia: The severity of premorbid course. *Journal of the American Academy of Child and Adolescent Psychiatry, 34:* 1273–1283.

American Psychiatric Association. (2000). *Diagnostic and Statistical Manual of Mental Disorders* (4th ed., text revision). Washington, DC: Author.

Andreasen, N., Rezai, K., Alliger, R., Swayze, V., Flaum, M., Kirchener, P., Cohen, G., & O'Leary, D. (1992). Hypofrontality in neuroleptic-naive patients and in patients with chronic schizophrenia: Assessment with xenon 133 single-photon emission computed tomography and the Tower of London. *Archives of General Psychiatry, 49:* 943–958.

Asarnow, J., & Asarnow, R. (1996). Childhood-onset schizophrenia. In E. Mash & R. Barkley (Eds.), *Child Psychopathology* (pp. 340–361). New York, NY: Guilford Press.

Arsarnow, J., & Goldstein, M. (1986). Schizophrenia during adolescence and early adulthood: A developmental perspective. *Clinical Psychology Review, 6,* 211–235.

Bleuler, E. (1950). *Dementia Praecox or the Group of Schizophrenias.* (J. Zinkin, Trans.). New York: International Universities Press. (Original work published 1911).

Bogerts, B., Lieberman, J., Ashtari, M., Bilder, R., Degreet, G., & Lerner, G. (1993). Hippocampus-amygdala volumes and psychopathology in chronic schizophrenia. *Biological Psychiatry, 33,* 236–246.

Bustillo, J., Lauriello, J., Horan, W., & Keith, S. (2001). The psychosocial treatment of schizophrenia: An update. *American Journal of Psychiatry, 158(2),* 163–175.

Campbell, M., Rapoport, J., & Simpson, G. (1999). Antipsychotics in children and adolescents. *Journal of the American Academy of Child and Adolescent Psychiatry, 38,* 537–545.

Carlsson, A. (1987). The dopamine hypothesis of schizophrenia 20 years later. In H. Hafner, W. Gattaz, & W. Janzarik (Eds.), *Search for the Causes of Schizophrenia* (vol. I, pp. 223–235). Berlin: Springer-Verlag.

Cornblatt, B., Obuchowski, M., Schnur, D., & O'Brien, J. (1998). Hillside study of risk and early detection in schizophrenia. *British Journal of Psychiatry, 172,* 26–32.

Dalman, C., Allebeck, P., Cullberg, J., Grunewald, C., & Koster, M. (1999). Obstetric complications and the risk of schizophrenia. *Archives of General Psychiatry, 56:* 234–240.

Dixon, L., Lehman, A., & Levine, J. (1995). Conventional antipsychotic medications for schizophrenia. *Schizophrenia Bulletin, 21,* 567–577.

Ernst, M., Malone, R., Rowan, A., George, R., Gonzalez, N., & Silva, R. (1998). Antipsychotics (neuroleptics). In J. Werry & M. Aman (Eds.), *Practitioner's Guide to Psychoactive Drugs for Children and Adolescents* (2nd ed., pp. 297–328).

Falloon, I. (2000). Problem solving as a core strategy in the prevention of schizophrenia and other mental disorders. *The Australian and New Zealand Journal of Psychiatry, 34* (Suppl.), 185–190.

Fromm-Riechmann, F. (1948). Notes on the development of treatment of schizophrenics by psychoanalytic psychotherapy. *Psychiatry, 11,* 263–273.

Goldstein, M. (1987). The UCLA high risk project. *Schizophrenia Bulletin, 13,* 505–514.

Gottesman, I. (1991). *Schizophrenia Genesis: The Origins of Madness.* New York: W.H. Freeman.

Gur, R., & Pearlson, G. (1993). Neuroimaging in schizophrenia research. *Schizophrenia Bulletin, 19:* 337–353.

Harrison, P. (1999). The neuropathology of schizophrenia: A critical review of the data and their interpretation. *Brain, 122,* 593–624.

Hollis, C. (1995). Child and adolescent (juvenile onset) schizophrenia: A case control study of premorbid developmental impairments. *British Journal of Psychiatry, 166,* 489–495.

Howard, R., Castle, D., Wessley, S., & Murray, R. (1993). A comparative study of 470 cases of early-onset and late-onset schizophrenia. *British Journal of Psychiatry, 163,* 352–357.

Inayama, Y., Yoneda, H., Sakai, T., Ishida, T., Nonomura, Y., Kono, Y., Takahata, R., Koh, J., Sakai, J., Takai, A., Inada, Y., & Asaba, H.. (1996). Positive association between a DNA sequence variant in the serotonin 2A receptor gene and schizophrenia. *American Journal of Medical Genetics, 67,* 103–105.

Kavanaugh, D., (1992). Recent developments in expressed emotion and schizophrenia. *British Journal of Psychiatry, 160,* 601–620.

Kendler, K., McGuire, M., Gruenberg, A., Spellman, M., O'Hare, A., & Walsh, D. (1993). The Roscommon family study: II. The risk of non-schizophrenic nonaffective psychoses in relatives. *Archives of General Psychiatry, 50,* 645–652.

Kety, S. (1987). The significance of genetic factors in the etiology of schizophrenia: Results from the national study of adoptees in Denmark. *Journal of Psychiatric Research, 21,* 423–429.

Kingdon, D., Turkington, D., & John, C. (1994). Cognitive behaviour therapy of schizophrenia. *British Journal of Psychiatry, 164,* 581–587.

Larson, T., Friis, S., Haahr, U., Joa, I., Johannessen, J., Melle, I., et al. (2001). Early detection and intervention in first-episode schizophrenia: A critical review. *Acta Psychiatrica Scandinavica, 103(5),* 323–334.

Leff, J., & Vaughn, C., (1985). *Expressed Emotion in Families.* New York: Guilford Press.

Lehman, A., & Steinwachs, D. (1998). Translating research into practice: The Schizophrenia Patient Outcomes Research Team (PORT) treatment recommendations. *Schizophrenia Bulletin, 24,* 1–10.

Lewis, G., Croft-Jeffreys, C., & Anthony, D. (1990). Are British psychiatrists racist? *British Journal of Psychiatry,* *171,* 410–415.

McClellan, J., & McCurry, C. (1998). Neurocognitive pathways in the development of schizophrenia. *Seminar in Clinical Neuropsychiatry, 3,* 320–332.

McClellan, J., Werry, J., Bernet, W., Arnold, V., Beitchman, J., Benson, S., et al. (2001). Practice parameter for the assessment and treatment of children and adolescents with schizophrenia. *Journal of the American Academy of Child and Adolescent Psychiatry, 40 (Supplement 7),* 4S–23S.

McGlashan, T. (1998). Early detection and intervention of schizophrenia: Rationale and research. *British Journal of Psychiatry Supplement, 172,* 3–6.

McGorry, P., & Jackson, H. (Eds.). (1999). *The Recognition and Management of Early Psychosis: A Preventive Approach.* New York, NY: Cambridge University Press.

Meltzer, H. (1997). Treatment-resistant schizophrenia—The role of clozapine. *Current Medical Research Opinion, 14,* 1–20.

Mueser, K., Bellack, A., Wade, J., Sayers, S., Tierney, A., & Haas, G. (1993). Expressed emotion, social skill, and response to negative affect in schizophrenia. *Journal of Abnormal Psychology, 102,* 339–351.

Mueser, K., Drake, R., & Bond, G. (1997). Recent advances in psychiatric rehabilitation for patients with severe mental illness. *Harvard Review of Psychiatry, 5,* 123–137.

Pallast, E., Jongbloet, P., Straatman, H., & Zielhuis, G. (1994). Excess seasonality of births among patients with schizophrenia and seasonal ovopathy. *Schizophrenia Bulletin, 20:* 269–276.

Patterson, P., Birchwood, M., & Cochrane, R. (2000). Preventing the entrenchment of high expressed emotion in first episode psychosis: Early developmental attachment pathways. *The Australian and New Zealand Journal of Psychiatry, 34* (Suppl.), 191–197.

Remschmidt, H., Schulz, E., Martin, Warnke, A., & Trott, G. (1994). Childhood-onset schizophrenia: History of the concept and recent studies. *Schizophrenia Bulletin, 20,* 727–746.

Schaeffer, J., & Ross, R. (2002). Childhood-onset schizophrenia: Premorbid and prodromal diagnostic and treatment histories. *Journal of the American Academy of Child and Adolescent Psychiatry, 41(5),* 538–545.

Schlaepfer, T., Harris, G., Tien, A., Peng, L., Lee, S., Federman, E., Chase, G., Barta, B., & Pearlson, G. (1994). Decreased regional cortical gray matter volume in schizophrenia. *American Journal of Psychiatry, 151:* 842–848.

Scott, J., & Dixon, L. (1995). Psychological interventions for schizophrenia. *Schizophrenia Bulletin, 21,* 621–630.

Tarrier N., Barrowclough, C., Porceddu, K., & Fitzpatrick, E. (1994). The Salford Family Intervention Project: Relapse rates of schizophrenia at five and eight years. *British Journal of Psychiatry, 165:* 829–832.

U.S. Department of Health and Human Services. (1999). *Mental Health: A Report of the Surgeon General.* Rockville, MD: Author.

Ventura, J., Nuechterlein, K., Lukoff, D., & Hardesty, J. (1989). A prospective study of stressful life events and schizophrenia relapse. *Journal of Abnormal Psychology, 98,* 407–411.

Weinberger, D. (1987). Implications of normal brain development for the pathogenesis of schizophrenia. *Archives of General Psychiatry, 44,* 660–669.

World Health Organization. (1997). Psychosocial rehabilitation: A consensus statement. *International Journal of Mental Health, 26,* 77–85.

Chapter 17

Eating Disorders

Michael P. Levine and Niva Piran

Introduction

This chapter focuses on the eating disorders that draw the attention of most clinicians and researchers: anorexia nervosa, bulimia nervosa, and eating disorders not otherwise specified. For information about other, less well-known eating problems in adolescents, and about the medical and nutritional effects of eating disorders in adolescents, see Lask and Bryant-Waugh (2000) and Fisher et al. (1995).

Anorexia Nervosa

DEFINITION. *Anorexia nervosa (AN)* is characterized by fierce and obsessive maintenance of an unduly low body weight or by a defiant refusal to achieve weight gains expected on the basis of height, age, and maturational status. Extreme weight management strategies include rigid forms of self-starvation, selective avoidance of many foods that are fattening or viewed as fattening, excessive exercising, and, in some instances, self-induced vomiting. These efforts are fueled by an over-valuation of shape, weight, and restrictive self-control as the principal determinants of self-worth (Fairburn & Harrison, 2003). The classic form of this disorder is called "restricting AN." The other recognized subtype combines AN with episodes of binge-eating and/or purging. These features predict more negative long-term outcomes (Steinhausen, 2003).

In western cultures, a phobic fear of fat is fundamental to the psychopathology of AN, but this is not the case universally. Many adolescents suffering from AN tend to have a "distorted body image" (e.g., overestimate their physical size), "deny" they are ill (i.e., stubbornly resist treatment), and are resistant to change, especially to weight gain (Fairburn & Harrison, 2003).

MALES WITH ANOREXIA NERVOSA. Muise, Stein, and Arbess (2003) report several significant differences. Adolescent girls often show bradycardia as part of a systemic response to starvation, but adolescent boys with AN are more likely to have an elevated heart rate and life-threatening cardiac complications. They are also more likely to be athletes obsessed with obtaining a masculine shape characterized by leanness and a narrow waist. Girls with AN are much more likely to have a high drive for thinness and a goal weight expressed precisely in pounds.

MORBIDITY, MORTALITY, AND PROGNOSIS.   Anorexia nervosa typically develops in early to mid-adolescence. It is a serious disorder that compromises physical, psychological, and interpersonal maturation. Preceding or following the development of AN, many adolescents are depressed, socially anxious, and/or obsessive. The course tends to be protracted and complicated. The outcome is favorable in only a third to two-thirds of juvenile-onset patients who are assessed 4 to 12 years later (Strober, Freeman & Morrell, 1997); and, for approximately 20%, AN will become a chronic, debilitating condition. Some adolescents with AN will eventually come to deal with hunger, eating, weight, and shape by developing *bulimia nervosa*, while the reverse is much less common. The presence of obsessive-compulsive personality symptoms is another predictor of less favorable prognosis (Steinhausen, 2003).

Anorexia nervosa is also a potentially deadly disorder. Nielsen et al. (1998) reviewed long-term follow-up studies of 829 patients who presented with AN before age 20. At a mean follow-up length of 12 years, 4.5% had died, i.e., 3.6 times the expected rate, adjusted for age and gender. The risk of death was greatest in the first year (a phenomenon that is especially true for males), but treatment appears to reduce the standardized mortality rate.

Nielsen et al.'s review strongly supports the need for immediate and vigorous treatment. Strober et al. (1997) found that, 12 years after adolescent patients with AN had received intensive, multimodal therapy, 75% had achieved full recovery in terms of weight restoration, hormonal functioning, and absence of pathological attitudes and behaviors. This figure is better than the expected favorable outcome for adults (Steinhausen, 2003), but it is consistent with a 70% recovery rate reported from five sites in Europe (Steinhausen, Boyadjieva, Griogoroiu–Serbanescu & Neumärker 2003). The need for support and patience, in addition to intensive and expert treatment, is seen in Strober et al.'s findings that 1 in 5 patients relapsed in the first year, and that the median time to full recovery was approximately 7 years.

EPIDEMIOLOGY AND COURSE.   A review by Hoek and van Hoeken (2003) indicates that the point prevalence of AN in the United States, the United Kingdom, and Europe is around 0.5% (1 in 200) in adolescent girls. The ratio of females to males with AN is, conservatively, 10:1. The rise in incidence of AN since the 1930s has disproportionately affected girls and women aged 15–24. Research reviewed by Hoek and van Hoeken (2003) estimates that in the 1980s the incidence for that gender and age cohort was 74 per 100,000. There also appears to be an upward trend in the incidence of AN for adolescent girls ages 10 through 14. Social class is no longer a major marker or predictor of risk for eating disorders. At any given time, about two-thirds of AN patients in the community are not receiving any mental health care.

Bulimia Nervosa

DEFINITION.   Bulimia nervosa (BN) is characterized by overvaluation of shape and weight and by cycles of binge-eating and purging. Binges are distinct, recurrent, out-of-control episodes of eating, during which the person consumes very large quantities (typically 1,000–2,000 kcal) of high-caloric food that she typically denies herself at other times. Purging includes use and abuse of self-induced vomiting, laxatives and diuretics, enemas, exercise, and brief periods of anorexic-like dietary restriction. Purging is an attempt to compensate for the aversive loss of control, the dissociative self-indulgence, and the anticipated weight gain from binge-eating,

The modal age of onset of BN is late adolescence or early adulthood. The body weight of adolescents with BN ranges from under- to overweight. While the binge-purge cycle is secretive and associated with the experience of shame, the experience of distress and the adverse impact of BN on health, relationships, and adjustment may motivate some adolescents with BN to seek help. A subgroup of adolescents with BN engages in substance abuse and self-injury. Research suggests that patterns of self-harm are more common in women with BN who have a history of trauma (Dansky, Brewerton, & Kilpatrick, 2000). Co-morbid substance abuse and self-injury are associated with poorer outcome.

MALES WITH BN.   Adolescent boys who develop BN tend to have a history of obesity or overweight (see Muise et al., 2003). There is often a long delay between onset of the BN and the seeking of treatment, because boys and young men may be ashamed of having a "female disorder" and because they are less troubled by binge-eating. In addition, boys are less invested in strict weight control toward a specific goal weight, so they are less likely to use extreme weight-loss techniques. These gender differences make it much more difficult to diagnose eating disorders in adolescent boys unless there is very salient weight loss (Ricciardelli & McCabe, 2004).

EPIDEMIOLOGY AND PROGNOSIS.   The prevalence of strictly defined BN in community samples of females ages 12 through 25 is approximately 1%. The incidence for adolescence is unknown. In the only two studies in which such data were available, the incidence for women aged 20–24 is about 82 per 100,000, while the incidence for males in general was less than 1 per 100,000 (Hoek & van Hoeken, 2003).

Bulimia nervosa, like AN, is often a chronic and debilitating condition. Several reviews have failed to identify any consistent predictors of good or poor outcome in BN (Gowers & Bryant-Waugh, 2004), but it appears that early detection of bulimia nervosa is associated with better outcomes following treatment (Keel, Mitchell, Miller, Davis & Crow, 1999).

Eating Disorders Not Otherwise Specified

The largest group of children and adolescents suffering from eating disorders have what the *Diagnostic and Statistical Manual of Mental Disorders* (4th ed., text revision; American Psychiatric Association, 2000) calls "Eating Disorder Not Otherwise Specified" or EDNOS (Gowers & Bryant-Waugh, 2004). In EDNOS there are significant problems with body image, eating, and weight management, but they do not meet all of the criteria for AN or BN. These "subclinical" or "subthreshold" forms of eating disorder are no less serious than the full-blown disorders.

One type of EDNOS that has recently received a lot of attention is binge-eating disorders (BED). People with BED have episodes of uncontrollable binge-eating that leave them feeling uncomfortably full, as well as ashamed, guilty, and depressed. However, they do not regularly compensate by purging, dieting, or abusing exercise. Very little is known about BED in adolescents, since those who present clinically with this disorder tend to be overweight or obese adults.

THE SPECTRUM OF EATING DISORDERS.   EDNOS puts one at risk for later development of AN or BN. This movement between categories (e.g., from AN to BN, from EDNOS to AN, and from BN to EDNOS), in combination with the high prevalence of body dissatisfaction, dieting, and binge-eating among adolescents, points to a "partial spectrum" of disordered eating and pathogenic weight-control attitudes and behaviors. This spectrum weaves together the strands of multiple continua (Levine, Piran & Irving, 2003). These "continua," which can be combined in many ways, are (1) internalization of the slender beauty ideal as a fundamental components of self-concept; (2) negative body image; (3) binge-eating; (4) restrictive dieting; (5) unhealthy forms of weight management such self-induced vomiting after eating, or abuse diet pills and exercise; and (6) negative emotions such as self-loathing, shame, social anxiety, and depression. Even the combination of body dissatisfaction and calorie-restrictive dieting is far from harmless. There is evidence that these phenomena predict increases over time in body weight, bulimic symptoms, and depressive symptoms (Field et al., 2003; Stice & Bearman, 2001). Less severe combinations along the eating disorders (ED) spectrum are also associated with poor nutrition, restricted physical and social activity, and abuse of tobacco, alcohol, and other drugs (Muise et al., 2003).

We qualify the spectrum as "partial" because the end-points—i.e., the severe syndromes of AN, BN, and BED—appear to be distinct from weight preoccupation or chronic dieting. The clinical syndromes, and especially the severe and potentially chronic cases, are intertwined with significant psychopathology (e.g., obsessive-compulsive disorder, post-traumatic stress disorder) and profound disturbances in personality.

EPIDEMIOLOGY AND COURSE.   Episodes of binge-eating are common among adolescent males and females, but at present, the prevalence of BED among adolescents is unknown. The prevalence of subclinical problems along the ED spectrum is, conservatively, 8% for adolescent girls and young women (Hoek & van Hoeken, 2003), and somewhere in the vicinity of 2–5% of adolescent boys (Ricciardelli & McCabe, 2004). Certainly, the female-to-male ratio is much less for EDNOS than it is for full-blown eating disorders (Muise et al., 2003).

MALES WITH DISORDERED EATING.   The prevalence of subclinical problems among adolescent males is a topic in need of further research and clarification. A subset of overweight adolescent boys is, at least occasionally, trying to lose weight by dieting and purging. These boys have low self-esteem and other features of depression, and they are prone to abuse of alcohol and other drugs (Muise et al., 2003). Future research on adolescent males and the ED spectrum will need to acknowledge that approximately 2–4% of boys suffer from significant anxiety about being too fat *and* not muscular enough. This form of negative body image increases the risk for steroid use and for a form of body dysmorphic disorder called muscle dysmorphia (Pope, Phillips & Olivardia, 2000; Ricciardelli & McCabe, 2004).

Individual Factors

According to Helena Kraemer (see Jacobi, Hayward, De Zwaan, Kraemer & Agras, 2004; Stice, 2002), "risk factor" clearly precedes, and has a potent statistical association with, the outcome of interest (e.g., bulimia nervosa or bulimic symptoms). A "causal risk factor" can be manipulated systematically in either direction so as to increase or decreases the outcome accordingly. Thus, longitudinal designs and prevention outcome research are both integral to establishing causal risk factors. Since causality does imply correlation, cross-sectional studies (e.g., retrospective case-controlled design) are a necessary, but ultimately ambiguous, first step.

At present the independent causal risk factors identified have a small-to-moderate effect size, and there is as yet an insufficient number of tests of multifactorial models.

A girl's perception of "social" pressures to be thin fosters internalization of the slender beauty ideal so prominent in the mass media. Social pressures also contribute to over-valuation of appearance and thinness as components of self-concept. There is substantial evidence that, for adolescent girls, perceived social pressure and internalization of the thin ideal are causal risk factors for increases over time in body dissatisfaction, unhealthy forms of dieting, negative emotions, binge-eating, and bulimic-type symptoms in the ED spectrum (Stice, 2002). The path linking these two factors to the spectrum of bulimic problems and, perhaps, to eating disorders in general is probably mediated by higher levels of two synergistic variables: body dissatisfaction and negative affect. Body dissatisfaction is one of the strongest predictors of subsequent eating pathology (Stice, 2002). Negative affect refers to "neurotic" moods and emotional states such as depression, anxiety, irritability, tension, etc. (Jacobi et al., 2004; Stice, 2002). Jacobi et al. (2004) highlight the role of "weight concerns" in predicting the development of the ED spectrum. The weight concerns syndrome includes body dissatisfaction, anxiety about fat and weight gain, drive for thinness, and dieting behavior.

While dieting is considered by many experts to comprise a risk factor for eating disorders, Stice (2002) does not consider dieting a *causal* risk factor because experiments assigning obese and non-obese adults to long-term low-calorie diets have resulted in reduced negative affect and/or decreased binge-eating. Although girls who have a greater body mass index (BMI = weight in kg/[height in m]^2) receive and perceive more social pressure to be thin, the prospective correlation between BMI and both body dissatisfaction and dieting behavior is small, and BMI consistently fails to predict later eating disorders (Jacobi et al., 2004). Similarly, although early pubertal development in girls is associated with increased adiposity, pubertal timing is not a risk factor for body dissatisfaction and eating pathology (Stice, 2002). However, early puberty in the context of other concurrent stressors (e.g., dating and beginning middle school) has a cumulative effect that increases the risk of eating disorders (Smolak & Levine, 1996).

Jacobi et al.'s (2004) review also *suggests* that early or concurrent presence of one or more of the following factors sets the stage for AN or BN: early childhood feeding problems (and the concomitant disruptions in parent-child interactions), sexual abuse, negative self-concept, generalized anxiety (overanxious) disorder, and low levels of interoceptive awareness (i.e., difficulties in interpreting and expressing internal stimuli such as hunger, anxiety, and anger). The correlates, risk factors, and causal risk factors for AN and BN reveal a great deal of overlap, although obsessive-compulsive symptoms or personality characteristics favor the development of AN, while social phobia favors the development of BN.

Risk Factors in Males

There are also some clear similarities between adolescent girls and adolescent boys in correlates and risk factors for the ED spectrum. In boys higher BMIs and increased perception of pressure from parents and peers to lose weight appear to be significant but not very potent risk factors. As is the case for females, adolescent and young adult males are at greater risk for the ED spectrum if they participate in competitive, high-level varsity sports that have weight restrictions (e.g., wrestling) or that emphasize body aesthetics (e.g., gymnastics and diving; Hausenblas & Carron, 1999). With respect to gender differences, the few available longitudinal studies indicate that several well-established risk factors in females (e.g., subjective pressure from mass media, body dissatisfaction and negative affect) are not risk factors for males.

THE DRIVE FOR MUSCULARITY.   "Body dissatisfaction" and "negative body image" appear to have a different meaning for adolescent boys than for adolescent girls. A majority of adolescent boys report being dissatisfied with their weight and shape, but, relative to females, males are much less likely to see thinness, weight, and control of hunger as key components of self-concept. Further, many boys and young men want to be heavier, larger, and more muscular without being fat. Pope et al. (2000) have documented the rise over the past 30 years of a masculine body ideal characterized by leanness and muscularity. Examples in the mass media are numerous, and include professional wrestler "The Rock" and a "buffed" Brad Pitt acting as Achilles in the movie *Troy*. This ideal proclaims (embodies) a number of highly valued masculine characteristics: strength and forcefulness, physical fitness, athletic prowess, and the potential to dominate, or at least not be controlled by, others.

The prevalence of adolescent boys who are dissatisfied with the salient discrepancy between their body shape and this ideal, and who are using various strategies to increase weight and muscle is somewhere between 20% and 50% (Ricciardelli & McCabe, 2004). A subset of these boys, such as those who are insecure, perfectionist, and/or involved in power sports, will be highly motivated to lose fat and build muscle mass by selective avoidance of certain foods, by working out excessively, and by (ab)using illegal anabolic steroids and legal nutritional supplements (Irving, Wall, Neumark-Sztainer & Story, 2002; Pope et al., 2000). Much more research is needed to support this sociocultural theory of the drive for muscularity in males and to understand the health implications of this motive. Nevertheless, its potential applicability to prevention and males is seen in a recent large-scale, well-designed, and very successful trial of the *Adolescents Training and Learning to Avoid Steroids* (ATLAS) program for male high school football players (Goldberg et al., 2000).

Race and Ethnicity

FEMALES.   This section draws on several excellent reviews of literature on body image and eating disorders in ethnicity minority groups in the United States (Dounchis, Hayden & Wilfley, 2001; Smolak & Striegel-Moore, 2001). No minority group status confers immunity to eating disorders, and across ethnic groups poor body image is the strongest correlate of dieting, binge-eating, and purging.

Anorexia nervosa is very rare among ethnic minorities, while the prevalence of BN is fairly equivalent across minority groups. Native American females and males report comparatively high rates of eating disordered behavior, including attempts to control weight by smoking cigarettes, taking diet pills, and vomiting (Croll, Neumark-Sztainer, Story & Ireland, 2002). Asian girls, as well as black girls, in the United States appear to have lower rates of eating disorders than whites, whereas Latina females have equivalent rates.

We illustrate the complexity of these comparisons by briefly examining the black–white difference. Compared to whites, blacks in the United States have lower rates of BN, lower levels of body dissatisfaction, and fewer weight concerns. Black girls are significantly more likely than white girls to want to gain weight in order to be (more) curvaceous. In fact, compared to whites, the African American community is more likely to choose a heavier, more rounded body as the ideal and to be more tolerant and flexible in defining ideal shapes. This evidence of a healthy resistance to weight control pressures has to be balanced against studies showing that black women and girls tend to be heavier (in part because they have an earlier onset of puberty), to have equivalent or greater rates of binge-eating and, perhaps, as a result, to have higher rates of obesity, fasting, and use of diuretics.

MALES.   The relationship between ethnicity and the ED spectrum in males is also poorly understood. Some evidence (e.g., Siegel, Yancey, Aneshensel & Schuler, 1999) indicates that African American boys are more satisfied with their bodies than white boys or other minority boys. Croll et al. (2002) found that, among 9th- and 12th-grade males, fewer black and white males reported at least one type of disordered eating in the past year, as compared with much higher rates in Asian, Hispanic, and Native American males. For all males the presence of disordered eating in the past year was associated with increased appearance concerns and the frequency of smoking cigarettes, and for all the groups except Native American males, disordered eating was also associated with increased use and abuse of alcohol.

Family Factors

Genetics

FAMILY AGGREGATION STUDIES.   Jacobi et al. (2004) reviewed studies based on clinical interviews of family members of individuals with an eating disorder and of community or psychiatric control groups. These studies indicated an aggregation in families of AN, BN, and EDNOS, as well as mood disorder, panic disorder, generalized anxiety disorder, and obsessive-compulsive disorder (OCD). Relatives of people with BN also have an elevated rate of substance abuse, social phobia, PTSD, and borderline personality disorder, although transmission of substance abuse and major depression are independent of an eating disorder. The relatives of patients with AN also have an increased prevalence of OCD and obsessive-compulsive personality disorder (OCPD), and there is a shared path of transmission between AN and OCPD.

TWIN STUDIES. The methodology and outcomes of twin research has been described in detail elsewhere (see, e.g., Bulik, 2004). To summarize, data from the relatively few existing studies suggest that somewhere between 40% and 80% of the variability in liability for AN and BN is attributable heritability, i.e., to cumulative genetic effects. The remainder of the variability in AN appears to be due to non-shared experiences (e.g., one twin, but not the other, has a traumatic experience or participates in gymnastics). With regard to BN, the remainder of the variability is accounted for primarily by non-shared experiences, although a small contribution of shared environment (e.g., social class or family rules) cannot be ruled out (Bulik, 2004). Together, the family aggregation and twin studies clearly indicate that girls who grow up in families where father, mother, or sister has an eating disorder constitute an at-risk population in terms of genetics and environments. Targeted prevention efforts may select this group for intervention.

Family Structure and Dynamics

Many prospective studies have found that general measures of family environment and family dynamics do not predict increases in disordered eating (Jacobi et al., 2004; Stice, 2002). On the other hand, several types of data indicate that teasing, direct critical comments, and weight loss advice from parents and family members contribute to negative body image and unhealthy weight management practices (Stice, 2002; Thompson, Heinberg, Altabe, & Tantleff–Dunn, 1999). Surprisingly, parents' attitudes and behaviors in regard to their own body image are probably not a potent or consistent source of influence on a son or daughter's body image or dieting. However, parental modeling (and peer modeling) of negative body and eating pathology does increase the risk of more pathological binge-eating and other bulimic symptomatology.

Social and Community Factors

To date most social research has focused on pressures for thinness. The impact of exposure to weight-related prejudice and teasing has also been explored (Thompson et al., 1999), but the impact of other discriminatory treatment has not been studied as extensively. Striegel-Moore, Dohm, Pike, Wilfley, and Fairburn (2002), found in a community study that *white* women with BED reported ethnically based discriminatory experiences more commonly than control women. Piran and Thompson (2004) found that exposure to both sexism and weight-related prejudice was related to ED symptoms in university and community samples of young women. These studies are in line with the findings of other qualitative studies that have reported an association between discriminatory experiences, negative body image, and disordered eating patterns (see, e.g., Piran, 2001b).

Examination of the impact of sexual and physical violations has comprised another line of investigation (Smolak & Murnen, 2002, 2004). A meta-analysis by Smolak and Murnen (2002) indicates that sexual abuse and physical abuse are non-specific risk factors for psychiatric symptomatology, including eating disorders broadly defined. The recent study by Striegel–Moore et al. (2002) reported a similar pattern of findings in their sample of White women with BED, although in a sample of black women there seemed to be a *specific* association between sexual abuse and BED. The study of violations and eating disorders has been extended to sexual harassment. For example, in a series of investigations Harned (2000) found that sexual harassment was significantly associated with disordered eating (see also Piran & Thompson, 2004). In further research Harned and Fitzgerald (2002) found a link between sexual harassment in the workplace and eating disorder symptoms that was mediated by psychological distress (negative affect).

A different line of inquiry has examined the relationships between the ED spectrum and various internalized constructs that are shaped by dominant social expectations in regard to the female gender. For example, Fredrickson and Roberts (1997) have developed scales of self-objectification to examine a girl's internalization of the masculine tendency to look at, talk about, and otherwise treat women and their bodies as sexual objects. Higher levels of self-objectification have consistently been found to be associated with negative body image, negative self-image, and disordered eating patterns (see review by Smolak & Murnen, 2004). In addition, several studies (e.g., Zaitsoff, Geller & Srikameswaran, 2002) have found a correlation between eating disordered beliefs and behaviors and the internalization by adolescent girls and women of the cultural expectation that they should silence their own needs in order to maintain close relationships.

Based on a qualitative study with adolescent school girls, Piran proposed and later tested, using structural equation modeling, a three-pathway model of social experiences related to development of eating disorders (Piran, 2001a; Piran & Cormier, 2004; Piran & Thompson, 2004). The pathways are the spectrum of violations of body ownership, exposure to discriminatory practices, and the social construction of women. This model integrates the lines of inquiry described above and offers a way to conceptualize the complexity of the social experiences related to eating symptomatology. The model's implications for prevention are discussed below under the new rubric of Critical Social Perspectives.

Resilience

Very little is known about the factors that provide resilience in the face of specific pressures that increase the risk of eating disorders (Shisslak & Crago, 2001). Much of the theorizing focuses on creating conditions that are the opposite of risk factors. Examples are (1) arranging for adult mentors (role models) or peer support groups that encourage girls to develop identities in which weight, shape, and body control are not the principal focus and (2) helping girls develop life skills that yield a sense of mastery and competence (vs. passivity and hopelessness) in meeting the many challenges of adolescence. Some sports (e.g., high school soccer) emphasize strength, skill, and stamina rather than weight and thinness, and participation in these sports seems to reduce the risk of eating disorders (Smolak, Murnen & Ruble, 2000).

In a cross-sectional study of over 80,000 adolescents, Croll et al. (2002) used logistic regression analysis to determine factors that reduced the odds that girls and boys had engaged in disordered eating and weight-management (e.g., self-induced vomiting or smoking cigarettes to manage weight) in the past 12 months. Without regard to ethnicity, four variables emerged as protective factors for both males and females: self-esteem, emotional well-being, higher GPA, and greater sense of connectedness to family. A fifth variable—greater sense of connectedness to school—also emerged as a protective factor for males. However, there were significant differences in protective factors across the minority groups and as a function of gender. For example, emotional well-being was a protective factor for Hispanic, black, and Asian girls, but not for Native American girls, while self-esteem was a protective factor for Hispanic and Asian girls only. Family connectedness was a protective factor for Native American girls but not for the other minorities. Among the boys, Native Americans were the only distinct minority in that there was but one protective factor: emotional well-being.

Eating disorders are the culmination of pathways that interweave risk factors specific to those disorders (e.g., body dissatisfaction and weight concerns) and risk factors implicated in the development of many disorders (e.g., negative affect). To analyze generic risk and protective factors, Durlak (1997) reviewed nearly 1,200 outcome evaluations of prevention and health. Across all eight major behavioral and health outcomes, five broad categories of variables emerged as consistent protective factors: (1) healthy social norms within the community (e.g., about cigarette smoking); (2) effective social policies (e.g., enforcement of laws governing non-sale of tobacco to minors); (3) good parent/child relationships; (4) personal and social competence; and (5) direct social support for children or for significant adults in children's lives. Other variables associated with positive outcomes in the behavioral realms (e.g., avoidance of drug use) were high-quality schools and positive peer models. Durlak's (1997) review and Croll et al.'s (2002) research strongly suggest that resilient children and adolescents have positive values and skills in several interlocking realms. These prosocial skills and interests are fostered by secure attachments within the family or with at least one person within the extended family or community.

Evidence-Based Treatment Interventions in Community Settings

What Works

Family therapy is the most studied and established form of treatment of adolescents with AN, with more limited data available to support its use in BN. Family therapy has been found quite consistently to result in positive outcome with adolescents with AN. There are three principal approaches to effective community-based family therapy: family therapy with a single family, multifamily family therapy, and parent counseling.

FAMILY THERAPY WITH A SINGLE FAMILY.   Effective family therapy for adolescents with AN, exemplified by the work of Dare and Szmukler (1991), mobilizes the family as a resource to help the anorexic adolescent. The family first works with the therapist to identify strategies for re-feeding. As the family learns and enforces these strategies, the therapist works with the parents to ensure consistent application. When eating patterns improve and weight restoration is in progress, therapy starts to address the common developmental challenges of adolescence. The last phase examines in synchrony the functioning of the parents as a couple and the individuation of the adolescent. This approach to therapy has been evaluated in several studies, starting with Russell, Szmukler, Dare, and Eisler's (1987) evaluation of 80 individuals with AN. These investigators found that adolescents under 18 assigned to family therapy had better outcomes and were less likely to drop out compared with the adolescents receiving individual therapy (see also Robin, Siegel, Koepke, Moye & Tice, 1994).

MULTIFAMILY THERAPY.   Multifamily therapy is typically applied as part of intensive management programs, often in partial hospitalization program (Dare & Eisler, 2000). This form of therapy engages up to six families simultaneously in day-long activities for at least one week, with continued intensive sessions for the following few months. As is the case for the single-family approach (Dare & Szmukler, 1991), the goals of the program are to support the parents' authority and skills in consistently managing the eating behavior of their adolescent, and later to address relational and structural issues in families, as well as examine the challenge of relapse prevention. In multifamily therapy, parents feel less marginalized and they can educate and support one another. Therapy unfolds in different formats, such as parent groups, adolescent groups, and letting parents supervise a teenager from another family. These different forums, combined with multiple experiential tasks and educational sessions, can create constructive shifts in the families' abilities to manage eating behavior, and also in addressing structural, relational and emotional issues in families. The multifamily approach to treatment has been found to be effective as an aspect of a group day-treatment program (Dare & Eisler, 2000).

PARENT COUNSELING.   In another approach to treatment, the parents are seen together without their child, but are given suggestions about helping their child with the eating problems, while the child is concurrently involved in individual therapy. Two research teams (Le Grange, Eisler, Dare & Russell, 1992; Robin et al., 1994) found in randomized controlled studies that the outcome of combined individual therapy and parent counseling is comparable to the outcome of family therapy. This suggests that conducting therapy with the entire family is not necessary. Indeed, family counseling may be preferable to family therapy when there is a high level of parental criticality, or when the family is chaotic or dealing with abuse issues.

PLANFUL MULTIMODAL/MULTIDISCIPLINARY INTERVENTIONS.   Treatment practices with adolescents who display the ED spectrum have also been guided by accumulated clinical wisdom. This is expressed in experience-based position papers put forward by different professional associations, and to a lesser degree by the limited outcome evaluation research (Robin et al., 1994). Various position papers show a general agreement about key aspects of treatment (Gowers & Bryant-Waugh, 2004). These include guidelines for assessment, for a multidisciplinary approach to treatment, and for individual and family therapy.

ASSESSMENT OF EATING DISORDERS.   Research has shown the importance of early diagnosis in adolescents. Yet, establishing a clinical diagnosis of an eating disorder in adolescence, and especially in early adolescence, is challenging. One obstacle is the limited applicability of adult clinical diagnostic criteria to children or younger adolescents (Lask & Bryant-Waugh, 2000). The criterion of weighing less than 85% of the expected weight can be difficult to assess with young adolescents. They may not present with weight loss and their expected weight may be difficult to determine. Similarly, for girls the menstruation criterion can be difficult to assess because of the irregularity, or absence, of menses in early adolescence. Further, the thinness schema, which involves a cluster of attitudinal factors that devalue fat and idealize thinness, is less consistent in children and early adolescents (Smolak & Levine, 1996), and therefore harder to assess. In addition, the frequency of both purging and binging tends to be lower in younger adolescents than in adults and therefore may not reach severity criteria.

All this emphasizes a point made earlier: Adolescents, and especially young adolescents, are much more likely to be diagnosed with EDNOS. Since it appears that eating disorder symptomatology is associated with more severe health consequences in children and younger adolescents, such as growth retardation and lower bone density, it is important to consider an eating disorder diagnosis and treatment whenever there is engagement in unhealthy weight control practices and severe preoccupation with body weight and shape.

In addition to establishing an eating disorder diagnosis, the assessment of eating disorders involves a comprehensive evaluation of medical, nutritional, psychological, and familial or other contextual factors (Katzman, 1999). All these factors are important in designing an individualized treatment plan, so it is advisable either that the evaluations are done concurrently by a multidisciplinary team, or that a health or mental health professional coordinates timely assessment by the different professionals (Michel & Willard, 2003). One important decision in a comprehensive assessment is whether the eating disorder can be managed on an outpatient basis or whether it requires partial or inpatient hospitalization.

A MULTIDISCIPLINARY APPROACH TO TREATMENT.   Kreipe et al. (1995), in a position paper of the Society for Adolescent Medicine, state that adolescents with eating disorders require management by an interdisciplinary team comprising physicians, nurses, dieticians, and mental health professionals. The multidisciplinary approach is practiced in most therapy centers specializing in the treatment of eating disorders in general, and in children and adolescents in particular (Lask & Bryant-Waugh, 2000).

MEDICAL MANAGEMENT.   Once a thorough physical examination, including a laboratory workup, has been conducted, frequency of medical follow-up will be determined by severity of the eating disorder and the individual's physical status. Thorough medical assessment helps determine the target weight. It also aids in deciding, based on weight and various health criteria, whether the treatment is effective, or, alternatively, whether an intensification of treatment or hospitalization is required in cases of medical destabilization.

NUTRITIONAL MANAGEMENT.   A nutritionist, who preferably is a registered dietitian, can work with the adolescent and the treatment team to help the individual in the challenging task of changing disordered eating patterns and adopting healthy and flexible approaches to eating. This usually requires re-education in the area of nutritional needs during adolescence, with a focus on food portions and food groups, costs of nutritional deprivation during adolescence, healthy eating and weight ranges, distorted ideas about food and body shape, and learning to listen over time to cues of hunger and satiety and to patterns of emotional eating, if relevant. The dietitian can also help evaluate the treatment progress of the individual.

FAMILY AND INDIVIDUAL THERAPY.   As described earlier in this chapter, family therapy has been successfully applied in three different formats: single family therapy, multifamily therapy, and parent counseling. Family therapy is synchronized with individual therapy as part of a collaborative, multidisciplinary team approach.

What Might Work

DYNAMIC SELF-PSYCHOLOGY.   Individual therapy has long been considered an essential component in community-based treatment of eating disorders. Although different therapeutic approaches for adults have been studied, there has been a paucity of research with adolescents (Robin, Gilroy & Dennis, 1998). One type of therapy recommended for adolescents is a dynamic approach that focuses on issues of identity, autonomy, accessing and processing emotional experiences, and addressing relational and developmental tasks, while emphasizing adolescents' strengths and coping skills. This approach, combined with parent counseling, was found at one-year follow-up to produce a favorable outcome comparable to the effects of family therapy, though weight gain was slower (Robin et al., 1994).

CBT AND IPT.   Cognitive-behavior therapy (CBT) for treatment of AN has not been systematically studied in adolescents. Cognitive-behavior therapy would likely focus on behavioral strategies such as meal plans and daily eating journals, and on countering distorted beliefs about the self, eating, and weight. Behavioral strategies have been often used with younger adolescents, but it is questionable whether younger adolescents have the level of abstract reasoning required for the cognitive restructuring employed in CBT.

There are also very limited data for deciding whether or not to use CBT in treating adolescents with BN, even though the approach has repeatedly been shown to be the most effective treatment for mixed samples of adults and older adolescents (Fairburn & Harrison, 2003). Similarly, to date, there is no outcome evaluation of the adolescent version of interpersonal psychotherapy (IPT). This treatment focuses on particular problem areas in the adolescent's interpersonal relationships. IPT has been found to effective in the treatment of BN with mixed samples of older adolescents and adults (Fairburn et al., 1995).

What Does Not Work

A non-monitored, one-dimensional approach to treatment is not recommended. The importance of employing a multidisciplinary approach to treatment has been emphasized. Research to date does not justify providing individual treatment for adolescents without involving the parents in treatment through family therapy or parent counseling (Robin et al., 1994). It is also a mistake not to involve medical and nutrition specialists while engaging the adolescent and the family in therapy, because these experts provide necessary care, psychoeducation, and ongoing assessment of outcome. Even subclinical levels of eating disorders can sometimes result in irreversible developmental damage in areas such as growth, fertility, or bone health, so close monitoring of treatment outcome is essential when treating adolescents (Katzman, 1999). Time-sensitive processes of development require a prompt intensification of treatment if no progress is achieved in treatment.

Evidence-Based Treatment Interventions in Residential Settings

What Works

Inpatient hospitalization is needed in the treatment of adolescents with eating disorders in situations of severe medical or psychiatric destabilization (Katzman, 1999). Inpatient programs are generally successful in leading to weight gain in anorexic patients or in arresting a bulimic pattern during the hospital stay (Dare & Eisler, 2000). Most inpatient programs employ a behavioral program with greater privileges accorded to patients as they meet weight and eating behavior goals. In an inpatient setting, where adolescents are very ill, it is even more important that a multidisciplinary team be involved in addressing medical, nutritional, psychological, and familial goals.

The post-discharge outcome of inpatient hospitalization is more questionable. As noted early in this chapter, studies of longer-term follow-up have found continued significant difficulties in approximately 50% of patients. Also, there have been no controlled outcome studies that have examined the impact on adolescents of particular components of inpatient treatment or ongoing outpatient care.

What Might Work

DAY HOSPITALIZATION. Day hospitalization programs have been designed to address the needs of those individuals with severe forms of eating disorders who require intensive treatment but are not under immediate medical or psychiatric destabliziation (Dare & Eisler, 2000; Piran, 1990; Robin et al., 1998). Given the managed care system in the United States, most individuals requiring intensive treatment will probably be treated using a partial hospitalization model. The potential clinical advantage of this model is its reliance on enhancing the skills and coping strategies of the patients and their families in achieving therapeutic goals, an approach that helps maintain gains following discharge (Dare & Eisler, 2000; Piran, 1990).

Day hospitalization programs for adolescents use a multidisciplinary approach involving medical, nutritional, individual and/or group psychotherapy, and family therapy, including multifamily group therapy (Dare & Eisler, 2000; Faith, Pinhas, Schmelefske & Bryden, 2003). However, in adolescent day hospital settings in particular, intensive work is conducted with parents, equipping them with strategies of managing their adolescent's eating behavior at home. Danziger, Carcl, Varsano, Tyano, and Mimouni (1988) involved parents in supervising their teenager's eating behavior during their daily attendance in the day hospital program. Follow-up assessment revealed maintenance of gains in 84% of the adolescents.

What Does Not Work

It is understandable that inpatient hospitalization may provide, at least temporarily, great relief for family and other individuals who are concerned about an adolescent with a severe eating disorder. However, those inpatient hospitalization programs that do not equip the adolescent and the family with strategies to maintain healthy weight and eating patterns upon discharge will probably not lead to the desired long-term gains (Dare & Eisler, 2000). Another challenging issue in intensive treatment settings for adolescents involves situations requiring an intensification of care that is not desired by a frightened or defiant adolescent and, sometimes, her family. These situations run the risk of disrupting the therapeutic alliance and of being experienced as punitive. It is a very positive sign that approaches to care and decision-making processes are being devised to address these treatment situations with adolescents while maintaining a relational model of high quality care (Faith et al., 2003; Manley, Smye & Srikameswaran, 2001).

Psychopharmacology

There are very few methodologically sound studies of pharmacotherapy in children and adolescents. Nevertheless, experts believe that very cautious use of medication has a place in a multidimensional, comprehensive treatment package for adolescents with eating disorders (Gowers & Bryant–Waugh, 2004; Roerig, Mitchell, Myers & Glass, 2002). Pharmacodynamics and pharmacokinetics are different in children and adolescents, who generally require *higher* doses of drug per kg of body weight in order to attain therapeutic blood levels. This is because at younger ages the kidneys and liver work more efficiently.

Anorexia Nervosa

Two placebo-controlled studies by Kaye and colleagues have shown that the SSRI fluoxetine (Prozac) can help prevent relapse in *adults* with AN who have been discharged from inpatient treatment after sufficient weight gain (de Zwaan, Roerig & Mitchell, 2004). But there is as yet no justification for use of antidepressants in treating adolescents with primary anorexia nervosa (Roerig et al., 2002). Adolescents and adults with AN, and thus with very low weight, have low levels of the serotonin precursor trytophan, so they probably cannot generate an adequate response to treatment with fluoxetine or other SSRIs (de Zwaan et al., 2004). If the adolescent with AN or BN presents with severe and deteriorating levels of anxiety, obsessionality, and depression—or with delusional thoughts about weight and body image—then pharmacotherapy may be warranted. Caution is still in order because there is a high probability of adverse effects when medications, including SSRIs, are administered to severely malnourished adolescents. Multidisciplinary treatment teams should be cautious, or even reluctant, in prescribing any drugs, including agents to facilitate gastric emptying during refeeding or to prevent osteoporosis caused by starvation-induced hormonal deficiencies (Gowers & Bryant–Waugh, 2004).

Bulimia Nervosa

A variety of different antidepressant drugs can, over two to four months at least, significantly improve mood and reduce the frequency of binge-eating in young and older *adults* with BN. This positive effect does not depend on whether the patient is currently depressed or has a history of depression (Roerig et al., 2002). The SSRI fluoxetine (Prozac) is the only drug approved by the FDA for the treatment of BN and/or depression in adolescents. Although a relatively high dose (60 mg/day) eliminates core symptoms of BN in less than one-third of adult cases, it does reduce the frequency of binge-eating and purging, while facilitating improvement of weight concerns. At this time it seems prudent to conclude that medication should never be used as the principal treatment for BN in adolescents, and that the immediate benefits of medication alone will likely not be sustained beyond four to six months (de Zwaan et al., 2004). Nevertheless, the pharmacotherapy literature, some of which subsumes samples including adolescent patients, indicates that antidepressant medication *may* be a useful adjunct to individual psychotherapy, including relapse prevention.

Binge-Eating Disorder

De Zwaan et al. (2004) reviewed six placebo-controlled, double-blind studies of medication in the treatment of *adults* with BED or "atypical eating disorders" marked by high binge-eating (and in some cases, overweight). In general, a variety of different drugs significantly reduced binge-eating; in half to two-thirds of these patients binge-eating was eliminated during the study period. Weight loss was excellent in some studies and poor in others. The implications of this research for treatment of adolescents are unknown, so once more caution is in order.

The Prevention of Eating Disorders

What Works

There are many reviews of programs designed to prevent the ED spectrum in children, adolescents, and young adults (see, e.g., Levine & Piran, 2004; Levine et al., 2003; Stice & Shaw, 2004). The vast majority of ED prevention programs for adolescents involve classroom curricula or other interventions in schools. On a continuum of prevention, school-based programs fall between universal (supported by public policy and intended for large groups within the general public) and selective (focused on adolescent girls as a high-risk population). Thus far, no prevention program for adolescents has been implemented successfully three or more times, so there is no clear standard for what works. Consequently, we draw on our previous work to review the models that have guided prevention, strategies that do not work, and strategies that represent, to date, the best practices with adolescent girls and boys.

What Might Work

SOCIAL COGNITIVE THEORY.   Most of the universal-selective and targeted prevention programs for adolescent girls have been guided by either Bandura's social cognitive theory or Fairburn's cognitive-behavioral theory (Stewart, 1998). According to these models, prevention should focus on (1) over-valuation of appearance in constructing one's identity; (2) the perception *and* feeling that one's body shape is quite discrepant from the culture's unrealistic beauty ideals; (3) maladaptive beliefs and negative feelings about body shape, eating, and weight loss; and (4) unhealthy or limited behaviors (e.g., calorie-restrictive dieting) motivated by body dissatisfaction and negative affect. These are learned through indirect and direct messages from a variety of social sources, including mass media, peers, and family members (Thompson et al., 1999). Cognitive processes are prominently involved in internalization of the slender beauty ideal, in the formation and organization of maladaptive beliefs about the meaning of "thin" and "fat" and "control" and "self," and in the tendency to compare one's weight and shape to the bodies of various other people, such as peers and celebrities (Smolak & Levine, 1996; Stewart, 1998; Thompson et al., 1999).

Social cognitive programs are designed to decrease cognitive-behavioral risk factors while increasing healthy attitudes and behaviors related specifically to body image and to healthy eating and exercising. Predetermined curricular lessons are implemented in the schools by classroom teachers or by mental health professionals. Social learning is fostered by brief lectures, observational learning, role-playing and rehearsal, social reinforcement, and guided discovery in group discussions and homework assignments.

NONSPECIFIC VULNERABILITY-STRESSOR MODE. Research indicates that a variety of different types of psychological and physical problems have similar risk factors: negative self-concept, lack of coping skills and other behavioral competencies, cumulative life stress, and lack of social support. This *nonspecific* relationship between vulnerability, stressors, and disorder implies that adolescents and their communities will be healthier when prevention specialists collaborate with adolescents and with community members to encourage the "5 C's" of youth development (Lerner, Fisher & Weinberg, 2000): Competence (life skills), Connection, Character, Confidence, and Caring (compassion). According to this nonspecific vulnerability-stressor (NSVS) model, adolescents need multiple opportunities to integrate social interest and social skills with a positive sense of the self as unique, competent, and connected to others. The NSVS model advocates the need for social changes that give adolescents a chance to succeed in building relationships and doing meaningful things.

CRITICAL SOCIAL PERSPECTIVES. The Critical Social Perspectives (CSP) model integrates Piran's three-pathway model of women's social experiences (see above) with her previous work on the participatory-ecological-empowerment-relational approach to prevention (Piran, 1999, 2001a, 2002; see also Levine & Piran, 2004). The CSP model has three basic principles. First, body image and body practices (how one dresses, how one eats and exercises, how one "manages" weight) are composed of learned meaning systems anchored in dominant cultural discourses and power structures. How a girl's cultures construct the meanings of male/female, white/black, social class, status, opportunity, and so forth will be an important determinant of what "fat" and "thin" and "control" and "good" mean to her. Second, girls' and women's experiences of their bodies are often disrupted by prejudice and other social inequities that are maintained by dominant ideologies. Third, *one must go beyond pressures for thinness* to conduct a critical analysis of the multiple pressures in particular social contexts that disrupts the adolescents' experiences of their bodies. This analysis should encompass other expressions of disrupted embodiment, such as self-harm behaviors or disregard for one's own safety and well-being (Piran, 2002).

The CSP approach to prevention is profoundly different from traditional curricular approaches derived from the social cognitive and NSVS models (Levine & Piran, 2004; Piran, 2001a). The CSP model encourages participants to engage in relational dialogues that are facilitated by an adult mentor. These discussions enable the girls (or boys, separately), individually and as a group, to explore and clarify their subjective experiences of context-specific factors shaping embodiment and disembodiment in their lives. This process of "consciousness-raising" provides critical knowledge that can be used to create healthier norms and practices within the group, and to establish objectives and strategies for changes within the larger school system. In this way, multiple discourses of analysis and of resistance become the foundation for collaborative efforts by the mentor and the program participants to transform not only how they are thinking and behaving, but also some of the significant contexts of their lives. Adolescent girls engaged in such a process were found to become embodied and empowered agents of constructive change, not disembodied vessels of shame and silence (Piran, 2001b).

A truly effective prevention program would reduce the number of new cases (the incidence, of eating disorders or problems within the ED spectrum) by minimizing the existence or impact of risk factors and by maximizing the power of protective factors. Compared to a similar group of healthy adolescents who did not receive the preventive intervention, valid assessment would reveal that program participants had fewer new cases of disordered eating over a meaningful, high-risk period of time (e.g., from ages 18 through 20). To date, only six universal-selective programs approached even a generous interpretation of these criteria for effectiveness. Five that have been reviewed in detail elsewhere (Levine et al., 2003; Levine & Piran, 2004) are summarized in Table 1. Here we concentrate on one universal-selective and one targeted program that are very recent and reflect a integration of several models.

UNIVERSAL-SELECTIVE PREVENTION: HEALTHY SCHOOLS–HEALTHY KIDS. Gail McVey and her colleagues in Toronto, Canada have conducted a project called

Table 1. Five Effective Prevention Programs

Social Cognitive Program: Neumark-Sztainer et al. (1995)—Ten-hour *Weigh to Eat* curriculum to help Israeli girls aged 15–16 resist and actively change sociocultural factors. At six-month follow-up, program participants had more regular eating and exercising patterns, and were less likely to begin unhealthy dieting and binge-eating.

Social Cognitive + NSVS Program: Santonastaso et al. (1999)—Engaged 16-year-old Italian girls in four 2-hour group discussions about, e.g., pubertal changes, body image, and challenges in coping with adolescence. At one-year follow-up program participants initially at risk had better body satisfaction and lower levels of bulimic behavior.

NSVS program: O'Dea & Abraham (2000)—*Everybody's Different* is a nine-lesson discovery-based program that promotes a multifaceted sense of uniqueness, self-respect, and self-worth (including healthy body esteem). At one-year follow-up, helped Australian middle school students to decrease concerns about physical appearance, athletic competence, and social acceptance.

CSP Program: Piran (1999)—Relational dialogues, consciousness-raising, and activism and advocacy by students and by Piran helped to reduce the incidence of eating disorders in adolescents attending an elite ballet school in Canada. Over time, across three different sets of students, the prevalence of AN was reduced ten-fold, new cases of BN were eliminated, and binge-eating and unhealthy weight management were significantly reduced.

CSP + NSVS + Social-Cognitive: Steiner-Adair et al. (2002)—The eight-unit *Full of Ourselves* curriculum helps girls ages 11 through 14 support each other as they think critically about, and take action in regard to, cultural messages concerning, e.g., gender, beauty, and weight-related prejudice. At six-month follow-up, program participants showed sustained improvement in body satisfaction and pre-post improvements in, e.g., internalization of the slender beauty ideal.

Healthy Schools–Healthy Kids (McVey, Tweed & Blackmore, 2004). This program combines elements of all three prominent models of prevention as it aims to increase positive self-esteem, body satisfaction, healthy eating, an active life-style, skills for coping with stress, and acceptance of diversity in size and shape. The eight-month intervention is designed specifically to affect multiple elements within the ecology of young adolescents by integrating general teacher and staff training, parent education, specific training of and feedback for teachers using the prevention curriculum, classroom lessons, support and consciousness-raising groups for girls (facilitated by school nurses), and positive messages conveyed throughout the school by posters and public service announcements.

Using a randomized (by school) controlled design, McVey et al. (2004) found that the *Healthy Schools–Healthy Kids* project had several positive effects on the girls (irrespective of grade), while it had no significant positive effects on the boys when their data were analyzed separately. At six-month follow-up, girls in the intervention schools reported greater reductions in awareness *and* internalization of the slender beauty-ideal than did girls in the control schools. Girls in the intervention schools also reported skipping fewer meals. Moreover, at post-test fewer girls in the intervention schools were trying to lose weight, but this expected difference was not maintained at follow-up. The intervention did not significantly improve body satisfaction for girls in general. However, when data for girls and boys were combined, there was a significant pre-to-post-to-follow-up increase in body satisfaction for the seventh-graders only.

This initial evaluation of the *Healthy Schools–Healthy Kids* ecological program (McVey et al., 2004) involved a short follow-up period, and there were no significant intervention effects for important variables such as body size acceptance, teasing, and appearance esteem. Further, serious ED symptoms were not assessed. Nevertheless, the preliminary evidence is encouraging because this ecological program appears to be effective in reducing one major risk factor for girls: internalization of the slender beauty ideal (Stice, 2002).

TARGETED PREVENTION: STUDENT BODIES.   Although there are a number of very promising targeted prevention programs for female college students (Levine & Piran, 2004; Stice & Shaw, 2004), precious few have been designed for adolescents. This is surprising, given the high rates of eating disorder symptoms among adolescents. *Student Bodies* is an eight-week computer-assisted psychoeducational program (CAPP) that has been shown to help college women reduce body dissatisfaction and weight concerns (Taylor, Winzelberg & Celio, 2001). Based on the social cognitive model and several elements of the CSP model, participants receive multimedia "psychoeducation" about body image, the development and consequences of eating disorders, cultural determinants of beauty, and healthy nutrition and exercise. Information is reinforced by cognitive-behavioral exercises, weekly readings, and short critical analyses. Moderated face-to-face discussions and computer-based "chats" are used to increase the experience of social support from, and connection with, other participants.

Using a pre-post only design, Abascal, Brown, Winzelberg, Dev, and Taylor (2003) evaluated the effects of internet delivery of a six-week version of *Student Bodies* on private school girls aged 15–16. Two classes of students were randomly selected for division into two groups: higher risk for ED/higher motivation for improvement in body image, or lower risk/lower motivation. The "high risk" for ED designation was based on a valid measure of weight concerns. In a third class all participants completed the curriculum as one "mixed" group. Girls in the lower risk/lower motivation group(s) benefited from the program in terms of increased knowledge and reduced shape concerns. However, the program was more effective for the higher risk/higher motivation groups, who showed improvements in knowledge and moderately large improvements (effect sizes range from .49 to .75) in shape concerns, weight concerns, drive for thinness, and dietary restraint. These data must be considered preliminary, especially since the program did not improve body image. Nevertheless, given the effectiveness of the *Student Bodies* program for college students, given the role of computers in the lives of today's adolescents, and given the desirability of a program that could be tailored to high- and low-risk populations, further development of the CAPP approach is certainly warranted.

What Does Not Work

The prevention outcome literature is marked by inconsistencies in outcomes, as well as the fact that that many different approaches produce improvements while the program is operating, only to see these positive effects dissipate at follow-up (Levine & Piran, 2004). Based on our experience and our reading of various prevention literatures, we strongly suggest that the following will be ineffective and even counterproductive: (1) "one shot" presentations emphasizing the lurid clinical details of eating disorders; (2) programs that are entirely didactic and do not engage adolescents in interesting activities aimed at critical analysis, constructive discussion, and meaningful preventive actions by the adolescents themselves; and (3) short-term, hastily conceived programs that have the tricky goals of preventing the *onset* of problems in the ED spectrum and of identifying and helping adolescents who have problems in that spectrum are *ongoing*.

Recommendations

The eating disorders classified as AN, BN, or EDNOS typically begin during adolescence and occur in about 10% of girls and young women and about 1% of boys and young men. All eating disorders are associated with significant morbidity and have the potential to become chronic debilitating conditions. While great progress has been made in discovering the genetic and neurophysiological mechanisms presumed to underlie disordered eating patterns and associated psychological phenomena, a critical look at cultural shifts and adverse social structures is necessary to explain the documented increase in eating disorders during the past few decades and to guide multidimensional treatment and prevention. Further research is required in all key areas, including epidemiology, assessment, diagnosis, treatment, and prevention of eating disorders in *adolescents* (Lask & Bryant-Waugh, 2000). The limited research available all areas is striking in relation to both the volume of research with adults and the volume of theory about adolescence as a high-risk period. Research is needed to assist in developing valid diagnostic systems with which to identify young adolescents with subclinical syndromes that create many different forms of developmental risk. Further, the approaches for therapy found to be efficacious with adults, such as cognitive behavior therapy and interpersonal psychotherapy, need to be adapted for and tested with adolescents with eating disorders.

Considering the mixed outcome of eating disorders, their morbidity, and the inherent inability of treatment to eradicate any disorder, there remains a need for substantial improvements in the prevention of eating disorders (Levine & Piran, 2004). Particular challenges in this field include the integration of specific and nonspecific changes in the ecology of adolescents with programs directed toward individuals and small group. This step itself will require an integration of approaches to different health promotion goals with youth. We believe that our field can draw upon a variety of prevention models and upon successful work in preventing substance use in order to meet these key challenges and one other—combining the prevention of eating disorders in children and adolescents with the prevention of obesity.

With regard to *best practice in treatment* of adolescents, we recommend that clinicians—

- Assess and treat eating disorders using a multidisciplinary team approach.
- Integrate individual therapy and nutritional counseling with established forms of family therapy; families do not cause eating disorders, but they play a critical role in sustained recovery.
- Use pharmacotherapy with great caution, particularly for adolescents with anorexia nervosa.
- Be well-informed, patient, and optimistic: The prognosis for eating disorders in adolescence is better than it is in adults, but it may take five to seven years or so for recovery to be complete and sustainable.

With regard to *best practice in prevention,* we recommend that—

- Education should focus on critical analysis of ways in which biology and culture interact to influence a spectrum of issues pertaining to gender, body image, embodiment, eating, and weight management.
- Each program should combine a general, research-based understanding of risk and protective factors with a contextual analysis of the particular factors operating in the lives of adolescents in that program.
- Programs should eschew didactic lessons and use a variety of techniques that engage adolescents and adults (e.g., mentors) in relational dialogues, consciousness-raising, life skill development, activism, and advocacy.
- Programs should adopt an ecological perspective in which efforts are made to change norms, values, practices, and other aspects of the environment so as to promote healthier attitudes and behaviors in regard to gender, weight, shape, eating, activity, etc.

References

Abascal, L., Brown, J.B, Winzelberg, A.J., Dev, P., & Taylor, C.B. (2003). Combining universal and targeted prevention for school-based eating disorder programs. *International Journal of Eating Disorders, 35,* 1–9.

American Psychiatric Association. (2000). *Diagnostic and Statistical Manual of Mental Disorders* (4th ed., Text revision). Washington, DC: Author.

Bulik, C.M. (2004). Genetic and biological risk factors. In J.K. Thompson (Ed.), *Handbook of Eating Disorders and Obesity* (pp. 3–16). Hoboken, NJ: Wiley.

Croll, J., Neumark-Sztainer, D., Story, M., & Ireland, M. (2002). Prevalence and risk and protective factors related to disordered eating behaviors among adolescents: Relationship to gender and ethnicity. *Journal of Adolescent Health, 31*, 166–175.

Dansky, B.S., Brewerton, T.D., & Kilpatrick, D.G. (2000). Comorbidity of bulimia nervosa and alcohol use disorders: Results from the National Women's Study. *International Journal of Eating Disorders, 27*, 180–190.

Danziger, Y., Carcl, C.A., Varsano, I., Tyano, S., & Mimouni, M. (January, 1988). Parental involvement in treatment of patients with anorexia nervosa in a pediatric day care unit. *Pediatrics, 81*, No. 1, 159–162.

Dare, C., & Eisler, I. (2000). A multi-family group day treatment programme for adolescent eating disorder. *European Eating Disorders Review, 8*, 4–18.

Dare, C., & Szmukler, G. (1991). The family therapy of short history early onset anorexia nervosa. In D.B. Woodside & L. Shekter-Wolfson (Eds.), *Family Approaches to Eating Disorders* (pp. 25–47). Washington, D.C.: American Psyciatric Press.

de Zwaan, M., Roerig, J.L., & Mitchell, J.E. (2004). Pharmacological treatment of anorexia nervosa, bulimia nervosa, and binge eating disorder. In J.K. Thompson (Ed.), *Handbook of Eating Disorders and Obesity* (pp. 186–217). Hoboken, NJ: Wiley.

Dounchis, J.Z., Hayden, H.A., & Wilfley, D.E. (2001). Obesity, body image, and eating disorders in ethnically diverse children and adolescents. In J.K. Thompson & L. Smolak (Eds.), *Body Image, Eating Disorders, and Obesity in Youth: Assessment, Prevention, and Treatment* (pp. 67–98). Washington, DC: American Psychological Association.

Durlak, J.A. (1997). Common risk and protective factors in successful prevention programs. *American Journal of Orthopsychiatry, 68*, 512–520.

Fairburn, C.G., & Harrison, P. (2003). Eating disorders [seminar]. *The Lancet, 361*, 407– 416.

Fairburn, C.G., Norman, P.A., Welch, S.L., O'Connor, M.E., Doll, H., & Peveler, R.C. (1995). A prospective study of outcome in bulimia nervosa and the long-term effects of three psychological treatments. *Archives of General Psychiatry, 52*, 304–312.

Faith, K., Pinhas, L., Schmelefske, J., & Bryden, P. (2003). Developing a feminist-informed model for decision making in the treatment of adolescent eating disorders. *Eating Disorders: The Journal of Treatment and Prevention, 11*, 305–315.

Field, A.E., Austin, S.B., Taylor, C.B., Malpeis, S.M., Rosner, B., Rockett, H.R., Gillman, M.W., & Colditz, G.A. (2003). Relation between dieting and weight change among preadolescents and adolescents. *Pediatrics, 112*, 900–906.

Fisher, M., Golden, N.H., Katzman, D.K., Kreipe, R.E., Rees, J., Schebendach, J., Sigman, G., Ammerman, S., & Hoberman, H.M. (1995). Eating disorders in Adolescents: A background paper. *Journal of Adolescent Health, 16*, 420–437.

Fredrickson, B., & Roberts, T. (1997). Objectification theory: Toward understanding women's lived experiences and mental health risks. *Psychology of Women Quarterly, 21*. 173–206.

Goldberg, L., MacKinnon, D.P., Elliot, D.L., Moe, E.L., Clarke, G., & Cheong, J. (2000). The Adolescents Training and Learning to Avoid Steroids Program: Preventing drug use and promoting healthy behaviors. *Archives of Pediatrics & Adolescent Medicine, 154*, 332– 338.

Gowers, S., & Bryant-Waugh, R. (2004). Management of child and adolescent eating disorders: The current evidence base and future directions. *Journal of Child Psychology and Psychiatry, 45*, 63–83.

Harned, M.S. (2000). Harassed bodies: An examination of the relationships among women's experiences of sexual harassment, body image, and eating disturbances. *Psychology of Women Quarterly, 24*, 336–348.

Harned, M.S., & Fitzgerald, L.F. (2002). Understanding a link between sexual harassment and eating disorder symptoms: A mediational analysis. *Journal of Consulting and Clinical Psychology, 70*, 1170–1181.

Hausenblas, H.A., & Carron, A.V. (1999). Eating disorder indices and athletes: An integration. *Journal of Sport and Exercise Psychology, 21*, 230–258.

Hoek, H.W., & van Hoeken, D. (2003). Review of the prevalence and incidence of eating disorders. *International Journal of Eating Disorders, 34*, 383–396.

Irving, L., Wall, M., Neumark-Sztainer, D., & Story, M. (2002). Steroid use among adolescents: Findings from Project EAT. *Journal of Adolescent Health, 30*, 243–252.

Jacobi, C., Hayward, C., de Zwaan, M., Kraemer, H.C., & Agras, W.S. (2004). Coming to terms with risk factors for eating disorders: Application of risk terminology and suggestions for a general taxonomy. *Psychological Bulletin, 130*, 19–65.

Katzman, D.K. (1999). Prevention of medical complications in children and adolescents with eating disorders. In N. Piran, M.P. Levine, & C. Steiner-Adair (Eds.), *Preventing Eating Disorders: A Handbook of Interventions and Special Challenges* (pp. 304–318). Philadelphia, PA: Brunner/Mazel.

Keel, P.K., Mitchell, J.E., Miller, K.B., Davis, T.L., & Crow, S.J. (1999). Long-term outcome of bulimia nervosa. *Archives of General Psychiatry, 56,* 63–69.

Kreipe, R.E., Golden, E.N.H., Katzman, D.K., Fisher, M., Rees, J., Tonkin, R.S., et al. (1995). Eating disorders in adolescents. A position paper of the Society for Adolescent Medicine. *Journal of Adolescent Health, 16,* 476–479.

Lask, B., & Bryant-Waugh, R. (Eds.). (2000). *Anorexia Nervosa and Related Eating Disorders in Childhood and Adolescence.* Hove: Psychology Press.

Le Grange, D., Eisler, I., Dare, C., & Russell, G.F.M. (1992). Evaluation of family therapy in anorexia nervosa. *International Journal of Eating Disorders, 12,* 347–357.

Lerner, R.M., Fisher, C.B., & Weinberg, R.A. (2000). Toward a science for and of the people: Promoting civil society through the application of developmental science. *Child Development, 71,* 11–20.

Levine, M.P., & Piran, N. (2004). The role of body image in the prevention of eating disorders. *Body Image, 1,* 57–70.

Levine, M.P., Piran, N., & Irving, L. (2003). Primary prevention of disordered eating behavior in adolescents. In T.P. Gullotta & M.Bloom (Eds.), *The Encyclopedia of Primary Prevention and Health Promotion* (pp. 423–428). New York: Kluwer Academic/Plenum Publishers.

Manley, R.S., Smye, V., & Srikameswaran, S. (2001). Addressing complex ethical issues in the treatment of children and adolescents with eating disorders: Application of a framework for ethical decision-making. *European Eating Disorder Review, 9,* 144–166.

McVey, G.L., Tweed, S., & Blackmore, E. (2004). *Evaluation of a comprehensive school-based program designed to increase healthy eating, active living and self-acceptance in middle school students.* Manuscript submitted for publication [contact *gail.mcvey@sickkids.ca*]

Michel, D.M., & Willard, S.G. (2003). *When Dieting Becomes Dangerous: A Guide to Understanding and Treating Anorexia and Bulimia.* New Haven: Yale University Press.

Muise, A.E., Stein, D.G., & Arbess, G. (2003). Eating disorders in adolescent boys: A review of the adolescent and young adult literature. *Journal of Adolescent Health, 33,* 427–435.

Neumark-Sztainer, D., Butler, R., & Palti, H. (1995). Eating disturbances among adolescent girls: Evaluation of a school-based primary prevention program. *Journal of Nutrition Education, 27,* 24–30.

Nielsen, S., MΘller-Madsen, Isager, T., JΘrgensen, J., Pagsberg, K., & Theander, S. (1998). Standardized mortality in eating disorders—A quantitative summary of previously published and new evidence. *Journal of Psychosomatic Research, 44,* 413–434.

O'Dea, J., & Abraham, S. (2000). Improving the body image, eating attitudes and behaviors of young and behaviors of young male and female adolescents: A new educational approach which focuses on self esteem. *International Journal of Eating Disorders, 28,* 43–57.

Piran, N. (1990). Treatment model and program overview. In N. Piran & A.S. Kaplan (Eds.), *A Day Hospital Group Treatment Program for Anorexia Nervosa and Bulimia Nervosa* (pp. 3– 19). New York, NY: Brunner/Mazel.

Piran, N. (1999). Eating disorders: A trial of prevention in a high risk school setting. *Journal of Primary Prevention, 20,* 75–90.

Piran, N. (2001a). A gendered perspective on eating disorders and disordered eating. In J. Worell (Ed.), *Encyclopedia of Gender* (pp. 369–378). San Diego, CA: Academic Press.

Piran, N. (2001b). Re-inhabiting the body from the inside out: Girls transform their school environment. In D.L.Tolman & M.Brydon-Miller (Eds.), *From Subjects to Subjectivities: A Handbook of Interpretative and Participatory Methods* (pp. 218–238). NewYork: NYU Press.

Piran, N. (2002). Embodiment: A mosaic of inquiries in the area of body weight and shape preoccupation. In S. Abbey (Ed.), *Ways of Knowing in and Through the Body: Diverse Perspectives on Embodiment* (pp. 211–214). Welland, Ontario: Soleil Publishing.

Piran, N., & Cormier, H. (2004). *On the social construction of gender and eating disorders in women.* Unpublished manuscript, OISE, University of Toronto, Canada.

Piran, N., & Thompson, S. (2004). *Expanding the social model of disordered wating patterns.* Unpublished mansucrtipt, OISE, University of Toronto, Canada.

Pope, H.G.Jr., Phillips, K.A., & Olivardia, R. (2000). *The Adonis Complex: The secret Crisis of Male Body Obsession.* New York : Free Press.

Ricciardelli, L.A., & McCabe, M.P. (2004). A biopsychosocial model of disordered eating and the pursuit of muscularity in adolescent boys. *Psychological Bulletin, 130,* 179–205.

Robin, A.L., Gilroy, M., & Dennis, A.B. (1998). Treatment of eating disorders in children and adolescents. *Clinical Psychology Review, 18,* 421–446.

Robin, A.L., Siegel, P.T., Koepke, T., Moye, A.W., & Tice, S. (1994). Family therapy versus individual therapy for adolescent females with anorexia nervosa. *Journal of Developmental and Behavioral Pediatrics, 15,* 111–116.

Roerig, J.L., Mitchell, J.E., Myers, T.C., & Glass, J.B. (2002). Pharmacotherapy and medical complications of eating disorders in children and adolescents. *Child & Adolescent Psychiatry Clinics of North America, 11,* 365.–385.

Russell, G.F.M., Szmukler, G.I., Dare, C., & Eisler, I. (1987). An evaluation of family therapy in anorexia nervosa and bulimia nervosa. *Archives of General Psychiatry, 44,* 1047–1056.

Santonastaso, P., Zanetti, T., Ferrara, S., Olivetto, M.C., Magnavita, N., & Favaro, A. (1999). A preventive intervention program in adolescent schoolgirls: A longitudinal study. *Psychotherapy and Psychosomatics, 68,* 46–50.

Shisslak, C.M., & Crago, M. (2001). Risk and protective factors in the development of Eeating disorders. In J.K. Thompson & L. Smolak (Eds.), *Body image, eating disorders, and obesity in youth: Assessment, prevention, and treatment* (pp. 103–125). Washington, DC: American Psychological Association.

Siegel, J.M., Yancey, A.K., Aneshensel, C.S., & Schuler, R. (1999). Body image, perceived pubertal timing, and adolescent mental health. *Journal of Adolescent Health, 25,* 155–165.

Smolak, L, & Levine, M.P. (1996). Developmental transitions at middle school and college. In L. Smolak, M.P.Levine, & R.H. Striegel-Moore (Eds.), *The Developmental Psychopathology of Eating Disorders: Implications for Research, Prevention, and Treatment* (pp. 207–233). Hillsdale, NJ: Erlbaum.

Smolak, L., & Murnen, S.K. (2002). A meta-analytic examination of the relationship between child sexual abuse and eating disorders. *International Journal of Eating Disorders, 31,* 136–150.

Smolak, L., & Murnen, S.K. (2004). A feminist approach to eating disorders. In J.K.Thompson (Ed.), *Handbook of Eating Disorders and Obesity* (pp. 590–605). Hoboken, NJ: Wiley.

Smolak, L., Murnen, S., & Ruble, A. (2000). Female athletes and eating disorders: A meta-analysis. *International Journal of Eating Disorders, 27,* 371–381.

Smolak, L., & Striegel-Moore, R.H. (2001). Challenging the myth of the golden girl: Ethnicity and eating disorders. In R.H. Striegel-Moore & L.Smolak (Eds.), *Eating Disorders: Innovative Directions in Research and Practice* (pp. 111–132). Washington, DC: American Psychological Association.

Steiner-Adair, C., Sjostrom, L., Franko, D.L., Pai, S., Tucker, R., Becker, A.E., & Herzog, D.B. (2002). Primary prevention of risk factors for eating disorders in adolescent girls: Learning from practice. *International Journal of Eating Disorders, 32,* 401–411.

Steinhausen, H-C. (2003). The outcome of anorexia nervosa in the 20th century. *American Journal of Psychiatry, 159,* 1284–1293.

Steinhausen, H-C., Boyadjieva, S., Griogoroiu-Serbanescu, M., & Neumärker, K.J. (2003). The outcome of adolescent eating disorders: Findings from an international collaborative study. *European Child & Adolescent Psychiatry, 12,* 91–98.

Stewart, A. (1998). Experience with a school-based eating disorders prevention programme. In W. Vandereycken & G.Noordenbos (Eds.), *The Prevention of Eating Disorders* (pp. 99–136). London: Athlone.

Stice, E. (2002). Risk and maintenance factors for eating pathology: A meta-analytic review. *Psychological Bulletin, 128,* 825–848.

Stice, E., & Bearman, S.K. (2001). Body-image and eating disturbances prospectively predict increases in depressive symptoms in adolescent girls: A growth curve analysis. *Developmental Psychology, 37,* 597–607.

Stice, E., & Shaw, H. (2004). Eating disorder prevention programs: A meta-analytic review. *Psychological Bulletin, 130,* 206–227.

Striegel-Moore, R.H., Dohm, F.A., Pike, K.M., Wilfley, D.E., & Fairburn, C. (2002). Abuse, bullying, and discrimination as risk factors for binge eating disorder. *American Journal of Psychiatry, 159,* 1902–1907.

Strober, M., Freeman, R., & Morrell, W. (1997). The long-term course of severe anorexia nervosa in adolescents: Survival analysis of recovery, relapse, and outcome predictors over 10–15 years in a prospective study. *International Journal of Eating Disorders, 22,* 339–360.

Taylor, C.B., Winzelberg, A., & Celio, A. (2001). The use of interactive media to prevent eating disorders. In R. Striegel-Moore & L. Smolak (Eds.), *Eating Disorders: Innovative Directions in Research and Practice* (pp. 255–270). Washington DC: American Psychological Association.

Thompson, J.K., Heinberg, L.J., Altabe, M., & Tantleff-Dunn, S. (1999). *Exacting Beauty: Theory, Assessment, and Treatment of Body Image Disturbance.* Washington, DC: American Psychological Association.

Zaitsoff, S.L., Geller, J., & Srikameswaran, S. (2002). Silencing the self and suppressed anger: Relationship to eating disorder symptoms in adolescent females. *European Eating Disorders Review, 10,* 51–60.

Chapter 18

Obesity

Jeanne Brooks-Gunn, Cassandra Fink, and Christina Paxson

Introduction

Rates of overweight and obesity for American children, adolescents, and adults have increased substantially over the last quarter-century. These increases cut across racial and socioeconomic lines and have been observed throughout the country. Nor are they confined to the United States: similar increases have been observed in a large number of industrialized and developing countries (Ebbeling, Pawlak & Ludwig, 2002). The rise in obesity has profound implications for health outcomes throughout life. Obesity is associated with a range of health problems, including cardiovascular disease, type 2 diabetes, and certain cancers. Obesity-related health problems not only increase mortality and reduce quality of life, but also result in high financial costs. A study based on data from NHANES III estimates that the direct health care costs of obesity represent 7% of all health care costs in the United States (Kiess et al., 2001).

Although rates have increased for all age groups, obesity among children and adolescents warrants special attention. Obese children and adolescents are more likely to develop health and psychosocial problems before adulthood than are those youth who are normal weight. In addition, obesity in adulthood is best predicted by adolescent obesity (Dietz & Gortmaker, 2001). A large literature based on longitudinal studies indicates that obese children and adolescents are at elevated risk of being obese as adults (Power, Lake & Cole, 1997; Strauss & Knight, 1999; Whitaker, Wright, Pepe, Seidel & Dietz, 1997; Williams, Davie & Lam, 1999). Obese adolescents are therefore at a higher risk of experiencing the adverse health and social consequences that attend adult obesity. Finally, obesity at young ages has been associated with adverse health outcomes in adulthood, even among those who lose weight in adolescence or young adulthood (Kiess et al., 2001). For all of these reasons, there are potentially large gains from preventing the development of obesity in children and adolescents.

The Definition and Measurement of Overweight and Obesity

Measures of overweight and obesity in children and adolescents often differ from those used for adults. For all groups, measures are based on body mass index

(BMI), defined as weight in kilograms divided by height in meters squared (kg/m^2). The Centers for Disease Control (CDC) classifies adults as "overweight" if BMI is 25 or above, and "obese" if BMI is 30 or above. Children aged 2–19 are defined to be "at risk for overweight" if BMI is greater than or equal to the 85th percentile but less than the 95th percentile for children of the same age and gender, where percentiles are based on pediatric growth charts developed by the CDC and National Center for Health Statistics (Kuczmarski et al., 2002). Similarly, "overweight" in children aged 2–19 is defined as BMI at or above the 95th percentile. Note that the CDC does not use the term *obese* for children and adolescents. However, the American Obesity Association and many published articles use the term *obese* for children above the 95th percentile and "overweight" for children between the 85th and 95th percentile, terminology we use in this chapter. It should also be noted that some studies of adolescents use the adult BMI cut-offs to define overweight and obesity rather than cut-offs based on growth chart percentiles.

Age-specific percentile cut-offs rather than absolute BMI levels are usually used to define overweight and obesity in children because body fatness changes over the years as children grow. Median BMI declines from age 2 to age 6, and then increases steadily into adulthood, a pattern that is also followed at higher percentiles of the distribution. For example, the 95th percentile of BMI for boys is 19.3 at 2 years, 17.8 at 4 years, 21.0 at 9 years, 25.1 at 13 years, and slightly over 30 (the adult cut-point for obesity) at age 20. Although the use of percentile cut-offs makes sense, it does imply that measures of the prevalence of overweight and obesity depend on the specific growth charts in use—and comparisons over time must be based on common growth charts. The CDC issued new growth charts in 2000 that are based on data from the National Health Examination Studies (NHES) and National Health and Nutrition Examination Studies (NHANES) which are conducted periodically (starting in 1964). The figures on prevalence that we cite below are based on these growth charts.

Studies differ in how data on height and weight are collected. Methods range from actual measurements using scales, stadiometers, and anthropometry to reports provided by parents or self-reports for older children. These different measurement methods can yield different rates of overweight and obesity in the same population. The prevalence rates cited below are based on the same data used to construct the CDC growth charts, which relied on actual measurements rather than self- or parental reports.

Prevalence of Overweight and Obesity

Table 1 provides information on changes in obesity (BMI $\geq$ 95th percentile) among 6–11 year-olds and 12–19-year-olds from the early 1960s through 2000, based on data from the NHES and NHANES. The table documents the rise in obesity among both children and adolescents. The obesity rate among all 6–11-year-olds rose from 4.3% in the 1960s to 15.3% in 1999–2000. The increase over this time period among adolescents was from 4.6% to 15.5%.

Rates of child and adolescent obesity vary across racial and ethnic groups, although comparisons over time are hampered by changes in racial and ethnic classifications between the 1960s and the present. In the 1960s, before Hispanic groups were classified separately, black adolescent boys had a lower rate of obesity than did

Table 1. Percent of Population with BMI > 95th Percentile for Age and Gender, by Sex, Age, Race, and Hispanic Origin, United States

	1963–65 1966–70	1971–74	1976–80	1988–94	1999–2000
6–11 years of age					
Both sexes	4.2	4.0	6.5	11.3	15.3
Boys	4.0	4.3	6.6	11.6	16.0
White	4.4	4.1	6.7	11.3	. . .
Black	1.6	5.3	6.7	12.3	. . .
White, non-Hispanic	. . .	. . .	6.1	10.7	*12.0
Black, non-Hispanic	. . .	. . .	6.8	12.3	17.1
Mexican	. . .	. . .	13.3	17.5	27.3
Girls	4.5	3.6	6.4	11.0	14.5
White	4.5	3.7	5.7	9.8	. . .
Black	4.5	3.3	11.1	16.7	. . .
White, non-Hispanic	. . .	. . .	5.2	*9.8	*
Black, non-Hispanic	. . .	. . .	11.2	17.0	22.2
Mexican	. . .	. . .	9.8	15.3	19.6
12–19 years of age					
Both sexes	4.6	6.1	5.0	10.5	15.5
Boys	4.5	6.1	4.8	11.3	15.5
White	4.7	6.3	4.7	12.1	. . .
Black	3.1	5.3	6.1	10.4	. . .
White, non-Hispanic	. . .	. . .	3.8	11.6	12.8
Black, non-Hispanic	. . .	. . .	6.1	10.7	20.7
Mexican	. . .	. . .	7.7	14.1	27.5
Girls	4.7	6.2	5.3	9.7	15.5
White	4.5	5.4	4.5	9.0	. . .
Black	6.4	10.1	10.7	16.3	. . .
White, non-Hispanic	. . .	. . .	4.6	8.9	12.4
Black, non-Hispanic	. . .	. . .	10.7	16.3	26.6
Mexican	. . .	. . .	8.8	*13.4	19.4

Source: National Center for Health Statistics (2002) Health, United States, 2002, table 71 (revised 1/14/2003). http://www.cdc.gov/nchs/data/hus/tables/2002/02hus071.
* Indicates that estimates are considered unreliable. The table gives no figure for the prevalence of overweight among non-Hispanic white girls 6–11 years of age.

white adolescent boys, and the rate for black adolescent girls was only two percentage points higher than that for whites. By the late 1970s, there were sharp racial and ethnic disparities in obesity rates. In 1976–80, the rate of obesity for black adolescent boys was 1.6 times that for white adolescent boys, and the rate for Mexican American adolescent boys was double that for white adolescent boys. For adolescent girls, the obesity rate for blacks was 2.3 times that for whites, and the rate of Mexican Americans was 1.9 that for whites. Between 1976–90 and 1999–2000, rates of obesity increased for all groups. Obesity rates for adolescent boys more than tripled, with Mexican American boys experiencing a 3.6-fold increase. Increases for adolescent girls were somewhat smaller: there was a 2.7-fold increase for whites, a 2.5-fold increase for blacks, and a 2.2-fold increase for Mexican Americans.

Table 2 shows adolescent prevalence rates of both overweight and obesity (BMI ≥ 85th percentile) and obesity alone (BMI ≥95th percentile) in 1999–2000, by race and ethnicity. This table documents the fact that patterns in overweight across genders

Table 2. Prevalence of Overweight and Obesity ≥BMI (85th Percentile) and Obesity
(BMI ≥ 95th Percentile): NHANES 1999–2000, Ages 12–19

	All	Non-Hispanic white	Non-Hispanic black	Mexican American
Percent overweight or obese (BMI ≥ 85th percentile)				
Both sexes	30.4 (1.9)	26.5 (2.4)	40.4 (2.2)	43.8 (2.6)
Male	30.5 (2.1)	27.4 (3.0)	35.7 (2.8)	44.2 (3.0)
Females	30.2 (2.8)	25.4 (3.3)	45.5 (3.0)	43.5 (4.2)
Percent obese (BMI ≥ 95th percentile)				
Both sexes	15.5 (1.6)	12.7 (1.7)	23.6 (2.1)	23.4 (2.1)
Male	15.5 (1.6)	12.8 (2.4)	20.7 (2.6)	27.5 (3.0)
Females	15.5 (1.6)	12.4 (2.1)	26.6 (2.7)	19.4 (2.8)

Source: Table 2 of Ogden, C.L, Flegal, K/M., Carroll, M.D., & Johnson, C.L. (2002). Prevalence and Trends in Overweight Among US Children and Adolescents, 1999–2000. *Journal of the American Medical Association* 288:1728–1732.
Notes: Standard errors in parentheses.

and racial groups are similar to those that appear for obesity. Rates of both overweight and obesity are similar for girls and boys when all racial and ethnic groups
are combined. The highest rates of both overweight and obesity are observed for
Mexican American boys and non-Hispanic black girls. Non-Hispanic whites—both
boys and girls—have the lowest rates of overweight and obesity in adolescence.

Physical and Emotional Consequences of Obesity in Adolescence

Obesity in childhood and adolescence is associated with a variety of physical
health problems (reviewed in Zametkin, Zoon, Klein & Munson, 2004). As discussed
above, a major health risk of obesity in childhood stems from the high persistence of
obesity from childhood into adulthood, coupled with obesity-related adult disease.
However, obese children and adolescents are also at greater risk of developing some
health problems while still young. Obese children are more likely to develop "adult"
disorders, including type 2 diabetes (previously called adult-onset diabetes), high
blood pressure, high cholesterol, and sleep disorders. Accumulating evidence indicates that the increase in child and adolescent obesity has been mirrored by an
increase in the prevalence of type 2 diabetes in these age groups (American Diabetes
Association, 2000; Rosenbloom et al., 1999). Sixty percent of overweight 5–10-year-
olds already have one associated cardiovascular disease risk factor and one-third of
obese children have symptoms of sleep apnea (Dietz & Gortmaker, 2001). Obesity in
childhood and adolescence has also been related to orthopedic problems and the
development of gallstones. However, no links have been found between childhood
obesity and asthma or cancer.

Although it is clear that child and adolescent obesity carries physical health
risks, less is known about the relationship between obesity and psychosocial problems. Research reviewed in Zametkin et al. (2004) indicates that obesity in adolescence has been associated with low self-esteem, poor body image, social stigma, and
social isolation. Other problems reported to be associated with obesity in children
and adolescents include elevated rates of loneliness, sadness, nervousness, smoking,
and drinking (DHHS, 2000). However, estimates of the strength of these associations
often vary across racial and ethnic groups, age groups, and across studies. And,

when positive associations between obesity and psychosocial problems are found, it often remains unclear whether obesity is the cause or consequence of these problems. For example, evidence from the National Longitudinal Study of Youth indicates that depressed mood in adolescents is associated with higher obesity after one year, controlling for baseline body mass (Goodman & Whitaker, 2002), suggesting that depressed mood may be a source of increases in body weight.

Individual Factors

Genetic Factors

Children with obese parents are at elevated risk of being obese as adults. Young children (aged 5 and under) are at a tenfold higher risk for becoming obese adults if both of their parents are obese compared to neither's is being obese (Whitaker et al., 1997). As children age, their own obesity (rather than that of their parents) becomes a better predictor of adult obesity. However, these results indicate that the early appearance of obesity has a familial component. A key question is whether the familial aggregation of obesity largely reflects genetic factors, environmental factors, or possibly gene-environment interactions.

The tendency toward overweight clearly has a heritable component. However, research has yielded a range of estimates of the degree of familial correlation in weight that is due solely to genetic make-up. Twin studies generally yield heritability estimates of BMI, measured as the fraction of the variance in BMI that can be attributed to genetic variation, of between 50% and 80%. Estimates of heritability decrease to between 25% and 50% when estimated from adoption studies or general family studies (Perusse & Bouchard, 1999). A useful review of these studies is Maes et al. (1997). One reason for the higher heritability estimates from twin studies is that monozygotic twins may share more environmental factors than dizygotic twins. However, studies of monozygotic twins reared separately and apart yield similar heritability estimates, on the order of 70%, providing evidence that the higher estimates may be more accurate (Allison et al., 1996). Even if a high estimate of heritability of BMI is accepted, it is important to note that there is still ample scope for environmental factors to influence obesity—as evidenced by the recent increase in obesity among stable populations.

Twin studies also provide evidence of gene-environment interactions, such that genetic make-up influences the response of body weight to environmental conditions. In one study, pairs of monozygotic male twins were fed a 1,000-calorie surplus for 100 days. At the end of this period, there was three times more variance in weight gain and six times more variance in abdominal visceral fat between pairs than within pairs, indicating significant genotype-overfeeding interactions. In the second study, seven pairs of adult male identical twins completed a protocol that increased their levels of exercise, holding energy and nutrient intake constant. Again, between-pair variance in loss of body fat was significantly greater than within-pair variance (Perusse & Bouchard, 1999). This evidence indicates that the susceptibility of individuals to adverse environmental factors and the effectiveness of prevention and treatment programs are likely to vary across individuals with different genetic make-ups.

The Prenatal Environment

Several aspects of the prenatal environment have been implicated as factors leading to increased risk of obesity among children. These include maternal diabetes, maternal nutrition and weight gain during pregnancy, and maternal smoking during pregnancy.

Among these factors, maternal insulin-dependent diabetes mellitus (IDDM) stands out as having the strongest association with obesity among offspring. Children born to mothers with IDDM have more body fat at birth and display higher weights throughout childhood and adolescence (Whitaker & Dietz, 1998). Although the mechanisms that link diabetes to overweight in offspring have not been completely identified, leading theories suggest that children with IDDM mothers have altered insulin production or insulin function. Less is known about the effects of gestational diabetes and non-insulin-dependent diabetes on obesity risk among offspring. Some research suggests that prenatal exposure to mild, diet-controlled gestational diabetes does not increase the risk of obesity among children (Whitaker et al., 1998). Other research found a small association between gestational diabetes and overweight in adolescence (Gillman et al., 2003). However, this association vanishes once controlling for maternal BMI.

High maternal weight gain during pregnancy has been considered a candidate for increased risk of childhood and adolescent obesity. Although there is evidence that maternal weight gain during pregnancy is associated with higher birth weight, little research has been conducted on whether children of mothers who gained more weight during pregnancy are more likely to become obese, and these studies are contradictory (Whitaker & Dietz, 1998).

Low birth weight, in and of itself, has been considered a risk factor for obesity later in life. There is a large body of evidence that low birth weight (2,500 or less) is associated with cardiovascular disease and type 2 diabetes in adulthood, especially among those who are obese as adults (Bhargava et al., 2004; Godfrey & Barker, 2000a,b). The evidence that low birth weight is associated with greater obesity risk among children and adolescents is less robust. Early research on the Dutch famine reported that 19-year-old men who were fetuses during the famine period were more likely to be obese than those men who were conceived earlier or later (Ravelli et al., 1976). Other research indicates that young children who display rapid "catch-up" growth in the first few years of life were smaller and thinner than their peers at birth, but were fatter by age five (Ong et al., 2000). However, research based on data from the National Collaborative Perinatal Project suggests that low birth weight is not itself a predictor of childhood obesity (Stettler et al., 2002). Although rapid weight gain in early life was associated with obesity at age 7, this effect was independent of birth weight. Furthermore, in this population, there was a positive association between birth weight and the risk of obesity at age 7.

Recent research has begun to examine whether prenatal smoking influences obesity risk among children (Toschke et al., 2003; von Kries et al., 2002). These studies, both of which are based on a sample of 5–6-year-old German children, indicate a positive association between prenatal smoking and child obesity, controlling for factors such as maternal education, parental obesity, the child's birth weight, breastfeeding, snacking behavior, and television and videogame use. However, it is possible that the association between maternal prenatal smoking and obesity reflects the effects of unmeasured socioeconomic factors that are associated with prenatal smoking.

Family Factors

Family Socioeconomic Status

While the data are fairly clear on the link between obesity and race/ethnicity, they are not as straightforward with regard to associations between obesity and family socioeconomic status (SES). In an early review article, Sobal and Stunkard (1989) concluded that while lower SES is strongly associated with higher rates of obesity among adult women from industrialized countries, evidence for children and adolescents of both genders was mixed. However, this review included studies from a long time span, many of which predated the recent increase in child and adolescent obesity. It is possible that the association between SES and obesity has changed over time, much as it has for racial and ethnic groups. More recent evidence typically finds inverse associations between child and adolescent obesity and SES (Dietz, 1991; Gerald et al., 1994; Wang, 2001). For example, Wang uses data from the NHANES III to document that there is a significant inverse association between adolescent obesity and SES, as measured by family income, even adjusting for race and ethnicity. However, the same is not true for younger children.

Recent research on maternal employment provides some insight into why the association between SES and childhood obesity is complex. Anderson, Butcher, and Levine (2003) hypothesize that the rise in maternal employment may have led to an increase in child obesity, since children with working mothers may consume more prepared or fast foods, receive less supervision after school (possibly increasing TV viewing or snack food consumption), have less time for outdoor play, or receive low-quality foods in child care settings. Using data from the National Longitudinal Study of Youth, they found that maternal employment was associated with obesity in children aged 3–11, but only for children of higher SES mothers. This research suggests that the factors leading to greater obesity and overweight among children and adolescents may vary across socioeconomic groups.

Family Eating Practices

Especially when children are young, their families influence the type and quantity of food to which they have access. However, despite the logic that family eating practices must in some way be related to the development of obesity in children and adolescents, the existing literature does not yield a simple story of how this association might work. Research reviewed in Birch and Fisher (1998) indicates that early repeated exposure to food influences the development of children's likes and dislikes: "children come to like and eat what is familiar" (p. 542). However, Birch and Fisher also caution that parents' attempts to exert control over their children's diets may backfire. Explicitly encouraging the consumption of specific foods (e.g., vegetables) may lead to a dislike for those foods. Likewise, restricting the consumption of unhealthy foods at home may result in higher consumption of those foods in unrestricted settings. This research suggests that parents should provide children with a healthy array of food choices but let children control the specific items and quantities consumed (Johnson & Birch, 1994). Although following this practice may reduce conflict around eating, there is not yet firm evidence that doing so prevents the development of child or adolescent obesity. We are not convinced that the current literature is strong enough to make any conclusions about the role of the family in influencing food preferences, although some of the prevention and treatment programs discussed in the following sections suggest that food choices of children and youth can be altered.

Social and Community

Societal Changes in Factors Influencing Obesity Risk

The fact that increases in obesity are observed for both children and adults, and across many countries, suggests that broad social and economic changes have created an environment that is more conducive to the development of obesity. A growing literature examines which social and economic factors have been most important, including reduced food prices, changes in food production, expansions of fast-food restaurants, and sedentary jobs. Cutler, Glaeser, and Shapiro (2003) hypothesize that the obesity epidemic is the result of technological changes in the production of food. Their argument is that innovations such as vacuum packaging, deep-freezing, and microwave ovens have reduced food preparation time, so that larger numbers of calories—mainly in the form of snacks—are more readily available. Lakdawalla and Philipson (2002) argue that the culprits are agricultural innovations that have reduced food prices and (for adults) increasingly sedentary jobs. Expansions of fast-food and full-service restaurants, and changes in prices of food at home and in restaurants, have been important factors in the rise in obesity among adults (Chou, Grossman & Saffer, 2004). Similar factors have been discussed as causes of the increase in childhood and adolescent obesity. The literature on children and adolescents has stressed changes in children's food consumption patterns, with an emphasis on "fast food," increases in television viewing and the use of video games and computers, and the role of the media in promoting the consumption of unhealthy foods. In what follows, we review evidence on the role of these factors in the development of obesity.

FAST FOOD.   Fast-food restaurants have expanded rapidly over the past three decades, and have become an increasingly important source of food for children and adolescents. A large-scale nutrition survey of children and adolescents conducted from 1994 to 1996 found that 30.3% of all subjects reported consuming fast food on a typical day (Bowman et al., 2004). Adolescents most often consumed "fast food," with 39% of 14–19-year-olds consuming "fast food" in a typical day. In results from multiple regressions, fast-food consumption was shown to be positively associated with being non-Hispanic black, with being male, with living in the South, and with having higher household income.

The consumption of "fast food" would not be a problem if it simply substituted for equally nutritious (and equal caloric) foods consumed at home or in full-service restaurants. However, some evidence suggests that this is not the case. Eating fast food is associated with higher total daily calorie consumption (Bowman et al., 2004). For example, 14–19-year-olds who consumed "fast food" on the first day of the survey (which covered two days spaced three to ten days apart) had total average daily caloric intake that was 379 calories higher than those who did not consume "fast food."

Fast-food consumers also ate significantly higher amounts of fats, carbohydrates, sugars, sweetened beverages, and significantly lower amounts of healthy foods such as milk, fruits, and vegetables.

These results, although suggestive, are not definitive. First, fast-food consumption may not be causally related to obesity: it could be that children and adolescents who visit fast-food restaurants more frequently would have consumed less healthy diets even if fast-food restaurants had not been available. The evidence that adults who live in areas that have experienced an increase in fast-food (and full-service) restaurants have experienced greater weight gain provides some evidence for causality. (Chou et al., 2004). However, more research on this issue targeted to children and adolescents is required.

Second, individuals vary in their response to "fast food." Given that adolescents are "exposed" to "fast food," why do some become obese while others do not? A recent study gave overweight (N = 26) and lean (N = 28) adolescents the opportunity to consume a large fast-food meal in a food court (Ebbeling et al., 2004). Calories consumed throughout the fast-food day and the next were measured. Despite the small samples, striking differences between the two groups were identified. The overweight participants consumed over 400 more calories of "fast food" than the lean participants, and appeared less likely to compensate for the extra calories at this meal by reducing consumption later in the day. As the authors note, these results suggest heterogeneity across individuals (genetic and/or environmental) in the association between exposure to "fast food" and obesity.

MEDIA USE.   Many believe that the rise in all forms of media equipment (televisions, VCR/DVDs, video games, and computers), underlie the rise in childhood obesity (Chen & Kennedy, 2001; Dietz, 2001). Almost half of all families with children have all four media staples in their homes, and according to parents, children spend over six hours each day using media equipment (Annenberg Public Policy Center, 2000). Several investigators have examined the link between media use and obesity in children; however, the results have been mixed. The absence of research consensus is due in part to (1) the lack of controls for confounding variables such as social class, age of child, family structure, etc., in many studies; (2) the (often untested) assumption that physical activity decreases as television viewing increases (the displacement effect, for which there is mixed evidence); and (3) the belief that children eat more while they are watching television than when they are doing other activities.

HOURS OF TELEVISION WATCHED.   Children spend on average 2 hours 46 minutes per day just watching television and 9–13-year-old children watch the most television of any age group except the elderly. The association between obesity and television viewing has been extensively studied (see Kohl & Hobbs, 1997, for a review). Much, although not all, of this research indicates that television viewing is associated with obesity. A recent study of children from age 4 through early adolescence indicates that children who watch in excess of three hours of television (or video) per day have an average higher BMI and skinfold thickness than those who spend less time in these activities (Framingham Children's Study—Proctor et al., 2003). The discrepancies in fatness across high- and low-television-viewing children increase with age, with the largest increases for children who are both sedentary and view more television. Television viewing may increase obesity by substituting for less sedentary activities;

by leading to increased snack consumption while watching television or by increasing children's exposure to advertising for unhealthy foods. Little work addresses these possible pathways through which television viewing might operate.

A link between hours of television viewed and prevalence of overweight was also found in older children (N = 746) aged 10–15 years old (Gortmaker et al., 1996). Children who watched more than five hours of television per day were 4.6 times more likely to be overweight than children watching zero to two hours of television per day. These results are contrary to a study of 6th- and 7th-grade girls (N = 971) in which hours of after-school television viewing was not significantly associated with change in body mass index or triceps skinfold thickness (Robinson et al., 1993).

TELEVISION IN THE BEDROOM.   A recent study by Knowledge Networks/SRI showed that 61% of children aged 8–17 have a television in their room. A survey of low-income preschool children found that the odds ratio for children being overweight was 1.06 for each additional hour per day of TV/video viewed. Among the families sampled (N = 2,761 adults with children aged 1–5) 40% of the children had a TV set in their bedroom. Children with a TV set in their bedroom spent 4.6 hours more per week watching TV and their odds ratio of being overweight was 1.31 versus children without a TV set in their bedroom (Dennison et al., 2002).

TELEVISION, EATING, AND COMMERCIALS.   The assumption mentioned earlier that links television viewing with food intake presumes two things: (1) that food advertising on television increases children's desire for high-calorie foods and thus influences children's caloric intake and (2) that children mindlessly eat while watching television. Children in the 3rd and 5th grades were asked to keep three 24-hour dietary recalls that included whether they were watching TV while eating (Matheson et al., 2004). On weekdays and weekend days, 18% and 26% of total daily energy, respectively, was consumed while viewing television. The fat content of food consumed while watching TV did not differ from food consumed at other times. This study suggests that a large proportion of children's daily energy intake is consumed while watching television, though the content of the food may not differ significantly from that consumed when not watching television.

Some studies have examined the impact television messages have on children. Sweets, snacks, convenience foods, soft drinks, and alcohol are among the most heavily advertised foods, whereas fruits and vegetables are among the least advertised (French et al., 2001). Earlier research emphasizes that advertising for children's television features foods high in sugar, fat, and salt (Cotugna, 1988). However, a direct link between the content of advertising and the development of childhood obesity has not been established.

An intriguing study exposed children aged 5–8 attending a summer camp to 14 consecutive days of television messages (Gorn & Goldberg, 1982). During their two-week stay at the camp, children viewed a half-hour videotaped cartoon program each afternoon. This was their only exposure to television while at camp. The half-hour program included 4.5 minutes of one of four types of messages: (1) candy commercials (N = 72), (2) no commercial messages (N = 72), (3) fruit commercials (N = 72), or (4) public service announcements (PSAs; N = 72). Following the half-hour cartoon program, children were given their choice of beverages (orange juice and Kool-Aid) and snacks (two fruits and two candy bars). Children exposed to the fruit commercials were most likely to select orange juice (45%), while those exposed to candy commercials were least likely to do so (25%). Children exposed to the candy commercials selected less fruit (25%) than the other three groups.

Another intriguing study on food messages on television shows targeted African Americans prime time television (Tirodkar & Jain, 2003). African Americans have a higher prevalence of obesity than the general population (27% versus 19% overall; 40.4% versus 30.4% among adolescents). Average hours of television watched per week is also greater than average among African American households (75 versus 52 hours per week). The four most-watched comedy television shows on black prime time were compared to the four most-watched comedy shows on general prime time. Prime time television consists of the shows airing between 8 PM and 11 PM on the six main television networks (ABC, NBC, FOX, UPN, WB, and CBS). Black prime time television consists of the prime time television shows with a cast made up of mainly African American actors. The UPN network has been the leader in airing black prime time television. Results showed that there were a greater number of food commercials on black prime time (4.8 per half-hour show versus 2.9 per half-hour show). Of the food commercials shown, black prime time had a greater percentage of candy/chocolate commercials (30% vs. 14%), soda commercials (13% vs. 2%), and other desserts (6% vs. 0%). General prime time had a greater percentage of food commercials containing alcohol (18% vs. 0%), bread/grains (12% vs. 6%), and other beverages (10% vs. 7%).

Evidence-Based Treatment Interventions in Community Settings

This section describes a number of community-based treatment interventions that have been evaluated. Rather than provide a comprehensive review—which would replicate an excellent recent Cochrane review article on the subject (Summerbell et al., 2004)—we instead discuss studies that represent the range of approaches to weight reduction for obese children and youth. Most of the treatments we discuss below were subject to randomized interventions, but we have included a few non-randomized programs for cases in which a particular approach has not been subject to appropriate evaluation yet. As is stressed in Summerbell et al., it is difficult to draw general conclusions about the best approaches to treat child and adolescent obesity. There are relatively few randomized studies, and those that exist often rely on small samples of (motivated) participants. The use of different follow-up periods and outcome measures makes it difficult to compare the effectiveness of different interventions. Furthermore, most of the randomized studies conducted to date have been done with younger children rather than adolescents. Finally, the majority of studies have relatively short follow-up periods, and little is known about the long-term effectiveness of treatment interventions. Despite these problems, there is some evidence that obesity among children and adolescents is amenable to treatment in community settings.

What Works

The most successful (and most often used) treatment programs for obese children are family-based (Epstein et al., 1990b). Parents are included in treatment programs since obesity runs in families and altering parental behaviors is probably central in the development and maintenance of healthy eating and activity practices. Several of the more rigorously evaluated programs are described in this section.

A Swedish clinical trial of family therapy combined with dietary counseling and medical checkups was evaluated for its effect on childhood obesity (Flodmark, Ohlsson, Ryden & Sveger, 1993). Forty-four obese children aged 10 and 11 were divided into two treatment groups: the family therapy group received dietary counseling and medical checkups coupled with family therapy; the conventional treatment group received only dietary counseling and medical checkups. The family therapy consisted of six sessions conducted by a pediatrician and a psychologist. Both groups lasted for 14–18 months and follow-up took place a year after the treatment phase ended. The third group, a comparison group (not randomized) was made up of 50 obese children who received no intervention. The family therapy group had significantly smaller increases in BMI than the conventional treatment group (0.7% versus 2.3%), and fewer children had severe obesity (BMI > 30) in the family therapy group than in the comparison group (5% versus 29%) at follow-up.

Perhaps the best-known treatments are those conducted by Epstein and colleagues (Epstein et al., 1990; Robinson, 1999a,b). This group has conducted five- and ten-year follow-ups in order to evaluate the effects of four different family-based behavioral treatment interventions on childhood obesity in 6–12-year-olds. Across the four studies, 185 families were randomized into alternative treatments. All children and youth were 20%–100% over their ideal weight based on height, age, and sex. Children in three of the four studies had obese parents. For all four studies, treatment lasted 8–12 weeks and monthly meetings continued for 6–12 months. All four studies used the Traffic Light Diet that assigns all foods a color based on their calorie content (green—go ahead and eat, yellow—proceed with caution, and red—stop) and provides a calorie range of 900–1,200 per day. According to the behavior-change perspective, the specific content of the diet may be less important than how it is defined, and the diet should be simple so that it is easy to implement and easy to monitor (Robinson, 1999a,b). The Traffic Light Diet fits this definition. Additionally, participants in all four studies filled out food diaries that were reviewed on a weekly basis.

In study I, 76 obese children and their families were randomized into one of three behavioral family-based treatment groups. In treatment one, both the obese child and parent were targeted and received positive reinforcement for weight loss and behavior change (parent–child group). In treatment two, only the child was targeted and reinforced for behavior change and weight loss (child-only group). In treatment three, families were reinforced for attendance but not for behavior change or weight loss (control group). All three groups participated in eight weekly treatment meetings, then six monthly meetings, and 21-, 60-, and 120-month follow-up meetings. The information provided at these meetings was identical for all three groups. The Traffic Light Diet (described briefly earlier) was used in this study. Parents in each of the three groups deposited $65 at the start of the study. The parent-child group received $5 back each week contingent on either parent or child losing weight for the week, the child-only group received $5 back contingent on the child's weight loss, and the control group received $5 back contingent on attendance. Another difference between the groups was the method of teaching used. The child-parent and child-only groups had to pass a review quiz from the preceding module before they could move on to the next module; the control group was taught in a more traditional lecture format.

Children in the parent-child group decreased percent overweight from baseline to five- and ten-year follow-up (−7.0%); however, children in the child-only group and the control group increased percent overweight from baseline to five- and ten-year follow-up (4.7% and 13.6%, respectively; Epstein et al., 1990, 1994). Parents in all groups significantly decreased percent overweight at the end of treatment, but these effects lasted only up to 21 months. This suggests that parent modeling cannot account for child outcome. Additionally, the lack of sustained parent weight loss suggests that the ideal behavioral treatment of obesity may differ for adults and children. The results from this study are very promising in that children in the family-based treatment were able to maintain the weight loss for 10 years.

In study II, 8–12-year-old children with at least one obese parent were randomly assigned to one of three groups: (1) diet-exercise group; (2) diet-alone group; (3) no-treatment control group. Contingencies were oriented toward the child in the diet-exercise and diet-alone groups. The exercise program increased energy expenditure through four miles of walking per day (2,800 kcal per week), with reinforcement for exercise change and child weight loss. The diet-alone group was instructed in calisthenics and stretching but was not reinforced for exercise changes, only child weight loss (Epstein et al., 1994). No significant differences for change in percentage overweight were observed between groups after five and ten years, though children in both treatment groups showed decreases (8.4% and 10.0%) in long-term percentage overweight.

In study III, 8–12-year-old children were reinforced for habit change. Parent obesity status was an independent variable. The first group of children had at least one obese parent and the second group had two parents who were not obese. During treatment, children with no obese parent had a greater decrease in percent overweight than children with an obese parent (−16.0% vs. −7.7%). At the ten-year follow-up, children with at least one obese parent increased their percent overweight 3.1%, while children with no obese parent decreased percent overweight by 11.1%. The finding that the outcome depended on parental obesity suggests that the treatment interacted with either aspects of the home environment or the child's genetic predisposition to obesity.

Study IV focused on reinforcing behavior change based on physical activity. Children with at least one obese parent (41 children aged 8 to 12 years) were randomized to one of three groups: (1) life-style exercise group, (2) programmed aerobic exercise group, or (3) calisthenics control group. Parents and children had reciprocal reinforcement contingencies, meaning they were instructed to support the behavior change of one another. The life-style exercise group decreased percent overweight significantly more than the calisthenics control group (child percent overweight −12% vs. 6.5%, and parent percent overweight −10.1% vs. −1%), while the programmed aerobic exercise group fell between the other two groups.

Combined five-year follow-up results for these four studies showed that four behavioral variables were related to child outcome: child report of selecting low calorie snacks, graphing weight, eating fewer red foods (based on the Traffic Light Diet), and parent-reported use of praise. At the ten-year follow-up, the results of the four studies were combined. Outcomes revealed that 34% of participants in the treatment groups had decreased percentage overweight by 20% or more, while 30% were no longer obese (Epstein et al., 1994), a remarkable finding.

Unlike most family-based interventions that target both the children and the parents, Golan and colleagues (1998) designed a randomized study that used the parents as the agents of change. Obese Israeli children aged 6–11 years participated in the one-year program (N = 60). All of the children were 20% or more above their expected weight and lived with both of their parents. The parents in the experimental group attended 14 one-hour group sessions held with groups of 15 other parents. In these sessions, parents were taught to alter the family's sedentary lifestyle, follow a healthy diet, decrease the family's exposure to food stimuli, and practice parenting skills (Golan et al., 1998). Additionally, the entire family attended five 15-minute individual sessions spaced out between the last six parent group sessions. Children were targeted in the conventional intervention group. They were prescribed a diet and participated in 30 one-hour group sessions. Both experimental and conventional treatment groups decreased the percentage of obese children overweight; however, the experimental group's decrease in degree overweight was significantly more than that of the conventional group (14.6% vs. 8.4%, respectively). Although both groups failed to increase significantly the amount of weekly physical activity in children, mothers in the experimental group significantly increased their mean physical activity while the mothers in the conventional group decreased their mean physical activity. The experimental group showed a significant reduction in four negative eating styles (eating while standing, eating with another action, eating between meals, and eating following stress), while the conventional group only reduced eating between meals. Although parents seemed to make a difference in their child's eating patterns and weight loss efforts, parental weight was not significantly reduced during the program and there was no association found between change in parental eating behavior and children's overweight reduction.

Brownell and colleagues (1983) evaluated three different methods of involving mothers in the treatment of obese adolescents. Obese (at least 20% more than the average weight for age, sex, and height) adolescents aged 12–16-years received the same 16-week treatment consisting of 45–60-minute weekly sessions (N = 42). Mothers and children were weighed before each session, and although mothers were encouraged to lose weight, they were not required to do so. Youth were randomized into three groups: (1) mother-child separately group, (2) mother-child together group, and (3) child-alone group. In the mother-child separately group, mothers and their children met at the same time but in different groups; the mother-child together group conducted the sessions with mothers and their children in the same group; the child-alone group provided group sessions for the children but the mothers did not attend or participate in any group. The mother-child separately group had greater decreases in percent overweight than the mother-child together group and the child-alone group (−17.1%, −7.0%, and −6.8%, respectively). The one-year follow-up showed that both the mother-child together and child-alone groups maintained their decrease in percent overweight (−5.5% and −6.0%, respectively) and the mother-child separately group decreased even more (−20.5%).

What Might Work

Very few individually based treatment programs for children exist, and the ones that do exist rely on unconfirmed report rather than objective evaluation. One individually based program, Committed to Kids, has been evaluated (Schumacher et al., 2002). Committed to Kids is a weight management program conducted with 13–17-year-olds in an outpatient, group setting. A physician, registered dietician, exercise physiologist, and behavior specialist are all involved in the weight management program. An efficacy study of Committed to Kids enrolled 93 adolescents, though only 56 participants completed the evaluations at the end of the year. More than 62% of participants experienced a decrease in body weight (from 177 ± 34.0 at baseline to 141.9 ± 20.1 at one-year follow-up) and BMI (from 32.3 ± 1.3 at baseline to 28.2 ± 1.2 at the one-year follow-up). Although this is promising, no randomized studies have been conducted.

Adolescents are often the focus for individual programs (DeWolfe & Jack, 1984). SHAPEDOWN is a fee-for-service obesity intervention program that was developed at the University of California, San Francisco (Mellin, Slinkard & Irwin, 1987). A 15-month randomized experimental study was conducted to determine the effectiveness of the SHAPEDOWN adolescent obesity intervention (N = 66). Those in the intervention group paid the normal service charge and attended 14 weekly sessions (their parents attended two sessions). The youth were voluntarily weighed at each group session. Those youth in the control group paid no fee and received no services. Relative weight (actual weight divided by expected weight and multiplied by 100) was measured at 3 and 15 months. The experimental group's weight significantly improved at the time of these measurements, as did their weight-related behavior (eating in front of the television, snacking, eating at the dinner table), self-esteem, and weight management knowledge. Overall, the SHAPEDOWN program seems successful in weight control for adolescents, but it is important to take into account that this is a fee-for-service program and not everyone is able to afford the program. Additionally, those who do participate may have more invested in the program (i.e., money) and are therefore more motivated to succeed. Finally, for both the SHAPEDOWN intervention and many of the other interventions discussed above, there is little evidence on how long the benefits of the intervention last. Given that a key aim of treating adolescent obesity is to reduce obesity in adulthood, more long-term follow-ups are required.

What Does Not Work

More research is required before firm conclusions can be drawn about what treatments do not work. A major drawback to existing studies, mentioned above, is that they are typically small and rely on samples of motivated individuals drawn from homogenous populations. Interventions that are promising for one population group may or may not be effective for other populations. For example, the conclusion that family involvement is important for the treatment of child obesity relies mainly on studies of younger children (with the exception of the studies by Brownell and colleagues). It may be that some family-based approaches become less effective at older ages. Additional research is also required on the effectiveness of different treatment programs across gender, racial, and socioeconomic groups.

Evidence-Based Treatment Interventions in Residential Settings

What Works

A search of the literature did not uncover residential treatments that had been tried successfully three times.

What Might Work

Summer camps for overweight children are becoming more common. Children generally go home thinner than they arrived, but there is debate about whether the weight stays off or is gained back once the child returns home to an uncontrolled environment. One such camp, the Carnegie International Camp, evaluated the change in body composition and activity during a camp session that took place July and August 2000 (Gately & Cooke, 2002; Walker et al., 2003). The camp used physical activity (six 1-hour sessions a day), diet (1,300, 1,800, or 2,300 kcals per day based on the individual) and education (weekly nutrition and life-style same-sex sessions). Participants' (N = 57) body mass, stature, percent body fat, aerobic fitness, exercise motivation, and self-esteem was measured at baseline and following the six-week camp. A normal weight comparison group (N = 38) also participated in these measurements.

The camp program was found to be effective in reducing risk factors for children's health with significant improvements in body weight (−5.6 kg), BMI (−2.1 kg/m^2), and psychometric variables. Weight and BMI of the comparison group increased significantly over the same time period (t(37) = 4.86 and t(37) = 4.51, respectively). Follow-up studies have shown successful management of percent body fat in approximately 71% of children who return to the camp each year. However, it should be kept in mind that those choosing to attend weight-loss camps may be more motivated than other obese children, and it is not clear whether the positive benefits generalize to broader populations.

A more intense residential program was conducted for severely obese children and adolescents at the Medical Pediatric Center Zeepreventorium in Belgium (Deforche et al., 2003). Subjects (N = 20) were randomly selected from 100 obese children and adolescents who participated in the ten-month residential treatment in 2000–2001. The mean BMI of subjects was 36.8 ± 4.3 kg/m^2 at baseline and subjects had to have a BMI greater than the 98th percentile (according to Flemish growth charts) to be admitted to the study. The residential program consisted of medical support, a 1,400–1,600-kcal per day diet, physical activity, psychological support, and limited parental involvement.

This program appears to have been highly effective. Subjects' height, weight, fat mass (FM), fat free mass (FFM), and aerobic fitness were assessed at baseline, week 11, week 24, and week 33. Following treatment, subjects were 46% less overweight (P < 0.001), BMI decreased 24% (P < 0.001), body mass decreased by 23 kg (P < 0.001), and FM decreased 8.9%.

What Does Not Work

Although residential treatment programs may be effective, they are not a realistic treatment option for most families. Summer camps and longer-term residential programs are costly. Longer-term programs separate children from their families and communities. More research is required to establish whether residential treatment programs for extremely obese children and adolescents are superior to those that that are community based.

Pharmacology

Pharmacological treatments are not generally prescribed for children, mainly because drugs that have been approved for use in adults have not been approved for pediatric use (Daniels, 2001). Four experimental drugs have produced weight loss in studies involving children; however, these drugs are designed for very specific cases: *metformin* for obese adolescents with insulin resistance and hyperinsulinaemia, *octreotide* for hypothalamic obesity, *growth hormone* in children with Prader–Willi syndrome, and *leptin* for congenital leptin deficiency. Pharmacological treatments are generally reserved for children with a biological cause of obesity or those presenting with severe obesity-related complications. Bariatric surgery has also been used for severely obese children in the last couple of decades, mainly the roux-en-y gastric bypass. This procedure results in dramatic weight loss; however, the side effects can be very severe, including death (Ebbeling et al., 2002).

Daniels (2001) presents a useful review of new developments in pharmacological interventions for pediatric patients. However, this article cautions that because existing treatments have not been approved for pediatric populations, physicians should be extremely conservative in their use. Behavioral interventions should be tried first. Pharmacological interventions should be used only for the most extremely obese children and adolescents for whom behavioral interventions do not work, and then only within the context of clinical trials with appropriate informed consent.

The Prevention of Obesity

A variety of approaches have been used to prevent obesity in children and adolescents. Not surprisingly, programs have focused on modifying the factors that are believed to account for obesity. Most are based in schools or community programs (Story, 1999). This is in contrast to treatment programs, which tend to focus on the family or, in a few cases, on just the child or adolescent.

What Works

A search of the literature did not uncover prevention programs that have been tried successfully three times.

What Might Work

The school setting is a good place to initiate programs aimed at preventing obesity. Multisite school programs using randomized designs are described in this section (Pathways, Reducing Children's Television Viewing to Prevent Obesity, Planet Health, Stanford Adolescent Heart Health Program, and KOPS). All had multiple components to their programs, and all measured weight as an outcome. Another small program (GEMS) for African American girls is also described.

Pathways (Caballero, Clay & Davis, 2003) focused on American Indian children in 41 elementary schools in three states (N = 1,704). Almost all (at least 90%) of the third-grade students in each school were American Indians. Overweight rates are very high in this population (25% to 46%). The intervention, lasting three years, included physical education, food service, classroom curriculum, and family involvement. Classroom curriculum consisted of two 45-minute lessons delivered by the teacher each week for 8–12 weeks depending on the age group. The goal for food service was to reduce the amount of fat in school meals. The physical education program implemented at least three 30-minute sessions per week of moderate to vigorous physical activity. Families were given take-home action packs that introduced them to the Pathways program and provided low-fat foods and ideas for healthful snacks. Additionally, families were invited to cooking demonstrations and other activities at school.

At baseline (end of second grade), 47% of the children had BMIs greater than the 85th percentile. No weight differences were seen at the end of the program (fifth grade) between the intervention and control groups. However, children in the 21 intervention schools reported lower daily caloric intake (about 250 fewer calories) and percentage of energy from total fat (about 2.5% lower). School lunches in the intervention schools did contain less fat (28% versus 32%), although the caloric values were similar in the two types of schools.

Reducing exposure to media may prevent childhood obesity, as demonstrated in a two-school study (Robinson, 1999a,b). Third and fourth grade students (N = 192) from two California elementary schools participated in the study. One school was randomized to the intervention (N = 92), which consisted of an 18-lesson curriculum aimed at reducing television, videotape, and video game use. The curriculum, implemented during regular class time, included lessons on self-monitoring and self-reporting of media use, a television turnoff event where children did not watch television or play video games for ten days, and lessons on how to follow a "television budget." The control school (N = 100) only participated in assessments.

The intervention group decreased television viewing time (−5.53 hours of television per week) and video game use (−2.54 hours of video game use per week) more than the controls. Children in the intervention group also had statistically significant relative decreases in BMI (−0.45 kg/m^2 adjusted difference), triceps skinfold thickness (−1.47 adjusted difference), waist circumference (−2.30 adjusted difference), and waist-to-hip ratio (−0.02 adjusted difference) compared to the controls. There were no effects on children's physical activity levels as a result of the intervention.

The Girls Health Enrichment Multi-Site Program (GEMS; Story et al., 2003) was a multicenter research program created to develop and test four interventions designed to prevent excess weight gain in African American girls as they enter and proceed through puberty. There were 240 girls at each of three sites and 360 girls at the fourth site (aged 8–10 years). Currently, only pilot data has been published with fifty four 8–10-year-old African American girls who were randomly assigned to one of two groups. Both groups participated in a 12-week program. The intervention group, "Girlfriends for KEEPS (Keys to Eating, Exercising, Playing, and Sharing)," met twice a week for one hour after school and focused on three factors: environmental, personal, and behavioral. Goals were set for physical activity, dietary changes, and family participation and reinforcement. Family packets were sent home each week and two family night events were held during the course of the 12-week program. Cultural sensitivity factors included providing African American session leaders, participating in ethnic and hip hop dance, and participating in active African American games. The control group met once a month for Saturday morning meetings where they participated in art and crafts, self-esteem, and other workshops. Nutrition and physical activity subjects were not included in the control group programming.

Weight, height, waist circumference, and BMI were measured at baseline and follow-up. Parental height and weight were also measured. Subjects also wore a Computer Science Application (CSA) accelerometer to measure their level of physical activity and completed surveys on physical activity, dietary intake, and self-efficacy. At the 12-week follow-up, there was no difference between the treatment and control group's BMI. However, physical activity levels were higher in the intervention group than in the control group (503.7 vs. 446.2 CSA-count/minute) and girls in the intervention group improved their behavioral intention for healthy eating and nutrition knowledge. Physical activity differences and dietary intake differences between the two groups were not statistically significant.

Planet Health, developed by Gortmaker and colleagues (1999), is a program for sixth and seventh graders (N = 1,295 in 10 schools using a randomized design). Program objectives included decreasing television viewing and fat intake, and increasing fruit and vegetable intake and physical activity. A significant reduction in the prevalence of obesity (BMI and tricep skinfold thickness greater than the 85th percentile) was observed in girls, but not in boys. Obesity declined from 23.6% to 20.3% among the girls in the intervention schools, while girls in the control group showed an increase of obesity from 21.5% to 23.7%. For girls, reducing television time by one hour predicted a reduction in obesity prevalence with an odds ratio of 0.85. The authors concluded that television viewing predicted change in obesity and accounted for the decrease in obesity among girls in the intervention schools.

The Stanford Adolescent Heart Health Program, which targeted Tenth-graders, was a multifaceted approach, not just focusing on obesity (Killen et al., 1998). The goals were to decrease dietary fat, smoking, and physical inactivity and increase aerobic fitness and selection of low-fat and high-fiber food. Four high schools in California were randomized to intervention or control, and baseline and follow-up data were collected from 1,130 students aged 14–16. The intervention schools followed a curriculum consisting of 20 classroom sessions. The youth in the intervention schools reported participating more in aerobic activity and were more physically fit (30.2% of students at the intervention schools who had not been regular exercisers at baseline were regular exercisers at the two-month follow-up, compared with 20% in the control group). This information was based on self-reported material.

The Kiel Obesity Prevention Study (KOPS; Muller et al., 2001) was an intensive program initiated with German 5–7- year-olds (N = 2,440). The design was a prospective cohort with intervention and control schools. On alternating years, schools changed and the control schools became the intervention schools and vice versa. Baseline measures included anthropometric measures, dietary assessment, and physical activity assessment. At baseline, 21 % of the children were overweight; 31% of the normal-weight children had parents who were overweight.

Intervention schools delivered behavioral and educational messages to children and their parents that included, eat fruits and vegetables, reduce the intake of high fat foods, be active at least an hour per day, and decrease TV viewing to less than one hour per day. Additionally, teachers were trained in a nutrition education program. For families with overweight or obese children and/or obese parents, three to five counseling sessions were offered and a six-month sports program was offered twice a week. The increase in skinfold thickness was lower for the intervention than the control classrooms (11.3 mm versus 13 mm) as was the percentage fat mass for the overweight children (0.4% in the intervention versus 3.6% in the control classrooms). Also, percentage increases were seen in the intervention classrooms in daily physical activity (12%), daily fruit and vegetable consumption (50%), nutrition knowledge (25%), and reduced daily television (1.6 vs. 1.9 hours).

In contrast to the other programs, KOPS did show weight reductions. KOPS, which focused on young elementary school children, provided more intensive services for those families with obese or overweight children (or parent), included parents in the intervention, and reduced time spent watching television.

Several school districts have also implemented comprehensive prevention programs. We describe two here. While intriguing, neither has been evaluated and neither used a randomized design. The Leaf Policy and Pilot Grant Program in California (Senate Bill 19; 2002, California Department of Education) was designed to provide school districts with the funds needed to develop district-wide comprehensive nutrition and physical activity policies. The objectives included promoting nutrition standards, encouraging consumption of California-grown fruits and vegetables, integrating nutrition education into the core curriculum, and encouraging physical activity.

Eligibility criteria for the grant differed for elementary, middle, and high schools. Elementary schools were only allowed to sell *full meals* during breakfast and lunch periods, with the exception of snacks that met the nutrient requirements: 35% or less fat, 10% or less saturated fat, and not more than 35% of total weight of the food item in sugar. Additionally, water, milk, 100% fruit juice, and fruit-based juice composed of no less than 50% fruit juice with no added sweeteners were the only beverages that could be sold on campus. Middle schools were allowed to sell carbonated drinks on campus; however, these drinks could not be sold from one-half hour before school started until after the end of the last lunch period. Vending machines that contained beverages that did not meet the requirements for elementary schools were locked one-half hour before school started until after the last lunch period. Middle schools and high schools had to ensure that all entrees and side dishes offered at school were the same portions as those served in the federal school meal program. Fruit and non-fried vegetables had to be sold at all food sale locations within the middle and high schools. Very primary data suggest that the sale of carbonated beverages and "junk food" in vending machines has been replaced with the sale of healthier alternatives such as juice, water, trail-mix, and pretzels. In May 2002, a total of $6,163 was spent on soda and junk food in the vending machines at Venice Health School; $7,358 was spent in May of 2003 after soda and junk food was replaced with healthy alternatives (Venice High School, California, 2003).

Another program, the 3C's (Cafeteria, Classroom, and Community) was initiated in a single California school district where 32% of the students are overweight (Baldwin, 2003). Learning about nutrition was integrated into existing curriculum and the cafeteria staff designed an attractive salad bar, promoted a new in-season fruit or vegetable each month, and highlighted new recipes. Additionally, a newsletter was provided to teachers and included recipes for the fruit or vegetable of the month and ideas for how to include nutrition education in their lesson plans. No evaluation data have been reported. However, both of these programs highlight the possibility of altering food choices in school settings as well as making healthy food choices more attractive.

What Does Not Work

Although the following programs, focusing on physical activity in schools, were well implemented, they did not produce desired results. Physical activity in schools may help prevent obesity when part of a more comprehensive program but it is not sufficient in and of itself as a prevention program. The Coordinated Approach to Child Health (CATCH; Hoelscher et al., 2001; Webber et al., 1996) targeted both dietary intake and physical activity as main components in the intervention. Study objectives included (1) reducing total fat, saturated fat, and sodium content of food served in school to 30%, 10% of calories, and 600–1,000 mg/serving, respectively; (2) increasing the amount of physical education class time that students spend in moderate to vigorous physical activity to 40%; and (3) reducing total cholesterol by 5 mg/dl in individuals.

In the intervention schools (N = 56), physical education teachers received special training, students participated in classes, and students and their parents did take-home assignments. The control schools (N = 40) did not receive programming. About 5,000 children in K through fifth grade participated, with follow-up (four years later) in sixth through eighth grade.

No effects were seen in BMI, skinfold thickness, blood pressure, or cholesterol for the CATCH intervention. Physical activity was increased (both in school and out-of-school), although fitness was not altered. The intensity of PE in the intervention schools increased compared to control schools ($P < 0.02$) and students in the intervention schools reported significantly more daily vigorous activity than controls (58.6 minutes vs. 46.5 minutes; $P < 0.003$).

The program Sports, Play, and Active Recreation for Kids (Project SPARK; Sallis et al., 1993) targeted physical activity, not specifically the prevention of obesity. Schools were assigned to a control condition (three schools), a teacher-led intervention (two schools), or a specialist-led intervention (two schools). Students in the fourth and fifth grades (N = 550) participated. Students in both intervention conditions received three 30-minute physical education classes per week as well as a self-management curriculum to encourage physical activity outside of school. Students in the control condition participated in regular physical education classes. No differences in BMI or skinfold thickness were seen after the intervention.

Recommendations

Obesity among children and adolescents is a growing problem with serious consequences for population health. The increase in obesity appears to result from broad societal changes in patterns of diet and physical activity. Although some groups within the population have been affected more than others, increases in obesity are widespread, appearing across racial, ethnic, and economic groups.

The large recent increase in the prevalence of child and adolescent obesity has heightened awareness of the need for effective prevention and treatment interventions. Yet we still have only limited knowledge of the best methods of intervention. Important priorities for future research include subjecting promising intervention and treatment methods to randomized evaluations using larger populations; studying how the efficacy of various interventions differs across children of different ages, genders, and socioeconomic groups; and conducting longer-term follow-ups to assess whether the effects of interventions persist through time. Despite the shortcomings of the existing literature, a few tentative conclusions can be drawn:

First, obesity treatment and prevention should begin earlier rather than later in childhood. Children seem to do better in obesity treatment interventions than older adolescents. This could be because eating and activity behaviors are not completely developed in children, whereas the habits of adolescents are more established. Younger children may also be more responsive to treatment interventions and have more support from their family. Similarly, it is important to begin treatment and prevention efforts early in childhood.

Second, family involvement appears to be a key factor in the treatment of obesity (with the caveat there is relatively little evidence on parental involvement in adolescent treatment programs). Involving parents may be easiest in treatment programs, which are usually implemented within medical settings, and more difficult in prevention programs which are typically school-based. It is interesting to note that several of the more successful school-based prevention programs that we reviewed, such as KOPS, included parent involvement. More research is needed on the benefits and best methods of involving parents in school-based prevention programs.

Third, successful treatment and prevention interventions tend to be multifaceted, focusing on broad changes in behaviors surrounding eating, television viewing and video game use, and physical activity. However, because nearly all interventions (both those that worked and those that did not) included multiple components, it is difficult to parse out which components are critical for success and which are less effective. One pattern in the prevention programs reviewed above is that those that focused on increasing physical education within schools did not work well, whereas those that focused on reducing television viewing and videogame use appeared to be more effective. However, more research on the optimal design of prevention programs is required before firm conclusions can be drawn.

Fourth, pharmacological interventions are not currently an option for the majority of obese children and adolescents. Although new research on pharmacological interventions may lead to treatments that are safe and effective for children, behavioral interventions currently hold the most promise. Similarly, although some residential programs have been shown to be effective, these are not viable options for the majority of children.

ACKNOWLEDGEMENTS.   We wish to thank the Center for Research on Health and Well-being at Princeton University and the National Institute for Child Health and Human Development (NICHHD) Research Network on Child and Family Well-being for their support of the writing of this chapter. This chapter will appear in T.P. Gullotta and G.R. Adams (Eds.), Handbook of Adolescent Behavioral Problems: Evidence-Based Approaches to Prevention. New York, NY: Springer.

References

Allison, D.B., Kaprio, J., Korkeila, M., Koskenvuo, M., Neale, M.C., & Hayakawa, K. (1996). The heritability of body mass index among an international sample of monozygotic twins reared apart. *International Journal of Obesity and Related Metabolic Disorders, 20*(6), 501–506.

American Diabetes Association. (2000). Type 2 diabetes in children and adolescents. Diabetes Care, 23 (3), 381–389.

Anderson, P., Butcher, K., & Levine, P. (2003). Maternal employment and overweight children. *Journal of Health Economics, 22*, 477–504.

Annenberg Public Policy Center of the University of Pennsylvania. (2000). *Media in the Home 2000 Report.*

Baldwin, S. Strategies to increase children's fruit and vegetable consumption: Using the 3C's approach (classroom, cafeteria, and community). Presented at the 131st Annual Meeting of the American Public Health Association, November, 2003.

Bhargava, S.K., Sachdev, H.S., Fall, C., Osmond, C., et al. (2004). Relation of serial changes in childhood body-mass index to impaired glucose tolerance in young adulthood. *The New England Journal of Medicine, 350*(9): 865.

Birch, L.L., & Fisher, J.O. (1998). Development of eating behaviors among children and adolescents. *Pediatrics 101*(3 Pt 2): 539–49.

Bowman, S.A, Gortmaker, S.L, Ebbeling, C.B., et al. (2004). Effects of fast-food consumption on energy intake and diet quality among children in a national household survey. *Pediatrics, 113*(1): 112–118.

Brownell, K.D., Kelman, J.H., & Stunkard, A.J. (1983). Treatment of obese children with and without their mothers: changes in weight and blood pressure. *Pediatrics, 71*(4), 515–523.

Caballero, B., Clay, T., Davis, S.M., et al. (2003). Pathways: a school-based, randomized controlled trial for the prevention of obesity in American Indian schoolchildren. *American Journal of Clinical Nutrition, 78*, 1030–1038.

Chen, J.L., & Kennedy, C.M. (2001). Television viewing and children's health. *Journal of Social Pediatric Nursing, 6*(1), 35–38.

Chou, S.Y., Grossman, M., & Saffer, H. (2004). An economic analysis of adult obesity: results from the Behavioral Risk Factor Surveillance System. *Journal of Health Economics, 23*(3), 565–58.

Cotugna. N. (1988). TV ads on saturday morning children's programming–what's new? *Journal of Nutrition Education 20*, 125–127.

Cutler, D.M., Glaeser, E.L., & Shapiro, J.M. (2003). Why have Americans become more obese? *The Journal of Economic Perspectives, 17*(1), 93–118.

Daniels, S. (2001). Pharmacological treatment of obesity in paediatric patients. *Paediatric Drugs, 3*(6), 405–410.

Deforche, B., De Bourdeaudhuij, I., Debode, P., Vinaimont, F., Hills, A.P., Verstraete, S., & Bouckaert, J. (2003). Changes in fat mass, fat-free mass and aerobic fitness in severely obese children and adolescents following a residential treatment programme. *European Journal of Pediatrics, 162*, 616–622.

Dennison, B.A., Erb, T.A., & Jenkins, P.L. (2002). Television viewing and television in bedroom associated with overweight risk among low-income preschool children. *Pediatrics, 109*(6), 1028–1035.

Department of Health and Human Services. (2000). *Healthy People 2010: Understanding and Improving Health* (second edition). Washington, D.C.: U.S. Government Printing Office.

DeWolfe, J.A., & Jack, E. (1984). Weight control in adolescent girls: a comparison of the effectiveness of three approaches to follow-up. *Journal of School Health, 54*(9), 347–349.

Dietz, W.H. (1991). Factors associated with childhood obesity. *Nutrition, 7*(4), 290–291.

Dietz, W.H. (2001). The obesity epidemic in young children. *British Medical Journal, 322*(7282), 313.

Dietz, W., & Gortmaker, S. (2001). Preventing obesity in children and adolescents. *Annu. Rev. Public Health, 22*, 337–53.

Ebbeling, C.B., Pawlak, D.B., & Ludwig, D.S. (2002). Childhood obesity: public-health crisis, common sense cure. *The Lancet, 360*, 473–482.

Ebbeling, C.B., Sinclari, K.B., & Pereira, M.A. et al. (2004). Compensation for energy intake from fast food among overweight and lean adolescents. *Journal of the American Medical Association, 291*(23), 2828–2833.

Epstein, L.H., McCurley, J, Wing, R.R., & Valoski, A. (1990a). Five-year follow-up of family-based behavioral treatments for childhood obesity. *Journal of Consulting and Clinical Psychology, 58*(5), 661–664.

Epstein, L.H., Valoski, A., Wing, R.R., & McCurley, J. (1990b). Ten-year follow-up of behavioral family-based treatment for obese children. *JAMA, 264*(19), 2519–2524.

Epstein, L.H., Valoski, A., Wing, R.R., & McCurley, J. (1994). Ten-year outcomes of behavioral family-based treatment for childhood obesity. *Health Psychology, 13*(5), 373–383.

Flodmark, C.E., Ohlsson, T., Ryden, O., & Sveger, T. (1993). Prevention of progression to severe obesity in a group of obese schoolchildren treated with family therapy. *Pediatrics, 91*, 880–884.

French, et al. (2001). Pricing and promotion effects on low-fat vending snack purchases: the CHIPS Study. *American Journal of Public Health, 91*(1), 112–117.

Gately P.J., & Cooke, C.B. (2002). School of Leisure & Sport, Leeds Metropolitan University, Leeds, LS6 3QS, UK.

Gerald, L.B., Anderson, A., Johnson, G.D., Hoff, C., & Trimm, R.F. (1994). Social class, social support and obesity risk in children. *Child Care Health Development, 20*(3), 145–163.

Gillman, M.W., Rifas-Shiman, S., Berkey, C.S., Field, A.E., & Colditz, G.A. (2003). Maternal Gestational Diabetes, Birth Weight, and Adolescent Obesity. *Pediatrics, 111*, e221–226.

Godfrey, K.M., & Barker, D.J. (2000a). Fetal nutrition and adult disease. *American Journal of Clinical Nutrition, 71*(5 Suppl), 1344S–1352S.

Godfrey, K.M., & Barker, D.J. (2000b). Fetal programming and adult health. *Public Health Nutrition, 4*(2B), 611–624.

Golan, M., Fainaru, M., & Weizman, A. (1998). Role of behavior modification in the treatment of childhood obesity with the parents as the exclusive agents of change. *International Journal of Obesity, 22*, 1217–1224.

Goodman, E., & Whitaker, R.C. (2002). A prospective study of the role of depression in the development and persistence of adolescent obesity. *Pediatrics, 110*(3), 497–504.

Gorn, G.J., & Goldberg, M.E. (1982). Behavioral evidence of the effects of televised food messages on children. *The Journal of Consumer Research, 9*(2), 200–205.

Gortmaker, S.L., Must, A., Sobol, A.M., Peterson, K., Colditz, G.A., & Dietz, W.H. (1996). Television viewing as a cause of increasing obesity among children in the United States, 1986–1990. *Archives of Pediatric and Adolescent Medicine, 150*(4), 356–362.

Gortmaker, S.L., et al. (1999). Reducing obesity via a school-based interdisciplinary intervention among youth: Planet Health. *Archives of Pediatrics and Adolescent Medicine, 153*(4), 409–418.

Hoelscher, D.M., Kelder, S.H., Murray, N., Cribb, P.W., Conroy, J., & Parcel, G.S. (2001). Dissemination and adoption of the Child and Adolescent Trial for Cardiovascular Health (CATCH): a case study in Texas. *Journal of Public Health Management Practice, 7*(2), 90–100.

Johnson, S.L., & Birch, I.L. (1994). Parents' and children's adiposity and eating style. *Pediatrics, 94*, 653–661.

Kiess, W., Galler, A., Reich, A., Muller, G., Kapellen, T., Deutscher, J., Raile, K., & Kratzsch, J. (2001). Clinical aspects of obesity in childhood and adolescence. *Obesity Reviews, 2*(1), 29–36.

Killen, J.D., Telch, M.J., & Robinson, J.N. et al. (1998). Cardiovascular disease reduction for tenth graders: A multiple factor school-based approach. *Journal of American Medical Association, 260*, 1728–33.

Kohl H.W., & Hobbs, K. (1997). Development of physical activity behaviors among children and adolescents. *Pediatrics, 101*, 549–554.

Kuczmarski, R.J., Ogden, C.L., Guo, S.S., Grummer-Strawn, L.M., Flegal, K.M., Mei, Z., Wei, R., Curtin, L.R., Roche, A.F., & Johnson, C.L. (2002). CDC growth charts for the United States: Methods and development. *Vital Health Statistics, 246*, 1–190.

Lakdawalla, D., & Philipson, T. (2002). The growth of obesity and technological change: A theoretical and empirical examination. National Bureau of Economic Research Working Paper W8946.

Maes, H.H.M., Neale, M.C., & Eaves, L.J. (1997). Genetic and environmental factors in relative body weight and human adiposity. *Behavior Genetics, 27*(4), 325–351.

Matheson, D.M., Killen, J.D., Wang, Y., Varady, A., & Robinson, T.N. (2004). Children's food consumption during television viewing. *American Journal of Clinical Nutrition, 79*(6), 1088–1094.

Mellin, L.M., Slinkard, L., & Irwin, C.E. (1987). Adolescent obesity intervention: Validation of the SHAPE-DOWN program. *Journal of the American Dietetic Association, 87*(3), 333–338.

Muller, M.J., Asbeck, I., Mast, M., Langnase, K., & Grund, A. (2001). Prevention of obesity- more than an intention. Concept and first results of the Kiel Obesity Prevention Study (KOPS). *International Journal of Obesity, 25*(1), 566–574.

Ogden, C.L., Flegal, K/M., Carroll, M.D., & Johnson, C.L. (2002). Prevalence and trends in overweight among US children and adolescents, 1999–2000. *Journal of the American Medical Association 288*, 1728–1732.

Ong, K., Ahmed, M.L., Emmett, P.M., Preece, M.A., & Dunger, D.B. (2000). Association between postnatal catch-up growth and obesity in childhood: prospective cohort study. *British Medical Journal, 320*(7240), 967–971.

Perusse, L., & Bouchard, C. (1999). Role of genetic factors in childhood obesity and in susceptibility to dietary variations. *Annals of Medicine, 31*(Suppl 1), 19–25.

Power, C., Lake, J.K., & Cole, T.J. (1997). Measurement and long-term health risks of child and adolescent fatness. *International Journal of Obesity, 21*, 507–526.

Proctor, M.H., Moore, L.L., Gao, D., Cupples, L.A., Brandlee, M.L., Hood, M.Y., & Ellison, R.C. (2003). Television viewing and change in body fat from preschool to early adolescence: The Framingham Children's Study. *International Journal of Obesity Related Metabolic Disorder, 27*(7), 827–833.

Ravelli, G. (1976). *Patterns of obesity and thinness prevalence in a national population of nineteen-year old men. Thesis.*

Robinson, T.N., Hammer, L.D., Killen, J.D., Kraemer, H.C., Wilson, D.M., Hayward, C., & Taylor, C.B. (1993). Does television viewing increase obesity and reduce physical activity? Cross-sectional and longitudinal analyses among adolescent girls. *Pediatrics, 91*(2), 499–501.

Robinson, T.N. (1999a). Behavioral treatment of childhood and adolescent obesity. *International Journal of Obesity, 23*(S2), S52–S57.

Robinson, T.N. (1999b). Reducing children's television viewing to prevent obesity. *Journal of American Medical Association, 282*(16), 1561–1567.

Rosenbloom, A.L., Joe, J.R., Young, R.S., & Winter, W.E. (1999). Emerging epidemic of type 2 diabetes in youth. *Diabetes Care, 22*(2), 345–354.

Sallis, J.F., McKenzie, T.L., Alcaraz, J.E., Kolody, B., Hovell, M.F., & Nader, P.R. (1993) Project SPARK: Effects of Physical Education on Adiposity in Children. *Annals New York Academy of Sciences, 699*, 127–136.

Schumacker, H., von Almen, T., Carlisle, L., & Udall, J. (2002). Committed to Kids: An integrated, 4-level team approach to weight management in adolescents. Journal of the American Dietetic Association. 102(3), S81–S85.

Sobal, J., & Stunkard, A.J. (1989). Socioeconomic status and obesity: a review of the literature. *Psychological Bulletin, 105*(2), 260–275.

Stettler, N., Zemel, B.S., Kumanyika, S., & Stallings, V.A. (2002). Infant weight gain and childhood overweight status in multicenter, cohort study. *Pediatrics, 109* (2), *194–199.*

Story, M. (1999). School Based approaches for preventing and treating obesity. *International Journal of Obesity,* 23(Suppl.2), S43–S51.

Story, M., Sherwood, N.E., et al. (2003). An after-school obesity prevention program for african-american girls: The minnesota GEMS pilot study. *Ethnicity & Disease, 13*, S1-54–S1-64.

Strauss, R., & Knight, J. (1999). Influence of the home environment on the development of obesity in children. *Pediatrics, 103*, e85.

Summerbell C.D., Ashton V., Campbell K.J., Edmunds L., Kelly, S., & Waters, E. (2004). Interventions for treating obesity in children (Cochrane Review). In: The Cochrane Library, Issue 3, 2004. Chichester, UK: John Wiley & Sons, Ltd.

Tirodkar, M.A., & Jain, A. (2003). Food messages on African American television shows. *American Journal of Public Health, 93*(3), 439–441.

Toschke, A.M., Montgomery, S.M., Pfeiffer, U., & von Kries, R. (2003). Early intrauterine exposure to tobacco-inhaled products and obesity. *American Journal of Epidemiology, 158*(11), 1068–1074.

von Kries, R., Toschke, A.M., Koletzko, B., & Slikker, W. (2002). Maternal smoking during pregnancy and childhood obesity. *American Journal of Epidemiology, 156*(10), 954–961.

Walker, L.L.M., Gately, P.J., Bewick, B.M., & Hill, A.J. (2003). Children's weight-loss camps: psychological benefit or jeopardy? *International Journal of Obesity, 27*, 748–754.

Wang, Y. (2001). Cross-national comparison of childhood obesity: the epidemic and the relationship between obesity and socioeconomic status. *International Journal of Epidemiology, 30*(5), 1129–1136.

Webber, L.S., Osganian, S.K., Feldman, H.A., et al. (1996). Cardiovascular risk factors among children after a 2 ½ year intervention- The CATCH Study. *Preventive Medicine, 25*(4), 432–441.

Whitaker, R.C., Pepe, M.S., Wright, J.A., Seidel, K.D., & Dietz, W.H. (1998). Early adiposity rebound and the risk of adult obesity. *Pediatrics, 101*(5).

Whitaker, R.C., & Dietz, W.H. (1998). The role of the prenatal environment in the development of obesity. *Journal of Pediatrics, 132*, 768–776.

Whitaker, R.C., Wright, J.A., Pepe, M.S., Seidel, K.D., & Dietz, W.H. (1997). Predicting obesity in young adulthood from childhood and parental obesity. *New England Journal of Medicine, 33*, 869–73.

Williams, S., Davie, G., & Lam, F. (1999). Predicting BMI in young adults from childhood data using two approaches to modeling adiposity rebound. *International Journal of Obesity and Related Metabolic Diosrders,* 23(4), 348–354.

Zametkin, A.J., Zoon, C., Klein, H., & Munson, S. (2004). Psychiatric aspects of child and adolescent obesity: A review of the past 10 years. *Journal of the American Academy of Child & Adolescent Psychiatry, 43*(2), 134–150.

Children, Teens, & Corporate America. Retrieved from—
http://www.angelfire.com/ms/MediaLiteracy/Demo.html
http://www.committed-to-kids.com/
www.cyberatlas.internet.com
http://members.aol.com/harx/child.html
http://www.nojunkfood.org/policy/success_snacks.html

Section III

Problem Behaviors

Chapter 19

Adolescent Delinquency
and Violent Behavior

Daniel J. Flannery, David Hussey, and Eric Jefferis

Introduction

Although juvenile arrests for violent crimes and victimization rates are on the decline, juveniles adjudicated as delinquent continue to be at substantial risk of perpetrating—and/or being the victims of—violent acts. In this chapter, we provide an overview of individual, family, and social factors related to risk for delinquency and violent behavior. This is followed by a summary of evidence-based treatment and preventive interventions. We begin with an overview of the scope of the problem followed by a developmental perspective on the etiology of delinquency and violence.

Juvenile Violence in Perspective

The United States is one of the more violent countries in the world, with a rate (1.66 per 100,000 population) for firearm-related deaths among children that is 2.7 times higher than the next closest country (Snyder & Sickmund, 1999). Increases through the mid-1990s in homicides were due mostly to increases in offending among males, and the increased use of firearms in the perpetration of homicide. Females, however, were not immune to the increase in violence, with arrests for violent crime increasing 125% among females between 1985 and 1991 (from 9,000 to 21,000 violent crime index arrests) compared to an increase of 67% for males during the same period.

Homicide by juveniles is most often committed with a gun. In 2001, the percentage of juvenile homicide victims older than 13 killed with a firearm was 72% (Snyder, 2003). For the period 1980–1997, a total of 88% of juvenile perpetrators of homicide were 15 years or older, 93% were male, and 56% were black. Over 90% of juvenile murderers kill someone of the same race. Males are much more likely to kill an acquaintance (54%) or a stranger (37%), while females are more likely to kill a family member (39% vs. 9%). Female adolescents are much more likely to use a knife (32%) or other violent means to kill (e.g., strangling) than use a gun (4%) (Snyder & Sickmund, 1999).

Since the early 1990s, violent crime rates in the United States have dropped significantly. Arrest rates for crimes perpetrated by juveniles have decreased 50% from 1993 to 2001, which includes a 10% reduction in the period 2000–2001 (Rennison, 2002). During 2001, the Violent Crime Index (consisting of murder and non-negligible manslaughter, forcible rape, robbery, and aggravated assault) fell to its lowest level since 1988, when arrests of youth between ages 10 and 17 dropped to 296 per 100,000 juveniles (Snyder, 2003). These significant declines have been linked to (1) reductions in violent crime in several large urban areas; (2) a decline in the use of firearms (down to 70% of all homicides from 82%); (3) a decrease in violent crime perpetrated by black males; and (4) declining rates of illicit substance use (Snyder & Sickmund, 1999). Though the declining trend appears to be promising, in 2001 juveniles still accounted for 12% of all violent crime arrests, 5% of arrests for murder, 12% of forcible rapes, 12% of aggravated assaults, and 14% of robberies (Snyder, 2003).

Blumstein (2002) and others (e.g., Cork, 1999; Lattimore et al., 1996) have attributed much of the rise and fall of homicide rates over the past two decades to the emergence and subsequent stabilization of the crack cocaine market in the 1980s and 1990s, and to a related increase in gun carrying by youth who were recruited into those crack markets. While the crack cocaine market may have stabilized, the increased lethality of firearms violence continues to plague youth in the United States (Fingerhut & Christoffel, 2002).

Etiology

The etiology of delinquent behavior and violence is complex and multidimensional. Current research suggests youth violence can best be understood from a developmental perspective because its origins are firmly rooted in early development and behavior (Tolan, Guerra & Kendall, 1995). These theoretical underpinnings also significantly influence the choice and type of treatment modality found to be effective. Three main findings consistently emerge in the literature on delinquency, crime, and violence:

1. Early onset of delinquency predicts later offending.
2. There is continuity in criminal behavior in that juvenile offenders are more likely to become adult offenders.
3. A small number of chronic juvenile offenders commit a significant portion of all crimes.

Early Onset

Early onset of childhood problems, specifically aggressive and disruptive behavior, is a significant and powerful risk factor for later antisocial behavior (Tremblay et al., 1992; Farrington, 1994). In fact, one of the most consistent findings throughout research is that aggression is a relatively stable and self-perpetuating behavior that often has origins in childhood (Olweus, 1979; Huesmann & Moise, 1999). Individual differences in social behavior related to aggression can be apparent before age 2 (Kagan, 1988) in the form of difficult temperament. By age 8, a child's aggressive behavior across situations can be relatively stable and predictive of adult aggression (Farrington, 1990) with the early onset of violent behaviors being predictive of similar or more serious behaviors over time (Farrington, 1991; Thornberry, Huizinga & Loeber, 1995).

Longitudinal research by Moffitt (1993) helped to conceptualize two types of delinquency patterns an early life-course persistent pattern and an adolescent-limited pattern. The early life-course group of children is characterized by early onset of delinquent behavior and persistent stability across time and settings. The adolescent limited pattern is characterized by both the onset and desistence of delinquent behaviors in adolescence. The *Diagnostic and Statistical Manual of Mental Disorders IV (DSM-IV)* makes a similar distinction in the childhood conduct disorder diagnosis by adding an early-onset specifier (i.e., childhood onset prior to age 10), calling attention to the particularly poor prognosis associated with the early onset of antisocial behaviors, and increased risk in adult life for antisocial personality disorder and substance-related disorders (APA, 1994). Since much behavioral consolidation takes place in the elementary school years, the early onset of childhood antisocial behavior is an important risk factor for prevention and intervention efforts.

Continuity

Habitual aggressive behavior is best understood as an interaction between individual predisposing factors and environmental influences often beginning early in development and continuing throughout adolescence and early adulthood. For example, boys who start their criminal careers in late childhood or early adolescence are at the greatest risk of becoming chronic offenders (Patterson, DeBarysne & Ramsey, 1989), with the continuity of childhood antisocial and aggressive behavior often continuing through adolescence and into adulthood (Farrington et al.,1990; Huesmann & Moise, 1999). Several longitudinal studies, spanning as much as 40 years across multiple western countries, lend support to the continuity of aggressive behavior (Farrington, 1990; McCord, 1983; Moffitt, 1990).

Chronicity

While researchers disagree on exact definitions and cut-off points for defining chronic juvenile offenders, evidence supports the basic assumption that chronic criminal behavior involves three related dimensions: (1) greater frequency of offending, (2) a wider variety or number of types of crimes, and (3) more serious acts (Farrington, 1991; Loeber, 1982). Many of the chronic, high-frequency offenders are also violent offenders (Loeber & Farrington, 1998). Those children displaying more frequent and serious antisocial behavior at younger ages tend to commit high numbers of offenses, including violent or serious offenses, over the longest periods of time (Farrington et al., 1990; Loeber, 1982; Tracy, Wolfgang & Figlio, 1990).

Developmental Pathways

Developmentally, the incidence and prevalence of serious delinquency and violence peak in adolescence and early adulthood and are more frequent among males than females (Elliott, 1994). A primary assumption of many delinquency theories is that serious problem behaviors unfold in an ordered fashion. Developmental pathway approaches help to link patterns such as early onset, continuity, and chronicity through conceptual formulations that integrate risk factors and problem behaviors with developmental sequences. Pathway research postulates that there is a series or trajectory of escalating behaviors leading from less serious to more serious offending. In analyzing the natural histories of children's antisocial and delinquent behavior, Loeber and colleagues have proposed three overlapping pathways of development toward delinquency—overt, covert, and the authority conflict pathway (Loeber et al., 1993; Loeber & Hay, 1994). The *overt pathway* involves acts that tend to be directly aggressive and include physical fighting and violence. The *covert pathway* involves acts that are less directly aggressive and more concealed such as stealing, lying, property damage, and theft. The *authority conflict pathway* is the earliest pathway, and involves such behaviors as defiance, disobedience, truancy, and running away. Pathway research supplies models for determining the relative risk for delinquent, antisocial behavior among subgroups of youth and helps in monitoring and evaluating interventions.

Risk and Resiliency Factors

The discussion now turns to individual, family, social, and community risk and resiliency factors. Risk factors are those aspects of an adolescent's life that are associated with an increased likelihood of poor outcomes, in this case risk of delinquency and violence, including behaviors that can threaten their overall health and well-being. Protective factors are those elements of a child's life that serve to increase the odds of a positive outcome such as not engaging in violent behavior (Blum, Beuhring & Rinehart, 2000). Protective factors are often simply the opposite of a risk factor. For example, having peers with pro-violence or delinquent attitudes is a risk factor for later delinquency. Conversely, associating with peers who exhibit anti-violence attitudes is a protective factor that reduces a youth's chance of later offending. Research has tended to focus on the risk factors associated with youth violence, and additional research is warranted into protective factors that mediate the effects of risk exposure (Hawkins et al., 1998). While it is often the case that risk and protective factors are mirror images of one another, the reader is cautioned against assuming that is always the case. Our understanding of protective factors and how they operate is still relatively new, particularly with respect to how these factors may mediate or moderate the effects of multiple risk factors and the developmental course of delinquent and violent behavior.

Individual Factors

Risk-factor explanations for delinquency and crime involve complex person–environment interactions across individual, family, peer, school, and community levels. Individual level factors for delinquency and criminal offending include psychological and biological characteristics identifiable in children at a young age. From the individual-level perspective, risk factors for delinquency and criminal offending include premature birth (Raine, Brennan & Mednick, 1994), male gender (Elliott, 1993), low verbal IQ (Huesmann, Eron, Leftkowitz & Walder, 1984), hyperactivity-impulsivity-and-attention-deficit constellations (HIA) (Farrington, et al., 1990), severe aggressiveness and early conduct problems (Thornberry, Huizinga & Loeber 1995), exposure to violence and victimization (Flannery, Singer & Wester, 2001; Thornberry, 1994; Widom, 1989), and substance use (Leukefeld et al., 1998).

Research on social-cognitive deficits has identified differences in how aggressive children encode and process information, including the attribution of hostile intent and lack of social-problem solving capacities (Huesmann et al., 1984; Lochman & Dodge, 1994). Children repeatedly exposed to violence may tend to be "hypervigilant," expect the worst, and respond aggressively to *perceived* hostility from peers or authority figures. Violence-exposed children may not have control of their reactions in situations in which they feel threatened or fearful. Consequently, they may act aggressively, without thinking, based on their misperceptions about the intentions of others.

Research on biological factors related to antisocial and aggressive behavior has examined several key factors, including genetics, hormones, and neurotransmitters. Antisocial personality seems to "run" in families, regardless of gender (Plomin, Nitz & Rowe, 1990) even without environmental transfer from parent to child. Hormone studies indicate that testosterone levels both influence and result from aggression for males (Susman & Ponirakis, 1997; Tremblay et al., 1997). Hormone levels act on sensory systems in the body, increasing or decreasing the potential for instigating a behavior. Social and physiological contexts can affect how hormones interact with behavior, such as environmental events that cause secretion of testosterone through arousal associated with stressful experiences. In a similar manner, low levels of the neurotransmitter serotonin seem to be associated with high levels of aggression, and adverse social environments may have a negative impact on serotonin function and aggression (Simon & Coccaro, 1999). As biological factors are beginning to be teased out with regard to aspects of delinquency, it is evident that more research is needed—especially on female adolescents.

Exposure to violence has been linked to a number of mental health and behavioral sequelae, including increased depression (Freeman, Mokros & Poznaski, 1993), stress (Lorion & Saltzman, 1993), fears and worries (Freeman et al., 1993), aggression (Rivera & Widom, 1990), anxiety (Singer et al., 1995), low self-esteem (Sturkie & Flanzer, 1987), post-traumatic stress (Davies & Flannery, 1998), and self-destructive behaviors (Rivara et al., 1992). These sequelae have significant effects on children's functioning at home and school, and can significantly impair a child's developmental course, adaptation, and functioning later in life.

Children and adolescents victimized by family violence are also at increased risk for perpetrating violence later in life. Thornberry (1994) showed that adolescents who had been direct victims of child maltreatment were more likely to report involvement in youth violence than non-maltreated subjects. Similarly, he showed that adolescents growing up in homes exhibiting partner violence, generalized hostility, or child maltreatment also had higher rates of self-reported violence.

Results from studies examining the relationship between violence exposure and delinquent behavior suggest that violent delinquents are more likely than nonviolent delinquents and controls to have experienced physical abuse (Rivara & Widom, 1990; Thornberry, 1994). One prospective study of young children demonstrated that the experience of physical abuse was a risk factor for the development of aggressive behaviors. Children exposed to such abuse were more likely to acquire deficient patterns of information processing compared to unexposed children (Dodge, Bates & Petit, 1990). Several other studies also concluded that being a witness or victim of violence, including intrafamilial abuse, was associated with self-reported violence and delinquency (Flannery, Singer, Williams & Castro, 1998; Kaufman & Cicchetti, 1989). Adolescents victimized by violence at home are also more likely to join a gang, especially for perceived protection (Chesney-Lind & Brown, 1999). Rather than serving as a vehicle for protection, being a member of a gang increases one's chances of being a victim of violence and increases an adolescent's opportunity to engage in delinquent activity (Huff, 1996a,b).

There is substantial comorbidity and overlap between antisocial behavior and delinquency and drug abuse, exposure to violence and victimization, mental health problems, and school problems (Thornberry, Huizinga & Loeber, 1995). Both delinquents and adolescent drug abusers are more likely to display low levels of educational achievement, disorganized family structure, and conflict problems (Hawkins, Catalano, & Brewer, 1995) and have histories of childhood aggression that are predictive of frequent drug use and delinquency (O'Donnell, Hawkins & Abbott, 1995). Children diagnosed with disruptive behavior disorders are at increased risk for aggressive behavior (Huesmann & Moise, 1999; Moffitt, 1990). In general, delinquents have a higher prevalence of psychological problems than non-delinquent youth (Flannery, Singer & Wester, 2001; Huizinga & Jakob-Chien, 1998), with the most violent delinquents scoring higher on externalizing symptoms and aggressive behavior.

The individual level effects of race and ethnicity on serious violent juvenile offending have long been debated by researchers (Hawkins, Laub, & Lauritsen, 1998). Significant racial and ethnic differences in the rates at which juveniles offend have been found since the early 1900s. The pattern that emerges from a review of studies that examined racial effects is that of a consistent difference in rates of violence (Lafree, 1995), with black juveniles offending at a much higher rate. While it is noteworthy that various measures of juvenile crime rates (i.e., official statistics, self-report, and victimization surveys) each have limitations, reporting differences alone cannot account for the fact that black youths were more than seven times more likely to be arrested for homicide in 1992 than were their white counterparts (Hawkins, Laub & Lauritsen, 1998). The disproportional nature of black to white violent crime arrest rates has declined significantly during the past two decades. In 1980, black juveniles' violent crime arrest rates were 6.3 times higher than those of their white juveniles counterparts. By 2001, the rate at which black youth were arrested for violent crimes had dropped to 3.6 times that of white youth (Snyder, 2003).

Although racial disparities in official reports of juvenile offending appear to be on the decline, differences remain that will likely continue to spur theoretical and policy debate. Current criminological theories of the causes of crime and criminal behavior have failed to address such differences adequately (Hawkins, Laub & Lauritsen, 1998). Explanations for the differences likely lie not only in substantial reporting differences across data sources (Hawkins et al., 1998), but also in the substantial interrelationships that exist amongst juveniles' race, income, and family structures (Blum et al., 2000). In their assessment of research regarding racial difference in serious juvenile offending, Hawkins et al. (1998) suggest that much extant literature is flawed because individual level correlations are often confounded with community level effects. Ecological conditions rather than individual differences can perhaps better explain the disproportionate rate at which black youth are committing serious delinquent acts. Individual-level economic disadvantage is often studied, for example, but it is an inappropriate proxy for community-level socioeconomic disparity, which is rarely measured. In sum, the extent to which black juveniles are disproportionately violent offenders has decreased in recent years, but they continue to be over-represented. Explanations for these disparities need additional research and more fully developed theoretical models. Well-constructed ecological factors are likely to reveal much about the causal mechanisms for this phenomenon.

Hawkins et al. (1998) provide us an important reminder that disparities in arrest rates historically have existed as other ethnic groups, including white ethnic groups from Europe, immigrated to the United States and became assimilated to the society. Blum et al. (2000) found that black male and Hispanic female youth wanting and expecting to attend college are protected from risk of involvement with weapon-related violence. This finding is consistent with earlier research that found educational expectations were a better predictor of delinquency than the difference between education aspirations and expectations (Farnworth & Lieber, 1989). Perhaps among these groups, belief in the ability to attain a higher social/economic status through higher education, which is vital to the "American dream," serves to partially mediate the wide-ranging risk factors discussed above.

Summary

Children and adolescents exposed to violence, particularly family violence, have an increased risk for becoming violent offenders. Juvenile delinquents, in general, have a higher prevalence of mental health problems than non-delinquents. Violent juvenile offenders are more likely to have been exposed to violence and physical abuse than non-delinquent and control adolescents. Although the disparity in arrest rates between black and white juveniles has been declining, the over-representation of minorities amongst violent offenders is still an important topic of discussion.

Family Factors

Family factors associated with the development of violent and offending behavior involve an array of characteristics and aggressive behaviors (McCord, 1979; Maguin et al., 1995). Since much of aggression is learned from interactions with others and the environment (Dodge et al., 1990; Huesmann & Eron, 1989), aggression can be taught by parents through models of behavior, reinforcement, and home conditions that frustrate or victimize the child (Patterson, DeBarysne & Ramsey, 1989). Family risk factors include child maltreatment, parental antisocial behavior and criminality, poor family management practices, harsh or inconsistent discipline, poor parent child relations, parental rejection, and having a delinquent sibling (Eron, Huesmann & Zelli, 1991; Maguin et al., 1995; Widom, 1989). Antisocial parents are at increased risk for rearing antisocial children and employing ineffective behavior management strategies that reward negative behavior (Patterson et al., 1989). Family stressors such as unemployment, family violence, marital discord, and divorce are also associated with delinquency (Patterson et al., 1989; McCord, 1979). Developmentally, much of learned aggression and behavior is established early on (Eron et al., 1991) and often nested in specific cultural and community contexts.

In an early study of children at risk who were resilient, or able to avoid serious trouble in the face of significant adversity, Masten (1994) found that the most important protective factor is a strong bond with a competent and caring prosocial adult. Blum et al. (2000) and colleagues (Resnick et al., 1997) provide strong evidence of the protective nature of positive youth–parent relationships using the nationally representative National Longitudinal Study of Adolescent Health data. While it is not surprising that strong positive relationships with a parent or caregiver serves to reduce an adolescent's chance of engaging in delinquency and violence, it is interesting that this factor was found the most consistent across sex, race, and ethnic groups, with white females being the exception. Other familial protective factors identified by Blum et al. (2000) include (1) joint decision-making for some black males and black females, (2) extended family in the homes for Hispanic males, and (3) frequency with which a parent is present at dinner for black males.

Social and Community Factors

Peers

Negative peer influences also contribute to the risk for aggressive, delinquent, and violent behavior. Children who display antisocial tendencies at an early age are more likely to be rejected by their peers because of their aggressive and coercive behaviors. Antisocial behavior and peer rejection then serve as risk factors for promoting later deviant peer associations (Patterson et al., 1989). As children age, peer versus family influences take on increasing importance in contributing to delinquency and criminal behavior. Peer groups appear to be a place for consolidation of negative and aggressive behaviors for youth already headed in that direction (Loeber & Hay, 1994). Association with antisocial peers may further contribute to the escalation of antisocial behaviors, including substance abuse, delinquency (Farrington & Hawkins, 1991), and school failure. Negative peer associations via gang involvement also significantly increase the possibility of more serious antisocial behavior (Huff, 1996b; Thornberry et al., 1995). Like positive parental relationships, positive peer relationships can also serve as a protective factor. Ageton (1983) and Elliott (1994) have found that having peers who disapprove of violence serves to inhibit youths' likelihood of committing violent acts.

School Factors

Eighty percent or more of serious delinquent youth had one or more school problems, including suspension, truancy, poor academic achievement, and drop out (Huizinga & Jakob-Chien, 1998). School problems are common and powerful correlates to delinquency, and their relationship has been well documented (Gottfredson, 1981; Maguin & Loeber, 1996). There is substantial overlap, for example, between truancy, suspension, and serious delinquency (Huizinga & Jakob-Chien, 1998). The nature and the direction of the relationship, however, between delinquency and poor academic achievement is unclear. Some longitudinal data have shown that poor school achievement predicts juvenile delinquency (Farrington, 1987), specifically through its association with disruptive behavior (Tremblay et al., 1992).

The school environment itself can also be a risk factor that fosters noncompliance, aggression, delinquency, and violence. Disorganized school structures with lax discipline and enforcement of rules, crowded physical space, and lack of conformity to behavior routines can increase the propensity toward aggression and violence (Flannery, 1997; Gottfredson, 1981; Guerra, Huesmann, Tolan, Acker & Eron, 1995). Outside of the school environment, unsupervised after-school time is a key risk factor that has been associated with increased delinquency, substance abuse, and association with deviant peers (Flannery, Williams & Vazsonyi, 1999).

Community Factors

Neighborhood and community factors that influence delinquency development include poverty, gang involvement, availability of drugs (Maguin et al., 1995), the presence of violence or high crime rates (Gottfredson & Hirschi, 1990; Sampson, Raudenbush & Earls, 1997), and low neighborhood attachment and social disorganization (Maguin et al., 1995; Sampson & Lauritsen, 1994). These factors can be addressed by large-scale multilevel programs that can effectively mobilize and organize community structures (Hawkins & Catalano, 1992).

While many factors are associated with youth violence and criminal activity, longitudinal research on risk factors and developmental pathways has helped to identify a common set of predictive factors associated with the etiology and progression of delinquent behaviors. The general goal of most prevention and intervention models is to reduce such risk factors and enhance protective factors across multiple life domains (i.e., individual, family, peer, situational, and community). Therefore, it is difficult to separate pure prevention strategies from intervention strategies because in theory as well as practice they are often integrated to address multiple-need populations across different contexts. Likewise, it is difficult to separate early aggressive behavior from delinquency because childhood aggression is one of the strongest antecedents of delinquency, and therefore is targeted by most delinquency prevention and intervention programs. In reviewing the evidence for effective delinquency intervention, we focus on community and residential settings, briefly describing programs or interventions that have the strongest empirical support, followed by those that are particularly promising, and then those that don't work. In addition, due to the strong developmental relationship between aggression and delinquency, and the need for early intervention, we will briefly discuss effective prevention programs.

Evidence-Based Treatment Interventions in Community Settings

What Works

Multisystemic Therapy (MST) is an intensive family- and community-based treatment that addresses the multiple determinants of serious antisocial behavior in juvenile offenders. The multisystemic approach views individuals within a complex network of interconnected systems that encompass individual, family, and community factors. Intervention may be necessary in any one or a combination of systems including peer and school networks.

Multisystemic Therapy targets chronic, violent, or substance-abusing male or female juvenile offenders, aged 12–17, at risk of out-of-home placement, and their families. Multisystemic Therapy is a family-based model that addresses multiple factors related to delinquency across the key ecological settings. It promotes behavior change in the youth's natural environment, using a strengths-based approach to facilitate change. Multisystemic Therapy interventions are based on nine core principles designed to empower parents with the skills and resources needed to address the difficulties that arise in raising youth and to empower youth to cope with family, peer, school, and neighborhood problems. The therapist helps the family to develop skills and supports to help the adolescent to behave responsibly. Intervention strategies are integrated into the social ecology of the youth and include strategic family therapy, behavioral parent training, and cognitive-behavioral approaches. Contingencies and incentives are established for appropriate peer relationships and behaviors, and specific evidence-based treatments can be integrated into the overall model to target discreet problem behaviors. Critical service characteristics include low caseloads (5:1 family to clinician ratio), intensive and comprehensive services (2–15 hours per week) available 24 hours per day 7 days a week, and time-limited treatment duration (four to six months) (Henggeler, 1999). Treatment adherence and fidelity are key ingredients for achieving long-term, sustained effects and decreasing drug use.

Evaluations of MST for serious juvenile offenders have demonstrated reductions in long-term rates of re-arrest, reductions in out-of-home placements, improvements in family functioning, and decreased mental health problems for serious juvenile offenders (Henggeler, 1999; Henggeler, Mihalic, Rone, Thomas & Timmons-Mitchell, 1998).

Functional Family Therapy (FFT) is a family-based intervention program that targets youth between the ages of 11 and 18 who are at risk for and/or presenting with delinquency, violent or disruptive behavior, or substance use. Functional Family Therapy has been successfully used as both a prevention and intervention model for at-risk adolescents. It is time limited, averaging 8–12 sessions for referred youth and their families, with generally no more than 30 hours of direct service time for more difficult cases. Functional Family Therapy is a flexible service-delivery model, utilizing one- and two-person teams to work with clients in the home, clinic, and juvenile court, and at time of re-entry from institutional placement. Functional Family Therapy has employed a wide range of practitioners, including paraprofessionals under supervision, trained probation officers, mental health technicians, and degreed mental health professionals. Over the past 30 years, FFT has evolved in several iterations. Like MST, FFT is multisytemic and multilevel in nature, addressing individual, family, and treatment system dynamics. Functional Family Therapy targets enhancing protective factors and reducing risk, including the risk of treatment termination. It is stepwise and has three specific intervention phases: engagement and motivation, behavior change, and generalization. Assessment is an ongoing and multifaceted part of each phase.

Aside from effectively treating aggressive, delinquent, and disruptive youth, FFT has also been successfully used for teens with substance abuse problems. Other notable effects relate to reducing youth's penetration and progression through other service systems, particularly more restrictive and higher-cost services (Alexander et al., 1998; Sexton & Alexander, 2000).

Multidimensional Treatment Foster Care (MTFC) is a cost-effective alternative to group or residential treatment, incarceration, and hospitalization for adolescents who have problems with chronic antisocial behavior, emotional disturbance, and delinquency. Community families are recruited, trained, and closely supervised to provide MTFC-placed adolescents with treatment and intensive supervision at home, in school, and in the community. Important elements of MTFC include the use of clear and consistent limits with follow-through on consequences, positive reinforcement for appropriate behavior, a relationship with a mentoring adult, and separation from delinquent peers.

MTFC targets teenagers with histories of chronic and serious criminal behavior at risk of incarceration. The program emphasizes behavior management methods to provide youth with a structured and therapeutic living environment. Parents receive pre-service training, supervision, and attend weekly group meetings run by a program case manager. Additional supervision and support is also given during daily telephone calls to check on youth progress and functioning. During placement, the youth's biologic (or adoptive) family maintains contact with their child through supervised home visits and frequent contact with the MTFC case manager regarding their child's progress. In addition, they also receive family therapy with the ultimate goal of returning the youth back to the home. Continuity is maintained because biologic parents are taught to use the same type of structured behavior management system being used in the MTFC home. Other important contacts are maintained between the MTFC case manager and teachers, probation officers, and other key individuals in the youth's life. Evaluations of MTFC have demonstrated that program youth compared to control group youth are stepped down from restrictive placements quicker, spend fewer days incarcerated at 12-month follow-up, and have fewer subsequent arrests (Chamberlain, 1998; Chamberlain & Reid, 1998).

What Might Work

Brief Strategic Family Therapy (BSFT) is a brief (approximately 12–15 sessions over three months) family-based intervention for children and youth aged 6–17 who are at risk for substance abuse and behavior problems. BSFT employs a structural family framework and focuses on improving family interactions. Therapists coach families to improve interactions contributing to youth problem behavior. Major techniques include joining the family and organizing a team; diagnosing family strengths, problem situations, and interactions; and restructuring these interactions to attain positive levels of family competence and functioning. Evaluation results demonstrate reductions in substance abuse, conduct problems, associations with antisocial peers, and improvements in family functioning (Robbins & Szapocznik, 2000).

What Does Not Work

Since probation is the major intervention tool of the juvenile court, it is important to discuss briefly intensive protective supervision models. Intensive protective supervision models remove or divert juvenile offenders from criminal justice institutions and provide them with more proactive and extensive community supervision than they would otherwise receive. While many different types of intensive juvenile supervision models exits, the results thus far have been disappointing to mixed. Clearly, further program development and research in this area is needed due to the prominence of this mode of intervention in managing juvenile delinquents.

Another, and perhaps one of the best-known, failed prevention efforts is "Scared Straight" and similar prison-based deterrence programs (Finckenauer, 1982; Petrosino, Turpin-Petrosino & Buehler, 2003). Scared Straight was started in the 1970s by a group of inmates in New Jersey who were serving life sentences. The program primarily involves a "scary" presentation by the inmates to youth who visit the facility, depicting various difficulties of prison life, including rape and other acts of violence. Despite a great deal of positive press coverage and anecdotal indicators of success, the program has been found ineffective in deterring juvenile delinquency among participating youth (Finckenauer, 1982).

Recently, Petrosino et al. (2003) conducted a meta-analysis of seven randomized studies of prison deterrence programs. Their meta-analysis revealed not only that these types of programs were ineffective, but that they were actually associated with *increases* in post-intervention offending rates (Petrosino et al., 2003). Findings such as these clearly demonstrate the need for rigorous evaluations of all prevention efforts to assure that the end result of the intervention is not more harm than good.

Evidence-Based Treatment Interventions in Residential Settings

What Works

Theoretically, rehabilitation has been the focus of correctional programs for juveniles. Yet, in general, treatment in public facilities and custodial institutions is less effective than other community alternatives. On a practice level, juvenile intervention programs are often poorly implemented, similar to adult correctional treatment programming. Additionally, given the large number of delinquents and offenders who pass through residential and institutional facilities, there are a relatively small number of evaluations that test appropriately matched treatments that have been clearly explicated and tested with sufficient research rigor. The majority of the program-specific studies that do exist are over 20 years old (Lipsey, Wilson & Cothern, 2000), and lack multiple replications with randomized control groups. Given this, it is more informative to identify general treatment principles that are useful in designing and evaluating rehabilitation programs in institutional settings. According to MacKenzie's review of crime prevention (1997), the following are principles of effective rehabilitation programs: structured and focused, use of multiple treatment components, focus on developing skills (social skills, academic, and employment skills) and use behavioral (including cognitive-behavioral) methods (with reinforcements for clearly identified, overt behaviors as opposed to non-directive counseling focusing on insight, self esteem, or disclosure), and provision of substantial, meaningful contact between qualified treatment personnel and the participants. The treatment provided to offenders must be of sufficient dosage (intensity) and integrity to insure that what is delivered is consistent with the planned design of a preferably theoretically based model. For example, with adults, prison-based therapeutic drug treatment is effective in reducing the future criminal activities of offenders. These intensive, behaviorally based substance abuse programs target offenders' drug use, a behavior that is clearly associated with criminal activities.

What Might Work

Two promising programs for juveniles that demonstrate the above principles are worth mentioning. First, the *Residential Student Assistance Program* (RSAP) is a residentially based substance abuse program for high-risk youth aged 14–17. This program uses trained professionals to provide individual and group substance abuse prevention and early intervention services to youth in residential facilities. This program has been recognized as a model program by the Substance Abuse and Mental Health Services Administration (SAMHSA), U.S. Department of Health and Human Services. Second, *Aggression Replacement Training* (ART), combines social skill training, or structured learning, with anger management training and moral education (Goldstein & Glick, 1987). ART has been used in schools as well as detention facilities. Therapist modeling and group role playing are used to observe and practice the development of social skills such as identifying problems, stating complaints, and resisting group pressure. Anger control training involves using self-talk to decrease aggressive and impulsive behaviors. Three randomized controlled studies found that youth improved social skills (Goldstein & Glick, 1987), however, behavioral improvement was mixed (Coleman, Pfeiffer & Oakland, 1992). A more recent model, *Equipping Youth to Help One Another Program* (EQUIP), combines ART with Positive Peer Culture (PPC). In one randomized controlled study, detention youth showed significant improvements in social skills and conduct and were less likely to recidivate within 12 months compared to controls (Leeman, Gibbs & Fuller, 1993).

What Does Not Work

Those involved in the treatment of adjudicated youth commonly encounter youth sentenced to traditional incarceration then parole as a path to rehabilitation. Lipsey (1992) noted that studies of poorly implemented rehabilitation programs given to low-risk offenders using vague behavioral targets were not found to be effective in reducing crime. Nor were programs that emphasized characteristics such as discipline, structure, challenge, and self-esteem that are not directly associated the offender's criminal behavior. These deterrence types of programs such as wilderness programs, boot camps, and Scared Straight, while popular with the media or the general public, do not generally guarantee lower recidivism rates for program participants (Flash, 2003; Lipsey, 1992; MacKenzie, 1997). *Boot camps* have a narrow focus on such things as physical discipline in a group environment where other delinquent youth may model and reinforce negative behaviors. As discussed earlier, Scared Straight involves brief encounters with inmates who detail the harshness and brutalities of prison life in order to deter youth from criminal behaviors. A reasonable number of evaluations demonstrate that these programs do not have an impact on the recidivism rates of offenders (MacKenzie, 1997).

Psychopharmacology

Juvenile aggressive behavior often overlaps with other problems such as drug addiction and mental health problems (Huizinga & Jakob-Chien, 1998; Tardiff, 1999). A single psychopharmacological remedy for juvenile violence does not exist, since there are various causes of violent behavior. The psychological disorders which are associated with youth violence are, however, often responsive to drug treatment.

Empirical studies have consistently found a co-occurrence between violent juvenile offending and drug use, with more violent offending being associated with more serious drug use (Huizinga & Jakob-Chien, 1998). Commonly abused substances which have been found to be associated with violent behavior include stimulants, hallucinogens, amphetamines, inhalants, and alcohol. For example, the stimulant cocaine causes intoxication which is initially manifested as euphoria, but can change to other states such as irritability and violent behavior. Chronic cocaine use can also result in paranoid delusional thinking, manic-like delirium, and severe violence (Tardiff, 1999).

Less is known empirically about the extent to which serious violent juvenile offending co-occurs with mental health problems. Of the few studies in this area, most have been hindered by unrepresentative samples (Huizinga & Jakob-Chien, 1998). Huizinga & Jakob-Chien (1998) addressed the problem of a representative sample with their analysis of Denver Youth Survey (DYS) data. They found significant co-occurrences of delinquency with psychological problems such as depression, obsessive-compulsiveness, and externalizing problems. Interestingly, both violent and non-violent juveniles demonstrated higher incidence of mental illness than did the non-delinquent group. Tardiff (1999) provides a concise review of psychiatric disorders associated with violence—including antisocial and borderline personality disorders, schizophrenia, and organic brain disorders such as temporal lobe epilepsy, head trauma, and various infections of the brain.

Short-term psychopharmacological treatments for psychotic patients who may need immediate treatment include a variety of antipsychotics and antianxiety drugs (Tardiff, 1999). Psychostimulants such as amphetamines have also shown promise in the long-term reduction of violence associated with attention-deficit/hyperactivity disorder. Several other long-term medications such as lithium, beta blockers, and anticonvulsants have tentatively proven effective in reducing violence amongst patients, particularly when paired with psychotherapy and social interventions.

The Prevention of Delinquency and Violent Behavior

What Works

Most prevention models are either family-based or school-based. A comprehensive review of all prevention programs is beyond the scope of this chapter, but we have included a table of key resources in this arena (Table 1). While there are a number of family-based home visitation models, the premiere model in terms of effectiveness is the *Nurse Family Partnership* (NFP). The Nurse Family Partnership consists of intensive home visitation by nurses for low-income, at-risk pregnant women during their first pregnancy and for the first two years after the birth of their child. The program is designed to help women improve pregnancy outcomes, infant and toddler care, and maternal health and development, including educational and vocational achievement, as well as prevent future unplanned pregnancies. NFP has demonstrated effectiveness in both white and African American families in rural and urban settings. A 15-year follow-up of low-income, teenage mothers in whom this

Table 1. Key Resources

Title	Authors & Institutions		URL
Blueprints for Violence Prevention	Center for the Study and Prevention of Violence	University of Colorado	http://www.colorado.edu/cspv/blueprints/
Exemplary and Promising Safe, Disciplined, and Drug-Free Schools Programs (U.S. Dept. of Education, 2001)	Safe, Disciplined, and Drug-Free Schools Expert Panel	U.S. Department of Education	*http://www.ed.gov/adminis/lead/safety/* exemplary01/exemplary01.pdf
Preventing Crime, What Works, What Doesn't, What's Promising	A Report to the United States Congress Prepared for the National Institute of Justice	Department of Criminology and Criminal Justice, University of Maryland	http://www.ncjrs.org/works/
SAMHSA Model Programs	Substance Abuse and Mental Health Services Administration	Department of Health and Human Services	*http://modelprograms.samhsa.gov/* template.cfm?page=default
Title V Model Programs Guide and Database	Development Services Group, Inc.		http://www.dsgonline.com/index.html
Youth Violence: A Report of the Surgeon General	U.S. Department of Health and Human Services, Centers for Disease Control and Prevention, National Center for Injury Prevention,	Substance Abuse and Mental health Services Administration, Center for Mental Health Services, and National Institutes of Health, National Institute of Mental Health	*http://www.surgeongeneral.gov/library/* youthviolence/toc.html

intervention was implemented in Elmira, New York, showed 69% fewer maternal arrests, 60% fewer instances of running away on the part of 15–year-old children, 56% fewer arrests on the part of the 15-year-old children, and 56% fewer days of alcohol consumption on the part of the 15-year-old children. (Olds, Hill, Mihalic & O'Brien, 1998).

Promoting Alternative Thinking Strategies (PATHS) is a multiyear, universal, school-based curriculum implemented by teachers and counselors. PATHS develops social and emotional competencies in elementary school-aged children ideally beginning at entry into school and involving and continuing through fifth grade. Teachers lead 20–30-minute sessions three times per week, helping children to identify, manage, and regulate feelings, while developing perspective-taking and problem-solving skills. PATHS has been effectively utilized with both regular education and special education students. Evaluation results have demonstrated reductions in childhood aggression, conduct problems, depression, and improved self-control (Greenberg, Kusché & Mihalic, 1998).

What Might Work

Fast Track is a comprehensive and long-term school-based intervention to reduce conduct disorders. Fast Track targets high-risk children identified in kindergarten for disruptive behavior and poor social skills. The program extends from first through tenth grade with a focus on transitions and the most intensive interventions taking place in first grade. Fast Track integrates five intervention components designed to promote competencies in the family, child, and school that deter subsequent delinquent behavior. The program involves training for parents in family management practices; frequent home visits by program staff to reinforce skills learned in the training, promote parental feelings of efficacy, and enhance family organization; social skills coaching for children delivered by program staff and based on effective models described earlier; academic tutoring for children three times per week; and a classroom instructional program focusing on social competency skills coupled with classroom management strategies for the teacher. Fast Track has demonstrated effectiveness in reducing aggression and conduct problems as well as associations with deviant peers for students of diverse demographic backgrounds, including sex, ethnicity, social class, and family composition (Conduct Problems Prevention Research Group, 2002; U.S. Department of Health and Human Services, 2001).

LINKING THE INTERESTS OF FAMILIES AND TEACHERS (LIFT)/GOOD BEHAVIOR GAME. Linking the Interests of Families and Teachers is an elementary school-based prevention program that targets antecedents of youth delinquency and violence. LIFT combines school-based skills training with parent training for 1st and 5th graders using twenty one-hour sessions over 10 weeks. LIFT utilizes a playground peer component to encourage positive social behavior and a 6-week group parent-training component. The program focuses on reducing antisocial behavior, alcohol and drug use, and involvement with delinquent peers (Eddy, Reid & Fetrow, 2000). A classroom-based component of LIFT is the Good Behavior Game. The Good Behavior Game uses classroom behavior management as the primary strategy to improve on-task behavior and decrease aggressive behavior. In short-term evaluations (Reid, Eddy, Fetrow & Stoolmiller, 1999; U.S. Department of Health and Human Services, 2001), LIFT decreased children's physical aggression on the playground, increased children's social skills, and decreased aversive behavior in mothers rated most aversive at baseline, relative to controls. Three years after participation in the program, 1st-grade participants had fewer increases in attention-deficit disorder-related behaviors (inattentiveness, impulsivity, and hyperactivity) than controls. At follow-up, 5th-grade participants had fewer associations with delinquent peers, were less likely to initiate patterned alcohol use, and were significantly less likely than controls to have been arrested. For the Good Behavior Game, teacher reports have identified positive reductions in aggressive and shy behaviors for first-graders (U.S. DHHS, 2001; Kellam, Ling, Merisca, Brown & Ialongo, 1998).

SEATTLE SOCIAL DEVELOPMENT PROJECT (SSDP). Seattle Social Development Project is a universal, multidimensional intervention that targets both general and high-risk youth in elementary and middle school. The program utilizes teacher and parent training, emphasizing classroom management for teachers, and conflict management, problem-solving, and refusal skills for children. Parents receive optional training programs targeting rules, communication, and strategies to support their child's academic success. Evaluations of the Seattle Social Development Project demonstrate reductions at the end of grade 2 in aggression, antisocial and externalizing behaviors, and self-destructive behaviors in children who participated in the program during the first and second grades. Other benefits of the program include lower rates of alcohol and delinquency initiation, improvements in family management practices and parent–child relationships, greater attachment and commitment to school, and less involvement with antisocial peers. Follow-up at age 18 shows that the Seattle Social Development Project significantly improves long-term attachment and commitment to school and school achievement and reduces rates of self-reported violent acts and heavy alcohol use. At follow-up, students who received the full intervention were also less likely than controls to be sexually active and to have had multiple sex partners. Replications of this program have confirmed its benefits in both general and high-risk populations of youths. (O'Donnell, Hawkins, Catalano, Abbot & Day, 1995; U.S. DHHS, 2001).

SECOND STEP: A VIOLENCE PREVENTION CURRICULUM. The Second Step is a classroom-based Curriculum for preschool through junior high school students (i.e., ages 4–14) that attempts to reduce impulsive, high-risk, and aggressive behaviors while increasing socioemotional competence and protective factors. The curriculum teaches three core competencies: empathy, impulse control and problem-solving, and anger management. Students participate in 20–50-minute sessions two to three times per week where they practice social skills. Elementary school parents can participate in a six-session training that familiarizes them with the content in the children's curriculum. Teachers also learn how to deal with disruptions and behavior management issues. Evaluation results demonstrate that preschool and elementary school students were less physically aggressive and displayed more positive social interactions than controls (Grossman et al., 1997; McMahon, Washburn, Felix, Yakin & Childrey, 2000).

The Strengthening Families Program for Parents Youth 10–14 is an adaptation of the Strengthening Families Program (ages 6–12) and was formerly called the Iowa Strengthening Families Program. The Strengthening Families Program is a universal family-based intervention designed to reduce substance abuse and behavioral problems with children aged 10–14. The curriculum concentrates on helping parents improve nurturing and child management skills, and helping youth to improve prosocial skills. The program consists of 7 two-hour sessions for parents and youth split between separate skill building sessions and combined (i.e., parent and child) family activities. Four booster sessions are added six months and one year after the initial series of seven sessions to reinforce previously learned skills. A five-year longitudinal evaluation found that experimental group youth had statistically significant reductions in conduct problems and substance abuse (Molgaard, Spoth & Redmond, 2000).

What Does Not Work

Like Scared Straight, some prevention programs are widely popular and persist despite substantial research evidence that they are ineffective. The *Drug Abuse Resistance Education (DARE) program* is a well-known example of a widely used school-based drug use prevention effort that has met with a lack of success (General Accounting Office, 2003). Although it has continuously expanded in scope, the original DARE program involved uniformed police officers teaching a core curriculum of 17 hour-long drug resistance lessons to fifth- and sixth-grade students (National Institute of Justice, 1994). The spread of DARE programs has been rapid: DARE programs were reportedly operating in 80% of United States School districts by 2002 (General Accounting Office, 2003).

Despite its enormous popularity, the DARE program has had little demonstrable effect on the long- or short-term drug use of participants. A meta-analyses of DARE programs reported by the National Institute of Justice in 1994 found that the programs were best at increasing students knowledge about drug use and improving their social skills, while short-term effects on actual substance use by students were not significant (National Institute of Justice, 1994; Lynam et al., 1999). Lynam et al. (1999) also conducted a ten-year follow-up of DARE participants and found that the DARE group did not perform any better than a comparison group in the long term. A recent report to Congress by the General Accounting Office (2003) examined six methodologically rigorous evaluations of the long-term effectiveness of DARE. The General Accounting Office (2003) reported that none of the studies found statistically significant differences between intervention and comparison groups in their levels of illicit drug use. Recognizing that the growing body of research has found little support for DARE, and despite its continued popularity, the DARE program has begun making changes to its curriculum in order to improve its efficacy. The revised curriculum will place more emphasis on normative beliefs about drug use, the consequences of drug use, and developing drug-use-resistance skills (General Accounting Office, 2003). In that the DARE program has recognized its limited impact, has sought to modify its curriculum to improve its efficacy, and has undertaken a serious evaluation of the new program, it has demonstrated promise as a potentially beneficial program.

Recommendations

Research has found that at least two important themes need to be taken into account when developing or implementing treatment programs for delinquent, violent youth. The first theme is that early, immediate intervention should be prioritized since behavioral problems, aggression, and other risk factors can be identified at an early age (Guerra et al., 1995; Tremblay, Kurtz, Masse, Vitaro & Phil, 1995). The second theme is the need for well-coordinated, multicomponent, prevention and intervention models that impact key risk and protective factors across multiple life domains (Henggeler et al., 1992; Tolan, et al., 1995). In general, comprehensive and multifactored interventions are superior to single-component interventions because they are able to address a range of delinquent behaviors by orchestrating different methodologies in an integrated and concerted fashion (Flannery & Huff, 1999). An additional benefit to such programming is that these types of interventions often address interrelated problem clusters, for example, drug abuse and delinquency, and therefore have additional positive benefits promoting healthy youth development and functioning.

Programs that seek to improve prosocial skills and competencies as well as to reduce aggressive or delinquent behavior are more effective than more limited efforts. Behavioral or cognitive-behavioral programs show the greatest treatment effect. Programs that include a family focus and attempt to change the environment that a child operates in (e.g., the school climate, the family, the peer group) are also more effective than programs that attempt to address factors solely at the level of the individual youth. We must keep in mind that delinquent, violent behavior is a complex phenomena with no single best-practice treatment identified that will benefit all youth who experience difficulty. None of the preventive or treatment strategies identified here are simple, cheap, or quick to implement effectively. Conversely, the most effective treatment programs address multiple risk factors in an intensive fashion with highly trained providers. Rigorous evaluation of behavior outcomes is a hallmark of best-practice programs, with findings used to modify treatment components as needed. The treatment of delinquent, violent behavior is costly and time-consuming but still pales compared to the cost of long-term incarceration.

References

Ageton, S.S. (1983). *Sexual Assault Among Adolescents*. Lexington, MA: Lexington Books.

Alexander, J.F., Barton, C., Gordon, D., Grotpeter, J., Hansson, K., Harrison, R., Mears, S., Sharon, F., Mihalic, F., Parsons, B., Pugh, C., Schulman, S., Waldron, H, & Sexton, T. 1998. *Blueprints for Violence Prevention, Book 3, Functional Family Therapy*. Boulder, Colo.: Center for the Study and Prevention of Violence.

American Psychological Association. (1994). *Diagnostic and statistical manual of mental disorders* (4th ed.). Washington, DC: Author.

Blum, R.W., Beuhring, T., & Rinehart, P.M. (2000). Protecting teens: Beyond race, income and family structure. Minneapolis, MN: Center for Adolescent Health, University of Minnesota.

Blumstein, A. (2002). Youth, guns, and violent crime. *Children, Youth, and Gun Violence*. 12(2):39–53. *www.futureofchildren.org*

Chamberlain, P. (1998). Treatment foster care. Juvenile Justice Bulletin, Office of Juvenile Justice and Delinquency Prevention. U.S. Department of Justice Clearinghouse, Rockville, MD.

Chamberlain, P., & Reid, J.B. (1998). Comparison of two community alternatives to incarceration for chronic juvenile offenders. *Journal of Consulting and Clinical Psychology, 66*, 624–633.

Chesney-Lind, M., & Brown, M. (1999). Girls and violence: An overview. In D. Flannery & R. Huff (Eds.), *Youth Violence: Prevention, Intervention, and Social Policy* (pp. 171–199). Washington, DC: American Psychiatric Press.

Coleman, M., Pfeiffer, S., & Oakland, T. (1992). Aggression replacement training with behaviorally disordered adolescents. *Behavioral Disorders, 18*(1), 54–66.

Conduct Problems Prevention Research Group. (2002). Using the Fast Track randomized prevention trial to test the early-starter model of the development of serious conduct problems. *Development and Psychopathology, 14*, 925–943.

Cork, D. (1999). Examining space-time interactions in city-level homicide data: Crack markets and the diffusion of guns among youth. *Journal of Quantitative Criminology, 15*, 379–406.

Davies, H., & Flannery, D.J. (1998). PTSD in children and adolescents exposed to community violence. *Pediatric Clinics of North America, 45*(2), 341–353.

Dodge, K., Bates, J., & Petit, G. (1990). Mechanisms in the cycle of violence. *Science, 250,* 1678–1683.

Eddy, J.M., Reid, J.B., & Fetrow, R.A. (2000). An elementary school–based prevention program targeting modifiable antecedents of youth delinquency and violence: Linking the Interests of Families and Teachers (LIFT). *Journal of Emotional and Behavioral Disorders, 8*(3):165–76.

Elliott, D.S. (1993). Longitudinal research in criminology: Promise and practice. In E. Weitekamp & H. Kerner (Eds.), *Cross-National Longitudinal Research on Human Development and Criminal Behavior.* Dordrecht: Klenner.

Elliott, D.S. (1994). Serious violent offenders: Onset, development, course, and termination. The American Society of Criminology 1993 presidential address. *Criminology, 32,* 1–21.

Eron, L.D., Huesmann, L.R., & Zelli, A. (1991). The role of parental variables in the learning of aggression. In D.J. Pepler & K.H. Rubin (Eds.), *The Development and Treatment of Childhood Aggression* (pp. 169–188). Hillsdale, NJ: Lawrence Erlbaum Associates, Inc.

Farnworth, M., & Lieber, M.J. (1989). Strain Theory Revisited: Economic Goals, Educational Means, and Delinquency. *American Sociological Review, 54,* 263–274.

Farrington, D.P. (1987). Early precursors of frequent offending. In J.Q. Wilson & G.C. Loury (Eds.), *From Children to Citizens* (pp. 27–50). New York: Springer-Verlag.

Farrington, D.P. (1990). Childhood aggression and adult violence: Early precursors and later-life outcomes. In D.J. Pepler & K.H. Rubin (Eds.), *The Development and Treatment of Childhood Aggression* (pp. 5–29). Hillsdale, NJ: Lawrence Erlbaum.

Farrington, D.P. (1991). Childhood aggression and adult violence: Early precursors and later-life outcomes. In D.J. Pepler & K.H. Rubin (Eds.), *The Development and Treatment of Childhood Aggression* (pp. 5–29). Hillsdale, NJ: Lawrence Erlbaum.

Farrington, D.P. (1994). Early developmental prevention of juvenile delinquency. *Criminal Behavior and Mental Health, 4,* 209–227.

Farrington, D.P., & Hawkins, J.D. (1991). Predicting participation, early onset and later persistence in officially recorded offending. *Criminal Behaviour & Mental Health, 1*(1), 1–33.

Farrington, D.P., Loeber, R., Elliott, D.S., Hawkins, J. D., Kandel, D.B., Klein, M.W., McCord, J., Rowe, D.C., & Tremblay, R.E. (1990). Advancing knowledge about the onset of delinquency and crime. In B.B. Lahey & A.E. Kazdin (Eds.), *Advances in Clinical Child Psychology* (Vol. 13, pp. 283–342). New York: Plenum.

Finckenauer, J. (1982). *Scared Straight and the Panacea Phenomenon.* Englewood Cliffs, NJ: Prentice-Hall.

Fingerhut, L.A., & Christoffel, K.K. (2002). Firearm-related death and injury among children and adolescents. *Children, Youth, and Gun Violence. 12,* 39–53. *www.futureofchildren.org*

Flannery, D.J., (1997). *School Violence: Risk, Preventive Intervention, and Policy.* Monograph for the Institute of Urban and Minority Education, Columbia University and the ERIC Clearinghouse for Education, Urban Diversity Series No. 109.

Flannery, D.J., & Huff, C.R. (1999). Implications for prevention, intervention, and social policy with violent youth. In D.J. Flannery & C.R. Huff (Eds.), *Youth violence: Prevention, Intervention, and Social Policy* (pp. 293–306). Washington, DC: American Psychiatric Press.

Flannery, D.J., Singer, M., & Wester, K. (2001). Violence exposure, psychological trauma, and suicide risk in a community sample of dangerously violent adolescents. *Journal of the American Academy of Child and Adolescent Psychiatry, 40*(4), 435–442.

Flannery, D.J., Singer, M., Williams, L., & Castro, P. (1998). Adolescent violence exposure and victimization at home: Coping and psychological trauma symptoms. *International Review of Victimology, 6,* 29–48.

Flannery, D.J., Williams, L., & Vazsonyi, A.T., (1999). Who are they with and what are they doing? Delinquent behavior, substance use, and early adolescents' after-school time. *American Journal of Orthopsychiatry, 69,* 247–253.

Flash, K. (2003). Treatment Strategies for Juvenile Delinquency: Alternative Solutions. *Child and Adolescent Social Work Journal, 20*(6) 509–527.

Freeman, L.N., Mokros, H., & Poznaski, E. (1993). Violent events reported by normal urban school-aged children: Characteristics and depression correlates. *Journal of the American Academy of Child and Adolescent Psychiatry, 32*(2), 419–423.

General Accounting Office. (2003). Youth Illicit Drug Use Prevention: DARE Long-Term Evaluations and Federal Efforts to Identify Effective Programs. Report number GAO-03-172R. Washington, DC: General Accounting Office.

Goldstein, A.P., & Glick, B. (1987). *Aggression Replacement Training.* Champaign, IL. Research Press.

Gottfredson, G.D. (1981). Schooling and delinquency. In S.W. Martin, L.B. Sechrest, & R. Rednez (Eds.), *New Directions in the Rehabilitation of Criminal Offenders* (pp. 424–469). Washington, DC: National Academy Press.

Gottfredson, M.R., & Hirschi, T. (1990). *A General Theory of Crime.* Stanford, CA: Stanford University Press.

Greenberg, M.T., Kusché, C., & Mihalic, S.F. (1998). *Blueprints for Violence Prevention, Book Ten: Promoting Alternative Thinking Strategies (PATHS).* Boulder, CO: Center for the Study and Prevention of Violence.

Grossman, D.C., Neckerman, H.J., Koepsell, T.D., Liu, P.Y., Asher, K.N., Beland, K., Frey, K., and Rivara, F.P. (1997). The effectiveness of a violence prevention curriculum among children in elementary school. *Journal of the American Medical Association, 277,* 1605–1611.

Guerra, N.G., Huesmann, L.R., Tolan, P.H., Acker, R., & Eron, L.F. (1995). Stressful events and individual beliefs as correlates of economic disadvantage and aggression among urban children. *Journal of Consulting and Clinical Psychology, 63,* 518–528.

Hawkins, D.F., Laub, J.H., & Lauritsen, J.L. (1998). Race, ethnicity, and serious juvenile offending. In R. Loeber, & D.P. Farrington (Eds.), *Serious & Violent Juvenile Offenders* (pp. 30–46). Thousand Oaks: Sage.

Hawkins, J.D., & Catalano, R.F. (1992). *Communities that Care.* San Francisco: Jossey-Bass.

Hawkins, J.D., Catalano, R.F., & Brewer, D.D. (1995). Preventing serious, violent, and chronic offending: Effective strategies from conception to age 6. In J.C. Howell, B. Krisberg, J.D. Hawkins, & J.Wilson (Eds.), *A Sourcebook: Serious, Violent, and Chronic Juvenile Offenders* (pp. 36–60). Thousand Oaks, CA: Sage.

Hawkins, J.D., Herrenkohl, T., Farrington, D.P., Brewer, D., Catalano, R.F., & Harachi, T.W. (1998). A review of predictors of youth violence. In R. Loeber & D.P. Farrington (Eds.), *Serious and Violent Juvenile Offenders: Risk Factors and Successful Intervention* (pp. 47–67). London: Sage Publications.

Henggeler, S. (1999). Multisystemic Therapy: An overview of clinical, procedures, outcomes, and policy implications. *Child Psychology and Psychiatry Review, 4*(1), 2–10.

Henggeler, S.W., Melton, G.B., & Smith, L.A. (1992). Family preservation using multisystemic therapy: An effective alternative to incarcerating serious juvenile offenders. *Journal of Consulting and Clinical Psychology, 60,* 953-961.

Henggeler, S.W., Mihalic, S.F., Rone, L.,Thomas, C., & Timmons-Mitchell, J. (1998). *Blueprints for Violence Prevention, Book Six: Multisystemic Therapy.* Boulder, CO: Center for the Study and Prevention of Violence.

Huesmann, L.R., & Eron, L.D. (1989). Individual differences and the trait of aggression. *European Journal of Personality, 3,* 95–106.

Huesmann, L.R., Eron, L.D., Leftkowitz, M.M., & Walder, L.O. (1984). Stability of aggression over time and generations. *Developmental Psychology, 20,* 1120–1134.

Huesmann, R.L., & Moise, J.F. (1999). Stability and continuity of aggression from early childhood to young adulthood. In D. Flannery & R. Huff (Eds.), *Youth Violence: Prevention, Intervention, and Social Policy* (pp.73–95). Washington DC: American Psychiatric Press.

Huff, C.R., (Ed.) (1996a). *Gangs in America* (2nd ed.). Thousand Oaks, CA: Sage.

Huff, C.R. (1996b). The criminal behavior of gang members and nongang at-risk youth. In C.R. Huff (Ed.), *Gangs in America* (2nd ed., pp. 75–102). Thousand Oaks, CA: Sage.

Huizinga, D., & Jakob-Chien, C. (1998). The contemporaneous co-occurrence of serious and violent juvenile offending and other problem behaviors. In R. Loeber & D.P. Farrington (Eds.), *Serious and Violent Juvenile Offenders: Risk Factors and Successful Intervention* (pp. 47–67). London: Sage Publications.

Kagan, J. (1988). Temperamental contributions to social behavior. *American Psychologist, 44,* 668–674.

Kaufman, A.E., & Cicchetti, D. (1989). Effects of maltreatment on school-age children's socioemotional development: Assessments in a day camp setting. *Developmental Psychology, 25*(4), 516–524.

Kellam, S.G., Ling, X., Merisca, R. , Brown, C.H., & Ialongo, N. (1998). The effect of the level of aggression in the first grade classroom on the course and malleability of aggressive behavior into middle school. *Development and Psychopathology, 10,* 165–85.

Lafree, G. (1995). Race and crime trends in the United States, 1946–1990. In D. Hawkins (Ed.), *Ethnicity, Race, and Crime: Perspectives Across Time and Place.* (pp. 169–193). Albany: State University of New York Press.

Lattimore, P.K., Trudeau, J., Riley, K.J., Leiter, J., & Edwards, S. (1996). *Homicide in Eight U.S. Cities: Trends, Context, and Policy Implications.* Washington, DC: NIJ.

Leeman, L.W., Gibbs, J.C., & Fuller, D. (1993). Evaluation of a multi-component group treatment program for juvenile delinquents. *Aggressive Behavior, 19,* 281–292.

Leukefeld, C.G., Logan, T.K., Clayton, R.R., Martin, C., Zimmerman, R., Cattarello, A., Milich, R., & Lynam, D. (1998). Adolescent drug use, delinquency, and other behaviors. In T.P. Gullatta, G.R. Adams, & R. Montemayor (Eds.), *Delinquent Violent Youth: Theory and Interventions [Advances in Adolescent Development, vol. 9]* (pp. 98–128). Thousand Oaks, CA: Sage Publications.

Lipsey, M. (1992). Juvenile delinquency treatment: a meta-analytic inquiry into the variability of effects. In T. Cook, et al. (Eds.). *Meta-analysis for Explanation: A Casebook.* New York: Russell Sage Foundation.

Lispsey, M.W., Wilson, D.B., & Cothern, L. (2000, April). *Effective intervention for serious juvenile offenders* (NCJ 181201). Washington, DC: U.S. Dept of Justice, Office of Justice Programs, Office of Juvenile Justice and Delinquency Prevention.

Lochman, J.E., & Dodge, K.A. (1994). Social-cognitive processes of severely violent, moderately aggressive, and nonaggressive boys. (1994). *Journal of Consulting and Clinical Psychology, 62*(2), 366–374.

Loeber, R. (1982). The stability of antisocial and delinquent child behavior: A review. *Child Development, 53,* 1431–1446.

Loeber, R., & Farrington, D.P. (1998). *Serious and Violent Juvenile Offenders: Risk Factors and Successful Intervention.* London: Sage Publications.

Loeber R., & Hay. D.F. (1994). Developmental approaches to aggression and conduct problems. In M. Rutter & D.F. Hay (Eds.), *Development Through the Life: A Handbook for Clinicians* (pp. 488–515). Oxford: Blackwell Scientific.

Loeber, R., Wung, P., Keenan, K., Giroux, B., Stouthamer-Loeber, M., Van Kammen, W.B., & Maughan, B. (1993). Developmental pathways in disruptive child behavior. *Development and Psychopathology, 5,* 101–133.

Lorion, R., & Saltzman, W. (1993). Children's exposure to community violence: Following a path from concern to research to action. *Psychiatry, 56,* 55–65.

Lynam, D.R., Milich, R., Zimmerman, R, Novak, S.P., Logan, T.K., Martin, C., Leukefeld, C., & Clayton, R. (1999). Project DARE: No effects at 10-year follow-up. *Journal of Consulting and Clinical Psychology, 67*(4), 590–593.

MacKenzie, D. (1997). Criminal justice and crime prevention. In Sherman, L.W., Gottfredson, D., MacKenzie, D., Eck, J., Reuter, P., & Bushway, S. (Eds.). *Preventing Crime: What Works, What Doesn't, What's Promising: A Report to the United States Congress.* National Institute of Justice (NCJ 165366). Washington, DC: U.S. Department of Justice, Office of Justice Programs.

Maguin, E., Hawkins, J.D., Catalano, R.F., Hill, K., Abbott, R., & Herrenkohl, T. (1995, November). *Risk factors measured at three ages for violence at age 17–18.* Paper presented at the meeting of the American Society of Criminology, Boston.

Maguin, E., & Loeber, R. (1996). Academic performance and delinquency. In M. Tonry (Ed.), *Crime and Justice: A Review of Research* (Vol. 20, pp. 145–264. Chicago: University of Chicago Press.

Masten, A.S. (1994). Resilience in individual development: Successful adaptation despite risk and adversity. In M.C. Wang & E.W. Gordon (Eds.), *Educational Resilience in Inner-City America,* (pp. 3–25). Hillsdale, NJ: Lawrence Erlbaum Associates.

McCord, J. (1979). Some child-rearing antecedents of criminal behavior in adult men. *Journal of Personality and Social Psychology, 37,* 1477–1486.

McCord, J. (1983). A forty year perspective on effects of child abuse and neglect. *Child Abuse & Neglect, 7*(3), 265–270.

McMahon, S.D., Washburn, J., Felix, E.D., Yakin, J., & Childrey, G. (2000). Violence prevention: Program effects on urban, preschool, and kindergarten children. *Applied and Preventive Psychology, 9,* 271–281.

Moffitt, T.E. (1990). Juvenile delinquency and attention deficit disorder: Boys' developmental trajectories from age 3 to age 15. *Child Development, 61,* 893–910.

Moffitt, T.E. (1993). Adolescence-limited and life-course persistent antisocial behavior: A developmental taxonomy. *Psychological Review, 100*(4), 674–701.

Molgaard, V.K, Spoth, R.I., & Redmond, C. (2000, August). *Competency Training The Strengthening Families Program: For Parents and Youth 10-14 (NCJ 182208).* Washington, DC: U.S. Department of Justice, Office of Justice Programs, Office of Juvenile Justice and Delinquency Prevention.

National Institute of Justice (1994). The DARE Program: A review of prevalence, user satisfaction, and effectiveness. Washington, DC: National Institute of Justice.

O'Donnell, J., Hawkins, J.D., & Abbott, R.D. (1995). Predicting serious delinquency and substance use among aggressive boys. *Journal of Consulting and Clinical Psychology, 63,* 529–537.

O'Donnell, J., Hawkins, J.D., Catalano, R.F., Abbot, R.D., & Day, E. (1995). Preventing school failure, drug use, and delinquency among low-income children: Long-term intervention in elementary schools. *American Journal of Orthopsychiatry, 65,* 87–100.

Olds, D., Hill, P., Mihalic, S., & O'Brien, R. (1998). *Blueprints for Violence Prevention, Book Seven: Prenatal and Infancy Home Visitation by Nurses.* Boulder, CO: Center for the Study and Prevention of Violence.

Olweus, D. (1979). Stability of aggressive reaction patterns in males: A review. *Psychological Bulletin, 86,* 852–875.

Patterson, G.R., DeBarysne, B.D., & Ramsey, E. (1989). A developmental perspective on antisocial behavior. *American Psychologist, 44*(2), 329–335.

Petrosino, A., Turpin-Petrosino, C., & Buehler, J. (2003). "Scared Straight" and other juvenile awareness programs for preventing juvenile delinquency (Updated C2 Review). In: The Campbell Collaboration Reviews of Intervention and Policy Evaluations (C2-RIPE), Philadelphia: Campbell Collaboration.

Plomin, R., Nitz, K., & Rowe, D.C. (1990). Behavioral genetics and aggressive behavior in childhood. In M. Lewis & S.M. Miller (Eds.), *Handbook of Developmental Psychopathology* (pp. 119–133). New York: Plenum Press.

Raine, A., Brennan, P., & Mednick, S. A. (1994). Birth complications combined with early maternal rejection at age 1 year predispose to violent crime at age 18 years. *Archives of General Psychiatry, 51*, 984–988.

Reid, J.B., Eddy, J.M., Fetrow, R.A. & Stoolmiller, M. (1999). Description and immediate impacts of a preventive intervention for conduct problems. *American Journal of Community Psychology, 27*(4):483–517.

Rennison, C. (2002). *Criminal Victimization 2001: Changes 2000–01 with Trends 1993–2001.* Washington, DC: Bureau of Justice Statistics.

Resnick, M.D., Bearman, P.S., Blum, R.W., Bauman, K.E., Harris, K.M., Jones, J., Tabor, J., Beuhring, T., Sieving, R.E., Shew, M., Ireland, M., Bearinger, L.H., & Udry, R. (1997). Protecting Adolescents From Harm: Findings From the National Longitudinal Study on Adolescent Health. *Journal of the American Medical Association, 278*(10): 823–32.

Rivara, F.P., Gurney, J.G., Ries, R.K., et al. (1992). A descriptive study of trauma, alcohol and alcoholism in young adults. *Journal of Adolescent Health, 13*, 663–667.

Rivera, B., & Widom, C.S. (1990). Childhood victimization and violent offending. *Violence & Victims, 5*(1), 19–35.

Robbins, M.S., & Szapocznik, J. (2000, April). *Brief Strategic Family Therapy.* (NCJ 179825). Washington, DC: U.S. Department of Justice, Office of Justice Programs, Office of Juvenile Justice and Delinquency Prevention.

Sampson, R., & Lauritsen, J. (1994). Violent victimization and offending: Individual-, ituational- and community-level risk factors. In A.J. Reiss & J.A. Roth (Eds.), *Understanding and Preventing Violence (Vol. 3) Social Influences* (pp. 1–115). Washington, DC: National Academy Press.

Sampson, R.J., Raudenbush, S.W., & Earls, F. (1997). Neighborhoods and violent crime: A multilevel study of collective efficacy. *Science, 277*, 918–924.

Sexton, T.L., & Alexander, J.A. (2000, December). *Functional Family Therapy.* Juvenile Justice Bulletin, Office of Juvenile Justice and Delinquency Prevention. U.S. Department of Justice Clearinghouse, Rockville, MD.

Simon, N.G., & Coccaro, E.F. (1999). Human aggression: What's animal research got to do with it? *The HFG Review, 3*(1), 13–20.

Singer, M.I., Anglin, T.M., Song, L., & Lunghofer, L. (1995). Adolescents' exposure to violence and associated symptoms of psychological trauma. *Journal of the American Medical Association, 273*(6), 477–482.

Snyder, H.N. (2003). Juvenile arrests 2001: Juvenile justice bulletin. Washington, DC: U.S. Department of Justice, Office of Juvenile Justice & Delinquency Prevention.

Snyder, H.N., & Sickmund, M. (1999). *Juvenile Offenders and Victims: 1999 National Report.* Washington, DC: Office of Juvenile Justice and Delinquency Prevention.

Sturkie, K., & Flanzer, J.P. (1987). Depression and self-esteem in the families of maltreated adolescents. *Social Work, 32*(6), 491–496.

Susman, E.J., & Ponirakis, A. (1997). Hormones-context interactions and antisocial behavior in youth. In A. Raine, P.A. Brennan, D.P. Farrington, & S.A. Mednick (Eds.), *Biosocial Bases of Violence* (pp. 251–269). New York: Plenum Press.

Tardiff, K. (1999). Psychopharmacological and neurobiological issues in the treatment of violent youth. In D.J. Flannery & C.R. Huff (Eds.), *Youth Violence: Prevention, Intervention, and Social Policy.* (pp. 275–290). Washington, DC: American Psychiatric Press, Inc.

Thornberry, T.P. (1994). *Violent Families and Youth Violence.* Washington, DC: U.S. Department of justice, National Institute of Justice, Office of Justice Programs.

Thornberry, T.P., Huizinga, R., & Loeber, R. (1995). The prevention of serious delinquency and violence: Implications from the Program of Research on the Causes and Correlates of Delinquency. In J.C. Howell, B. Krisberg, J.D. Hawkins, & J.J. Wilson (Eds.), *A Sourcebook: Serious, Violent, and Chronic Juvenile Offenders* (pp. 213–237). Thousand Oaks, CA: Sage.

Tolan, P.H., Guerra, N.G., & Kendall, P. (1995). A developmental-ecological perspective on antisocial behavior in children and adolescents: Towards a unified risk and intervention framework. *Journal of Consulting and Clinical Psychology, 63*, 579–584.

Tracy, P.E., Wolfgang, M.E., & Figlio, R.M. (1990). *Delinquency Careers in Two Birth Cohorts.* New York: Plenum.

Tremblay, R.E., Kurtz, L., Masse, L.C., Vitaro, F., & Phil, R.O. (1995). A bimodal preventive intervention for disruptive kindergarten boys: Its impact through adolescence. *Journal of Consulting and Clinical Psychology, 63,* 560–568.

Tremblay, R.E., Masse, B., Perron, D., Le Blanc, M., Schwartzman, A.E., & Ledingham, J.E. (1992). Early disruptive behavior, poor school achievement, delinquent behavior and delinquent personality: Longitudinal analyses. *Journal of Consulting and Clinical Psychology, 60,* 64–72.

Tremblay, R.E., Schaal, B., Boulerice, B., Arseneault, L., Soussignan, R., & Perusse, D. (1997). In A. Raine, P.A. Brennan, D.P. Farrington, & S.A. Mednick (Eds.), *Biosocial Bases of Violence* (pp. 271–291). New York: Plenum Press.

U.S. Department of Education. (2001) *Safe, Disciplined, and Drug-Free Schools Programs.* Washington, D.C.: U.S. Department of Education, Office of Special Educational Research and Improvement, Office of Reform Assistance and Dissemination.

U.S. Department of Health and Human Services (2001). *Youth Violence: A Report of the Surgeon General.* Rockville, MD: U.S. Department of Health and Human Services, Centers for Disease Control and Prevention, National Center for Injury Prevention and Control; Substance Abuse and Mental Health Services Administration, Center for Mental Health Services; and National Institutes of Health, National Institute of Mental Health.

Widom, C. (1989). The cycle of violence. *Science, 244,* 160–166.

Chapter 20

Substance Misuse and Abuse

Carl G. Leukefeld, Hope M. Smiley McDonald,
William W. Stoops, LaDonya Reed, and Catherine Martin

Introduction

Adolescent substance misuse and abuse have been the changing focus of the popular press in the United States and the general public since the late 1970s. In fact, it was in the late 1970s when the United States first became aware of the widespread use of alcohol and drugs among adolescents in the general population. The high levels of drug and alcohol use were reported by the national Monitoring the Future Study. Although the overall rates of alcohol and drug misuse and abuse have changed over time and decreased from the highest levels in the late 1970s, substance misuse and abuse continue to be problems among U.S. adolescents.

Findings from the 2002 Monitoring the Future Study (Johnston, O'Malley & Bachman, 2003a) indicate that by eighth grade 47.0% of students have tried alcohol and 21.3% say they had been drunk at least once. Marijuana was tried by 19.2% of eighth-graders, and it had been used by 8.3% of eighth-graders in the previous month. Likewise, 15.2% of eighth-graders said they had used inhalants, 8.7% had tried amphetamines, and 31.4% said they had tried cigarettes. Most students had tried alcohol, with 66.9% of tenth-graders and 78.4% of twelfth-graders reporting that they had tried alcohol. There was more limited use of marijuana: 38.7% of tenth-graders and 47.8% of twelfth-graders had tried marijuana. Overall trends in substance use among eighth- to twelfth-graders showed fluctuations over the past years, with current decreases in use. For high school seniors, drug use remained fairly stable over the past year with overall decreased use. However, these data suggest that adolescents remain at high risk for drug misuse as well as for progressing into abuse.

Adolescent interventions in the United States have targeted risk and protective factors as well as problems associated with use. Risk and protective factors are grounded in resiliency and invulnerability studies (see Hawkins, Catalano & Miller, 1992) as well as public health approaches designed to focus on risk factors, which include behaviors, attitudes, and knowledge, in addition to factors that protect individuals from problems associated with substance use and misuse. Risk and protective factors have been defined by Clayton (1992) to include individual characteristics, attributes, situational conditions, or environmental contexts that increase the probability of drug use or misuse or transition to another level of use. Protective factors inhibit, reduce, or buffer the probability of drug use and misuse or a transition to further drug involvement. However, risk and protective factors cannot always be differentiated at the individual level. For example, a protective factor for one adolescent could be a risk factor for another adolescent. Specifically, family involvement could be protective if a family promotes health and no substance use, but family involvement could be high-risk if family members use and "encourage" substance use with their own use and related behaviors. Substance use also can change the balance of risk and protective factors, which may change the level of substances used.

A bio/psycho/social/spiritual theoretical perspective (Leukefeld & Leukefeld, 1999) has been proposed as a way of thinking about substance abuse. This framework presents theoretically grounded approaches and incorporates the interaction of behavior, environment, spirituality, and biology. It is also compatible with a public health focus on the interaction of the agent (substance), the host (the adolescent), and the environment (the setting that brings the two together) (see Daugherty & Leukefeld, 1998). The bio/psycho/social/spiritual theoretical perspective incorporates four possible pathways or combinations of pathways to substance abuse: (1) *Biology or genetic* pathways include heritability and biologically based theories of substance abuse, which are commonly depicted as the disease model of addiction. (2) *Psychological* pathways incorporate individual characteristics that contribute to the motivation to use substances, expectancies to use, personality factors, and thinking that substance abuse is a learned behavior that can be unlearned. (3) *Social and environmental* pathways include laws, culture, family norms, customs, and peer associations which are related to substance abuse. (4) *Spirituality* incorporates the idea that a belief in something is a protective factor from substance abuse as well as being important for recovery from substance abuse. Although the clinical literature is fairly consistent in the idea that spirituality is related to recovery, it is not without controversy since the focus can be on the idea that spirituality and religiosity are similar.

This chapter provides an overview of selected factors related to adolescent substance misuse and abuse etiology, prevention, and treatment. *Primary prevention* is defined in this chapter to include planned actions that help adolescents prevent predictable problems, protect existing states of health as well as healthy functioning, and promote desired goals for adolescents. *Treatment* is defined as activities and actions that are focused on helping adolescents reduce problems associated with substance use/misuse and that change individual substance abuse behavior and enhance social functioning. This chapter provides an overview of selected factors at the individual level, family level and social/community level which have been found to be associated with adolescent substance use and misuse. In addition, promising adolescent drug abuse prevention and treatment interventions are presented.

Individual Factors

Many individual factors have been associated with adolescent drug misuse and abuse. Examples of these factors include childhood conduct disorder problems (Lynam, 1996); low self-esteem (Kaplan, Martin & Robbins, 1982; Overholser, Adams,

Lehnert & Brinkman, 1995); sensation-seeking (Beck, Thombs, Mahoney & Fingar, 1995); and—from a literature review by Hawkins, Catalano & Miller's (1992)—poor impulse control, genetic predisposition to alcoholism, low family bonding, antisocial behavior, aggressiveness, academic failure, low commitment to school, early peer rejection, drug-using peers, alienation, early drug use, and favorable attitudes to drug use.

Variability in acute drug effects, individual differences in the adolescent drug user, and differences in social context when the drug is ingested must be taken into account when assessing individual factors and vulnerabilities as well as developing an individualized treatment plan for each adolescent. For example, drug effects can range from decreasing anxiety seen in a group of socially anxious friends who smoke cigarettes before school in order to moderate dysphoria and disinhibition to an adolescent who gets a family message that he or she is a failure, begins drinking alcohol, and decides to kill him/herself using a father's gun. When assessing ways to assist adolescents who are abusing substances, issues associated with immediate morbidity must be addressed first and then the complex system in which the abuse occurs can be addressed.

Psychiatric disorders and psychological symptoms may be associated with the likelihood with which an individual initiates drug use, continues drug use following the initial exposure, and/or continues to use drugs despite adverse social or health consequences (de Wit & Bodker, 1994). A possible determinant of drug use risk is the discriminative, reinforcing, and/or behavioral effects of a drug (e.g., Brady & Lukas, 1984). In addition, the interaction of individual differences and the unique drug properties impact initial and continued use. For example, psychiatric comorbidity may impact adolescent drug use in several ways, which includes "self-medication" in association with attention-deficit/hyperactivity disorder (ADHD), nicotine use, social phobia, and alcohol use. A direct effect of nicotine is enhanced concentration (Conners et al., 1996) and a direct effect of alcohol is decreased anxiety (Kushner et al., 1996). Thus, these drugs would have strong reinforcing and behavioral effects for vulnerable adolescents.

The contributions of psychiatric disorders and/or personality traits on unique drug use choices have been examined in adults. For example, Chait (1994) reported that normal subjects who chose methylphenidate over placebo scored higher on the *extroversion* and *impulsivity subscales of the Eysenck Personality Inventory* and the experience-seeking subscale of the *sensation-seeking (SS) scale* when compared to subjects who did not choose either methylphenidate or placebo. Martin and colleagues (1999) demonstrated that the interaction of conduct disorder and sensation-seeking (SS) scale was associated with the reinforcing effects of amphetamines in young adults. Sensation-seeking also has been correlated with drug use in adolescents (Andrucci, Archer, Pancoast & Gordon, 1989; Martin et al., 2002). Thus, it appears that drugs have unique reinforcing properties in high sensation-seekers.

Psychiatric disorders that are common among youth with substance use disorders include disruptive disorders (conduct disorder, oppositional defiant disorder, and ADHD), mood disorders (major depression and bipolar disorder), anxiety disorders (generalized anxiety disorder, social phobia, and post-traumatic stress disorder), and bulimia nervosa (Biederman, Wilens, Mick, Faraone & Spencer, 1998; Bukstein, Brent & Kaminer, 1989; Howard, Walker, Walker, Cottler & Compton, 1999; Hser, Grella, Collins & Teruya, 2003; Kilpatrick, Ruggiero, Acierno, Saunders & Resnick, 2003;

Kuperman et al., 2001; Milberger, Biederman, Faraone, Chen & Jones, 1997; Molina, Bukstein & Lynch, 2002; O'Brien & Vincent, 2003; Riggs, 2003; Whitmore, Mikulich, Thompson, Riggs, Aarons & Crowley, 1997; Windle & Windle, 2001). In addition to the general association of substance use disorders with psychiatric comorbidity, there appear to be selected disorders that have particular risk for specific substance use, which as noted above include ADHD, which has been linked to cigarette smoking (Milberger et al., 1997), as well as social phobia and panic attacks, which have been associated with alcohol use disorders in adolescents (Zimmermann, Wittchen, Hofler, Pfister, Kessler & Lieb, 2003).

Specific disorders can be exacerbated by drug use or by drug withdrawal. For example, untreated comorbidity has been associated with treatment failure and untreated comorbidities which are likely to persist after successful substance abuse treatment (Bukstein et al., 1992; Grella, Hser, Joshi & Rounds-Bryant, 2001; Riggs et al., 1996; Wise, Cuffe & Fischer, 2001). There may be a spectrum of psychiatric disorders among adolescents that if treated could decrease drug use. Table 1 presents a summary of disorders that are commonly comorbid with substance abuse in addition to pharmacological treatment strategies. It is important to emphasize that treating psychiatric disorders alone has not been associated with significant improvement in substance use and that psychiatric medications are not the first line of treatment but should be considered part of treatment (Riggs, Mikulich & Hall, 2001).

Acute drug effects and withdrawal have not received rigorous laboratory assessments in adolescents. Although drug withdrawal symptoms may be less frequent in adolescents when compared to chronic adult users, withdrawal symptoms and syndromes should be assessed and treated in the same way as adult treatment (Bukstein, 1997). An exception may be nicotine dependence since there is no evidence that nicotine substitution is effective in maintaining abstinence among adolescent smokers (Hanson, Allen, Jensen & Hatsukami, 2003; Smith et al., 1996). However, the use of adolescent nicotine substitution is in the early stages of evaluation. Table 2 presents a summary of acute effects and withdrawal symptoms associated with drugs of abuse.

Early substance abuse can change the developmental trajectory of an adolescent who is undergoing dramatic physiological, social, and interpersonal changes which are likely to exacerbate preexisting psychiatric disorders (Crowley & Riggs, 1995; Rutter, Giller & Hagell, 1998). Adolescents who engage in high-risk behavior because of disinhibition and high sensation-seekers may be particularly vulnerable under the influence of disinhibiting drugs like alcohol. In general, high-risk behaviors that increase under the influence of alcohol and other drugs include aggression, violence, and risky behaviors like unprotected sex (see Jessor and Jessor, 1977). For example, adolescents under the influence of alcohol and other drugs are more likely to be in car accidents, be raped, or drown (Lescohier & Gallagher, 1996; Windle, Shope & Bukstein, 1996). Marijuana use has been associated with increased risk for motor vehicle accidents, assault, and self-inflicted injuries (Gerberich, Sidney, Braun, Tekawa, Tolan & Quesenberry, 2003). Although adolescents with conduct disorder may display bravado initially, adolescents with conduct disorder and depression are at highest risk for a lethal suicide attempt, particularly under the influence of an illicit drug (Fergusson, Woodward & Horwood, 2000; Kelly et al., 2002). Individual vulnerability to depression and disinhibition may be aggravated by acute drug effects which can propel an adolescent into dangerous behavior that can include harm to self and others.

Table 1. Psychiatric Disorders, Substance Use, and Promising Pharmacological Treatment Strategies

Comorbidity	Medication	Impact on Psychiatric Symptoms	Changes in Substance Use
Mood disorders			
Bipolar, aggression	Lithium	Stabilizes mania	Decreases substance abuse (Geller et al., 1998)
Major depression, dysthymia	Fluoxetine SSRIs	Decreases depression, good safety profile (Deas et al., 2000; Deas and Thomas, 2001; Riggs et al., 1997)	
Anxiety			
Post-traumatic stress disorder (PTSD)	SSRIs	Assists with sleep difficulties, depressive symptoms, intrusive memories, hyperarousal (March and Wells, 2002)	
Social anxiety	SSRIs, Paxil	Decreases social anxiety in adults (Liappas et al., 2003; Randall et al., 2001)	
Disruptive Disorders			
Attention-deficit/hyperactivity disorder (ADHD)	pemoline	Pemoline has been associated with decreased ADHD symptoms at the same level as adolescents who were not abusing stimulants but no accompanying decrease in substance use; note that concerns regarding liver toxicity require careful selection of patients and liver enzyme monitoring. (Riggs et al., 1996, 2001; Safer et al., 2001)	None
ADHD	Stimulants	Stimulant use (methylphenidate, dexedrine short and long acting) is associated with decreases in inattention and impulsivity	Decreased use of all substances abuse other than nicotine; increases nicotine use in laboratory setting (Henningfield and Griffiths, 1981; Wilens et al., 2003)
ADHD + depression	Bupropion	Since bupropion is effective for both depression and ADHD it may be considered when the disorders occur together; has good safety profile in substance users; there is an increased risk for seizure in patients with bulimia and bulimic is associated with alcohol abuse; note that: tricyclics are contraindicated in adolescents using substances because of potential for interactions with drugs of abuse and lethality associated with a tricyclic overdose. (Daviss et al., 2001; Haney et al., 2001; Riggs and Davies, 2002; Riggs et al., 1998; Wilens et al., 1997)	
Bulimia nervosa	Antidepressants	Antidepressants (tricyclic, serotonergic uptake inhibitors, monoamine oxidase inhibitors) were effective in decreasing bulimia nervosa (Ahu and Walsh, 2002; Bacaltchuk and Hay, 2003)	
Conduct disorder (CD)	Stimulants	Decreases CD symptoms (Klein et al., 1997)	

Table 2. Drugs of Abuse: Acute Effects and Withdrawal Symptoms

Drug	Pharmacological Effects	Withdrawal Symptoms	Management
Nicotine	Euphoria, increased heart rate and blood pressure, weak analgesia, nausea and vomiting, increased attention	Anxiety, irritability, decreased concentration, restlessness, hunger, tremor, heart racing, sweating, craving, insomnia, drowsiness, headaches, depression, digestive disturbances	
Alcohol/Sedative Hypnotics	**100 mg/ml** blood alcohol level (BAL): mild sedation and intoxication (slurred speech; staggering gait; slowed reflexes) **100–200 mg/ml:** impairment of visual-motor skills and integration of sensory information **>200 mg/ml:** severe intoxication and sedation **>450 mg/ml:** stupor and coma personality change (belligerence, irritability, dysphoria, social disinhibition)	**Acute:** Increased heart rate and blood pressure, agitation, tremors, increased reflexes, auditory and visual hallucinations **12–14 hours:** seizures (infrequent) **72–96 hours:** Delirium tremens with confusion, disorientation, severe agitation, visual and tactile hallucinations, severe autonomic hyperactivity with hyperthermia, medical emergency requiring hospitalization	Withdrawal: Hospitalization is often required; sedative-hypnotics **Major health risk:** delirium tremens; hospitalization, as this may be life-threatening
Marijuana	Euphoria, relaxation, and disinhibition; impaired problem-solving skills and difficulty organizing thoughts and conversing; impaired cognitive function and motor coordination	Irritability, restlessness, nervousness, loss of appetite, weight loss, insomnia, chills, tremors, and sleep disturbance "Amotivational syndrome"; depression in some	
Stimulants (amphetamines)	Restlessness, dizziness, tremor, irritability, insomnia, weakness, hyperactive reflexes, headache, chills, flushing, excessive sweating, palpitations, increased blood pressure and heart rate , anorexia, nausea, and vomiting, diarrhea. Acute toxicity: paranoid symptoms and panic, hyperthermia, and seizures	Crash (9 hours to 4 days): acute sadness leading to agitation, depression, and drug craving followed by fatigue and exhaustion Withdrawal (1 to 10 weeks): less drug craving, more normal sleep, depressed or anxious mood Extinction (Indefinite): Mood normalizes but episodic drug craving persists, especially with certain cues (i.e., alcohol use)	Intoxication: support and benzodiazepines to calm Chronic use: hospitalization is often required because of withdrawal depression
Cocaine	(See stimulants) More risk for cardiac complications	(See stimulants)	(See stimulants) **Major health risk:** hospitalization for medical conditions if necessary

Drugs of abuse without withdrawal symptoms

Inhalants (glues, aerosols, solvents)	Disinihibition, disorientation, dizziness, headache, red, watery eyes, respiratory problems High dose: confusion, impaired judgment, memory difficulties, seizure, coma, slowed heart rate **Major health risk:** sudden death (either via cardiopulmonary arrest or respiratory depression)	Acute effects: delirium requiring hospitalization with supportive care
Hallucinogens (PCP, LSD)	Increased blood pressure and heart rate, confusion, sweating, agitation, visual hallucinations, nausea and vomiting PCP: More likely to cause acute psychotic reactions	
Ecstasy (MDMA)	Confusion, depression, insomnia, anxiety, paranoia, hangover 24 hours later, increased heart rate and blood pressure, dehydration, heart failure, kidney damage, malignant hyperthermia, bruxism, euphoria, comfort and empathy, connecting with others, decreased inhibitions **Major health risk:** Suicide Sunday (suicidal the following day)	Acute intoxication: safe environment with reassurance; benzodiazepines for agitation

Cambor & Millman, 1996; Friedman et al., 1996.

Family Factors

A number of familial factors have been identified that play a role in risk and resiliency to adolescent substance use and abuse (Cattarello, Clayton & Leukefeld, 1995; Clayton, Leukefeld, Donohew, Bardo & Harrington, 1995; Leukefeld et al., 1998; Patton, 1995). These factors include family structure, history, and relationships, as well as parenting styles and parental drug use (Brook, Cohen, Whiteman & Gordon, 1992; Dube, Felitti, Dong, Chapman, Giles & Anda, 2003; Ensminger, Juon & Fothergill, 2002; Gil, Vega & Turner, 2002; Guo, Hill, Hawkins, Catalano & Abbott, 2002; Kellam, Brown, Rubin & Ensminger, 1983; Li, Pentz & Chou, 2002; Sale, Sambrano, Springer & Turner, 2003; Swadi, 1999). According to Cattarello and colleagues (1995), a factor may add to risk or resiliency depending on its direction. For example, although being in a single-parent home may be a risk factor for adolescent substance abuse, having both parents at home may be a protective/resiliency factor against adolescent substance abuse. Ethnicity and gender also have been shown to play a complex role in adolescent substance use and abuse (Beauvais and Oetting, 2002; de Wit, Offord & Wong, 1997; Guo et al., 2002).

Family structure plays an important role in risk or resiliency for adolescent substance abuse (Dube et al., 2003; Gil et al., 2002; Kellam et al., 1983). For example, in one study, students in the Miami-Dade county school district were interviewed concerning substance use and risk/resiliency factors during their middle-school years and then later (Gil et al., 2002). The results of this study demonstrate that for European Americans, but not African Americans, parental divorce significantly increased the risk for marijuana use and dependence.

A study by Dube and colleagues (2003) demonstrated that a family history of abuse, neglect, and dysfunction contribute to adolescent substance use and abuse. In this study, adverse childhood events (ACEs) and substance abuse variables were examined among adult members of the Kaiser Health Plan. Study findings suggest that ACEs increase the risk of initiation of illicit drug use by age 14 and the prevalence of lifetime drug use. That is, respondents who reported histories of emotional, physical/sexual abuse, or emotional or physical neglect were more likely to report adolescent substance use.

The interaction and relationships within a family is another factor that can contribute to the risk for and resiliency to adolescent substance abuse (e.g., Denton and Kampfe, 1994; Guo et al., 2002; Reardon and Griffing, 1983). For example, in families with higher levels of rules and monitoring, there were significantly lower levels of drug use initiation in a sample of Seattle students which was followed over an 11-year period (Guo et al., 2002). The results of this study indicate that increased levels of involvement, bonding, and discipline within a family contributed to resiliency to not use drugs. Increased levels of family conflict also contribute to risk of using drugs. Other family factors that can contribute to the risk and resiliency include rules and parental expectations (Denton and Kampfe, 1994), since parents of adolescents who use drugs are more likely to set unclear rules and have unrealistic parental expectations.

Parenting style also can play a role in adolescent substance use (Brook et al., 1992; Cohen and Rice, 1997). Specifically, adolescent drug use initiation or increased drug use have been associated with paternal permissiveness and maternal low attachment (Brook et al., 1992). When eighth- and ninth-grade students and their parents were examined on parenting style, academic achievement, tobacco use, and alcohol use, perceived parenting style significantly differed between parents and their children (Cohen and Rice, 1997). In addition a child's perception of lower parental authoritativeness was associated with alcohol and tobacco use, while parent perception of parenting style was not associated with adolescent drug use.

Parental substance use has been identified as one of the most common risk factors for adolescent substance use (Cattarello et al., 1995; Leukefeld et al., 1998; Li et al., 2002). For example, longitudinal data from Indianapolis students over 18 months clearly demonstrated the impact of parental substance use on adolescent substance use (Li et al., 2002). Specifically, parents' tobacco and marijuana use was significantly associated with tobacco, alcohol, and marijuana use by their children. Parents' alcohol use also predicted alcohol use by their children. This effect was also increased when both parents reported using a substance.

Gender and ethnicity also contribute to the influence of family factors on adolescent substance use (i.e., Ensminger et al., 2002, Gil et al., 2002). For African American women, family poverty was associated with lower occurrence of lifetime marijuana and cocaine use, although this relationship was not evident in African American men (Ensminger et al., 2002). As mentioned above, the number of parents at home differentially modifies the risk to use drugs, which varied by ethnicity (Gil et al., 2002). Another study reported that the prevalence of marijuana in the United States is lower in most minority groups, when compared to whites (Beauvais and Oetting, 2002). However, the effects of gender upon risk and resiliency to substance use are complex and variable. For example, the higher prevalence of drug use in males may in part be accounted for by greater numbers of opportunities to use drugs for males than for females (e.g., Van Etten & Anthony, 2001). However, research has shown that once an opportunity to use drugs has occurred, males and females do not generally differ in their likelihood of transition to drug use (e.g., Van Etten & Anthony, 2001).

In addition to gender, ethnicity can play a complex and variable role in risk and resiliency to use drugs. For example, African Americans report exposure to a larger number of risk factors than European Americans (Gil et al., 2002). However, risk factors to drug use within an ethnic group have at times not been predictive of actual prevalence of drug use (Vega et al., 1993). This difference in the predictive value of risk factors within an ethnic group may be due in part to cultural differences within particular ethnic groups (Vega et al., 1993).

Other family factors also have been associated with adolescent substance use and abuse; these include family relationships and history as well as parenting style and parental substance use. The direction (either positive or negative) of each of these factors may contribute to risk or resiliency, and the effects of these factors vary depending upon gender and ethnicity.

Social and Community Factors

Social and community factors can have a role in risk and resiliency for adolescent substance misuse and abuse (for reviews, see Cattarello et al., 1995; Clayton et al., 1995; Leukefeld et al., 1998). These factors include peer attitudes toward substance use, school environment, prevention efforts, and multiple community factors like cultural norms, population mobility, neighborhood deviance, and poverty (Brook, Kessler & Cohen, 1999; Guo et al., 2002; Harrison & Narayan, 2003; Johnston, O'Malley & Bachman, 2003b; Novak, Reardon & Buka, 2002; Oetting, Donnermeyer & Deffenbacher, 1998a; Sale et al., 2003; Swadi, 1999; Trudeau, Spoth, Lillehoj, Redmond & Wickrama, 2003; Yamaguchi, Johnston & O'Malley, 2003). Like family factors, social and/or community factors can also add to risk or resiliency, depending on the direction. For example, associating with peers who use drugs may be a risk factor for drug use; associating with peers who do not use drugs may be a resiliency factor, which "protects" against drug use. Ethnicity and gender also play a complex role in social and community factors that contribute to adolescent substance use and abuse (Guo et al., 2002; Harrison & Narayan, 2003; Oetting, Donnermeyer, Trimble & Beauvais, 1998b; Perry et al., 2003). Practitioners should be aware that gender and ethnicity influence risk and resiliency to drug abuse and should thus not take a "one size fits all" approach to prevention and treatment of adolescents.

Peer attitudes and substance use can influence adolescent substance use or misuse (Brook et al., 1999; Guo et al., 2002; Sale et al., 2003; Swadi, 1999). For example, in a sample of Seattle youth followed over 11 years, high levels of peer prosocial activity was protective against drug use initiation, while antisocial peer activity was a risk factor for drug use over time (Guo et al., 2002). In another longitudinal study, New York youth who associated with peers who smoked cigarettes or used marijuana were more likely to initiate marijuana use during their lifetimes (Brook et al., 1999). Peer influence appears to be age dependent, because in adolescents older than 12, peer attitudes and drug use were better predictors of substance use than they were for children (Sale et al., 2003). Practitioners should thus be mindful of age when considering treatment and prevention strategies.

School environment and prevention efforts can also contribute to risk and resiliency for adolescent substance use (e.g., Harrison & Narayan, 2003; Perry et al., 2003; Trudeau et al., 2003; Yamaguchi et al., 2003). For example, in a sample of ninth-grade Minnesota students, adolescents who actively participated in sports or other extracurricular activities were less likely to smoke cigarettes or use marijuana (Harrison & Narayan, 2003). Thus, a school environment that encourages participation in extracurricular activities may be protective against adolescent drug use. It should be noted, however, that involvement in activities was not protective against alcohol use in this study. School prevention activities also contribute to risk and resiliency for substance abuse (Trudeau et al., 2003). For example, results from a sample of rural seventh-graders from a Midwestern state showed that students involved in a *Life-Skills Training* (LST) program (Botvin, 1996, 2000) were slower to initiate substance use than students who received minimal contact. These results are consistent with other LST approaches (Botvin, Baker, Dusenbury, Tortu & Botvin, 1990; Botvin, Griffin, Diaz, Scheier, Williams & Epstein, 2000). However, not all school prevention efforts influence risk to use substances. In fact, one study suggested that schools which used drug testing to curb drug use did not have lower rates of student self-reported drug use (Yamaguchi et al., 2003).

It should be noted that social behaviors, including drug taking, are learned through cultural influences, and are influenced by culture and community norms (Oetting et al., 1998a). In fact, Oetting and colleagues (1998a) describe numerous cultural/community factors, which include population mobility, neighborhood deviance, and poverty, that can influence adolescent substance use (1998a). Although a full discussion of these factors is beyond the scope of this chapter, one critical community factor that may influence adolescent substance use is neighborhood environment. Novak and colleagues (2002) recently reported that neighborhood environment significantly contributed to beliefs about substance use among urban youth. That is, perceived risk of hard drug use on the part of adolescents was influenced by their residential neighborhood, which was in addition to individual variables like past experiences with drug and alcohol. Perceived risk of drug use also can contribute to adolescent substance use (Johnston et al., 2003b).

Like family factors, gender and ethnicity also contribute to the way that social and community factors can influence adolescent substance use (Harrison & Narayan, 2003; Oetting et al., 1998b; Perry et al., 2003). Perry and colleagues (2003) reported a significant difference in self-reported substance use for boys following the *Drug Abuse Resistance Education* (DARE) Plus prevention program.[1] However, differences were not found among girls. Clearly, gender and ethnicity are associated with risk and resiliency with regard to substance use (Oetting et al., 1998b; O'Malley, Johnston, & Bachman, 1995; Patton, 1995). Consequently, practitioners should tailor prevention and treatment strategies to individuals because risk and resiliency factors vary with a person's gender and ethnicity. Thus, a number of social and community factors have been associated with adolescent substance misuse and abuse, which include peer attitudes toward drug use, school environment and prevention efforts, and other community factors like population mobility, neighborhood deviance, and poverty. The direction of these factors also may contribute to risk or resiliency and vary depending upon gender and ethnicity.

Evidence-Based Treatment Interventions in Community Settings

Program characteristics have been associated with successful treatment outcomes among adolescents as well as particular treatment programs. Overall, there are three types of adolescent substance abuse treatment interventions: (1) community-based outpatient treatment, (2) residential treatment, and (3) therapeutic community treatment. The varied types of programs reflect efforts to target risk factor antecedents (Paglia & Room, 1999), which include the *individual*, with genetic susceptibility and general demographics; *schools*, with school alienation and poor academic performance; the *family*, with familial conflict and family disruption; *peers* who befriend peer substance users; and the *community*, with cultural norms and substance availability (Dakof, Tejeda & Liddle, 2001; Hogue & Liddle, 1999; Lowry, Kann, Collins & Kolbe, 1996; Resnick et al., 1997; Roberts, 1997).

What Works

Current research shows that the most effective adolescent substance abuse intervention programs integrate multiple approaches, which include individual and group counseling, behavioral therapy, education, specialist services like case management, and specialized family therapy to address adolescent characteristics, which

---

[1]The DARE Plus program includes increased parent participation, community involvement, and extracurricular activities in addition to the regular DARE curriculum.

include an adolescent's development and maturation, and patterns that link drug use with other problem behaviors (Crome, 1999; Hogue & Liddle, 1999; Jainchill, Bhattacharya & Yagelka, 1995; McLellan, Alterman, Cacciola, Metzger & O'Brien, 1992; Nutt, 1997).

Family-based adolescent interventions have been shown to be effective in changing adolescent substance use, particularly interventions that target multiple facets of the youth's life (Friedman, Terras & Kreisher, 1995). For example, *Multisystemic Therapy* (MST) was developed as an alternative to incarceration, hospitalization, or residential treatment for serious juvenile offenders (Henggeler, Schoenwald, Liao, Letourneau & Edwards, 2002). A primary feature of this home-based treatment includes case management with intensive individual and family counseling by clinical psychologists, who are available 24 hours a day, seven days a week. Evaluations of this program indicate that adolescents who complete treatment have decreased re-arrest and substance use rates when compared to adolescents in the control groups (Borduin, Henggeler, Blaske & Stein, 1990; Borduin, Mann, Cone, Henggeler, Fucci, Blaske & Williams, 1995), even four years after treatment in the areas of aggressive criminal activity and selected illicit drug use (Henggeler, Clingempeel, Brondino, & Pickrel, 2002).

Similarly, the family-based *Multidimensional Family Therapy* (MDFT), a three-phase treatment program, which addresses social competence, pro-social behaviors, anti-drug use attitudes and behaviors, the peer network, family relationships, problem-solving, and life-style changes, has been found to be effective (Liddle, Dakof, Parker, Diamond, Barrett, & Tejeda, 2001). In a randomized clinical study (Liddle et al., 2001), the MDFT proved efficacious in comparison to two peer-led interventions—the *Multifamily Educational Intervention* (MEI) and *Adolescent Group Therapy* (AGT), —which are mentioned in the paragraphs below. Treatment gains for the MDFT treatment group were maintained with decreased substance use, enhanced academic performance, and family functioning one year after treatment completion (Liddle et al., 2001). Other studies suggest that MDFT is a cost-effective treatment modality when compared to usual community treatment (Liddle, Rowe, Quille, Dakof, Mills, Sakran & Biaggi, 2002). Thus, family-based substance abuse treatment interventions, such as MST and MDFT, show promise in decreasing substance use and increasing important protective factors in the adolescent's life.

What Might Work

Motivational Enhancement Therapy (MET) and *Cognitive-Behavioral Therapy* (CBT) have shown success with adults (Carroll, 1996; Miller, Brown, Simpson, Handmaker, Bien, Luckie, Montgomery, Hester & Tonigan, 1995). In addition, smaller clinical trials indicate that these approaches might be effective for adolescents (Colby, Monti, Barnett, Rohsenow, Weissman, Spirito, Woolard & Lewander, 1998; Kaminer, Burleson, Blitz, Sussman & Rounsaville, 1998; Monti, Colby, Barnett, Spirito, Rohsenow, Myers, Woolard & Lewander, 1999; Waldron, Slesnick, Brody, Turner & Peterson, 2001). With MET, a client's motivation is considered to be internal rather than external. Consequently, the clinician guides a client toward change through listening and reflection, goal-setting, non-confrontational therapy sessions, and by increasing the client's self-efficacy with past successes (for a description of MET, see Miller & Rollnick, 1991). Cognitive-Behavioral Therapy is structured to build coping skills through group discussions, behavioral modeling, and role play (for a description of CBT, see Monti, Abrams, Kadden & Cooney, 1989). However, adolescent-specific research on MET and CBT is limited (Diamond, Godley, Liddle, Sampl, Webb, Tims & Meyers, 2002).

A potential approach for treating drug-involved adolescents is the *Family Empowerment Intervention* (FEI), tested in Florida (Dembo, Livingston & Schmeidler, 2002). FEI treatment goals aim to enhance family functioning, family communication, parenting skills, and increase involvement in social support networks, such as in schools (Dembo, Ramirez-Garnica, Rollie, Schmeidler, Livingston & Hartsfield, 2000). Treatment is provided at home through a trained paraprofessional who delivers three 1-hour meetings per week. The 12-month outcomes from this home-based program yielded fewer drug sales, decreased episodes of intoxication, diminished marijuana use, better psychosocial outcomes, and lower hair-test positive rates for marijuana use when compared to the controls (Dembo et al., 2000, 2002).

The emphasis of delivering treatment to the family is a common denominator among the MST, MDFT, and FEI programs. Clearly, treating the family is an important aspect of enhanced treatment outcomes for adolescents; however more evaluations are needed to determine which particular aspects of these therapies are more efficacious and more cost-effective.

What Does Not Work

Two peer-led interventions, the *Multifamily Educational Intervention* (MEI) and the *Adolescent Group Therapy* (AGT), were tested against the efficacy of MDFT treatment intervention described above (Liddle et al., 2001). The MEI combined psychoeducational and family interventions for troubled adolescents and their families (Liddle et al., 2001). Families were encouraged to help each other during group therapeutic discussions, which focused on stress reduction, improving family organization/communication, and problem-solving. The AGT intervention incorporated adolescent therapy groups to address issues, which included stress management, developing social skills (e.g., communication, self-control, and problem-solving), and building social support among group members. Didactic presentations, group discussions, intense individual sessions, and group skill-building exercises were used to establish participation and trust (Liddle et al., 2001).

Although all of the adolescents in these three treatment modalities demonstrated at least some improvement, the adolescents in the AGT and MEI treatments had higher drop-out rates, higher substance use, lower academic performance, and showed less family functioning in comparison to the MDFT groups following treatment (Liddle et al., 2001). From intake to follow-up, AGT had no effect on family functioning and the MEI group showed deteriorated family relations (Liddle et al., 2001). One year after treatment, 76% of the youths in the MDFT treatment condition had a C average or better, while 60% of AGT and 40% of MEI youths had a C average or better. The AGT treatment group showed better substance abuse outcomes than the MEI group, although these treatment gains were not realized until a year after treatment (Liddle et al., 2001). Given the efficacy of MDFT and the more limited success of AGT in comparison to MEI, the authors concluded that a critical aspect of successful adolescent substance abuse treatment is the concurrent focus on the adolescent and his/her family in an individualized-tailored manner (Liddle et al., 2001).

Evidence-Based Treatment Interventions in Residential Settings

Among criminal justice system-involved adolescents, national studies of substance abuse treatment have shown that residential treatment is an effective approach for treating chemically dependent adolescents and reducing their criminality (Hubbard, Cavanaugh, Craddock & Rachal, 1985; Sells & Simpson, 1979), despite long histories of violent crime, child maltreatment, and personal and/or family dysfunctions (see reviews by Hawkins, Herrenkohl, Farrington, Brewer, Catalano, & Harachi, 1998; Williams & Chang, 2000).

What Works

Given the successes of *adult therapeutic communities* (TCs) when combined with aftercare (De Leon, 1995, 2000; Inciardi, Surratt, Martin & Hooper, 2002; Wexler, 1995), the TC has been modified to address adolescent-specific needs. Jainchill and her colleagues (Jainchill et al., 1995; Jainchill, Hawke, De Leon & Yagelka, 2000) describe the treatment modifications made to the TC model for adolescents, which included a shorter length of stay, family participation in the process, limited use of peer pressure since pretreatment peer influences have generally been negative, a more vertical authority structure, and adolescent clients' having less input than their adult counterparts in TC management. Work is secondary to pursuing a GED or academic achievement. The average length of stays for adolescent TCs are between 6 and 18 months (Jainchill, Bhattacharya & Yagelka, 1995).

The TC model has been shown to be effective for treating adolescents, with decreased drug use across most drug categories, even among high-risk adolescent offenders (Hawke, Jainchill & De Leon, 2000). Despite these successes, only 31% of the youth completed treatment, 52% dropped out, and the rest of the youth were terminated for other reasons (Jainchill, Hawke, De Leon & Yagelka, 2000). However, it is important to note that treatment entry and treatment retention are significant obstacles in treating adolescents in general (Dembo, et al., 2002), particularly those in residential treatment (Orlando, Chan & Morral, 2003).

What Might Work

Although TCs have been the residential treatment modality that have received the most attention in the literature, other residential programs have been evaluated with mixed outcome results. Sealock, Gottfredson, and Gallagher (1997) evaluated a short-term residential program for drug-involved juvenile offenders in Baltimore. The two-month residential treatment included Alcoholics Anonymous group sessions, academic courses, recreation, vocational education, work assignments, and social activities. Before the juveniles were released into the community, a family therapist provided an assessment, developed a treatment plan, and provided family therapy. The intensive phase of treatment was delivered in the community following residential treatment, which included daily communication with youth, regular support group meetings, and family support sessions (Sealock et al., 1997). This evaluation demonstrated problems with treatment fidelity and integrity during the intensive treatment, and the quality and intensity of services delivered were questionable (Sealock et al., 1997). Although there were no differences in the rates of alleged or adjudicated offenses between the aftercare clients and the control group, the aftercare youth reported that they committed fewer new crimes than the controls (Sealock et al., 1997). There was little evidence that the program impacted family involvement and communication, but the youth were less likely to report drug use (Sealock et al., 1997).

In another study, adolescents received residential treatment for ten weeks and participated in group sessions focusing on social development (e.g., self-control, consequential thinking, developing positive social networks, and problem-solving) and substance refusal (Hawkins, Jenson, Catalano & Wells, 1991). Residential treatment was followed by six months of aftercare (Hawkins et al., 1991). This study demonstrated an indirect relationship between social skills and drug use outcomes at the one-year follow-up; improvements in male subjects' social skills lowered intentions to use drugs, and decreased intentions to use were associated with positive drug and alcohol outcomes (Jenson, Wells, Plotnick, Hawkins & Catalano, 1993).

What Does Not Work

Shorter treatment lengths associated with residential programs, such as the two-month Baltimore study described above, have reduced outcomes. National studies have shown that treatment duration is critical, since adolescents require longer time in treatment than adults (Hubbard et al., 1985; Sells & Simpson, 1979; Jainchill et al., 2000). Thus, time in treatment has been positively associated with residential adolescent treatment (Hubbard et al., 1985). Clearly, time in treatment and aftercare are important components of adolescent residential substance abuse treatment. Defining how much attention, time, and resources should be devoted to these areas is a gap in the literature because few treatment programs earmark monies for evaluation (Dembo et al., 2002).

Adolescents are also less likely to complete treatment when they perceive diminished control over treatment entry and level of autonomy while in treatment (Crome, 1999). The literature suggests that adolescent relapse is closely associated with social pressure, so the formation of positive peer groups is important during and after adolescent treatment (Brown, Vik & Creamer, 1989; Dembo, et al., 2002; Kandel, 1985).

Psychopharamacology

Although the use of medications in adolescent treatment is more limited than adult treatment, a basic understanding about the effects, both psychologically and physiologically, that various drugs can have in adolescent treatment is important. Withdrawal from some substances such as alcohol and opioids can require hospitalization initially for safe detoxification. Table 2 provides a summary of drug effects, withdrawal, and management of the most widely used substances by adolescents.

Overall, one of the most important aspects of successful adolescent treatment involves providing multiple interventions that can target multiple facets of an adolescent's life, growth, and development. These components can include family functioning, peer networks, social competence, problem-solving, vocational development, and educational development. Targeted therapy that addresses these areas, in concert with family involvement in treatment, has shown promise in promoting successful treatment outcomes for adolescents.

The Prevention of Substance Abuse

Recent literature reviews have identified characteristics that are associated with effective prevention programs that target low- and high-risk youth (Kumpfer & Alvarado, 2003; Nation et al., 2003; Paglia & Room, 1999; Tobler, Roona, Ochshorn, Marshall, Streke & Stackpole, 2000). While earlier prevention programming focused on single behaviors (Catalano, Hawkins, Berglund, Pollard & Arthur, 2002), recent substance use prevention interventions focus on schools, communities, mass media, policy changes, and enforcement (Bauman & Phongsavan, 1999). Prevention interventions are successful when they incorporate broad health-promotion and competence-enhancement strategies, targeting reductions in risk factors and enhancing protective factors (Durlak & Wells, 1997; Kumpfer & Alvarado, 2003; Taylor & Biglan, 1998; Nation et al., 2003; Tobler, Roona, Ochshorn, Marshall, Streke & Stackpole, 2000; Webster-Stratton & Hammond, 1997; Weissberg, Kumpfer & Seligman, 2003).

Studies also indicate that prevention programs must be age-appropriate (Kumpfer & Alvarado, 2003; Nation et al., 2003; Webster-Stratton & Taylor, 2001) and socioculturally relevant to be successful (Nation et al., 2003; Kumpfer, Alvarado, Smith & Bellamy, 2002). Studies have also shown that an anti-drug program's message to adolescents is effective when discussion is focused on the short-term effects of substance use such as diminished attractiveness rather than the long-term adverse effects, such as poor health (Paglia & Room, 1999).

What Works

One example of a successful comprehensive prevention program is the *Midwestern Prevention Project* (Pentz, 1998, 1989). Initially implemented in Kansas City, Missouri and later in Indianapolis, Indiana, this program included mass media, school-based skills training, parent programming, school policy changes, and community organization to address changing local ordinances on the availability of alcohol and tobacco products. Adolescent alcohol, cigarette, and marijuana use decreased significantly from baseline to the one-year follow up, and reduced rates of cigarette and marijuana use among high- and low-risk youth were maintained over three years (Chou et al., 1998).

Family participation in treatment is another cornerstone of an effective prevention program (Nation et al., 2003; Tobler et al., 2000). Research consistently suggests that strategies for improved family relations, communication, and parental supervision are critical links to improved outcomes (Ary, Duncan, Biglan, Metzler, Noell & Smolkowski, 1999; Taylor & Biglan, 1998). The National Institute on Drug Abuse endorses family interventions/therapy because family relationships are associated with risk factors, mediators, or protective factors in the literature (Swadi, 1999). Programs like *Preparing for the Drug Free Years* (Kosterman, Hawkins, Haggerty, Spoth & Redmond, 2001) and the *Strengthening Families Program* (Kumpfer & Alvarado, 2003) which target parents of 6–10-year-old children of substance abusers and families of young children and preteens are examples of family-based prevention programs.

Both of these family preventive programs (1) target reducing familial risk factors, such as poor familial communication; (2) provide parenting skills training; and (3) enhance protective factors associated with teen substance use. An evaluation of the Preparing for the Drug Free Years reported significant reductions in teen alcohol use at 1-, 2-, and 3½-year follow-ups (Kosterman et al., 2001; Park et al., 2000). Several evaluations have reported the efficacy of enhanced parenting skills and family communication and reduced family conflict across ethnic groups, in rural and urban settings (Aktan, Kumpfer & Turner, 1996; Kumpfer, Molgaard & Spoth, 1996).

What Might Work

A school-based project with multiple prevention activities called *Project Northland* targeted middle school-aged children with four program components—parental involvement, educational activities, peer leadership, and community task force activities—that were implemented in randomized school districts (Perry, Williams, Veblen-Mortenson, Toomey, Komro, Anstine et al., 1996). By the end of eighth grade, intervention participants showed decreased alcohol use, even among the regular drinkers, as well as reduced cigarette and marijuana use (Perry et al., 1996). Similarly, one experimental tobacco trial of the *Program to Advance Teen Health* (PATH) found that the school- and community-based program was more successful in decreasing tobacco use among teens than its school-only counterpart (Biglan, Ary, Smolkowski, Duncan & Black, 2000). Thus, comprehensive prevention programs that use consistent messages from multiple social contexts, show efficacy in delaying adolescent substance use and abuse (Paglia & Room, 1999).

Other studies have shown that sufficient intervention dosage, such as the quantity and quality of intervention contact hours, is a critical part of successful prevention interventions (Kumpfer & Alvarado, 2003; Nation et al., 2003). In a longitudinal, randomized trial of a school-based prevention program, Botvin and colleagues (1995) reported that a multicomponent approach in the seventh grade with booster sessions in the eighth and ninth grades reduced alcohol and drug use for the intervention group, and these gains were maintained at a six-year follow-up. Another school-based program, *Project ALERT*, used booster sessions in the eighth grade to reinforce what youth had learned in the previous year and demonstrated, in a large randomized study in 30 schools in California and Oregon, reduced drug use among high- and low-risk students (Ellickson & Bell, 1990). The school-based *Reconnecting Youth program* targeted high school students at risk of dropping out and with behavioral problems (Eggert, Thompson, Herting, Nicholas & Dicker, 1994). Reductions in substance use and involvement with deviant peers were reported at the follow-up (Eggert et al., 1994); however, further research is needed to see if these results can be replicated.

What Does Not Work

Prevention researchers advocate using varied, interactive teaching methods to enhance important life skills, which include assertiveness, communication, and coping (Nation et al., 2003; Tobler et al., 2000). However, educational approaches alone, particularly those that use didactic teaching methods, have demonstrated limited decreases in drug use among youth (Paglia & Room, 1999). In a meta-analysis of 207 school-based programs, Tobler et al. (2000) found that program type (interactive) and size (smaller programs) were significant predictors for effectiveness. In contrast, non-interactive prevention programs, which used lectures to deliver drug knowledge or affective development, demonstrated small effects (Tobler et al., 2000).

A popular, but ineffective, prevention program that uses didactic teaching is *DARE*. Fifteen evaluation studies report that DARE does not have long-term effects on adolescent drug use (Clayton, Leukefeld, Harrington & Cattarello, 1996; Clayton, Cattarello & Johnstone, 1996; Ennett, Tobler, Ringwalt & Flewelling, 1994; Lynam et al., 1999; Ringwalt, Green, Ennett, Lachan, Clayton & Leukefeld, 1994). The proliferation of the DARE program exemplifies the need for theory and research support before program implementation (Nation et al., 2003). Effective prevention programs have been developed and identified, but recent studies show that effective programs are rarely implemented (Ennett et al., 2003; Kumpfer, 2002; Ringwalt, Ennett, Vincus, Thorne, Rohrbach & Simons–Rudolph, 2002). Although DARE is widely regarded as ineffective, DARE Plus has been revised to include increased parental participation, community involvement, and extracurricular activities, which are key elements of effective prevention programs (Perry et al., 2003). Initial findings of DARE Plus are discussed earlier. It is important to emphasize that the DARE program changed in response to evaluation data.

Finally, rural communities might be in low stages of prevention program readiness (Plested, Smitham, Jumper-Thurman, Oetting & Edwards, 1999). Consequently, rural practitioners in "low prevention readiness" areas should be sensitive to historical and cultural issues that support drug use and should use local information. In rural communities that are "prevention ready," practitioners should identify effective and feasible program models, target local resources, and plan staff training (Plested et al., 1999).

Recommendations

The adolescent substance abuse literature has expanded over the past years in the areas of etiology, treatment interventions, and prevention approaches. The etiological literature embraces the importance of risk and protective factors within the public health framework. We know that certain factors have been associated with drug misuse and abuse. These factors are individual factors, which include poor school attendance, low grades, delinquency, low self-esteem; family factors, which include disorganized families, lack of family cohesion, and poor parenting; peer factors, which include peer substance use and peer problem behaviors; and social/community factors, which include inconsistent messages.

One of the first steps in understanding and helping an adolescent drug abuser is being aware of the direct effects of the drugs on an adolescent and the associated withdrawal symptoms. This information will help identify problems, avert medical emergencies, and will inform the next step, whether it is pharmacologically assisted withdrawal or placement on a medication that might help decrease relapse. Another key component in helping an adolescent drug abuser is knowledge about comorbidities associated with drug abuse liability. This knowledge can increase sensitivity to understand the unique problems that an adolescent drug abuser with comorbidity may encounter when experiencing the effects of a drug and/or relapsing. Key to managing the adolescent drug abuser is knowledge about acute drug effects, drug withdrawal, and comorbidity. A critical adjunct to this sensitivity is a relationship with a clinician who can assess and treat drug toxicity, drug withdrawal, and/or comorbidity.

Family factors associated with resiliency to adolescent drug use include consistent rules, monitoring, and increased parental involvement. Family factors which have been consistently related to risky adolescent drug use include more adverse childhood events and parental substance use. Thus, parents should take a positive and active part in the lives of their children, maintain consistent rules with follow-up, not use illicit drugs, and promote no drug use. Social and community factors that have been associated with resiliency to drug use include prosocial peer interactions, participation in positive activities, and community/school prevention activities. Social and community factors related to risk to drug use include peers and communities that accept substance use. Thus, to decrease drug use among adolescents, communities should discourage drug use and encourage positive extracurricular activities. Schools should also adopt effective substance use prevention interventions.

When adolescent treatment interventions are examined, the most promising approaches target multiple domains within an adolescent's life, which include their family, an adolescent's development and maturation, adolescent peer networks, and behavioral patterns that are linked to drug abuse and other problem behaviors. More effective drug abuse treatment programs incorporate several therapeutic approaches, including individual counseling, group sessions, structure, and case management. Regardless of where adolescents receive treatment, from a community-based program or a residential program, adolescents benefit most from treatment when their families are active participants in the therapeutic process. For high-risk youth who require residential treatment, a modified therapeutic community has shown promise in decreasing substance use and criminality while increasing pro-social behaviors. The amount of time devoted to length of stay and aftercare are areas that warrant future attention.

Prevention interventions, which target families, schools, and communities with consistent "no use" messages are more effective, particularly when planned booster sessions are used after treatment. Rather than using didactic teaching methods and focusing on single behaviors, the hallmarks of effective prevention programs are interactive educational approaches, which include targeting multiple behaviors, specific ages, and culturally appropriate values. Finally, given the number of adolescents who continue to experiment with drugs, additional research is needed to understand better adolescence issues and to examine innovative approaches to prevent and treat drug misuse and abuse.

Support is acknowledged from grants Nos. DA 13076 and DA11580 from the National Institute on Drug Abuse.

References

Ahu, A.J., & Walsh, B.T., (2002). Pharmacologic treatment of eating disorders. *Canadian Journal of Psychiatry, 47,* 227–234.

Aktan, G.B., Kumpfer, K.L., & Turner, C.W. (1996). Effectiveness of a family skills training program for substance use prevention with inner city African-American families. *Substance Use and Misuse, 31,* 157–175.

Andrucci G.L., Archer R.P., Pancoast D.L., & Gordon R.A. (1989). The relationship of MMPI and sensation seeking scales to adolescent drug use. *Journal of Personality Assessment, 53,* 253–266.

Ary, D.V., Duncan, T.E., Biglan, A., Metzler, C.W., Noell, J.W., & Smolkowksi, K. (1999). Development of adolescent problem behavior. *Journal of Abnormal Child Psychology, 27,* 141–150.

Bacaltchuk, J., & Hay, P. (2003). Antidepressants versus placebo for people with bulimia nervosa. Cochrane Database System Review (4):CD003391.

Bauman, A. & Phongsavan, P. (1999). Epidemiology of substance use in adolescence: prevalence, trends and policy implications. *Drug and Alcohol Dependence, 55,* 187–207.

Beauvais, F., & Oetting, E.R., (2002). Variances in the etiology of drug use among ethnic groups of adolescents. *Public Health Records, 117*(S1), S8–S14.

Beck, K., Thombs, D., Mahoney, C., & Fingar, K. (1995). Social context and sensation seeking: Gender differences in college student drinking motivations. *International Journal of Addictions, 30,* 1101–1115.

Biederman, J., Wilens, T.E., Mick, E., Faraone, S.V., & Spencer, T. (1998). Does Attention Deficit Hyperactivity Disorder impact the developmental course of drug and alcohol abuse and dependence? *Biological Psychiatry, 44,* 269–273.

Biglan, A., Ary, D.V., Smolkowski, K., Duncan, T., & Black, C. (2000). A randomized controlled trial of a community intervention to prevent adolescent tobacco use. *Tobacco Control, 9,* 24–32.

Borduin, C.M., Henggeler, S.W., Blaske, D.M. & Stein, R.J. (1990). Multisystemic treatment of adolescent sexual offenders. *International Journal of Offender Therapy and Comparative Criminology, 34,* 105–113.

Borduin, C.M., Mann, B.J., Cone, L.T., Henggeler, S.M., Fucci, B.R., Blaske, D.M., & Williams, R.A. (1995). Multisystemic treatment of serious juvenile offenders: Long-term prevention of criminality and violence. *Journal of Consulting and Clinical Psychology, 63,* 569–578.

Botvin G.J., (1996). *Life Skills Training: Promoting Health and Personal Development.* Princeton, N.J.: Princeton Health Press.

Botvin, G.J., (2000). *Life Skills Training.* Princeton, N.J.: Princeton Health Press.

Botvin, G.J., Baker, E., Dusenbury, L., Botvin, E.M., & Diaz, T. (1995). Long-term follow-up results of a randomized drug abuse prevention trial in a white middle-class population. *The Journal of the American Medical Association, 273,* 1106–1112.

Botvin, G.J., Baker, E., Dusenbury, L., Tortu, S., & Botvin, E., (1990). Preventing adolescent drug abuse through a multi-modal cognitive-behavioral approach: Results of a 3-year study. *Journal of Consulting and Clinical Psychology, 58*(4), 437–446.

Botvin, G.J., Griffin, K.W., Diaz, T., Scheier, L., Williams, C., & Epstein, J.A., (2000). Preventing illicit drug use in adolescents: Long-term follow-up data from a randomized control trial of a school population. *Addictive Behaviors, 5,* 769–774.

Brady J., & Lukas S.E. (1984). Testing drugs for physical dependence potential and abuse liability. NIDA Monograph 52, Washington, DC: US Government Printing Office.

Brook, J.S., Cohen, P., Whiteman, M., & Gordon, A.S., (1992). Psychosocial risk factors in the transition from moderate to heavy use or abuse of drugs. In M.D. Glantz & R.W. Pickens (Eds.). *Vulnerability to drug abuse* (pp. 359–388). Washingon, DC: American Psychological Association.

Brook, J.S., Kessler, R.C., & Cohen, P. (1999). The onset of marijuana use from preadolescence and early adolescence to young adulthood. *Development and Psychopathology, 11,* 901–914.

Brown, S.A., Vik, P.W., & Creamer, V.A. (1989). Characteristics of Relapse following adolescent substance abuse treatment. *Addictive Behavior, 14,* 291–300.

Bukstein O. (1997) Practice parameters for the assessment and treatment of children and adolescents with substance use disorders. *Journal of the America Academy of Child and Adolescent Psychiatry, 36*(10 Suppl), 140S–156S.

Bukstein, O.G., Brent, D.A., & Kaminer, Y. (1989) Comorbidity of substance abuse and other psychiatric disorders in adolescents. *American Journal of Psychiatry, 146,* 1131–1141.

Bukstein, O.G., Glancy, L.J., & Kaminer, Y. (1992) Patterns of affective comorbidity in a clinical population of dually diagnosed adolescent substance abusers. *Journal of the America Academy of Child and Adolescent Psychiatry, 31*(6), 1041–1045.

Cambor, R.L., & Millman, R.B. (1996). Alcohol and drug abuse in adolescents. In M. Lewis (Ed.), *Child and Adolescent Psychiatry: A Comprehensive Textbook* (2nd ed., pp. 736–752). Baltimore, MD: Williams & Wilkins.

Carroll, K.M. (1996). Relapse prevention as a psychosocial treatment: a review of controlled clinical trials. *Experimental and Clinical Psychopharmacology, 4,* 46–54.

Catalano, R.F., Hawkins, J.D., Berglund, M.L., Pollard, J.A., and Arthur, M.W. (2002). Prevention Science and Positive Youth Development: Competitive or Cooperative Frameworks? *Journal of Adolescent Health, 31,* 230–239.

Cattarello, A.M., Clayton, R.R., & Leukefeld, C.G., (1995). Adolescent alcohol and drug abuse. In J.H. Oldham & M.B. Riba (Eds.), *Review of Psychiatry Volume 14* (pp. 151–168). Washington, DC: American Psychiatric Press.

Chait, L.D. (1994) Reinforcing and subjective effects of methylphenidate in humans. *Behavioral Pharmacology, 5*, 281–288.

Chou, C.P., Montgomery, S., Pentz, M.A., Rohrbach, L.A., Anderson Johnson, C., Flay, B.R., & MacKinnon, D.P. (1998). Effects of a Community-Based Prevention Program on Decreasing Drug Use in High-Risk Adolescents. *American Journal of Public Health, 88*(6), 944–948.

Clayton, R.W. (1992). Transitions in drug use: Risk and protective factors In M.D. Glantz & R.W. Pickens (Eds.), *Vulnerability to Drug Abuse* (pp. 15–52). Washington, DC: American Psychological Association.

Clayton, R.R., Cattarello, A.M., & Johnstone, B.M. (1996). The effectiveness of Drug Abuse Resistance Education (Project DARE): Five year follow-up results. *Preventive Medicine, 25*, 307–318.

Clayton, R.R., Leukefeld, C.G., Donohew, L., Bardo, M., & Harrington, N.G., (1995). Risk and protective factors: A brief review. In C.G. Leukefeld & R.R. Clayton (Eds.). *Prevention Practice in Substance Abuse* (pp. 7–14). Binghamton, NY: Haworth.

Clayton, R.R., Leukefeld, C.G., Harrington, N., Cattarello, A. (1996). DARE (Drug Abuse Resistance Education): Very Popular but Not Very Effective. In C.B. McCoy, L.R. Metsch, & J.A. Inciardi (Eds.). *Intervening with Drug-Involved Youth* (pp. 101–109). Thousand Oaks, CA: SAGE Publications

Cohen, D.A., & Rice, J., (1997). Parenting styles, adolescent substance use, and academic achievement. *Journal of Drug Education, 27*(2), 199–211.

Colby, S.M., Monti, P.M., Barnett, N.P., Rohsenow, D.J., Weissman, K., Spirito, A., Woolard, R.H., & Lewander, W.J. (1998). Brief motivational interviewing in a hospital setting for adolescent smoking: a preliminary study. *Journal of Consulting and Clinical Psychology, 66*, 574–578.

Conners, C.K., Levin, E.D., Sparrow, E., Hinton, S.C., Erhardt, D., Meck, W.H., Rose, J.E., & March, J. (1996) Nicotine and attention in adult attention deficit hyperactivity disorder. *Psychopharmacology Bulletin, 32*(1), 67–73.

Crome, I.B. (1999). Treatment interventions – looking towards the millennium. *Drug and Alcohol Dependence, 55*, 247–263.

Crowley, T.J., & Riggs, P.D. (1995) Adolescent substance use disorder with conduct disorder and comorbid conditions. *Adolescent Drug Abuse: Clinical Assessment and Therapeutic Interventions. NIDA Research Monograph 156. (NIH Publication No. 95-3908.)* (pp. 49–111). Rockville, MD: U.S. Department of Health and Human Services.

Dakof, G.A., Tejeda, M., & Liddle, H.A. (2001). Predictors of Engagement in Adolescent Drug Abuse Treatment. *Journal of the American Academy of Child and Adolescent Psychiatry, 40*(3), 274–281.

Daugherty, R.P. & Leukefeld, C.G. (1998). *Preventing Alcohol and Drug Problems Across the Life Span.* New York: Plenum

Daviss, W.B., Bentivoglio P., Racusin R., Brown K.M., Bostic J.Q., & Wiley L. (2001) Bupropion sustained release in adolescents with comorbid attention-deficit/hyperacivity disorder and depression. *Journal of the American Academy of Child and Adolescent Psychiatry , 40*(3), 307–314.

Deas, D. Randall, C.L., Roberts, J.S., & Anton, R.F. (2000). A double-blind, placebo-controlled trial of sertraline in depressed adolescent alcoholics: a pilot study. *Human Psychopharmaocology, 15* (6), 461–469.

Deas, D., & Thomas, S.E., (2001) An overview of controlled studies of adolescent substance abuse treatment. *American Journal on Addictions, 10*(2), 178–189.

De Leon, G. (1995). Therapeutic communities for addictions: A theoretical framework. *The International Journal of the Addictions, 30*, 1603–1645.

De Leon, G. (2000). *The Therapeutic Community: Theory, Model, and Method.* New York: Springer Publishing Company.

Dembo, R., Livingston, S., & Schmeidler, J. (2002). Treatment for Drug-Involved Youth in the Juvenile Justice System. In: C.G. Leukefeld, F. Tims, & D. Farabee (Eds.), *Treatment of Drug Offenders: Policies and Issues.* New York: Springer Publishing Company.

Dembo, R., Ramirez-Garnica, G., Rollie, M., Schmeidler, J., Livingston, S., & Hartsfield, A. (2000). Youth recidivism 12 months after a family empowerment intervention: Final report. *Journal of Offender Rehabilitation, 31*, 29–65.

Denton, R., & Kampfe, C. (1994). The relationship between family variables and adolescent substance abuse: A literature review. *Adolescence, 29*(114), 475–495.

de Wit, H., & Bodker, B. (1994) Personality and drug preference in normal volunteers. *International Journal of Addiction, 20*, 1617–1630.

de Wit, D.J., Offord, D.R., & Wong, M. (1997). Patterns of onset and cessation of drug use over the early part of the life course. *Health Education & Behavior, 24,* 746–758.

Diamond, G., Godley, S.H., Liddle, H.A., Sampl, S., Webb, C., Tims, F.M., & Meyers, R. (2002). Five outpatient treatment models for adolescent marijuana use: a description of the Cannabis Youth Treatment Interventions. *Addiction,* 97 (Suppl 1), 70–83.

Dube, S.R., Felitti, V.J., Dong, M., Chapman, D.P., Giles, W.H., & Anda, R.F. (2003). Childhood abuse, neglect, and household dysfunction and the risk of illicit drug use: The adverse childhood experiences study. *Pediatrics, 111*(3), 564–572.

Durlak, J.A. & Wells, A.M. (1997). Primary prevention mental health programs for children and adolescents: A meta-analytic review. *American Journal of Community Psychology, 25,* 115–152.

Eggert, L.L., Thompson, E.A., Herting, J.R., Nicholas, L.J., & Dicker, G.C. (1994). Preventing adolescent drug abuse and high school dropout through an intensive school-based social network development program. *American Journal of Health Promotion, 8(3),* 202–215.

Ellickson, P.L., & Bell, R.M., (1990). Drug prevention in junior high: A multi-site longitudinal test. *Science, 247,* 1299–1305.

Ennett, S.T., Ringwalt, C.L., Thorne, J., Rohrbach, L.A., Vincus, A., Simons-Rudolph, A., & Jones, S. (2003). A Comparison of Current Practice in School-Based Substance Use Prevention Programs with Meta-Analysis Findings. *Prevention Science, 4*(1), 1–14.

Ennett, S.T., Tobler, N., Ringwalt, C., & Flewelling, R. (1994). How effective is drug abuse education? A meta-analysis of Project DARE outcome evaluations. *American Journal of Public Health, 84,* 1394–1401.

Ensminger, M.E., Juon, H.S., & Fothergill, K.E., (2002). Childhood and adolescent antecedents of substance use in adulthood. *Addiction, 97*(7), 833–844.

Fergusson, D.M., Woodward, L.J., & Horwood, L.J. (2000) Risk factors and life processes associated with the onset of suicidal behavior during adolescence and early adulthood. *Psychological Medicine, 30*(1), 23–39.

Friedman, L., Hyman, S.E., Roberts, D.H., & Fleming, N.F. (1996). *Source Book of Substance Abuse and Addiction.* Baltimore: Lippincott, Williams and Wilkins.

Friedman, A.S., Terras, A., & Kreisher, C. (1995). Family and client characteristics as predictors of outpatient treatment outcome for adolescent drug abusers. *Journal of Substance Abuse, 7,* 345–356.

Geller, B., Cooper, T.B., Sun K., Zimerman B., Frazier J., Williams M., & Heath J. (1998) Double-blind and placebo-controlled study of lithium for adolescent bipolar disorders with secondary substance dependency. *Journal of the American Academy of Child and Adolescent Psychiatry, 37*(2), 171–178.

Gerberich, S.G., Sidney, S., Braun, B.L., Tekawa, I.S., Tolan, K.K., & Quesenberry, Jr, C.P. (2003) Marijuana use and injury events resulting in hospitalization. *Annals of Epidemiology, 13,* 230–237.

Gil, A.G., Vega, W.A., & Turner, R.J. (2002). Early and mid-adolescence risk factors for later substance abuse by African Americans and European Americans. *Public Health Reports, 117*(S1), S15–S29.

Grella, C.E., Hser YI, Joshi V., & Rounds-Bryant J. (2001) Drug treatment outcomes for adolescents with comorbid mental and substance use disorders. *Journal of Nervous and Mental Disease, 189*(6), 384–392.

Guo, J, Hill, K.G., Hawkins, J.D., Catalano, R.F., & Abbott, R.D. (2002). A developmental analysis of sociodemographic, family, and peer effects on adolescent illicit drug initiation. *Journal of the American Academy of Child and Adolescent Psychiatry, 41*(7), 838–845.

Haney, M., Ward A.S., Comer S.D., Hart C.L., Foltin R.W., & Fischman M.W. (2001). Bupropion SR worsens mood during marijuana withdrawal in humans. *Psychopharmacology, 155*(2), 171–179.

Hanson, K., Allen, S., Jensen, S., & Hatsukami, D. (2003) Treatment of adolescent smokers with the nicotine patch. *Nicotine and Tobacco Research, 5*(4), 515–526.

Harrison, P.A., & Narayan, G. (2003). Differences in behavior, psychological factors, and environmental factors associated with participation in school sports and other activities in adolescence. *Journal of School Health, 73*(3), 113–120.

Hawke, J.M., Jainchill, N., & De Leon, G. (2000). Adolescent Amphetamine Users in Treatment: Client Profiles and Treatment Outcomes. *Journal of Psychoactive Drugs, 32*(1), 95–105.

Hawkins, J.D., Catalano, R.D., & Miller, J.Y. (1992): Risk and protective factors for alcohol and other drug problems in adolescence and early adulthood: Implications for substance abuse prevention. *Psychological Bulletin, 112,* 64–105.

Hawkins, J.D., Herrenkohl, T., Farrington, D.P., Brewer, D., Catalano, R.F., & Harachi, T.W. (1998). A review of Predictors of Youth Violence. In R. Loeber & D.P. Farrington (Eds.), *Serious Violent Juvenile Offenders.* Thousand Oaks, CA: Sage.

Hawkins, J.D., Jenson, J.M., Catalano, R.F., & Wells, E.A. (1991). Effects of a skills training intervention with juvenile delinquents. *Research on Social Work Practice, 1,* 107–121.

Henggeler, S.W., Clingempeel, W.G., Brondino, M.J., & Pickrel, S.G. (2002). Four-Year Follow-up of Multi-systemic Therapy with Substance-Abusing and Substance-Dependent Juvenile Offenders. *Journal of the American Academy of Child and Adolescent Psychiatry, 41*(7), 868–874.

Henggeler, S.W., Schoenwald, S.K., Liao, J.G., Letourneau, E.J., & Edwards, D.L. (2002). Transporting Efficacious Treatments to Field Settings: The Link between Supervisory Practices and Therapist Fidelity in MST Programs. *Journal of Clinical Child Psychology, 31*(2), 155–167.

Henningfield, J.E., & Griffiths, R.R. (1981) Cigarette smoking and subjective response: Effects of d-amphetamine. *Clinical Pharmacology and Therapeutics, 30*, 497–505.

Hogue, A. & Liddle, H.A. (1999). Family-based Preventive Intervention: An Approach to Preventing Substance Use and Antisocial Behavior. *American Journal of Orthopsychiatry, 69*(3), 278–293.

Howard, M.O., Walker, R.D., Walker, P.S., Cottler, L.B., Compton, W.M. (1999) Inhalant use among urban American Indian youth. *Addiction, 94*(1), 83–95.

Hser, Y.I., Grella, C., Collins, C., Teruya, C. (2003) Drug-use initiation and conduct disorder among adolescents in drug treatment. *Journal of Adolescence, 26*(3): 331–45.

Hubbard, R.L., Cavanaugh, E.R., Craddock, S.G., & Rachal, J.V. (1985). Characteristics, behaviors, and outcomes for youth in the TOPS. In A.S. Friedman & G.M. Beschner, (Eds.). *Treatment Services for Adolescent Substance Abusers* (pp. 49–65)., Rockville, MD: National Institute on Drug Abuse. NIDA-DHHS Publication No. ADM 85–1342.

Inciardi, J.A., Surratt, H.L., Martin, S.S., & Hooper, R.M. (2002). The Importance of Aftercare in a Corrections-Based Treatment Continuum. In: C.G. Leukefeld, F. Tims, & D. Farabee (Eds.). *Treatment of Drug Offenders: Policies and Issues.* New York: Springer Publishing Company.

Jainchill, N., Bhattacharya, G., & Yagelka, J. (1995). Therapeutic Communities for Adolescents. In E. Rahdert & D. Czechowicz (Eds.). *Adolescent Drug Abuse: Clincial Assessment and Therapeutic Interventions* (pp. 190–217). *NIDA Research Monograph 156 (NIH Publication No.: 95-3908).* Rockville, MD: National Institute on Drug Abuse, Division of Clinical and Services Research.

Jainchill, N., Hawke, J., De Leon, G., & Yagelka, J. (2000). Adolescents in Therapeutic Communities: One-Year Posttreatment Outcomes. *Journal of Psychoactive Drugs, 32*, 81–94.

Jenson J.M., Wells, E.A., Plotnick, R.D., Hawkins, J.D., & Catalano, R.F. (1993). The effects of skills and intentions to use drugs on posttreatment drug use of adolescents. *American Journal of Drug and Alcohol Abuse, 19*(1), 1–18.

Jessor, R. & Jessor, S. (1977). *Problem Behavior and Psychosocial Development: A Longitudinal Study of Youth.* New York: Academic Press.

Johnston, L.D., O'Malley, P.M., & Bachman, J.G. (2003a). *Monitoring the Future National Results on Adolescent Drug Use: Overview of Key Findings, 2002. (NIH Publication No. 03-5374).* Bethesda, MD: National Institute on Drug Abuse.

Johnston, L.D., O'Malley, P.M., & Bachman, J.G. (2003b). *Monitoring the Future National Survey Results on Drug Use, 1975–2002. Volume I: Secondary School Students (NIH Publication No. 03-5375).* Bethesda, MD: National Institute on Drug Abuse.

Kaminer, Y., Burleson, J.A., Blitz, C., Sussman, J., & Rounsaville, B.J. (1998). Psychotherapies for adolescent substance abusers: a pilot study. *Journal of Nervous and Mental Disorders, 186*, 684–690.

Kandel, D.B. (1985). On processes of peer influences in adolescent drug use: A developmental perspective. In: J. Brook, D. Lettieri, D. Brook; & B. Stimmel (Eds.). *Alcohol and Substance Abuse in Adolescence.* New York: Haworth Press.

Kaplan, H.B., Martin, S.S., & Robbins, C. (1982). Application of a general theory of deviant behavior: Self-derogation and adolescent drug use. *Journal of Health and Social Behavior, 23*, 274–294.

Kellam, S.G., Brown, C., Rubin, B., & Ensminger, M. (1983). Paths leading to teenage psychiatric symptoms and substance abuse: Developmental epidemiological studies in Woodlawn. In S. Guze, F. Earls, & J. Barrett (Eds.). *Childhood Psychopathology and Development* (pp. 17–51). New York: Raven.

Kelly, T.M., Cornelius, J.R., Lynch, K.G. (2002) Psychiatric and substance use disorders as risk factors for attempted suicide among adolescents: a case control study. *Suicide and Life Threatening Behaviors, 32*(3), 301–12.

Kilpatrick, D.G., Ruggiero, K.J., Acierno, R., Saunders, B.E., Resnick, H.S., & Best, C.L. (2003) Violence and risk of PTSD, major depression, substance abuse/dependence, and comorbidity: results from the National Survey of Adolescents. *Journal of Consulting and Clinical Psychology, 71*(4), 692–700.

Klein, R.G., Abikoff, H. Klass, E., Ganeles, D., Sees, L.M., & Pollack, S. (1997) Clinical efficacy of methylphenidate in conduct disorder with and without attention deficit hyperactivity disorder. *Archives of General Psychiatry, 54*(12), 1073–80.

Kosterman, R., Hawkins, J.D., Haggerty, K.P., Spoth, R., & Redmond, C. (2001). Preparing for the Drug Free Years: Session-Specific Effects of a Universal Parent-Training Intervention with Rural Families. *Journal of Drug Education, 31*(1), 47–68.

Kumpfer, K.L. (2002). Prevention of alcohol and drug abuse: What works? *Journal of Substance Abuse, 23* (Suppl. 3), 25–44.

Kumpfer, K.L., & Alvarado, R. (2003). Family-Strengthening Approaches for the Prevention of Youth Problem Behaviors. *American Psychologist, 58*, 457–465.

Kumpfer, K.L., Alvarado, R., Smith, P., & Bellamy, N. (2002). Cultural sensitivity and adaptation in family-based interventions. *Prevention Science, 3*, 241–246.

Kumpfer, K.L., Molgaard, V., & Spoth, R. (1996). Family interventions for the prevention of delinquency and drug use in special populations. In R. Peters & R. McMahon (Eds.). *Preventing Childhood Disorders, Substance Abuse, and Delinquency* (pp. 241–267). Thousand Oaks, CA: Sage.

Kuperman, S., Schlosser, S.S., Kramer, J.R., Bucholz, K., Hesselbrock, V., Reich, T., & Reich, W., (2001). Developmental sequence from disruptive behavior diagnosis to adolescent alcohol dependence. *American Journal of Psychiatry, 158*, 2022–2026.

Kushner, M.G., Mackenzie, T.B., Fiszdon, J. Valentiner, D.P., Foa, E., Anderson, N., & Wangensteen, D. (1996). The effects of alcohol consumption on laboratory-induced panic and state anxiety. *Archives of General Psychiatry, 53*(3), 264–270.

Lescohier, I., & Gallagher, S.S. (1996). Unintentional Injury. in R.J. DiClemente, W.B. Hansen, & L.E. Ponton (Eds). *Handbook of Adolescent Health Risk Behavior* (pp. 225–258). New York: Plenum Press.

Leukefeld, C.G., & Leukefeld, S. (1999). Primary socialization theory and a bio/psycho/social/spiritual practice model for substance use. *Substance Use & Misuse, 34*(7), 983–991.

Leukefeld, C.G., Logan, T.K., Clayton, R.R., Martin, C., Zimmerman, R., Cattarello, A., Milich, R., & Lynam, D. (1998). Adolescent drug use, delinquency, and other behaviors. In T.P. Gullotta, G.R. Adams, & R. Montemayor (Eds.). *Delinquent Violent Youth: Theory and Interventions* (pp. 98–128). Thousand Oaks, CA: Sage.

Li, C., Pentz, M.A., & Chou, C.P. (2002). Parental substance use as a modifier of adolescent substance use risk. *Addiction, 97*(12), 1537–1550.

Liappas, J., Paparrigopoulos, T., Tzavellas, E., & Christodoulou, G., (2003) Alcohol detoxification and social anxiety symptoms: a preliminary study of the impact of mirtazapine administration. *Journal of Affective Disorders, 76*, 279–284.

Liddle, H.A., Dakof, G.A., Parker, K., Diamond, G.S., Barrett, K., & Tejeda, M. (2001) Multidimensional Family Therapy for Adolescent Drug Abuse: Results of a Randomized Clinical Trial. *American Journal on Drug and Alcohol Abuse, 27*(4), 651–688.

Liddle, H.A., Rowe, C.L., Quille, T.J., Dakof, G.A., Mills, D.S., Sakran, E., & Biaggi, H. (2002). Transporting a research-based adolescent drug treatment into practice. Journal of *Substance Abuse Treatment, 22*, 231–243.

Lowry, R., Kann, L., Collins, J., & Kolbe, L. (1996). The effect of socioeconomic status on chronic disease risk behaviors among US adolescents. *Journal of the American Medical Association, 276* (10), 792–797.

Lynam, D. (1996). The early identification of chronic offenders: Who is the fledgling psychopath? *Psychological Bulletin, 120*, 209–234.

Lynam, D., Milich, R., Zimmerman, R. Logan, TK, Martin, C., Leukefeld, C., Clayton, R. (1999). Project DARE demonstrates no effects at 10-year follow-up. *Journal of Consulting and Clinical Psychology, 67*, 590–593.

McLellan, A.T., Alterman, A.I., Cacciola, J.S., Metzger, D., & O'Brien, C.P. (1992). A new measure of substance abuse treatment: initial studies of the Treatment Survey Review. *Journal of Nervous and Mental Disorders, 180*, 101–110.

March, J., & Wells, K. (2002) Combining medications and psychotherapy. In J.F. Leckman, L. Schill, & D.S. Charney (Eds.). *Pediatric Psychopharmacology: Principles and Practice* (pp. 426–446). London: Oxford University Press.

Martin, C.A., Kelly, T.H., Delzer, T., & Rayens, M.K. (1999) The interaction between sensation seeking and conduct disorder symptoms predicts drug use and amphetamine response, abstracted, in L.S. Harris, (Ed.). *Problems of Drug Dependence, National Institute on Drug Abuse Research Monograph.* Washington: U.S. Government Printing Office, 1999. (June 12–17; Presented at the College on Problems of Drug Dependence Annual Meeting).

Martin C.A., Kelly T.H., Rayens M.K., Brogli B.R., Brenzel A., Smith J.W., & Omar H.A. (2002). Sensation Seeking, Puberty, and Nicotine, Alcohol and Marijuana Use in Adolescence. *Journal of the American Academy of Child and Adolescent Psychiatry, 41*(12, 1495–1502.

Milberger, S., Biederman,J., Faraone, S.V., Chen, L., & Jones, J. (1997) Further evidence of an association between Attention-Deficit/Hyperactivity Disorder and cigarette smoking. *American Journal on Addictions, 6,* 205–217.

Miller, W.R., Brown, J.M., Simpson, T.L., Handmaker, N.S., Bien, T.H., Luckie, L.F., Montgomery, H.A., Hester, R.K., & Tonigan, J.S. (1995). What works? A methodological analysis of the alcohol treatment literature. In R.K. Hester, & W.R. Miller (Eds.), *Handbook of Alcoholism Treatment Approaches: Effective Alternatives* (pp. 12–44). Boston: Allyn & Bacon.

Miller, W.R. & Rollnick, S. (1991). *Motivational Interviewing: Preparing People to Change Addictive Behavior.* New York: Guilford Press.

Molina, B.S.G., Bukstein, O.G., & Lynch, K.G., (2002) Attention-deficit/hyperactivity disorder and conduct disorder symptomology in adolescents with alcohol use disorder. *Psychology of Addictive Behaviors, 16*(2), 161–164

Monti, P.M., Abrams, D.B., Kadden, R.M., & Cooney, N.L. (1989). *Treating Alcohol Dependence: A Coping Skills Training Guide.* New York: Guilford.

Monti, P.M., Colby, S.M., Barnett, N.P., Spirito, A., Rohsenow, D.J., Myers, M., Woolard, R., & Lewander, W. (1999). Brief intervention for harm reduction with alcohol-positive older adolescents in a hospital emergency department. *Journal of Consulting and Clinical Psychology, 67,* 989–994.

Nation, M., Crusto, C., Wandersman, A., Kumpfer, K.L., Seybolt, D., Morrissey-Kane, E., & Davino, K. (2003). What Works in Prevention. *American Psychologist, 58,* 449–456.

Nutt, D. (1997). 'Tis a wonder that it works at all!. *Addiction, 92,* 958–959.

Novak, S.P., Reardon, S.F., & Buka, S.L. (2002). How beliefs about substance use differ by socio-demographic characteristics, individual experiences, and neighborhood environments among urban adolescents. *Journal of Drug Education, 32*(4), 319–342.

Oetting, E.R., Donnermeyer, J.F., & Deffenbacher, J.L. (1998a). Primary socialization theory: The influence of community on drug use and deviance. III. *Substance Use and Misuse, 33*(8), 1629–1665.

Oetting, E.R., Donnermeyer, J.F., Trimble, J.E., & Beauvais, F. (1998b). Primary socialization theory: Culture, ethnicity, and cultural identification. The links between culture and substance use. IV. *Substance Use and Misuse, 33*(10), 2075–2107.

O'Brien, K.M., & Vincent, N.K. (2003) Psychiatric comorbidity in anorexia and bulimia nervosa: nature, prevalence and casual relationships. *Clinical Psychology Review, 23*(1),57–74.

O'Malley, P.M., Johnston, L.D., & Bachman, J.G. (1995). Adolescent substance use: Epidemiology and implications for public policy. *Pediatric Clinics of North America, 42,* 241–260.

Orlando, M., Chan, K.S., & MOrral, A.R. (2003). Retention of court-referred youths in residential treatment programs: client characteristics and treatment process effects. *American Journal of Drug and Alcohol Abuse, 29*(2), 337–357.

Overholser, J., Adams, D., Lehnert, K., & Brinkman, D. (1995). Self-esteem deficits and suicidal tendencies among adolescents. *Journal of the American Academy of Child and Adolescent Psychiatry, 34,* 919–928.

Paglia, A., & Room, R. (1999). Preventing Substance Use Problems Among Youth: A Literature Review and Recommendations. *The Journal of Primary Prevention, 20,* 3–50.

Park, J., Kosterman, R., Hawkins, J.D., Haggerty, K.P., Duncan, T.E., Duncan, S.C., & Spoth, R. (2000). Effects of the "Preparing for the Drug Free Years" Curriculum on Growth in Alcohol Use and Risk for Alcohol Use in Early Adolescence. *Prevention Science, 1*(3), 125–138.

Patton, L.H. (1995). Adolescent Substance Use: Risk Factors and Protective Factors. *Pediatric Clinics of North America, 42,* 283–293.

Pentz, M.A. (1998). Preventing drug abuse through the community: Multicomponent programs make the difference. In A. Sloboda & W.B. Hansen (Eds.), *Putting Research to Work for the Community. NIDA Publication No. 98-4293* (pp. 73–86). Rockville, MD: National Institute on Drug Abuse.

Pentz, M.A., Dwyer, J.H., MacKinnon, D.P., Flay, B.R., Hansen, W.B., Wang, E.Y., & Johnson, C.A. (1989). A multicommunity trial for primary prevention of adolescent drug abuse: Effects on drug use prevalence. *Journal of the American Medical Association, 261,* 3259–3266.

Perry, C.L., Komro, K.A., Veblen-Mortenson, S., Bosma, L.M., Farbakhsh, K., Munson, K.A., Stigler, M.H., Lytle, L.A. (2003). A randomized controlled trial of the middle and junior high school D.A.R.E. and D.A.R.E. Plus programs. *Archives of Pediatric and Adolescent Medicine, 157,* 178–84.

Perry, C.L., Williams, C.L., Veblen-Mortenson, S., Toomey, T.L., Komro, K.A., Anstine, P.S., McGovern, P.G., Finnegan, J.R., Forster, J.L., Wagenaar, A.C., & Wolfson, M. (1996). Project Northland: Outcomes of a communitywide alcohol use prevention program during early adolescence. *American Journal of Public Health, 86,* 956–965.

Plested, B., Smitham, D.M., Jumper-Thurman, P., Oetting, E.R., & Edwards, R.W. (1999). Readiness for Drug Use Prevention in Rural Minority Communities. *Substance Use and Misuse, 34* (4&5), 521–544.

Randall C.L., Johnson M.R., Thevos A.K., Sonne S.C., Thomas S.E., Willard S.L., Brady K.T., & Davidson J.R. (2001) Paroxetine for social anxiety and alcohol use in dual-diagnosed patients. *Depression and Anxiety, 14* (4), 255–62.

Reardon, B., & Griffing, P., (1983). Factors related to the self-concept of institutionalized, white, male, adolescent drug abusers. *Adolescence, 18*(69), 29–41.

Resnick M.D., Bearman, P.S., Blum, R.W., Bauman, K.E., Harris, K.M., Jones, J., Tabor, J., Beuhring, T., Sieving, R.E., Shew, M., Ireland, M., Bearinger, L.H., & Udry, J.R. (1997). Protecting adolescents from harm: findings from the National Longitudinal Study on Adolescent Health. *Journal of the American Medical Association, 278*(10), 823–865.

Riggs, P.D (2003) Treating adolescents for substance abuse and comorbid psychiatric disorders. *Scientific & Practice Perspectives, 2*(1), 18–29.

Riggs, P.D., & Davies, R.D. (2002). A clinical approach to integrating treatment for adolescent depression and substance abuse. *Journal of the American Academy of Child and Adolescent Psychiatry, 41*(10), 1253–1255.

Riggs, P.D., Thompson, L.L., Mikulich, S.K., Whitmore, E.A., & Crowley, T.J. (1996). An open trial of pemoline in drug-dependent delinquents with attention-deficit hyperactivity disorder. *Journal of the American Academy of Child and Adolescent Psychiatry 35*(18), 1018–1024.

Riggs, P.D., Leon S.L., Mikulich S.K., & Pottle L.C. (1998). An open trial of bupropion for ADHD in adolescents with substance use disorders and conduct disorder. *Journal of the American Academy of Child and Adolescent Psychiatry, 37*(12), 1271–1278.

Riggs, P.D., Mikulich S.K., Coffman L.M., & Crowley T.J. (1997) Fluoxetine in drug-dependent delinquents with major depression: An open trial. *Journal of Child and Adolescent Psychopharmacology , 7*(2), 87–95.

Riggs, P.D., Mikulich, S.K., & Hall, S. (2001) Effects of Pemoline on ADHD, antisocial behaviors and substance use in adolescents with conduct disorder and substance use disorder. In *College on Problems of Drug Dependence: 63rd Annual Scientific Meeting*. Rockville, M.D.: National Institute on Drug Abuse.

Ringwalt, C.L., Ennett, S., Vincus, A., Thorne, J., Rohrbach, L.A., & Simons-Rudolph, A. (2002). The Prevalence of Effective Substance Use Prevention Curricula in U.S. Middle Schools. *Prevention Science, 3*(4), 257–265.

Ringwalt, C.L., Green, J., Ennett, S., Lachan, R., Clayton, R., & Leukefeld, C.G. (1994). *Past and Future Directions of the D.A.R.E. Program: An Evaluation Review*. Washington, DC: U.S. Department of Justice, Office of Justice Programs, National Institute of Justice.

Roberts, H. (1997). Children, inequalities, and health. *British Medicine Journal, 314*, 1122–1125.

Rutter, M., Giller, H., & Hagell, A. (1998). *Antisocial Behavior by Young People*. Cambridge, UK: Cambridge University Press.

Safer, D.J., Zito, J.M., & Gardner, J.F. (2001). Pemoline hepatotoxicity and post marketing surveillance. *Journal of the American Academy of Child and Adolescent Psychiatry, 40*(6), 622–629.

Sale, E., Sambrano, S, Springer, J.F., & Turner, C.W. (2003). Risk, protection, and substance use in adolescents: A multi-site model. *Journal of Drug Education, 33*(1), 91–105.

Sealock, M.D., Gottfredson, D.C., & Gallagher, C.A. (1997). Drug treatment for juvenile offenders: Some good and bad news. *Journal of Research in Crime and Delinquency, 34*, 210–236.

Sells, S.B. & Simpson, D.D. (1979). Evaluation of treatment outcome for youths in the drug abuse reporting program (DARP): a follow-up study. In Friedman, A.S., Beschner, G.M. (Eds.), *Youth Drug Abuse* (pp. 571–628). Lexington, MA: Lexington Books.

Smith, T.A., House, R.F.J., Croghan, I.T., Gauvin, T.R., Colligan, R.C., Offord, K.P., Gomez-Dahl, L.C., & Hurt, R.D. (1996) Nicotine patch therapy in adolescent smokers. *Pediatrics, 98*(4 Pt 1), 659–667.

Swadi, H., (1999). Individual risk factors for adolescent substance use. *Drug and Alcohol Dependence, 55*(3), 209–224.

Taylor, T.K., & Biglan, A. (1998). Behavioral family interventions for improving child-rearing: A review for clincians and policy makers. *Clinical Child and Family Psychological Review, 1*, 41–60.

Tobler, N.S., Roona, M.R., Ochshorn, P., Marshall, D.G., Streke, A.V., & Stackpole, K.M. (2000). School-Based Adolescent Drug Prevention Programs: 1998 Meta-Analysis. *The Journal of Primary Prevention, 20*, 275–336.

Trudeau, L., Spoth, R., Lillehoj, C., Redmond, C., & Wickrama, K.A.S. (2003). Effects of a preventive intervention on adolescent substance use initiation, expectancies, and refusal intentions. *Prevention Science, 4*(2), 109–122.

Van Etten, M.L., & Anthony, J.C. (2001). Male-female differences in transitions from first drug opportunity to first use: Searching for subgroup variation by age. *Journal of Womens Health and Gender Based Medicine,* 10(8), 797–804.

Vega, W.A., Zimmerman, R.S., Warheit, G.J., Apospori, E., & Gil A.G. (1993). Risk factors for early adolescent drug use in four ethnic and racial groups. *American Journal of Public Health,* 83(2), 185–189.

Waldron, H.B., Slesnick, N., Brody, J.L., Turner, C.W., & Peterson, T.R. (2001). Treatment outcomes for adolescent substance abuse at 4- and 7- month assessments. *Journal of Consulting and Clinical Psychology,* 69, 802–813.

Webster-Stratton, C., & Hammond, M. (1997). Treating children with early-onset conduct problems: A comparison of child and parent training interventions. *Journal of Consulting and Clinical Psychology,* 65, 93–109.

Webster-Stratton, C. & Taylor, T. (2001). Nipping early risk factors in the bud: Preventing substance abuse, delinquency, and violence in adolescence through interventions targeted at young children (0–8 years). *Prevention Science, 2,* 165–192.

Weissberg, R.P., Kumpfer, K.L., & Seligman, M.E.P. (2003). Prevention that Works for Children and Youth: An Introduction. *American Psychologist, 58,* 425–432.

Wexler, H.K. (1995). The success of therapeutic communities for substance abusers in American prisons. *Journal of Psychoactive Drugs,* 27, 57–66.

Whitmore, E.A., Mikulich, S.K., Thompson, L.L., Riggs, P.D., Aarons, G.A., & Crowley, T.J. (1997). Influences on adolescent substance dependence: conduct disorder, depression, attention deficit hyperactivity disorder and gender. *Drug and Alcohol Dependence, 47,* 87–97.

Wilens, T.E., Biderman, J., & Spencer, T.J., (1997). Case study: adverse effects of smoking marijuana while receiving tricyclic antidepressants. *Journal of the American Academy of Child and Adolescent Psychiatry,* 36(1), 45–48.

Wilens, T.E., Faraone, S.V., Biederman, J., & Gunawardene, S. (2003). Does stimulant therapy of attention-deficit/hyperactivity disorder beget later substance abuse? A meta-analytic review of the literature. *Pediatrics,* 111(1),179–185.

Williams, R.J., & Chang, S.Y. (2000). A comprehensive and comparative review of adolescent substance abuse treatment outcome. *Clinical Psychology: Science and Practice,* 7(2), 138–166.

Windle, M., Shope, J.T., & Bukstein, O. (1996). Alcohol use. In R. DiClemente, W. Hansen & L. Ponton (Eds.), *Handbook of Adolescent Health* (pp. 115–159) New York, NY: Plenum.

Windle, M., & Windle, R.C. (2001) Depressive symptoms and cigarette smoking among middle adolescents: prospective associations and intrapersonal and interpersonal influences. *Journal of Consulting and Clinical Psychology,* 69(2), 215–226

Wise B.K., Cuffe S.P., & Fischer T. (2001). Dual diagnosis and successful participation of adolescents in substance abuse treatment. *Journal of Substance Abuse Treatment,* 21 (3), 161–165.

Yamaguchi, R., Johnston, L.D., & O'Malley, P.M., (2003). Relationship between student illicit drug use and school drug-testing policies. *Journal of School Health,* 73(4), 159–164.

Zimmermann, P., Wittchen, H.U., Hofler, M., Pfister, H., Kessler, R.C., & Lieb, R. (2003). Primary anxiety disorders and the development of subsequent alcohol use disorders: a 4-year community study of adolescents and young adults. *Psychological Medicine, 33*(7), 1211–22.

Chapter 21

Gambling

Tobias Hayer, Mark Griffiths, and Gerhard Meyer

Introduction

For most people, gambling is an enjoyable and harmless activity. However, for a small minority, gambling can become both addictive and problematic.[1] *Pathological gambling* appears in the fourth edition of the *Diagnostic and Statistical Manual of Mental Disorders* (*DSM-IV*) in the category "impulse control disorder not elsewhere classified" along with other disorders such as kleptomania or pyromania (American Psychiatric Association, 1994). Generally, pathological gambling can be described as a persistent and recurrent maladaptive gambling behavior that disrupts personal, family, or vocational pursuits. The *DSM-IV* criteria highlight loss of control, withdrawal symptoms, tolerance as well as relapse and suggest a strong similarity to substance abuse disorders, although unique (gambling-specific) characteristics are also evident (e.g., chasing).

Due to the increase in accessibility and opportunities to gamble, a large body of research has shown that increasing numbers of adolescents engage in gambling (e.g., Griffiths, 1995; Jacobs, 2000). Surveys in the United States reveal that participation in card games, sports betting, games of skills, and video lottery terminals are most common in youth (e.g., National Research Council, 1999). In order to determine the extent of problem gambling in different population segments, Shaffer and Hall (2001) conducted a meta-analysis and summarized 139 distinct estimates from North American prevalence studies, including 32 samples with adolescents. Their calculations demonstrate a lifetime rate for pathological gambling (level 3 gambling) in adolescence of 3.38% (past-year prevalence: 4.8%) and a lifetime level of adolescent

---

[1]There is still much controversy about terminological issues. In general, "pathological gambling" refers to a diagnosable psychiatric disorder and thus to clinically significant symptoms and is limited to the far end of a continuum of gambling involvement. However, the term "problem gambling" is used in two different ways: (a) to describe solely less serious (mild to moderate) problems associated with gambling activities on a subclinical level or (b) to encompass all levels of gambling problems without distinguishing between different severities. Throughout this chapter, we will use the term "problem gambling" to refer to all gambling behavior associated with harmful effects.

problem gambling (level 2 gambling) of 8.4% (past-year prevalence: 14.6%). European prevalence studies also have identified small but significant number of adolescents can be classified as problem gamblers (e.g., Becoña Iglesias, del Carmen Míguez Varela & Vázquez González, 2001 [Spain]—5.6%; Johansson & Götestam, 2003 [Norway]—1.8%; Fisher, 1999 [UK]—5.6%; Lupu, Onaca & Lupu, 2002 [Romania]—6.8%). Despite methodological inconsistencies, these prevalence studies highlight the growing need (a) to introduce effective prevention programs for adolescents to diminish the incidence of problem adolescent gambling and (b) to implement appropriate treatment facilities for adolescents to avert further maladaptive outcomes and foster a behavioral change.

Individual Factors

The empirical foundation of preventive action and intervention efforts arises from research determining risk and protective factors. Risk factors are defined as conditions associated with an increased likelihood of a negative outcome (e.g., gambling problems). Protective factors are those conditions that reduce the potential of developing symptoms of psychosocial maladjustment or moderate the effect of exposure to risk factors (e.g., Coie et al., 1993). In accordance with other problem behaviors, the development and maintenance of problem gambling cannot be explained by a single factor. Within the individual domain, several risk factors such as demographic features (gender, age, ethnicity), biological/biochemical, personality, cognitive, gambling-related factors, and factors related to the engagement in other problem behaviors seem to be associated with adolescent problem gambling. These are briefly examined in turn.

Gender

More boys are regular gamblers than girls (Griffiths, 1991; Gupta & Derevensky, 1998). Furthermore, they are more likely to be classified as problem gamblers (e.g., Fisher, 1999; Griffiths, 1995; Ladouceur et al., 1999; Poulin, 2000; Winters, Stinchfield & Fulkerson, 1993). Jacobs (2000) summarizes gender differences among juvenile players and draws the following conclusions: Male juveniles tend to spend more time and money when gambling, initiate gambling earlier, enjoy more skill-based games, and gamble on a greater number and variety of games. However, there are studies that do not show these general trends (e.g., Volberg, 2002).

Age

While preferences for gambling forms differ according to developmental level, age does not constitute a solid predictor of problem gambling during adolescence in most studies (e.g. Fisher, 1999; Poulin, 2000). Thus, in general, there seems to be no association between age and prevalence rates of problem gambling—although there are exceptions (e.g. Ladouceur et al., 1999; Shapira et al., 2002; Volberg, 2002). More important than the link between age and problem gambling appears to be the age of onset. The sooner the initial contact into gambling, the higher the risk of developing gambling problems upon reaching adulthood. For instance, Shaffer et al. (1994)

reported pathological gamblers first gambled at an age of 9.7 years, whereas the average age of onset for their non-pathological counterparts was 11.6 years. Such findings have been reported consistently by other researchers (e.g. Griffiths, 1990; Volberg, 2002; Winters et al., 1993).

Ethnicity

Although research findings have been conflicting, several studies suggest ethnic minorities are at greater risk to develop problems related to gambling, for example, Aboriginals (Alberta Alcohol and Drug Abuse Commission, 2003a) and American Indians (Zitzow, 1996). Likewise, Volberg (2002) found higher prevalence rates among black and Asian adolescents with gambling-related problems compared to adolescents from other racial groups. Shapira et al. (2002) noted that African American adolescents are the population most likely to be pathological gamblers in Florida, as measured by the *DSM-IV* criteria. In the UK, Fisher (1999) reported ethnic background did not correlate with problem gambling. However, Griffiths (2000) found a high rate of problem scratchcard gambling amongst a population consisting almost entirely of Asian (Muslim) adolescent gamblers.

Genetics

Genetic factors may influence pathological gambling by multiple pathways. It is unlikely that a single gene is responsible for pathological gambling. Genetic studies with adults may provide insight into the genetic basis of pathological gambling. Evidence has come from twin studies (Eisen et al., 1998; Winters & Rich, 1998), showing that inherited and/or shared environmental experiences explain approximately half of the variance associated with pathological gambling in males. Comings et al. (1996) conducted a molecular genetic study providing further support for a shared genetic component for pathological gambling linking the Taq A1 allele, a specific variant of the human dopamine D2 receptor gene (DRD2), to pathological gambling. More recently, Comings et al. (2001) demonstrated that several genes for dopamine, serotonin, and norepinephrine metabolism contributed significantly to the risk of pathological gambling. However, further evidence is needed to monitor the relative importance and changes of genetic effects during the lifespan.

Biology/Biochemistry

Neurotransmitter genes are believed to play a significant role in mediating reinforcement effect in the brain. Thus, recent theoretical models of the development and maintenance of pathological gambling highlight the significance of neurobiological mechanisms (e.g., Potenza, 2001). Furthermore, brain monoamines such as dopamine, norepinephrine, and serotonin seem to underlie certain behavioral patterns. Several functions important in pathological gambling are worth noting: (a) abnormalities in the reward mechanisms related to the mesocorticolimbic dopamine circuitry, (b) a behavioral inhibition and disinhibiton mechanism mediated by the serotonergic system (serotonin dysfunction is associated with impulsive disorders and thus implies a deficit in cerebral inhibition), and (c) abnormalities in an arousal mechanism related to the dorsal tegmental noradrenergic system (e.g., Potenza, 2002).

A recent study using functional magnetic response imaging suggests similarities in the brain processes involved in the anticipation and experience of monetary gains and losses and those of euphoria-inducing drugs (Breiter et al., 2001), whereby the ventromedial cortex has been implicated in the processing of monetary gains and losses (Gehring & Willoughby, 2002). Also, the first functional magnetic resonance imaging (fMRI) study of exclusively male pathological gamblers confirm that gambling cues elicit gambling urges and leads to a temporally dynamic pattern of brain activity changes (Potenza, et al., 2003). Finally, a number of studies have found associations with frontal lobe dysfunctions and pathological gambling, in particular regarding decision-making impairment (e.g., Cavedini et al., 2002) and exceptionally high rates of EEG abnormalities among pathological gamblers (e.g., Regard et al., 2003). Next to these results based on adult samples, Chambers and Potenza (2003) propose that during adolescence, normative neurodevelopment involves a relative immaturity of frontal cortical and subcortical monoaminergic systems that underlies impulsive behavior and thus can be responsible for an increased vulnerability to addictive behaviors among youths.

Personality/Emotional or Mental State

Numerous studies have tried to identify core personality traits or factors related to the emotional/mental state of adolescent problem gamblers. Based on previous reviews of the empirical research literature (Derevensky et al., 2003; Dickson, Derevensky & Gupta, 2002), the most important factors can be summarized as follows: adolescent problem gamblers have lower self-esteem and higher rates of depression, including a heightened risk for suicide ideation and suicide attempts; show poor or maladaptive general coping skills; and tend to use more emotion and avoidant coping styles. In addition, youth with gambling problems score high on measures of risk-taking, sensation-seeking, excitability, extroversion, anxiety, and low on measures of conformity and self-discipline.

Cognitions

Cognitive biases also play a significant role in the development and maintenance of problem gambling among adolescents (e.g., Griffiths, 1994; Ladouceur, Ferland & Fournier, 2003). In particular, young men seem to have overinflated views about their chances of winning and the influence of their own behavior in controlling chance outcomes (Moore & Ohtsuka, 1999). Such cognitive distortions reflect a normative phenomenon when gambling and thus do not provide a sufficient explanation of why individuals gamble in excess. However, cognitive biases are more prevalent among adult problem gamblers when gambling involvement increases (Ladouceur & Walker, 1996).

Engagement in Other Problem Behaviors

Research clearly demonstrates that adolescent problem gamblers engage in other potentially addictive behaviors, such as use of tobacco, alcohol, and illegal drugs to a greater extent than non-problem gamblers (Griffiths & Sutherland, 1998; Vitaro et al., 2001; Winters et al., 2002). In addition, they are prone to be involved in delinquent behaviors (e.g., Gupta & Derevensky, 1998; Ladouceur et al., 1999; Winters et al., 1993). Yeoman and Griffiths (1996) report that approximately 4% of juvenile crime was associated with gaming machine use and further provide limited evidence that a minority of juveniles aged 10–17 years commit crimes in order to supplement their gambling. According to Stinchfield et al. (1997), antisocial behavior, gender (i.e., being male), and lifetime alcohol use explained 25% of the variance in highest level of gambling frequency. Compared to their peers, adolescent problem gamblers also show a wide range of school-related difficulties. Differences between groups were obtained for being expelled from class by a teacher, failing a course or academic year, academic achievement, and time spent studying on homework (Ladouceur et al., 1999). Furthermore, young problem gamblers are more likely to truant from school, argue, lie, and steal in relation to their gambling (Fisher, 1999; Griffiths, 1995).

In addition to the bulk of correlation studies, very few studies with longitudinal designs investigated the predictive links shared by (problem) gambling, substance use/abuse, and delinquency. The abuse of alcohol among male adolescents represents a predictor for a subsequent increase in gambling over time or a pattern of stability of regular gambling activities, respectively (Barnes et al., 2002). Higher parental monitoring of the leisure activities of adolescents operates as a puffer between alcohol abuse and frequent gambling participation. For females, alcohol misuse predicts an increasing pattern of gambling only when additional factors were present. Thus, alcohol abuse seems to be a causal risk factor for high rates of gambling (see also Vitaro et al., 2001).

Summarizing the literature, Winters and Anderson (2000) suggest three possible developmental pathways for risk status, substance use disorders, and problem gambling that warrant further investigation. Pathway 1 reflects an indirect process—a high-risk status may contribute to a developmental disorder (e.g., conduct disorder), which in turn predicts problem gambling or other substance use disorder. Alternatively, pathway 2 suggests that belonging to a high-risk group enhances vulnerability for both disorders directly and independently. In contrast, pathway 3 implies that a high-risk status leads to a substance use disorder. Adolescent gambling problems may result from a substance use disorder. We also suggest a fourth plausible pathway that must be addressed empirically in future—can (problem) gambling function as a "gateway drug" that makes a substance use disorder more likely during the course of development?

Family Factors

Youth problem gambling is strongly related to how the adolescents perceive parental gambling. Many researchers (e.g., Fisher, 1999; Gupta & Derevensky, 1998; Ladouceur et al., 1999; Winters et al., 1993) have shown that adolescent pathological gamblers are more likely to have a mother or father with gambling problems than adolescents who have not been classified as pathological gamblers. Some parents even purchase lottery tickets and scratchcards for their children (Wood & Griffiths, 1998). Furthermore, a majority of adolescents tend to gamble with family members, with most parents unconcerned with their children's gambling participation or lacking knowledge about adolescent problem gambling (Fisher, 1999; Ladouceur et al., 1998). Family structure also seems to be linked to adolescent problem gambling, even though research findings are not straightforward. Fisher (1999) and Volberg (2002) have found that young people from single-parent families are at greater risk to be classified as problem gamblers. Winters et al. (1993) could not confirm these associations—neither to family composition, nor to family closeness.

Social and Community Factors

Addictions always result from an interplay of multiple factors, including the individual, the social environment, and the nature of the activity itself—a paradigm that resembles the public health triad of host, environment, and agent (Korn & Shaffer, 1999). Focusing on the gambling activity, Griffiths (e.g., 1999, 2003) has consistently argued that situational and structural characteristics can play an important contributory factor in gambling acquisition, development, and maintenance. For instance, situational or ecological determinants of gambling are important in the initial decision to start gambling. These characteristics are primarily environmental features, such as the location of the gambling venue, the number of gambling venues in a specific area, or advertisements that stimulate people to gamble and thus encompass important dimensions such as availability, acceptability, and accessibility of gambling. For example, an active promotion combined with an easy accessibility of gambling outlets may foster the initial contact with gambling, and thus the risk of maladaptive developmental courses. Structural characteristics have implications for the gamblers' motivation by reinforcing their gambling activities and satisfying their needs. They also have the potential to induce excessive gambling. Griffiths (e.g., 1999, 2003) has summarized the most important structural characteristics (see below).

Structural Characteristics of Gambling that Increase the Attractiveness of Gambling for Adolescents and Thus Its Addiction Potential (Griffiths, 1999, 2003)

Variable stake size (including issues around affordability, perceived value for money)
Event frequency (time gap between each gamble)
Amount of money lost in a given period of time, which is important in chasing behavior
Prize structures (number and value of wins)
Probability of winning
Size of jackpot
Skill and pseudo-skill elements (actual or perceived)
Opportunities of "near misses" (number of failures that are close to being successful)
Lights, color and sound effects
Social or asocial nature of the game
Rules of the game
Use of tokens, chips or credit cards (which temporarily disrupts the financial value system)

As Griffiths (1999) points out, the most important factors appear to be the accessibility of gambling and the event frequency. When these characteristics are combined, the greatest problems occur. Not surprisingly, juveniles reporting gambling problems prefer rapid, continuous, and interactive games (Jacobs, 2000). Relationships between regulatory policy and (problem) gambling behavior in adolescence have not been explored. Given the research, it is necessary to gain further insight into the effect of gambling policy and adolescent engagement in gambling (e.g., investigate the impact of restrictions or number of gambling venues). Concurrent with the implementation of policy intervention, research has to monitor and evaluate their effects systematically in order to adjust policies accordingly.

Summary

Nearly all the risk factors outlined above stem from epidemiological research and are correlative in nature. The underlying mechanisms, precursors, and consequences of gambling problems as well as the causal nature of these relationships still need to be confirmed empirically. Furthermore, no established peer-reviewed research literature on protective factors exist with respect to problem gambling in adolescence. A selection of protective factors that minimize the occurrence of problem behaviors or mental disorders during adolescence and childhood are listed in Table 1 and may also be applicable for problem gambling.

Overall, these findings could be taken as a starting point and may foster research, eventually delineating discrete pathways leading to the development of distinct subgroups (e.g., adolescence-limited versus life-course persistent problem gambling).

Table 1. Conditions that Minimize the Risk of Occurrence of Problem Behaviors or Mental Disorders in Childhood and Adolescence (Adapted from Scheithauer et al., 2004)

Protective factors with regard to the individual/resiliency	Protective factors with regard to the family and environment
Positive temperament (flexible, active)	Stable emotional relation to a caregiver (emotional support)
Adequate impulse control	
Intelligence (better-than-average)	Supporting family climate
Special abilities and interests in hobbies	Family cohesion/positive bonding
Prosocial behavior	**Parental monitoring/supervision**
Communication skills (speech)	**Adaptive school performance/school-Connectedness**
Positive self-esteem	Clear, prosocial normative expectations
Social skills*	Positive role models in terms of coping (e.g.,
Sense of self-efficacy	Relations to peers having prosocial norms and
Active coping strategies	who are not drug users)
Internal locus of control	Social support networks
Anticipating behavior	Girls: support and autonomy
Self-confidence	Boys: structure and rules at home
Strong ethnic identity	**Availability of and participation in prosocial activity**
	High social and academic expectations
	Perceived connectedness with school and participation in extracurricular activity

* Note: Protective factors for which first empirical evidence exists with respect to problem gambling in adolescence are bold (see Alberta Alcohol and Drug Abuse Commission, 2003b).

Nower and Blaszczynski (2004) propose such a pathways model of pathological gambling as a harm-minimization strategy to guide educators in assessing, discriminating, and managing discrete subgroups of youth problem gamblers and referring them to appropriate services. The pathways model takes a multiple range of interacting risk factors into account. Furthermore, it suggests three distinct routes leading to adolescent problem gambling, implying three clinically different subgroups (i.e., behavioral-conditioned, emotionally vulnerable, and antisocial impulsivist youth gamblers). Although phenomenologically similar, etiological differences suggest a differentiated application of intervention and prevention strategies. However, the causal pathways of this model have to be tested empirically.

Evidence-Based Treatment Interventions in Community Settings

What Works

Treatment approaches cover a wide ride of activities and are based on various theoretical foundations. However, there is a sparse description of treatment studies in the literature related to adolescent pathological gambling. In fact, no controlled studies with random assignment and comparison groups could be found that provided empirical evidence for the effectiveness of treatment approaches related to adolescent pathological gambling. Thus, a review of the literature did not reveal a program that met the standard for what works.

What Might Work

Only two empirically evaluated therapeutic approaches to treat adolescent pathological gambling have been reported in the literature. Ladouceur, Boisvert, and Dumont (1994) conducted a study evaluating the effectiveness of cognitive-behavioral treatment with four male pathological videopoker players aged 17–19 years. This multimodal treatment approach consisted of five components: (a) information about problem gambling, (b) cognitive interventions, (c) problem-solving training, (d) social skills/assertiveness training, and (e) relapse prevention. Individual treatment lasted approximately three months; after treatment was completed, clinically significant improvements for the perception of control as well as reductions in the perception of the severity of gambling problems were found. At two follow-ups after three and six months, respectively, all participants had ceased their gambling.

Gupta and Derevensky (2000) introduced an eclectic therapy to treat 36 male adolescent problem gamblers. The participants were 14–21 years old and sought treatment over a five-year period. Individual therapy was provided weekly and consisted of detailed intake assessment, establishing acceptance of the problem, identification of underlying problems and addressing personal issues, development of adequate coping skills, restructuring of free time, involvement of family and social support, cognitive restructuring, establishing debt repayment plans, and relapse prevention. During one-year follow-up, 35 adolescent gamblers were abstinent and also improved on measures of depression, drug and alcohol use, and peer/family relationship. Due to the individual (and thus heterogeneous) approaches including variability in number of sessions and the high motivational base (adolescents actively seeking treatment), the efficacy cannot be adequately determined.

Taken together, these two studies suggest that a cognitive-behavioral approach, including cognitive restructuring, problem-solving, social skills training, and relapse prevention might effectively treat adolescent problem gamblers. Although cognitive-behavioral strategies have been most effective in treating adults (e.g., Meyer & Bachmann, 2000), further randomized studies are necessary to confirm this for the adolescent population. Cognitive-behavioral treatments appear to pay insufficient attention to motivational factors, as many gamblers are ambivalent about stopping with an activity that has been both a source of excitement and likewise a source of great suffering. The *stages of change* derived from the transtheoretical model of intentional behavior change provide a valuable theoretical framework (Prochaska, DiClemente & Norcross, 1992) for understanding the motivational processes underlying behavioral change for individuals struggling with addictions. According to this model, individual progress occurs not necessarily in a linear way. Rather, for most addicted people, change is a dynamic process with fluctuating motivations. There are thus identifiable stages, including resistance (precontemplation), contempletation, preparation, action, and maintenance (and relapse). Consequently, DiClemente, Story, and Murray (2000) have suggested the applicability of this model for gambling problems in youth, with empirical research currently underway.

Further valuable ideas can be derived from Bellringer (1992), who outlined a non-theoretical treatment approach for young problem gamblers with ten key aspects that fall into two categories: preparation (P) and action (A). These key aspects can be used as guidelines and be viewed as a supplement to other treatment techniques as a process of therapy itself (see below).

General Guidelines in Treating the Adolescent Problem Gambler (Bellringer, 1992)

Preparation$_1$: understanding the issues and gaining insight;

P$_2$: structuring change (setting up a plan with realistic short-, medium-, and long-term goals and measurable objects);

Action$_3$: assessing the problem in detail (including the gambler's motivation to stop gambling);

A$_4$: providing counseling (empowering the adolescent to change, agreeing on boundaries, creating the right atmosphere and appropriate involvement of family or other helping agencies);

A$_5$: establishing trust and confidentiality, helping the gambler to be open and honest (and coming back);

A$_6$: building self-esteem, which is important in restoration of self-confidence;

A$_7$: providing support—should involve a support agency, including the practitioner, the practitioner's agency, other agencies, and the adolescent gambler's family, friends, and significant others (strengthening of relationships with family members is particularly important after treatment termination and/or as a tool of relapse prevention; eventually recommending group and attendance of self-help groups);

(continued)

A_8: assessing the adolescent gambler's financial situation (debt counseling: talking to creditors, cutting up credit cards, drawing up budget plans), gradually give back financial responsibility to the gambler as long-term goal;

A_9: developing alternative interests and replacing the time spent for gambling with a range of activities that are rewarding themselves;

A_{10}: measuring progress (provide effective feedback to the adolescent gambler, revising or resetting assessment and/or goals).

Another important issue is to identify why so few adolescents enroll in treatment programs. Griffiths (2001) reviewed many plausible explanations (e.g., there may be insufficient treatment opportunities specifically available for adolescents, available treatment programs may not be appropriate and/or suitable for adolescents, adolescent problem gamblers may undergo spontaneous remission and/or mature out of problems, the negative consequences may be attributed to other problem behavior, etc.). Although not every assertion made has been empirically tested, the list serves as a starting point for further research.

What Does Not Work

Given the paucity of scientifically validated evidence in this area, it is difficult to specify approaches that definitely do not work in treating adolescent gamblers. However, after reviewing the literature that deals with the treatment of adult problem gamblers (e.g., Meyer & Bachmann, 2000), we can infer that unimodal models ignoring the complex interaction of several risk and protective factors in the initiation, development, maintenance, and recovery of problem gambling will most likely lead to treatment failures.

Summary

Treatment paradigms must be adopted to the developmental needs, interests, concerns, behaviors, and difficulties that adolescents typically experience (Gupta & Derevensky, 2000). In general, health care systems have to adopt a multiple-option approach, including diverse treatment programs. These range from low-threshold (e.g., minimal intervention) to high-threshold (e.g., inpatient hospitals) approaches. Two important clinical issues still are unresolved: (1) how to make adolescents more motivated to seek treatment and (b) to define the type of therapeutic approach that is most effective in reducing adolescent gambling problems. Cognitive-behavioral approaches seem to be the most promising treatment alternative so far.

Evidence-Based Treatment Interventions in Residential Settings

What Works/What Might Work/What Does Not Work

To our knowledge, no trials have been published that empirically evaluate treatment approaches of pathological gambling in adolescence (either in inpatient hospitals, group homes, or residential schools). Thus, no statement can be made as to the effectiveness of evidence-based treatment interventions for pathological gambling in residential settings. Based on the absence of empirical evidence, it is speculative to discuss effective components of treatment interventions for problem gambling in residential settings. As with treatment interventions in community settings, it seems important not only to tackle the gambling behavior itself, but also issues such as the identification of underlying problems that are producing stress (e.g., severed familial relationships), the restructuring of free time and the development of alternative (healthy) life-styles, establishing debt repayment strategies (where necessary), and relapse prevention (see Gupta & Derevensky, 2000).

Psychopharmacology

Neuro/biological studies suggest the involvement of various neurotransmitters in the etiology of pathological gambling. Medication that targets neurotransmitter systems appear to be successful in treating pathological gamblers. However, no study to date has examined pharmacological treatment of adolescent problem gambling. The use of three classes of drugs seem to be promising approaches to treat adult pathological gambling: selective serotonin reuptake inhibitors, opioid receptor antagonists, and mood stabilizers (e.g., Grant, Kim & Potenza, 2003; Pietrzak, Ladd & Petry, 2003; Potenza, 2002).

Of the medication tested, several selective serotonin reuptake inhibitors demonstrate preliminary evidence for their efficacy. Fluvoxamine and paroxetine have been shown to be superior to placebo in the short-term treatment of adults. But before recommendations can be made for adolescent pathological gamblers, long-term efficacy in treating adult pathological gamblers are needed. Additionally, despite preliminary evidence suggesting the usefulness of clomipramine, citalopram, and fluoxetine, it is premature to use these selective serotonin reuptake inhibitors in the treatment of adolescents—particularly because their safety in pediatric populations has not yet been determined. Aside from selective serotonin reuptake inhibitors, studies with naltrexone (an opioid receptor antagonist) has led to positive results in the treatment of adult pathological gamblers. Naltrexone directly blocks the transmission of dopamine in the nucleus accumbens and modulates dopaminergic paths that seem to be implicated in the etiology of addictions. However, possible side effects in the treatment of adolescents need to examined before recommending trials in populations with minors.

Summary

In general, systematic research in the area of psychopharmacology and problem gambling is recent and limited to small adult sample studies. Double-blind, placebo-controlled studies are required to assess efficacy for use with adolescents.

The Prevention of Problem Gambling

What Works

To date, little information exists concerning the effectiveness of programs for the prevention of problem gambling. All published and evaluated studies have used a universal approach, regardless of the gambling habits of the students before starting the intervention. Correspondingly, these studies focused mainly on increasing knowledge and correcting misconceptions about gambling, but did not measure or obtain meaningful behavioral changes. General evidence shows that accurate knowledge about healthy and unhealthy behaviors (including, to some degree, attitudes toward these behaviors) does not necessarily affect the behavior itself (e.g., Durlak, 2003; Botvin, 2001, for the prevention of substance abuse in adolescents in particular). Thus, it is premature to draw a definite conclusion as to what type of preventive intervention works in terms of behavioral change related to problem gambling (e.g., age of onset, amount of money bet or time spent on gambling).

What Might Work

Due to the fact that certain cognitive factors play a key role in the development and maintenance of problem gambling or persistent gambling participation, prevention programs are mainly designed to target these cognitive misconceptions and/or to deliver accurate information about gambling. Gaboury and Ladouceur (1993) conducted the first gambling prevention study and created a mainly information-based prevention program in a classroom setting for high school students. The program consisted of three sessions covering several topics, such as providing general information about gambling, possible negative consequences of enduring gambling activities, the explanation of automatic behavior in gambling, and possible strategies to control gambling behavior. Results indicated that the experimental group improved their knowledge about gambling significantly. This difference was also evident at a six-months follow-up measurement. However, at six-month follow-up, no influence on actual gambling behavior, newly known coping strategies to control gambling behavior, or attitudes related to gambling could be observed.

A further study by Ferland, Ladouceur, and Vitaro (2002) targeted misconceptions about gambling with an amusing 20-minute video. According to the authors, the video captures the students' attention and interest in a cost- and time-effective way and probably does so better than traditional teaching. Seventh- and eighth-graders were randomly assigned to three experimental conditions and a control condition. Results showed that (a) the video session only, (b) the provision of information in combination with interactive learning elements (presentation of information), as well as (c) an integrated approach of both conditions are useful in increasing knowledge and correcting erroneous cognitions about gambling. Furthermore, the integrated approach (video plus presentation of information) provided the best approach in giving the students a more realistic view of gambling and in reducing their misconceptions about gambling. A study by Lavoie and Ladouceur (2004) confirmed the effectiveness of a video as a meaningful medium in order to achieve two goals: (a) to increase knowledge about gambling and (b) to decrease gambling-related attitudinal errors with Canadian students from grades 5 and 6. However, an information session that preceded watching the video did not turn out to be superior to the "video-only" condition.

Similarly, a youth gambling prevention program introduced by Ferland, Ladouceur, and Jacques (2000) shared the main characteristics of the Gaboury and Ladouceur (1993) program but added an interactive learning element. Students actively tested the concepts and ideas outside of the classroom using take-home activities. The learning portion of the prevention program consisted of three sessions that (a) explained what gambling activities are, discussed the pitfalls of gambling, and helped to understand the concept of randomness; (b) put into practice a problem-solving strategy for resisting social pressures; and (c) addressed issues related to problem gambling. Preliminary results indicated a significant improvement of the students' knowledge and a decrease of misconceptions about gambling activities. However, behavioral data revealed that students did not succeed in improving their ability to solve problems.

More recently, Ladouceur et al. (2003) published a study that evaluated the effectiveness of gambling prevention activities for primary school students (first phase of the study) as well as comparing the relative effectiveness of two different prevention programs administered by a gambling expert and regular teacher, respectively (second phase of the study). This second phase of the study comprised three experimental conditions. For two experimental conditions, program components were drawn from the "Count me out" awareness program (see below), and provided by both the teacher and gambling expert. For the third experimental condition, three other interactive exercises were created and conducted by the gambling expert. These exercises were already used in the first phase of the study in order to target the modification of erroneous perceptions. Results supported the notion that erroneous perceptions among primary school students (fifth- and sixth-graders) can be reduced by a prevention program specifically designed to explain the concepts of chance and randomness. Furthermore, preventive exercises developed by the gambling experts had a bigger impact than elements drawn from the "Count me out" program. In addition, students benefitted more from a program delivered by an expert than by a regular teacher.

A more comprehensive approach was evaluated by Williams (2002), who designed a broad-spectrum school-based prevention program as an attempt to prevent problem gambling. The program contains five elements, both gambling-specific (e.g., information of gambling and problem gambling, correction of cognitive errors) and gambling-unspecific (teaching and rehearsal of decision-making and social problem-solving skills as well as adaptive coping skills). The program was implemented at a Canadian high school in order to advocate responsible gambling and enhance certain key life skills, but not necessarily to reduce gambling participation or even encourage abstinence from gambling. Control group comparisons took place one week and three months after the intervention had been completed. At both points, significant group differences were evident: increase of gambling-related knowledge, more negative attitudes towards gambling, and decrease of cognitive errors. However, no differences were evident with regard to the ability to calculate true gambling odds. Furthermore, the study did not find significant changes in gambling behavior due to the fact that gambling behavior decreased within both (experimental and control) groups.

Overall, very few controlled prevention studies have been published in peer-reviewed journals. Results obtained thus for display the usefulness of prevention programs to modify erroneous cognitions. However, robust and sustained behavior changes have not been demonstrated. There are several reasons why the results should be treated with caution. Firstly, the prevention of (adolescent) problem gambling is quite a recent area of research and still in its infancy. Secondly, the existing programs mainly promote knowledge about gambling-related issues and therefore are limited in scope. Thirdly, small sample sizes, short-term approaches, and restrictions to the North

American culture limit generalizations. Fourthly, most of the research was carried out by the same team; thus the findings need to be replicated by others.

What Does Not Work

Research from other areas clearly demonstrates that fear-inducing approaches techniques and information-only techniques are not successful in altering behavior (e.g., Durlak, 2003; Evans, 2003; Griffiths, 2003). In particular, these programs do not consider developmental tasks such as coping with social influences, which may effect health-threatening behaviors. Simply scaring young people is an ineffective way of preventing later problem behavior and should be avoided when designing programs to prevent problem gambling in adolescence. In a similar way, information-only approaches (e.g., the dissemination of information about psychoactive substances) have little positive effects on behavioral change. Furthermore, delivering information in the form of abstract and non-interactive teacher sessions may not be an optimal method to increase factual knowledge and as a consequence to prevent health-damaging behaviors such as problem gambling.

Summary

It is still unresolved what type of prevention program works with regard to enduring behavioral changes or if the positive effects reported have any long-lasting effect. Nevertheless, findings from universal cognitive-based approaches demonstrate that inappropriate perceptions related to gambling activities can be corrected among students at least in the short term, especially when not relying solely on a didactic, non-interactive approach. In addition, multiple non-evaluated programs exist, which may serve as a basis for an innovative and effective conception of a preventive program for adolescents or young adults, respectively. The list below gives insight into the range of efforts being made to address these populations in assumedly appropriate ways (see also Dickson et al., 2002; Nower & Blaszczynski, 2004; Williams, 2002, for further activities addressing problem and underage gambling, although these have not yet formally assessed and/or published in a peer-reviewed journal).

Promising but Not (Yet) Formally Evaluated Prevention Programs For Adolescents—A Selective Overview

1. "Don't bet on it" comprises a classroom-based prevention program developed for students from grades 9 to 12. The module consists of several interactive elements, curricular activities, and teaching units related to gambling issues (teacher reference materials and student handouts as well as an equivalent program for seventh–eighth graders called "All bets are off!" also are available from the Michigan Model for Comprehensive School Health Education).

(continued)

2. A creative effort to promote awareness and deliver the message that gambling participation can lead to negative consequences are plays like "After the Beep" or "Three-of-a-Kind," designed for high school students. In addition, discussing the content of the play may subsequently increase the awareness of high school students better than didactic approaches. (Source: Responsible Gambling Council Ontario).

3. Curricular activities as provided by Crites (2003), who suggested educating children in the area of probabilities and statistics using gambling-related scenarios. The range of specific innovative hands-on activities gives insight into the workings of the lottery and the games of keno, roulette, and craps and can be easily integrated into mathematic lessons. Such approaches may promote critical thinking among the students and equip children and adolescents with knowledge about the nature of random events or the expected monetary value when participating in gambling.

4. "Count me out" ("*Moi, je passe*") is another school-based program awareness program addressed to students in the last three years of primary school and in high school. The program has already been applied in Quebec. Its components include information about gambling in general, erroneous beliefs and inaccurate cognitions, and the promotion of personal/social skills. Material resources include a CD-ROM and a video, among other things, and the program explicitly offers activities that correspond to the students' stage of development (Le Group Jeunesse, 2000).

5. An example of an interactive opportunity to deal with gambling-related issues can be found online at http://www.youthbet.net. This page was developed by the TeenNet Gambling Project (Department of Public Health Sciences, University of Toronto) and provides a virtual neighborhood environment with several locations that encompasses gambling settings (casino, store) where informal gambling activities take place (playground) and information resources (library, community centre) developed with teenagers for teenagers.

Recommendations

To date, the paucity of knowledge about the pathogenesis of problem gambling makes it difficult to develop and implement comprehensive prevention and intervention actions for adolescents. Therefore, in the first instance, gambling research needs to establish a comprehensive multicausal etiological and testable model including causal pathways (e.g., Nower & Blaszczynski, 2004) with modifiable risk as well as protective factors. The small body of gambling research (e.g., with regard to protective factors or the exact mechanisms of action for specific risk factors) does not permit us to draw conclusions in terms of best practices so far. Nevertheless, prevention studies of alcohol, tobacco, and other drugs provide valuable insights and useful information on how to design effective prevention programs for problem gambling in adolescence (e.g., Evans, 2003). Strategies that encompass motivational issues, resisting peer group pressures (including adequate responses to common advertising appeals), and correcting erroneous social perceptions seem to be the most promising approaches to successfully alter behavior.

Evidence from related disciplines strongly suggests that fear or scaring strategies display an ineffective and insufficient way of yielding positive (behavioral) outcomes. Instead of labeling gambling as deviant, evil, or even sinful, (gambling) prevention programs must offer young people a way to develop adequate personal skills and social competencies. One of the most important issues encompasses the concept of social inoculation—inoculating adolescents with the knowledge and skills necessary to resist social pressures with regard to risk behaviors to which they may be exposed. According to Gupta and Derevensky (2000) prevention models must (a) increase awareness of adolescent problem gambling, (b) enhance knowledge about youth problem gambling, (c) change attitudes toward gambling and encourage adoption of a more balanced view, (d) teach effective coping and adaptive skills, and (e) correct inappropriate cognitions related to gambling activities (i.e., role of skill, illusion of control, gambler's fallacy, assessment of the odds of winning). Eventually, prevention and especially treatment efforts should recognize the striking link between problem gambling and substance abuse and thus the possibility of "switching addictions."

In the future, one of our main goals must be to connect research findings, theory, and prevention science with practice. More research is needed that evaluates methods and materials of gambling prevention programs in order to support the effective implementation of empirically based practices. Important key actions, research, and practical challenges around adolescent gambling are summarized in below. How we meet these challenges will determine the extent to which future generations throughout the world will develop gambling-related problems.

Key Actions, Research, and Practical Challenges Around Adolescent Gambling (Dickson et al.; 2002; Korn & Shaffer, 1999; National Research Council, 1999; Shaffer et al., 2003; Stinchfield & Winters, 1998)

A. Risk and protective factors

- Conduct a more rigorous comparison between risk factors of adolescent problem gambling and other problem domains and translate empirical knowledge into science-based prevention and treatment initiatives
- Arrange studies with longitudinal designs to determine causal risk factors and protective factors preceding the outcome of problem gambling and highlight typical developmental pathways
- Confirm study findings with different study methods and designs, across populations, and in other cultures
- Identify whether certain gambling forms serve as a "gateway drug"

B. Prevention and treatment

- Raise public awareness about the extent of adolescent problem gambling, especially among parents and educators (see Shaffer et al., 2000)

- Incorporate gambling-related information and prevention efforts quickly and economically into already existing and effective mental health and education programs
- Establish primary prevention programs within the curricula of elementary, middle, and high schools
- Provide well-timed, long term, and sufficient-dosage actions and consider the evolving needs of adolescents and issues like transitions or certain developmental tasks (including age-, gender- and culture-specific approaches in terms of program materials and intervention techniques)
- Stimulate high-quality research related to the treatment of adolescent pathological gamblers
- Carefully evaluate the effectiveness of prevention programs and treatments in inpatient and outpatient settings for different types of adolescent problem gamblers
- Include family members or associates as a continuing supportive resource
- Reach young people who are absent from school (e.g., truancy, school drop-out), who are more likely to be engaging in gambling and other potentially addictive behaviors

C. Policy

- Determine the utility of regulatory gambling policy and subsequent proliferation of gambling
- Raise the minimum age of all forms of commercial gambling to 18 years and impose stricter penalties for gambling operators who allow children and adolescents to gamble illegally
- Assure the consistency of public policies strategies, ensure that laws, policies and the content of prevention programs need to be coherent
- Evaluate the impact of structural characteristics of gambling technologies with regard to the needs of adolescents
- Evaluate the impacts of the evolvement of new gambling opportunities (e.g., internet gambling, interactive TV gambling, betting with mobile phones)
- Install task forces to monitor problem gambling issues explicitly, including adolescent problem gambling
- Foster collaboration among researchers, policy makers, program advocates, and community leaders to produce rigorous and useful research evidence (input from all stakeholders is necessary to form synergetic effects and bring research into practice)

References

Alberta Alcohol and Drug Abuse Commission (Eds.). (2003a). *Summary report: The Alberta Youth Experience Survey 2002.* [Online]. Available: http://corp.aadac.com/programsservices/research/pdf/Tayes_overview.pdf.

Alberta Alcohol and Drug Abuse Commission (Eds.). (2003b). *An Overview of Risk and Protective Factors: The Alberta Youth Experience Survey 2002.* [Online]. Available: http://corp.aadac.com/programsservices/research/pdf/Tayes-SumReportBook.pdf.

American Psychiatric Association (1994). *Diagnostic and Statistical Manual of Mental Disorders* (4th ed.). Washington, DC: APA.

Barnes, G.M., Welte, J.W., Hoffman, J.H., & Dintcheff, B.A. (2002). Effects of alcohol misuse on gambling patterns in youth. *Journal of Studies on Alcohol, 63,* 767–775.

Becoña Iglesias, E., del Carmen Míguez Varela, M., & Vázquez González, V. (2001). El juego problema en los estudiantes de Enseñanza Secundaria [Problem gambling in secondary school students]. *Psicothema, 13*, 551–556.

Bellringer, P. (1992). *Working with Young Problem Gamblers: Guidelines to Practice.* Leicester: UK Forum on Young People and Gambling.

Botvin, G.J. (2001). Prevention of substance abuse in adolescents. In N.J. Smelser & P.B. Baltes (Eds.), *International Encyclopedia of the Social and Behavioral Sciences* (pp. 15255–15259). Oxford: Pergamon Press.

Breiter, H.C., Aharon, I., Kahneman, D., Dale, A., & Shizgal, P. (2001). Functional imaging of neural responses to expectancy and experience of monetary gains and losses. *Neuron, 30*, 619–639.

Cavedini, P., Riboldi, G., Keller, R., D'Annucci, A., & Bellodi, L. (2002). Frontal lobe dysfunction in pathological gambling patients. *Biological Psychiatry, 51*, 334–341.

Chambers, R.A., & Potenza, M.N. (2003). Neurodevelopment, impulsivity, and adolescent gambling. *Journal of Gambling Studies, 19*, 53–84.

Coie, J.D., Watt, N.F., West, S.G., Hawkins, J.D., Asarnow, J.R., Markman, H.J., Ramey, S.L., Shure, M.B., & Long, B. (1993). Prevention science: A conceptual framework and some directions for a national research program. *American Psychologist, 48*, 1013–1022.

Comings, D.E., Gade-Andavolu, R., Gonzales, N., Wu, S., Muhleman, D., Chen, C., Koh, P., Farwell, K., Blake, H., Dietz, G., MacMurray, J.P., Lesieur, H.R., Rugle, L.J., & Rosenthal, R. (2001). The additive effect of neurotransmitter genes in pathological gambling. *Clinical Genetics, 60*, 107–116.

Comings, D.E., Rosenthal, R., Lesieur, H.R., Rugle, L.J., Muhleman, D., Chiu, C., Dietz, G., & Gade, R. (1996). A study of the dopamine D2 receptor gene in pathological gambling. *Pharmacogenetics, 6*, 223–234.

Crites, T. (2003). What are my chances? Using probability and number sense to educate teens about the mathematical risks of gambling. In H.J. Shaffer, M.N. Hall, J. Vander Bilt & E.M. George (Eds.), *Futures at Stake: Youth, Gambling, and Society* (pp. 63–83). Reno: University of Nevada.

Derevensky, J.L., Gupta, R., Dickson, L., Hardoon, K., & Deguire, A.-E. (2003). In D. Romer (Ed.), *Reducing Adolescent Risk: Toward an Integrated Approach* (pp. 239–246). Thousand Oaks: Sage.

Dickson, L.M., Derevensky, J.L., & Gupta, R. (2002). The prevention of gambling problems in youth: A conceptual framework. *Journal of Gambling Studies, 18*, 97–159.

DiClemente, C.C., Story, M., & Murray, K. (2000). On a roll: The process of initiation and cessation of problem gambling among adolescents. *Journal of Gambling Studies, 16*, 289–313.

Durlak, J.A. (2003). Effective prevention and health promotion programming. In T.P. Gullotta & M. Bloom (Eds.), *Encyclopedia of Primary Prevention and Health Promotion* (pp. 61–69). New York: Kluwer.

Eisen, S.A., Lin, N., Lyons, M.J., Scherrer, J.F., Griffith, K., True, W.R., Goldberg, J., & Tsuang, M.T. (1998). Familial influence on gambling behavior: An analysis of 3359 twin pairs. *Addiction, 93*, 1375–1384.

Evans, R.I. (2003). Some theoretical models and constructs generic to substance abuse prevention programs for adolescents: Possible relevance and limitations for problem gambling. *Journal of Gambling Studies, 19*, 287–302.

Ferland, F., Ladouceur, R., & Jacques, C. (2000, June). *Evaluation of a Gambling Prevention Program for Youths.* 11th International Conference on Gambling and Risk-Taking, Las Vegas, Nevada.

Ferland, F., Ladouceur, R., & Vitaro, F. (2002). Prevention of problem gambling: Modifying misconceptions and increasing knowledge. *Journal of Gambling Studies, 18*, 19–29.

Fisher, S. (1999). A prevalence study of gambling and problem gambling in British adolescents. *Addiction Research, 7*, 509–538.

Gaboury, A., & Ladouceur, R. (1993). Evaluation of a prevention program for pathological gambling among adolescents. *The Journal of Primary Prevention, 14*, 21–28.

Gehring, W.J., & Willoughby, A.R. (2002). The medial frontal cortex and the rapid processing of monetary gains and losses. *Science, 295*, 2279–2282.

Grant, J.E., Kim, S.W., & Potenza, M.N. (2003). Advances in the pharmacological treatment of pathological gambling. *Journal of Gambling Studies, 19*, 85–109.

Griffiths, M.D. (1990). The acquisition, development and maintenance of fruit machine gambling. *Journal of Gambling Studies, 6*, 193–204.

Griffiths, M.D. (1991). Amusement machine playing in childhood and adolescence: A comparative analysis of video games and fruit machines. *Journal of Adolescence, 14*, 53–73.

Griffiths, M. (1994). The role of cognitive bias and skill in fruit machine playing. *British Journal of Psychology, 85*, 351–369.

Griffiths, M. (1995). *Adolescent Gambling.* London: Routledge.

Griffiths, M. (1999). Gambling technologies: Prospects for problem gambling. *Journal of Gambling Studies, 15*, 265–283.

Griffiths, M. (2000). Scratchcard gambling among adolescent males. *Journal of Gambling Studies, 16*, 79–91.

Griffiths, M. (2001, October). Why don't adolescent problem gamblers seek treatment? *Electronic Journal of Gambling Issues, 5*. [Online]. Available: http://www.camh.net/egambling/issue5/opinion/index.html.

Griffiths, M. (2003). Adolescent gambling: Risk factors and implications for prevention, intervention, and treatment. In D. Romer (Ed.), *Reducing Adolescent Risk: Toward an Integrated Approach* (pp. 223–238). Thousand Oaks: Sage.

Griffiths, M., & Sutherland, I. (1998). Adolescent gambling and drug use. *Journal of Community and Applied Social Psychology, 8*, 423–427.

Gupta, R., & Derevensky, J.L. (1998). Adolescent gambling behavior: A prevalence study and examination of the correlates associated with problem gambling. *Journal of Gambling Studies, 14*, 319–345.

Gupta, R., & Derevensky, J.L. (2000). Adolescent with gambling problems: From research to treatment. *Journal of Gambling Studies, 16*, 315–342.

Jacobs, D.F. (2000). Juvenile gambling in North America: An analysis of long term trends and future prospects. *Journal of Gambling Studies, 16*, 119–152.

Johansson, A., & Götestam, K.G. (2003). Gambling and problematic gambling with money among Norwegian youth (12–18 years). *Nordic Journal of Psychiatry, 57*, 317–321.

Korn, D.A., & Shaffer, H.J. (1999). Gambling and the health of the public: Adopting a public health perspective. *Journal of Gambling Studies, 15*, 289–365.

Ladouceur, R., Boisvert, J.M., & Dumont, J. (1994). Cognitive-behavioral treatment for adolescent pathological gamblers. *Behavior Modification, 18*, 230–242.

Ladouceur, R., Boudreault, N., Jacques, C., & Vitaro, F. (1999). Pathological gambling and related problems among adolescents. *Journal of Child & Adolescent Substance Abuse, 8*, 55–68.

Ladouceur, R., Ferland, F., & Fournier, P.M. (2003). Correction of erroneous perceptions among primary school students regarding the notions of chance and randomness in gambling. *American Journal of Public Health, 34*, 272–277.

Ladouceur, R., Jacques, C., Ferland, F., & Giroux, I. (1998). Parents' attitudes and knowledge regarding gambling among youth. *Journal of Gambling Studies, 14*, 83–90.

Ladouceur, R., & Walker, M. (1996). A cognitive perspective on gambling. In P.M. Salkovskis (Ed.), *Trends in Cognitive Behavioural Therapies* (pp. 89–120). New York: Wiley.

Lavoie, M.P., & Ladouceur, R. (2004, february). Prevention of gambling among youth: Increasing knowledge and modifying attitudes toward gambling. *Electronic Journal of Gambling Issues, 10*. [Online]. Available: http://www.camh.net/egambling/issue10/ejgi_10_lavoie_ladoueceur.html.

Le Group Jeunesse (2000). *Count Me Out (Moi, je passe): Awareness Program for the Prevention of Gambling Dependency.* Montreal, QC: Le Group Jeunesse.

Lupu, V., Onaca, E., & Lupu, D. (2002). The prevalence of pathological gambling in Romanian teenagers. *Minerva Medica, 93*, 413–418.

Meyer, G., & Bachmann, M. (2000). *Spielsucht. Ursachen und Therapie [Gambling Addiction: Causes and Treatment].* Berlin: Springer.

Moore, S.M., & Ohtsuka, K. (1999). Beliefs about control over gambling among young people, and their relation to problem gambling. *Psychology of Addictive Behaviors, 13*, 339–347.

National Research Council (1999). *Pathological Gambling: A Critical Review.* Washington, DC: National Academic Press.

Nower, L., & Blaszczynski, A. (2004). The pathways model as harm minimization for youth gamblers in educational settings. *Child and Adolescent Social Work Journal, 21*, 25–45.

Pietrzak, R.H., Ladd, G.T., & Petry, N.M. (2003). Disordered gambling in adolescents: Epidemiology, diagnosis, and treatment. *Pediatric Drugs, 5*, 583–595.

Potenza, M.N. (2001). The neurobiology of pathological gambling. *Seminars in Clinical Neuropsychiatry, 6*, 217–226.

Potenza, M.N. (2002). A perspective on future directions in the prevention, treatment, and research of pathological gambling. *Psychiatric Annals, 32*, 203–207.

Potenza, M.N., Steinberg, M.A., Skudlarski, P., Fulbright, R.K., Lacadie, C.M., Wilber, M.K., Rounsaville, B.J., Gore, J.C., & Wexler, B.E. (2003). Gambling urges in pathological gambling: A functional magnetic resonance imaging study. *Archives of General Psychiatry, 60*, 828–836.

Poulin, C. (2000). Problem gambling among adolescent students in the Atlantic provinces of Canada. *Journal of Gambling Studies, 16*, 53–78.

Prochaska, J.O., DiClemente, C.C., & Norcross, J.C. (1992). In search of how people change: Applications to addictive behaviors. *American Psychologist, 47*, 1102–1114.

Regard, M., Knoch, D., Gütling, E., & Landis, T. (2003). Brain damage and addictive behavior: A neuropsychological and electroencephalogram investigation with pathologic gamblers. *Cognitive and Behavioral Neurology, 16*, 47–53.

Scheithauer, H., Petermann, F., Meyer, G., & Hayer, T. (2004). Entwicklungsorientierte Prävention von Substanzmissbrauch und problematischem Glücksspielverhalten im Kindes- und Jugendalter [Developmental prevention of substance abuse and problem gambling in childhood and adolescence]. In R. Schwarzer (Hrsg.), *Gesundheitspsychologie. Reihe: Enzyklopädie der Psychologie*. Göttingen: Hogrefe.

Shaffer, H.J., Forman, D.P., Scanlan, K.M., & Smith, F. (2000). Awareness of gambling-related problems, policies and educational programs among high school and college administrators. *Journal of Gambling Studies, 16*, 93–101.

Shaffer, H.J., & Hall, M.N. (2001). Updating and refining prevalence estimates of disordered gambling behaviour in the United States and Canada. *Canadian Journal of Public Health, 92*, 168–172.

Shaffer, H.J., Hall, M.N., Vander Bilt, J., & Vagge, L. (2003). Youth and gambling: Creating a legacy of risk. In H.J. Shaffer, M.N. Hall, J. Vander Bilt & E.M. George (Eds.), *Futures at Stake: Youth, Gambling, and Society* (pp. 3–24). Reno: University of Nevada.

Shaffer, H.J., LaBrie, R., Scanlan, K.M., & Cummings, T.N. (1994). Pathological gambling among adolescents: Massachusetts Gambling Screen (MAGS). *Journal of Gambling Studies, 10*, 339–362.

Shapira, N.A., Ferguson, M.A., Frost-Pineda, K., & Gold, M.S. (2002, december). *Gambling and problem gambling prevalence among adolescents in Florida*. [Online]. Available: http://psych.med.ufl.edu/aec/research/abstracts/childgambling.pdf.

Stinchfield, R., Cassuto, N., Winters, K., & Latimer, W. (1997). Prevalence of gambling among Minnesota public school students in 1992 and 1995. *Journal of Gambling Studies, 13*, 25–48.

Stinchfield, R., & Winters, K.C. (1998). Gambling and problem gambling among youths. *Annals of the American Academy of Political and Social Science, 556*, 172–185.

Vitaro, F., Brendgen, M., Ladouceur, R., & Tremblay, R.E. (2001). Gambling, delinquency, and drug use during adolescence: Mutual influences and common risk factors. *Journal of Gambling Studies, 17*, 171–190.

Volberg, R.A. (2002, march). *Gambling and problem gambling among adolescents in Nevada*. [Online]. Available: http://www.hr.state.nv.us/directors/NVGamblingAmongAdolescents_Nevada.pdf.

Williams, R. (2002, December). *Prevention of problem gambling: A school-based intervention*. [Online]. Available: http://www.abgaminginstitute.ualberta.ca/documents/research/Williams_prevention.pdf.

Winters, K.C., & Anderson, N. (2000). Gambling involvement and drug use among adolescents. *Journal of Gambling Studies, 16*, 175–198.

Winters, K.C., & Rich, T. (1998). A twin study of adult gambling behavior. *Journal of Gambling Studies, 14*, 213–225.

Winters, K.C., Stinchfield, R.D., Botzet, A., & Anderson, N. (2002). A prospective study of youth gambling behaviors. *Psychology of Addictive Behaviors, 16*, 3–9.

Winters, K.C., Stinchfield, R., & Fulkerson, J. (1993). Patterns and characteristics of adolescent gambling. *Journal of Gambling Studies, 9*, 371–386.

Wood, R.T.A., & Griffiths, M. (1998). The acquisition, development and maintenance of lottery and scrachtcard gambling in adolescence. *Journal of Adolescence, 21*, 265–273.

Yeoman, T., & Griffiths, M. (1996). Adolescent machine gambling and crime. *Journal of Adolescence, 19*, 183–188.

Zitzow, D. (1996). Comparative study of problematic gambling behaviors between American Indian and non-Indian adolescents within and near a Northern Plains reservation. *American Indian & Alaska Native Mental Health Research, 7 (2)*, 14–26.

Chapter 22

Adolescent Sex Offenders

Christina M. Camp, Laura F. Salazar, Ralph J. DiClemente, and Gina M. Wingood

Introduction

Sexual assault is one of the fastest growing violent crimes in the United States (Shaw, 1999). Around the country, police, prosecutors, mental health professionals, and probation officers continue to struggle to deal with the rise in the number of juvenile sex offenders. It is estimated that in the United States, juveniles commit almost half of all child molestations and about 20% of all rapes (Federal Bureau of Investigation, 2002). Among adult sexual offenders, nearly 50% have reported that they began their history of offenses during adolescence (Abel, Mittelman & Becker, 1985; Groth, Longo & McFadin, 1982). Moreover, during adolescence many offenders exhibit patterns of non-violent sexual offending and progress to more serious sexual offenses as adults (Longo & Groth, 1983). Additional evidence suggests that juvenile sex offenders may go on to commit over 380 sexual offenses during their lifetime (Ertl & McNamara, 1997). Although these statistics indicate that juvenile sex offenses are more prevalent than was once thought, estimates are likely to be low due to issues of secrecy and under-reporting.

The consequences of sex offending are substantial for victims, society, perpetrators, and their families. In addition to the human costs in terms of emotional and physical suffering, significant financial costs are incurred as a function of child welfare, juvenile justice system involvement, and therapeutic intervention (Prentsky & Burgess, 1990). Statistics such as those mentioned earlier, and the high risk that perpetrators pose to their victims and the community at large, support the need for and increased understanding of factors influencing the development of sexually aggressive behavior, reliable assessment strategies, and effective treatment programs. Attention directed to these areas will assist with early intervention and may decrease the likelihood that offenders will continue such destructive patterns of behavior.

Sexual offending, a legal term, refers to a broad range of behaviors, yet is generally defined by any sexual contact which involves coercion, manipulation of power, or is committed against individuals who are unable to give informed consent. Ertl and

McNamara (1997) provide descriptions of three categories of sexual offenses: those which are referred to as *hands-off* offenses, which include voyeurism, making obscene phone calls, and exhibitionism; *hands-on* offenses, which usually include some type of force, aggression, or coercion, such as fondling or rape; and *pedophiliac offenses*, in which the victim is at least four years younger than the perpetrator. It should be noted that offenders may also select victims who are significantly lower functioning than themselves, putting them in a position of power so that they can manipulate their victim.

Adolescent sex offenders have also been classified as a function of their motives and other factors that mediate their pattern of offending. Becker (1988) provides an overview of four types of sexual abusers, with most offenders displaying features of each: (1) the true paraphiliac with a well-established pattern of deviant sexual arousal; (2) an antisocial youth who not only sexually offends, but exploits people in other ways as well when the opportunity presents itself; (3) an adolescent with a psychiatric or neurological/biological disorder that affects his/her ability to control aggressive and sexual impulses; and (4) an adolescent that does not have adequate social and interpersonal skills, who seeks sexual gratification from younger children because it is unavailable from peer groups (p. 327).

Adolescent sexual offending is a complex phenomenon that defies a simplistic explanation. As such, many theories have been proposed to explain why some children and teens sexually abuse others. However, to date there is no empirically derived and tested model to explain why adolescents commit sexual crimes. The most widely accepted theory that provides an explanation for sexually abusive behavior in children is learning theory. *Learning theory* is based on the concept that all behavior and knowledge is learned through experience. In using this theoretical framework to explain sexually abusive behavior in children, theorists purport that sexually abusive behavior in children is linked to many factors, including exposure to sexuality and/or violence, early childhood experiences (e.g., sexual victimization), exposure to child pornography, substance abuse, and exposure to aggressive role models or family violence (Ryan & Lane, 1997).

Early theories about children who sexually abuse others proposed that these individuals move through a predictable progression or a *"sexual abuse cycle."* Theorists supporting this perspective suggest that the pathway to the development of sexually aggressive behaviors begins with the adolescent's having a negative self-image, which results in an increased probability of maladaptive coping strategies when confronted with negative responses to himself or herself. The negative self-image also leads the individual to predict a negative reaction from others. To protect against this anticipated rejection, the adolescent will become socially isolated and withdrawn and will begin to fantasize to compensate for his or her feelings of powerlessness. Finally, the sexual offense is carried out, leading to more negative self-imaging and thoughts of rejection, facilitating a repetitive cycle (Ryan & Lane, 1997). More recently this cycle has been criticized as too rigid—interviews with offenders reveal that life problems (at school, in the family) and any number of thoughts or feelings can trigger an offending behavior as well (Longo, 2002). The literature in this area is lacking, and more comprehensive information regarding these theories is desperately needed in order to assist with early detection and risk identification and to provide adequate services prior to the occurrence of more serious sexual offenses.

The current chapter provides an overview of individual, familial, and behavioral characteristics of adolescents who have sexually offended. This chapter also reviews common approaches to treating and preventing recurrent sexually aggressive behavior in juveniles.

Individual Factors

While some researchers have conducted descriptive studies in an effort to develop a clinical picture of juvenile sexual offender characteristics and behaviors, the limited frequency of such behaviors identified within research studies makes it difficult to distinguish unique features between offending and non-offending adolescents. Thus, to date, there is no clear, meaningful, and responsible way to distinguish between actual and potential juvenile sexual offenders (Becker & Hunter, 1997). Additionally, while we can describe features characteristic of many sexual offenders, they do not apply to all of them; many do not possess all or any of these characteristics. Hence, traits and behavior may vary from one individual and another, and currently we only have the ability to classify a juvenile sex offender after he or she has offended or been discovered (Rich, 2003).

Nonetheless, descriptive studies indicate that the majority of sex offenders are male, and that their most likely victims have been noted to be female, followed by young boys. The average offender is 14 years of age, and possesses a low to average IQ. Nearly half of all juvenile sexual assaults are contact offenses, are committed under the threat of force, and are inclusive of vaginal or anal penetration or sodomy. Histories of physical and sexual abuse and exposure to domestic violence have also been noted to be prevalent among this population. Additionally, many juvenile offenders have been exposed to pornography as early as age 7 (Center for Sex Offender Management, 1999; Ryan, 1999; Ryan, Miyoshi, Metzner, Krugman & Fryer, 1996; Weinrott, 1996).

Graves, Openshaw, Ascione, and Ericksen (1996) incorporated meta-analysis in evaluating 20 years (1973–1993) of empirical data stemming from demographic research on juvenile sex offenders. Through their analysis, three categorical subtypes of offenders emerged: (a) pediophilic offender, (b) sexual assault offender, and (c) mixed offense offender. The *pedophilic offenders* were identified as youth demonstrating limited confidence in their ability to engage in social interactions and being socially isolated from their peers. Findings further indicated that the youth in this group consistently molested children who were significantly younger than themselves as well as a strong preference for female victims. The subgroup of *sexual assault offenders* were juveniles whose first offense was reported when they were between the ages of 13 and 15. They were more likely to victimize females, and they committed offenses against victims of various ages. *Mixed offense offenders* were described as youth who had committed a variety of offenses, including exhibitionism, voyeurism, frotteurism (frotteurism involves actual touching and rubbing of the genitalia against a non-consenting person, in association with sexual arousal) as well as other offenses involving physical contact. These youth were identified as having the most severe degree of social and psychological difficulty. The majority of these youth committed their first offense between the ages of 6 and 15, and their usual victim was female.

Relative to other demographic characteristics, the meta-analysis yielded results indicating that a greater proportion of youth sexual offenders come from middle to lower socioeconomic status familial backgrounds, 59% and 44%, respectively. As it pertains to race, 60% of the sexual assault subgroup and 59% of the pedophilic and mixed offenders were Caucasian. Similar to the mixed offender group, sexual assault offenders were more likely to be Caucasian rather than black or Hispanic. Findings related to religious affiliation among these groups were limited—38% of the adolescent offenders reported that they were Catholic, while 62% did not identify a religious affiliation.

There are a broad range of factors that may contribute to the development of sexually abusive behavior. At the individual level factors that have been associated with adolescent sexual aggression include a history of sexual and or physical abuse; social isolation, poor impulse control or impulse conduct disorder, and limited cognitive abilities.

Rates of juvenile sex offenders who have experienced sexual abuse as children range from 40% to 80%, while proportions of juvenile sex offenders who were victims of physical abuse range from 25% to 50% (Becker and Hunter, 1997). It is important to note that the abusive experiences of juvenile sex offenders have not been found to differ consistently from those of non-sex-offending juveniles (Knight & Prentsky, 1993). Thus, the role of child maltreatment in the etiology of sexual aggression remains unclear. However, these trends indicate the importance of considering the extent to which a history of childhood sexual or physical abuse plays a role in the development of the sexual offender. Additionally, theoretical models of sexually abusive behavior have been developed that support the ideology that the experience of victimization is a significant influential factor in the development of sexually offending behavior (Becker & Kaplan, 1993; Ryan & Lane, 1997).

Many researchers have observed significant deficits in social competence among adolescent sex offenders (Becker, 1990; Knight & Prentsky, 1993). Inadequate social skills, poor peer relationships, and social isolation are some of the difficulties that have been identified among this group (Katz, 1990; Miner & Crimmins, 1995). For example, Katz (1990) evaluated social competence among non-sex-offending juvenile delinquents, adolescent "child molesters," and a high school comparison group. Findings revealed that juveniles who had child molestation offenses were more socially maladjusted when compared to the two other groups. Beckett (1999) provides additional support for this finding in stating that "particularly for adolescent child abusers, poor social competency and deficits in self-esteem rather than paraphilic interests in the psychopathic tendencies currently appear to be the best explanation as to why they commit sexual assaults" (p. 224). Additionally, Miner and Crimmins (1995) reported that juveniles in their study who had committed sexual offenses exhibited fewer peer attachments and felt less positive attachments to their schools when compared with other delinquent and nondelinquent juveniles.

These findings highlight the important relationship between a child's psychosocial environment and their ability to meet developmental milestones associated with social competence. Marshall and Eccles (1993) provide an example of this in suggesting that it is through the social environment that developmental vulnerabilities have the opportunity to develop and grow into risk factors or into the assets and strengths that serve as protective factors against risk for sexually deviant behavior. They further indicate that it is through the social environment that

> children find (or fail to find) love, attention, emotional bonding and attachment, role modeling, structure, supervision, guidance, social relationships, physical and emotional security, wisdom and mentoring, information, ideas, and encouragement. Hence, the

availability of these critical factors promote optimal development and resiliency to risk factors among adolescents by fostering trust, independence, self-esteem, social mastery and competence, motivation, intimacy, knowledge, morals, satisfaction, and a healthy personal identity (Rich, 2003, p. 62).

Alternatively, the absence of these factors can facilitate an environment in which a child can develop developmental vulnerabilities and experience significant difficulty in succeeding.

Overall, it is suggested that adolescent sexual offenders lack appropriate social skills, and that this may be associated with their behavior. As a result of research findings that provide support for considering social skill deficits in the development of sexually abusive behaviors among adolescents, many treatment programs have incorporated social skills training as one component of intervention (Becker & Kaplan, 1993; Davis & Leitenberg, 1987).

Behavioral and cognitive disorders are commonly diagnosed in children and adolescents who sexually abuse others (Center for Sex Offender Management, 1999). Kavoussi, Kaplan, and Becker (1988) reported that the most common psychiatric diagnosis in their sample of male juvenile sex offenders was a conduct disorder (48%). Moreover, a much higher rate was revealed among adolescents who had raped or attempted to rape adult women (75%). It should be further noted that many offenders are provided with a diagnosis of conduct disorder due to the fact it provides the very best description of behaviors associated with sexual offending.

The incidence of attention deficit hyperactivity disorder (ADHD) has not yet been adequately explored among juveniles with sexual aggression. Yet, attention deficit hyperactivity disorder has been found in up to 22% samples, with more than one-third of offenders exhibiting some traits of ADHD (Becker & Kaplan, 1993; Becker, Kaplan, Cunningham-Raither & Kavoussi, 1986; Kavoussi, Kaplan & Becker, 1988). Kavoussi and colleagues (1988) also found that out of their sample of 58 juvenile sex offenders in outpatient treatment, nearly 7% met the full criteria for attention-deficit disorder. Close to 38% of the juveniles revealed some symptoms of attention-deficit disorder. Similarly, Miner, Siekert, and Ackland (1997) found that more than 60% of their sample of incarcerated juvenile sex offenders in their sample exhibited hyperactive and restless behaviors, and 75% were identified as having attention problems, behavior problems, a learning disability or all three. Additionally, few differences were found between sex-offending and non-sex-offending delinquents relative to these patterns of behavior (Awad et al., 1984; Gilby, Wolf & Goldberg, 1989). Given the commonalities in attention deficits, behavior problems, and school difficulty across both juvenile sex-offender and non-sex-offending delinquent populations, some researchers conclude that attention problems and social and general behavioral difficulties are factors that are common to most troubled youth.

The literature related to the intellectual and cognitive levels of juveniles who have committed sexual offenses is also limited. However, existing studies examining this phenomenon suggest that the prevalence of intellectual and cognitive impairments among juvenile sex offenders is an area worthy of further exploration. For example, Ferrera and McDonald (1996) conducted a review of the literature and determined that approximately 33% of juvenile sex offenders have some form of neurological impairment. Additionally, more than one-quarter (25.2%) of juvenile sex offenders had IQ scores below 80, in contrast to 11.1% of non-sex-offending adolescents who scored in this range of functioning. The presence of cognitive and behavioral disorders in the background of juvenile sex offenders carries significant implications for treatment. It is noted that the neurologically impaired juvenile offender who goes undetected in treatment settings is not likely to benefit significantly from treatment due to difficulties associated with concentration, comprehension, and memory (Ferrera & McDonald, 1996).

Family Factors

According to the literature, a strong relationship exists between dysfunctional families and the incidence of delinquent behavior in children of such families. Specifically, descriptive studies indicate that adolescent sexual offenders demonstrate the tendency to have high rates of family instability, parent–child separation, exposure to violence, and parental psychopathology (Miner, Siekert, and Ackland, 1997; Van Ness, 1984). Lee and colleagues (2002) provide support for this perspective in indicating that family dysfunction often goes hand in hand with childhood difficulties among sexual offenders and further state that childhood sexual, physical, and emotional abuse and family dysfunction are general developmental risk factors for sexually aggressive behavior.

Studies that have evaluated family instability as a function of parent–child separation vary in percentages of juveniles who are from intact families. For example, Kahn and Chambers (1991) found that less than one-third of the juvenile sex offenders in their sample stemmed from intact families. Additionally, Graves et al. (1996) used meta-analysis to analyze the findings of multiple studies examining characteristics of juvenile sex offenders that were conducted over a 20 year period. The findings from this analysis suggested that juveniles who committed sexual assaults against victims who were their peers or older were more likely to come from single-parent homes (78%) than those who committed "pedophilic" offenses (44%) or mixed offenses (37%). Pedophilic offenders more frequently stemmed from foster or blended families (53%). Conversely, Miner, Siekert, and Ackland (1997) conducted a study among incarcerated offenders which revealed that only 16% of the juveniles in their sample came from intact families. It is important to take into account, however, that the low rate of intact families reported in this study may reflect the nature of the sample evaluated (i.e., incarcerated juveniles). Nevertheless, in contrast to this study, Cellini (1995) reported that approximately 70% of juvenile sex offenders lived in two-parent homes at the time their abusive behavior was discovered. It was not clear, however, whether the two parents in these homes were both birth parents.

Collectively, these studies suggest that many adolescent offenders have experienced physical or emotional separation from their parents. The cause of this separation may be family instability, parental separation or divorce, or residential placement of the juvenile. However, despite the causes it is clear that parent–child separation may mediate a significant disruption in emotional and personality development among adolescents who commit sexual offenses.

Histories of maltreatment that are inclusive of neglectful or inadequate parenting, as well as dysfunctional child-rearing environments are also prevalent among both juvenile sexual offenders and non-sexual offenders (Hunter and Figueredo, 1999). The literature indicates that parents of sexual offenders have been noted to experience difficulties with substance abuse, psychological impairments, and involvement in the criminal justice system (Awad et al., 1984; Kaplan, Becker & Martinez, 1992). Each of these factors can influence the extent to which children receive adequate parenting. Miner, Siekert, and Ackland (1997) conducted a study among juvenile sex offenders and reported that nearly 60% of the biological fathers had substance abuse histories and 28% had criminal histories. Biological mothers, when compared to fathers, were less likely to have substance abuse histories (28%) or criminal histories (17%). The mothers, however, were more likely than the fathers to have a history of psychiatric treatment (23% versus 13%, respectively). Moreover, Smith and Israel (1987) found that some parents of juveniles who sexually abused their siblings were physically and/or emotionally inaccessible and distant. It was further indicated that some parents evidenced sexual pathology and exposed the juveniles to their sexual behaviors.

Exposure to family violence has also been identified as a common risk factor in the development of sexual violence among adolescents. Van Ness (1984) yielded results indicating that 41% of adolescent sex offenders in his sample had experienced intra-familial violence or neglect during childhood. In contrast, only 15% of the non-sex-offender sample reported histories of abuse or neglect. In a more recent study, Ryan and colleagues (1996) reported that 63% of their sample of 1,000 juveniles witnessed family violence, while Skuse et al. (2000) found that male victims of sexual abuse were more likely to sexually victimize others if they had witnessed family violence. It was further suggested that "it may be more appropriate to view a climate of violence conferring an increased risk, despite whether or not the boy is a direct victim of physical abuse" (p. 229). Similarly, Bentovin (2002) identified family violence as one of three distinguishing factors associated with juvenile sex offenders who are also sexual abuse victims. These findings highlight the significant contribution of exposure to violence and history of sexual abuse in the development of sexually deviant behavior.

These studies indicate that a large proportion of adolescents who sexually abuse others experience significant care deficits and commonly grow up in families in which they experience and/or witness violence, lack of empathy, as well as a lack of sexual boundaries. Recently, the manner in which these factors influence the development and progression of sexually deviant behavior in adolescents has been explored by researchers. Davis and Leitenberg (1987) theorize that the manner in which familial dysfunction influences the development of sexual offending behavior may be explained in one of the following ways: (1) when physical aggression or marital violence are tolerated, the adolescent learns that this is acceptable behavior; (2) neglect and abuse may predispose the adolescent to seek revenge on substitute targets, (3) parental abuse may lower self-esteem and the sexual offense may be a way of restoring self-worth; and finally (4) parental abuse may sensitize a child to more intimate relationships with peers, and consequently, he may socialize and then sexualize relationships with much younger children. Given this information, the cause of juvenile sex offending is more likely to be associated with a combination of factors, including a history of sexual and or physical abuse, family dysfunction, neglect, exposure to violence, and maltreatment. Additionally, Skuse et al. (2000) argues that a history of childhood sexual abuse is most likely to be a significant factor only when other risk factors indirectly related to the abuse are present. As Rich (2003), suggests "juvenile sexual offending is one possible result of multiple causes that come together in the social environment in which children develop and learn (p. 47)."

Evidence-Based Treatment Interventions in Community Settings

What Works

Due to ethical and methodological limitations, studies documenting evidence-based treatment strategies for adolescent sex offenders are nonexistent in the literature.

What Might Work

Community-based treatment is generally offered to juveniles who are enrolled in outpatient groups and/or day programs at a local mental health clinic for their sex-offense-specific treatment. Careful screening of all potential participants is essential to the success of community-based programming. Generally, thorough assessments take into account issues related to dangerousness as well as severity of psychiatric and psychosexual disturbance. Furthermore, adolescents who are appropriate for community-based outpatient treatment must be deemed to be at a "low risk" for re-offending, as a function of demonstrating increased accountability for their sexual offenses, motivation for change, and an increased level of receptiveness for professional help.

Relative to the structure and duration of treatment, in outpatient care, on a weekly basis, on average juveniles participate in one session of individual therapy, a maximum of two group therapy sessions, and approximately one 60-minute session of family therapy. Additionally, similar to the treatment course described in residential settings, the outpatient treatment trajectory is approximately 18 months (Rich, 2003). While the level of treatment may vary between residential and community programs, interventions for adolescent sex offenders in community-based treatment settings do not differ significantly in treatment modality and content when compared to programs implemented in residential facilities. A community-based treatment setting is distinct in that this level of treatment provides a forum that assists the juvenile in structuring his or her life to better follow relapse prevention plans, develop and maintain a positive range of activities, and to avoid future incidents of acting out or re-offending (Lundrigan, 2001).

Finally, a common belief about juvenile sexual offenders is that even after treatment, most will offend again. However, juveniles who participate in treatment programs have relatively low sexual recidivism rates—between 7% and 13% over follow-up periods of two to five years—when compared to recidivism rates that range between 25% and 50% for nonsexual juvenile offenders (Hunter & Figueredo, 2000). Despite these findings, it has been consistently documented in the literature that a large proportion of adult sex offenders initiate their history of offenses during adolescence (Abel, Mittelman & Becker, 1985; Groth, Longo & McFadin, 1982). Therefore, the concept of relapse prevention is a key issue in working with adolescent sex offenders.

Relapse prevention strategies are utilized in both residential and outpatient treatment programs as well as among probation officers as a methodology for supervision of sexual offenders once they re-enter the community. Relapse prevention is an approach borrowed from treatment programs for addictions (Becker & Kaplan, 1993). Individuals in recovery learn to identify situations that increase their risk of relapse and then rehearse techniques to reduce or avoid such risks. Through this approach, the sexual offender identifies similar situations and their accompanying thoughts and behaviors that make up the sequence of events leading to the offense. Situations such as being alone with a child, feeling lonely or sexually aroused, or masturbating to thoughts of children increase the risk of relapse. The offender then learns and rehearses coping strategies such as avoidance of at risk situations, cognitive techniques such as thinking of the consequences of further offenses, and ongoing behavioral techniques such as avoiding thoughts of children when masturbating. The goal is to teach the adolescent that the risk to commit additional sexual assaults persists for a prolonged period and that he must learn management strategies that can be used long after therapy and probation has ended.

What Does Not Work

To date, specialized treatment strategies for adolescent sex offenders that have been tried and identified as ineffective have yet to be documented in the literature.

Evidence-Based Treatment Interventions in Residential Settings

What Works

Due to ethical and methodological limitations, studies documenting evidence-based treatment strategies for adolescent sex offenders are nonexistent in the literature.

What Might Work

Settings for juvenile sex offender treatment generally consist of inpatient residential treatment or outpatient community-based facilities. When determining whether a juvenile sex offender should receive residential or outpatient services, two factors should be considered. The first issue is that the safety of the community is of primary concern. The second consideration is related to ensuring that youth be placed in the least restrictive environment possible (Ertl & McNamara, 1997). Residential and community-based treatment centers have been designed to balance both the needs of the community and juvenile sex offenders (Shaw, 1999).

According to Bourke and Donohue (1996), residential treatment or inpatient care is recommended for juvenile sex offenders with the following characteristics: (1) the offenses have been numerous and involved more than one individual; (2) violence or aggression was used during the assault (s); (3) severe and emotional behavior problems are present; (4) antisocial attitudes are demonstrated; (5) there is poor motivation for treatment; (6) suicidal or homicidal ideation is present; (7) a volatile relationship at home threatens the safety of the individual; (8) or lastly, the victim is present in the juvenile sex offenders home (p. 57). Residential programs offer intensive approaches to treatment within a controlled setting for an extended period in time. These programs have higher levels of treatment consistency. In addition, some residential treatment programs encompass offense-specific treatment staff that can enhance safety, increase the efficacy of therapy, and reduce sexual acting out (Lundrigan, 2001).

While enrolled in residential care or inpatient care, on a weekly basis, juveniles attend approximately two sessions of individual psychotherapy, a maximum of four group therapy sessions, and extended (60–70 minutes) family sessions. The average length of residential treatment is approximately 18 months (Rich, 2003). There are specific goals associated with the treatment of adolescent sex offenders. These goals include but are not limited to accepting responsibility for behavior, identifying a cycle or pattern of offending, acquisition of skills through learning methods to disrupt the cycle of abuse, developing empathy for the victim, increasing the use of appropriate social skills, addressing one's own history of sexual abuse, decreasing deviant forms of sexual arousal, increasing accurate sexual knowledge, improving family relationships, and relapse prevention (Ertl & McNamara, 1997; Ryan, 1999; Shaw, 1999; Worling & Curwen, 2000).

The most common treatment models associated with facilitating the aforementioned goals are cognitive-behavioral and psychodynamic therapy. A major goal of *cognitive-behavioral therapy* is to identify core beliefs about self and others that lead to automatic thoughts that influence emotional, physiological, and behavioral responses. Once irrational beliefs are identified and disputed by the client an effective new philosophy can then be created that in turn influences behavior change (Beck, 1979, 1995). Conversely, the goal of *psychodynamic therapy* is to facilitate an understanding of unconscious motivations and past experiences that shape and drive emotion, cognition, and relationships, and behaviors (Rich, 2003). Unfortunately, it has been noted that while these treatments are theoretically sound they have not been empirically related to sexual recidivism (Weinrott, 1998). Moreover, Duncan (2001) conducted a review of the literature and suggests that, "no solid evidence exists to demonstrate that any specific treatment models have unique effects, or that any therapeutic approach is superior to another" (p. 31).

Despite the extent to which each of these modalities of treatment have failed to be empirically validated, cognitive behavioral therapy maintains its position as the leading form of treatment when working with this particular population. The attention that cognitive behavioral treatment receives in the field as the primary choice of intervention in working with juvenile offenders stems from the extent to which it lends itself to an evidence-based model and manualized treatment. Relative to sexual offender treatment, cognitive behavioral therapy offers a framework for the development of common goals, language, and concepts regarding what the juvenile is expected to learn in order to facilitate rehabilitation or to maintain the safety of the community. In addition, it enables both the client and the practitioner to make treatment ideas and goals concrete, easily defined, and measurable over time. This allows for treatment goals to be operationalized, incorporated into a model, and empirically proven. Each of these factors has great implications for manualized treatment and evidence-based practices. Alternatively, psychodynamic treatment is abstract in that it focuses on minor shifts in the conscious and unconscious over time, is devoid of manualized guidelines, requires more supervision and training of clinicians, and does not consistently garner observable results.

Nonetheless, while cognitive behavioral therapy has unique features associated with evidenced-based model development and manualized treatment, evidence-based interventions in the treatment of juvenile sex offenders have yet to be established in the literature. Chambless et al. (1998) (as cited in Rich, 2003) offers insight into the methodological limitations of conducting such research in noting that evidence-based designs must be replicable and require random selection and random assignment to cohorts. It is difficult to establish each of these conditions with forensic populations.

Moreover, Chambless et al. (1998) cites specific concerns related to the ethical implications of conducting research that would require the provision of pseudo-treatment to a cohort of juvenile sex offenders and then releasing them into the community to observe the outcomes of a comparison group. Overall, a significant amount of literature has been devoted to treatment approaches and modalities related to juvenile sex offending, with little focus on evaluating the efficacy of these forms of intervention. The paucity in the literature pertaining to evidence-based practices in treating juvenile sex offenders can best be explained by ethical and methodological limitations of conducting randomized control research within this population.

What Does Not Work

To date, specialized treatment strategies for adolescent sex offenders that have been tried and identified as ineffective have yet to be documented in the literature.

Psychopharmacology

The use of hormonal agents or antiandrogens as the primary approach to psychopharmacological treatment for paraphilic disorders in adult populations has been well documented in the literature (Bradford, 1995). Antiandrogen medications serve to block the action of testosterone in male offenders. Clinically, these medications eliminate or reduce the sex drive and assist the sexual offender in controlling sexual fantasies, thoughts, arousal, and behavior. Unfortunately, antiandrogens do not discriminate deviant from normal arousal, thereby leading to the suppression of all sexual functioning. As a result, antiandrogen treatment is commonly referred to as chemical castration and is inclusive of the following hormonal medications: medroxyprogesterone (Provera and Depo-Povera), cyproterone (Androcur), and leuprolide acetate (Lupron).

Alternatively, among adolescents the overall effectiveness of hormonal treatment as an approach to treating paraphillias is neither clear nor universally accepted. Although psychopharmacological interventions, including sex-drive-hormone-reducing medications such as medroxyprogesterone, have been found to be effective in reducing sex offending in adult offenders, they can have serious side effects. Such medications, when used with juveniles, may significantly affect the body and negatively impact normal growth and development. It is further suggested that the long-term use of antiandrogens in adolescents has been noted to be questionable psychologically and medically (O'Shaughnessey, 2002). Thus, ethical concerns related to the use of these medications with juveniles are substantial (Hunter and Lexier, 1998). The clinical indication for the use of antiandrogens in the 16–17-year age group is the presence of very serious sexual deviation.

Given the documented concerns regarding the use of antiandrogens or hormonal medications when treating adolescent paraphilias, many researchers and professionals have begun to explore the use of psychotropic medications within this population. For example, Hunter and Lexier (1998) noted reports from the professional literature that describe the utility of selective serotonin reuptake inhibitors (SSRIs). It is suggested that SSRIs often have sexual dysfunction side effects such as suppressed sexual desire and delayed ejaculation. However, these researchers further noted that the role of serotonin in regulating sexual behavior is not fully understood. Many questions concerning psychopharmacological approaches remain. These questions include which juveniles are likely to benefit from such an approach and at what dosages. Nevertheless, these psychotropic medications provide potential promise given that they are better tolerated than antiandrogens and they do not disrupt normal development. There has been no research to date that documents the relative efficacy of this form of medication in adolescents. Therefore, the treatment literature will benefit from research in this area.

The Prevention of Adolescent Sex Offenses

What Works

More theoretical and empirical research is needed before evidenced-based primary prevention strategies can be developed and implemented.

What Might Work

According to the literature, little attention has been devoted to the development, implementation, and evaluation of programs that promote primary prevention of antisocial sexual behaviors among adolescents. However, as previously stated, a series of risk factors, including poor familial relationships, sexual victimization, a history of physical abuse or maltreatment, exposure to violence, and a lack of social competence, may interact to mediate the development of sexually aggressive behaviors. Therefore, programs targeted at preventing the development of antisocial sexual behaviors in youth would benefit from core components that seek to facilitate healthy family functioning, promote coping skills that increase one's ability to overcome adversity prosocially, increase social ties and school bonding, and offer the provision of support and guidance. Programming should also assist in the development of social skills, facilitate personal identity development, teach problem-solving skills, and encourage children to avoid sexual risk through education. Each of these components protects against developmental risk factors and is key in building developmental strengths and prosocial teen sexual values. They also have the potential to neutralize troubled behaviors, and buffer against behaviors that may be harmful to self or others (Rich, 2003).

Additionally, the role that the media plays in portraying sexual values, behavior, and aggressiveness cannot be overlooked. In noting that sexual aggression occurs within developmental and sociocultural learning environments, it is important to account for the extent to which many children are introduced to sex through inappropriate exposure via the media and internet. Brown and Keller (2000) report that many adolescents rank the media as their major source for sexual ideas and information. They also purport that there is a strong association between exposure to sexual content in the media and sexual beliefs and behaviors. Acquisition of inappropriate sexual behaviors associated with exposure to the media may be facilitated through learning and behavioral rehearsal. The difficulties that teens face in interpreting and acting on the messages that they receive from the media has been addressed by Brown and Keller (2000). These researchers state that "a clash between the media's depiction of sexual relationships and the real life experiences of youth contributes to their difficulty in making healthy sexual decisions." Thus, the incorporation of programming associated with healthy sexual education is essential. Healthy sexual education allows youth to have access to countervailing information or ideas that will assist them in making sense of the information that they receive through media outlets. Furthermore, healthy sexual education can also assist adolescents in developing healthy sexual decision-making and problem-solving skills. Mastery of both of these components are key in facilitating successful transitions throughout the stages of adolescent development.

What Does Not Work

Evaluation research indicating that there are ineffective primary prevention programs in the literature have not yet been documented.

Recommendations

Despite the fact that research conducted to date has large gaps, there are findings which are noteworthy: (a) Adolescents commit a significant proportion of sexual offenses in the Unites States, the most conservative estimates suggest about 20% of all cases. (b) The majority of perpetrators are male and their victims are primarily female. (c) A significant proportion of adolescent sex offenders have a history of being physically or sexually abused. (d) Social skill deficits as reflected in poor relationships and social isolation have been demonstrated in several samples. (e) Adolescent sex offenders, like juvenile delinquents, exhibit high rates of family instability and psychopathology with frequent separations from family of origin. (g) Recidivism rates for juvenile sex offenders are relatively low, ranging between 7% and 13%.

Several individual, familial, behavioral, and environmental factors have been explored in association with the development of adolescent sexual offending behavior. There is strong evidence that supports the contribution of childhood histories of maltreatment, family, and social relationship variables. Studies have also evaluated childhood sexual histories and intellectual functioning with inconclusive results. However, it has been determined that there is not a single factor common to all sexual offenders or one theory that explains the etiology of sexually aggressive behavior. Juvenile sex offenders are a heterogeneous group with a variety of antecedents and consequences influencing their behavior (Rich, 2003). Juvenile sexual offending behavior is more than likely caused by multiple causation and interactive factors (O'Shaughnessey, 2002). Therefore, research will benefit from the development of a comprehensive model of sexually deviant behavior which takes into account and explains the interaction of individual, social, and environmental factors. An effective model will demonstrate the ability to predict future occurrences of sexual offending as well as foster the development of effective intervention and prevention strategies.

The most important conclusion to be highlighted from this review is that research on adolescent sexual offenders is still in the early stages of development. The majority of the research to date has been exploratory, descriptive, and theoretical. Moreover, evidenced-based treatment strategies for adolescent sex offenders have not yet been documented in the literature. The lack of controlled treatment outcome studies is due in part to the ethical and methodological limitations of randomly assigning offenders who may be of danger to the general population to a wait list control or no treatment control group. Nevertheless, it remains essential for treatment components to be isolated and tested to determine which factors contribute to positive treatment outcomes and which factors do not. To the extent possible, these studies need to be conducted among homogenous subgroups of sex offenders with specification of treatment conditions. Currently the most appropriate forms of treatment seemingly available to this population include individual and group-based intervention strategies that are cognitive behavioral in nature. These therapies should address critical factors associated with offending behavior, which include accepting responsibility for behavior, identifying a cycle of offending, learning specific behavioral techniques to disrupt the cycle of abuse, increasing the use of appropriate social skills, addressing one's own history of sexual abuse, and relapse prevention. Given the extent to which familial instability has been implicated in the development sexually offending behavior among adolescents, significant attention should be devoted to conducting thorough family assessments and family therapy with this population.

Antiandrogens have commonly been used in treating sexual offending adults for a significant period of time. However, these particular treatments have been noted to have a negative impact on the physical growth and development of adolescents. More recently, serotonin reuptake inhibitors (SSRIs) have been identified as a more promising strategy in treating adolescent sex offenders yet additional research is needed to document dosage and the type of juvenile sex offender who will receive the greatest benefit from this level of treatment.

Finally, relapse prevention, a strategy through which adolescents are trained to recognize and cope with situations that may serve to threaten their control over inappropriate sexual arousal, has been identified as an integral component to the successful treatment of adolescent sex offenders. This is an effective method of secondary prevention. Yet, given the significant incidence of children who are sexually victimized by adolescents, it is important to define this issue as a public health concern and devote additional attention to the development of primary prevention programs. Appropriate programming promoting the importance of healthy sexuality in schools as well as in the home may play a critical role in deterring sexually deviant behavior among juveniles. This programming may benefit from incorporating key components that serve to counteract against potential harmful effects of developmental risk factors associated with sexual offending behaviors. These components include healthy sexual education; the facilitation of healthy family functioning and adaptive coping skills; the enhancement of social ties, social skills, and school bonding; personal identity development; and problem-solving skills. Only when a concerted effort has been made in each of these areas we will be able to make progress in prevention, early detection, and treatment of adolescent sex offenders.

References

Abel, G.G., Mittelman, M.S., & Becker, J.V. (1985). Sex offenders: Results of assessment and recommendations for treatment in clinical criminology. In M.H. Ben-Aron, S.J. Hucker, and C.D. Webster (Eds.), *The Assessment and Treatment of Criminal Behavior*. Toronto, Canada: M and M Graphic.

Awad, G.A., Saunders, E., & Levene, J. (1984). A clinical study of male adolescent sexual offenders. *International Journal of Offender Therapy and Comparative Criminology*, 20, 105–116.

Beck, A.T. (1995). Cognitive Therapy. In H.I. Kaplan & B.J. Sadock (Eds.). *Comprehensive Textbook of Psychiatry: Vol. 6* (pp. 2167–2177). Baltimore, MD: Wiliams & Wilkins.

Beck, A.T. (1979). Cognitive therapy and the emotional disorder. New York : Meridian Book.

Becker, J.V. (1988). What we know about the characteristics and treatment of adolescents who have committed sexual offenses. *Child Maltreatment 3,* 317–329.

Becker, J.V. (1990). Treating adolescent sexual offenders. *Professional Psychology: Research and Practice, 5,* 362–365.

Becker, J.V., & Hunter, J.A. (1997). Understanding and treating child and adolescent sexual offenders. In T.H. Ollendick and R.J. Prinz (Eds.), *Advances in Clinical Child Psychology.* New York, NY: Plenum Press.

Becker, J.V., & Kaplan, M.S. (1993). Cognitive behavioral treatment of the juvenile sex offender. In H.E. Barbaree, W.L. Marshall & S.M. Hudson (Eds.),*The Juvenile Sex Offender.* New York, NY: Guilford Press.

Becker, J.V., Kaplan, M.S., Cunningham-Rathner, J., & Kavoussi, R. (1986). Characteristics of adolescent incest sexual perpetrators: Preliminary findings. *Journal of Family Violence, 1*(1), 85–97.

Beckett, R. (1999). Evaluation of adolescent sexual abusers. In M. Erooga & H. Mason (Eds.), *Children and Young People Who Sexually Abuse Others: Challenges and Responses* (pp. 204–224). London: Routledge.

Betovim, A. (2002). Research on the development of sexually abusive behavior in sexually abusive males: The implications for clinical practice. In M.C. Calder (Ed.), *Young People Who Sexually Abuse: Building the Evidence Base for Your practice* (pp. 204–224). London: Routledge.

Bourke, M.L., & Donohue, B. (1996). Assessment and treatment of juvenile sex offenders: An empirical review. *Journal of Child Sexual Abuse, 5*(1), 47–70.

Bradford, J.M.W. (1995). *Pharmacological Treatment of the Paraphilias: In Review of Psychiatry.* Washington (DC): American Psychiatric Press.

Brown, J., & Keller, S. (2000). Can the mass media be healthy sex educators? *Family Planning Perspectives, 32,* 255–257.

Cellini, H.R. (1995). Assessment and treatment of the adolescent sexual offender. In B.K. Schwartz and H.R. Cellini (Eds.), *The Sex Offender: Corrections, Treatment and Legal Practice* (Vol. 1). Kingston, NJ: Civic Research Institute.

Center for Sex Offender Management. (1999). *Understanding Juvenile Sexual Offending Behavior.* Silver Spring, MD: Center for Sex offender Management.

Chambless, D.L., Baker, M.J., Baucom, D.H., Beutler, L.E., Calhoun, K.S., Crist–Cristoph, P., Daiuto, A., DeRubeis, R., Detweiler, J., Haaga, D.A., Johnson, S.B., McCurry, S., Mueser, K.T., & Pope, K.S. (1998). Update on empirically validated therapies, II. *The Clinical Psychologist, 51,* 3–16.

Davis, G.E., & Leitenberg, H. (1987). Adolescent sex offenders. *Psychological Bulletin 101, 3,* 417–427.

Duncan, B. (2001). The future of psychotherapy. *Psychotherapy Networker, 25*(4), 24–33.

Ertl, M.A., & McNamara, J.R. (1997). Treatment of juvenile sex offenders: A review of the literature. *Child and Adolescent Social Work Journal, 14*(3), 199–221.

Federal Bureau of Investigation. (2002). *Uniform Crime Reports for the United States.* Washington, DC: U.S. Department of Justice.

Ferrera, M.L., & McDonald, S. (1996). *Treatment of the Juvenile Sex Offender: Neurological and Psychiatric Impairments.* Northvale, NJ: Jason Aronson.

Gilby, R., Wolf, L., & Goldberg, B. (1989). Mentally retarded adolescent sex offenders: A survey and pilot study. *Canadian Journal of Psychiatry, 34*(6): 542–548.

Graves, R.B, Openshaw, D.K., Ascione, F.R., & Ericksen, S.L. (1996). Demographic and parental characteristics of youthful sexual offenders. *International Journal of Offender Therapy and Comparative Criminology, 40,* 300–317.

Groth, N.A., Longo, R.E., & McFadin, J.B. (1982). Undetected recidivism among rapists and child molesters. *Crime and Delinquency, 28*(3), 450–458.

Hunter, J.A., Jr., & Figueredo, A.J. (1999). Factors associated with treatment compliance in a population of juvenile sexual offenders. *Sexual Abuse: A Journal of Research and Treatment, 11*(1), 49–67.

Hunter, J.A., & Figueredo, A.J. (2000). The influence of personality and history of sexual victimization in the prediction of juvenile perpetrated child molestation. *Behavior Modification, 24*(2), 241–263.

Hunter, J.A., Jr., & Lexier, L.J. (1998). Ethical and legal issues in the assessment and treatment of juvenile sex offenders. *Child Maltreatment, 3*(4), 339–348.

Kahn, T.J., & Chambers, H.J. (1991). Assessing reoffense risk with juvenile sexual offenders. *Child Welfare LXX, 3,* 333–345.

Kaplan, M.S., Becker, J.V., & Martinez, E.H. (1992). Adolescent perpetrators of incest. In R.T. Ammerman & M. Hersen (Eds.), *Assessment of Family Violence*. New York: Wiley.

Katz, R.C. (1990). Psychosocial adjustment in adolescent child molesters. *Child Abuse and Neglect, 14*(4), 567–575.

Kavoussi, R.J., Kaplan, M. & Becker, J.V. (1988). Psychiatric diagnoses in adolescent sex offenders. *Journal of the American Academy of Child and Adolescent Psychiatry, 27*(2), 241–243.

Knight, R.A., & Prentsky, R.A. (1993). Exploring characteristics for classifying juvenile sex offenders. In E. Barbaree, W.L. Marshall, and S.M. Hudson (Eds.), *The Juvenile Sex Offender*. New York: Guilford Press.

Lee, J.K.P., Jackson, H.J., Pattison, P., & Ward, T. (2002.). Developmental risk factors for sexual offending. *Child Abuse and Neglect, 26*, 73–92.

Longo, R.E. (2002). A holistic approach to treating young people who sexually abuse. In M.C. Calder (Ed.), *Young People Who Sexually Abuse: Building the Evidence Base for Your Practice* (pp. 218–230). Dorset, England: Russell House.

Longo, R.E., & Groth, A.N. (1983). Juvenile sexual offenses in the histories of adult rapists and child molesters. *International Journal of Offender Therapy & Comparative Criminology, 27*(2), 150–155.

Lundrigan, P.S. (2001). The outpatient program. In P.S. Lundrigan (Ed.), *Treating Youth Who Sexually Abuse* (pp. 65–79). New York: Hawthorne.

Marshall, W.L, & Eccles, A. (1993). Pavlonian conditioning processes in adolescent sex offenders. In H.E. Barabee, W.L. Marshall, & S.M. Hudson (Eds.), *The Juvenile Sex Offender* (pp. 118–142). New York: Gilford Press.

Miner, M.H., & Crimmins, C.L.S. (1995). Adolescent sex offenders: Issues of etiology and risk factors. In B.K. Schwartz and H.R. Cellini (Eds.), *The Sex Offender: Vol. 1. Corrections, Treatment and Legal Practice*. Kingston, NJ: Civic Research Institute.

Miner, M.H., Siekert, G.P., & Ackland, M.A. (1997). *Evaluation: Juvenile Sex Offender Treatment Program, Minnesota Correctional Facility—Sauk Centre*. Final report—Biennium 1995–1997. Minneapolis, MN: University of Minnesota, Department of Family Practice and Community Health, Program in Human Sexuality.

O'Shaughnessey, R.J. (2002). Violent adolescent sexual offenders. *Child and Adolescent Psychiatric Clinics, 11*(4), 749–765.

Prentsky, R., & Burgess, A.W. (1990). Rehabilitation of child molesters: A cost-benefit analysis. *American Journal of Orthopsychiatry, 60*(1), 108–117. *Behavior, 21*(6), 635–660.

Rich, P. (2003). *Juvenile Sexual Offenders: Understanding, Assessing and Rehabilitating*. Hoboken, NJ: John Wiley and Sons.

Ryan, G. (1999). Treatment of sexually abusive youth. *Journal of Interpersonal Violence, 14*(4), 442–436.

Ryan, G.D., & Lane, S.L. (1997). *Juvenile Sexual Offending: Causes, Consequences and Correction*. Lexington, MA: Lexington Books.

Ryan, G., Miyoshi, T.J., Metzner, J.L., Krugman, R.D., & Fryer, G.E. (1996). Trends in a national sample of sexually abusive youths. *Journal of the American Academy of Child and Adolescent Psychiatry, 35*(1), 17–25.

Skuse, D., Betovim, A., Hodges, J., Stevenson. J. Andreou, C., Lanyado, M. New, M. Williams., B., & McMillian, D. (2000) Risk factors for the development of sexually abusive behavior in sexually victimized adolescent boys. In C. Itzen (Ed.), *Home Truths About Child Sexual Abuse: Influencing Policy and Practice* (pp. 222–231). London: Routledge.

Shaw, J.A. (1999). Practice parameters for the assessment and treatment of children and adolescents who are sexually abusive of others. *Journal of American Academy of Child and Adolescent Psychiatry, 38*(12), (Suppl.), 55S–76S.

Smith, H., and Israel, E. (1987). Sibling incest: A study of dynamics of 25 cases. *Child Abuse and Neglect, 11*(1):101–108.

Van Ness, S.R. (1984). Rape as instrumental violence: A study of youth offenders. *Journal of Offender Counseling, Services and Rehabilitation, 9*, 161–170.

Weinrott, M. (1998, August). *Empirically-based treatment interventions for juvenile sex offenders*, Paper presented at the Child Abuse Action Network and the State Forensic Service, Augusta, Maine.

Weinrott, M.R. (1996) *Juvenile Sexual Aggression: A Critical Review*. Boulder, CO: Center for the Study and Prevention of Violence, University of Colorado.

Worling, J.R., & Curwen, T. (2000). Adolescent sexual offender recidivism: success of specialized treatment and implications for risk prediction. *Child Abuse and Neglect, 24*(7), 965–982.

Chapter 23

Sibling Incest Offenders

Laura F. Salazar, Christina M. Camp, Ralph J. DiClemente, and Gina M. Wingood

Introduction

Nearly every known society has some form of "incest taboo" or rules of behavior that prohibit sexual relationships and marriage between certain specified relatives (Henslin, 2001). In the United States, for example, it is illegal for certain specified relatives to interact sexually. The list of specified relatives includes parents and children; brothers and sisters; and in some states, first cousins. It has been only in the last 30 years that the issue of incest started receiving attention in the United States (Gupta & Cox, 1988). Even so, the origins and scope of incest are still not well understood.

Some researchers assert that the origin of the incest taboo is "instinctual": where humans inherently feel and demonstrate an aversion for engaging in sex with a parent or sibling. Freud (1955b) postulated that the incest taboo has its roots in early human patriarchal society where men held absolute power and control over their family members, which extended to include a sexual right to their daughters. Sons revolted against their fathers and set up an incest taboo as a form of protection from future revolts against themselves. Some sociologists, however, generally concur that the incest taboo has a social basis. If societies allowed incest, then disruptions in the socialization of a group's children would occur (Malinowski, 1927), and the proscribed role of family members would be conflicted. Parents who violate the taboo and have sex with their children may be unable to determine the best interests of their children, be appropriate role models to them, or pass down family values. Moreover, the incest taboo may serve a specific social function in that children are steered to marry outside the nuclear family, resulting in the forming of new families and enhanced social networks (Henslin, 2001). Thus, having an incest taboo serves the best interests of the family, of the children, and of society.

The *Westermarck theory* is another theoretical perspective regarding the incest taboo. This theory is based on an evolutionary paradigm and has been applied specifically to sibling incest—one form of incest (Westermarck, 1889). According to this theory, incest avoidance rather than being socially constructed evolved in humans because of the ostensibly harmful effects of close inbreeding. Through the process of natural selection, humans developed an aversion to incest. Early association between siblings is critical to the establishment of incest avoidance; it is thought that children raised in close proximity are less likely to develop later sexual interest (Bevc & Silverman, 1993). The theory further posits that incest avoidance between siblings can be disrupted if siblings are separated at birth or separated for a significant period of time. Some evidence to support the Westermarck theory has been provided by research that shows children who were not siblings but were raised together (e.g., in communes) were less likely to select each other as marital partners (Shepher, 1983), or if they did marry, then their marriages were characterized as sexually dysfunctional with high rates of divorce (Wolf, 1995). Research among 500 college students that examined the Westermarck hypothesis among sibling relationships found that separation of siblings of a year of more in early childhood was positively related to completed or attempted genital, oral, or anal intercourse postchildhood (Bevc & Silverman, 1993). However, separation was not related to whether siblings engaged in other less extreme forms of sexual activity (i.e., touching, fondling, exhibitionism). Thus, based on these findings, close proximity may not inhibit sexual interest per se, but may serve to inhibit sexual reproduction, which is considered an adaptive function from an evolutionary perspective.

In the United States and in other societies, violating the incest taboo is considered a form of family sexual abuse. But, what constitutes a violation? As far as behaviors are concerned, a violation would occur by engaging in a sexual relationship (i.e., having anal, oral, or vaginal intercourse) or partaking in sexual activities such as exposure, fondling of breasts and genitals, and oral-genital contact. In addition to the specified "blood relation," violating the incest taboo can also occur when sexual activity happens between family members who are not blood relatives (e.g., stepfather and stepdaughter; stepbrother and stepsister, an uncle through marriage and his niece) and between quasi-family members (e.g., foster parent and foster child, godparent and godchild).

Although these violations are unequivocal when the abuse involves an adult and a child, there are fewer consensuses however when the violation of the taboo involves siblings. For example, is "sex play" considered sibling incest? When the sex play entails the showing or touching of each other's genitals (e.g., "I'll show you mine if you show me yours") and is harmless, then it is generally not considered sibling incest. Harmless sex play is characterized as of short duration and excludes sex engaged in by force, sex among older children or among children of significant age differentials (Finkelhor, 1980). Thus, some aspects of the definition of what constitutes a violation of the incest taboo mentioned previously may not be applicable to sibling incest.

To distinguish between age-appropriate curiosity or sex-play and sibling incest, some researchers and practitioners have redefined sibling incest more specifically as "sexual interaction beyond age-appropriate exploration such that older siblings, who differ significantly in age or by virtue of their power and resources, may also be considered abusive" (Tower, 1996, p. 134). Yet, what age is considered "beyond age-appropriate exploration," and what is the number of years that should be considered as a significant difference in age? Some researchers and professionals have attempted to use Freud's (1955a) stages of psychosexual development as a guide (Finkelhor,

1980) by characterizing any sexual activity over the age of eight as inappropriate while also operationalizing the age differential as five or more years (see de Jong, 1989). Furthermore, other professionals have taken a more simplistic albeit extreme view and feel that sibling incest should be defined only in terms of its effects on the victim. If the victim views the experience as traumatic or harmful, then the event should be considered sibling incest. Conversely, if the experience is viewed as positive, then it should not be taken seriously. This latter perspective, however, has been criticized by many clinicians for several reasons: (1) adults may not be able to rate accurately experiences that happened to them as children; (2) it does not account for perpetrator-victim status; (3) it fails to consider power differentials, age differentials, and consensual vs. coercive; and (4) it does not determine the level of denial associated with the experience. For example, Finkelhor (1980) conducted a study of 796 undergraduates and found that 15% of the women and 10% of the men reported retrospectively a sexual experience with a sibling. Overall, 30% of the respondents rated their experiences of sibling incest as "positive," 30% as "negative," and the remaining were indifferent. However, closer examination of the data revealed that women more often than men were coerced, were the junior "partner," and rated the experience as unpleasant or negative, bringing into question how the topic should be defined and assessed. Recently the definition has been expanded to also incorporate non-contact behaviors that are meant to sexually stimulate either the sibling victim or the offender. These non-contact behaviors would include the taking of pornographic pictures, forcing the sibling to view pornography, unwanted sexual references in conversation, and forcing the sibling to masturbate or to watch the offender masturbate (Haskins, 2003).

Unfortunately, many times in our society, the incest taboo is broken. Some research has shown that there may be as many as 15 million victims of incest in the United States (Stark, 1984). The associated negative psychological sequelae can be deemed traumatic (Canavan, Meyer & Higgs, 1992; Cole, 1982) and may create an immense burden for a victim that continues through adulthood (Rudd & Herzberger, 1999). For example, research has provided evidence to suggest that victims of incest may suffer from lowered self-esteem (Finkelhor, 1980; Laviola, 1992), higher rates of sexual activity (i.e., "promiscuity) (Finkelhor, 1980; Rudd & Herzberger, 1999), sexual dysfunction (Laviola, 1992), adult victimization (Russell, 1986), intrusive thoughts of the incest (Laviola, 1992), flashbacks and nightmares (Rudd & Herzberger, 1999; Tsun, 1999), as well as suicidality, depressive symptomatology, eating disorders, and substance abuse (Rudd & Herzberger, 1999).

Although boys and girls may both be victims, evidence suggests that girls are far more likely to be victimized than boys (Finkelhor & Araji, 1986; Risin & Koss, 1987). For example, in a large school-based study of 89,000 adolescents in a Midwestern state in the U.S., a 10% random subsample was generated to investigate the relation between childhood sexual abuse and adult sexual victimization. The results indicated that for extrafamilial abuse (i.e., perpetrated by individual outside the family), intrafamilial abuse (i.e., incest—perpetrated by family member), or both forms of child sexual abuse, a greater proportion of girls were victims than boys. For intrafamilial sexual abuse only, girls were 5 times as likely as boys (3.5% vs. .7%) to report victimization (Lodico, Gruber, & DiClemente, 1996). Similar findings were found in a study involving a clinical sample of 73 adult survivors of sibling incest and sibling assault. Caffaro and Conn-Caffaro (1998) found that of the 39% (n = 29) that had experienced sibling incest, the largest majority (63%) of the victims (n = 18) were women who had been molested by an older brother (male-on-female incest). The next largest category comprised 20% of the sample (n = 6) and was men who had been molested by an older brother (male-on-male incest). Only 10% of the sample (n = 3) were men who had been molested by an older sister (female-on-male incest). Two women (7%) reported that they had been molested by an older sister (female-on-female incest).

Much of the research on incest has focused on the etiology and epidemiology of father–daughter or older male relative –younger female relative incest (Cole, 1982; Laviola, 1992; Worling, 1995), with comparatively less research on sibling incest (Ascherman & Safier, 1990; Caffaro & Conn-Caffaro, 1998). Results of sibling incest research are somewhat mixed. For example, some research has estimated a high prevalence rates of sibling incest among abuse victims and suggests that sibling incest may be more common than other forms of child sexual abuse (Cawson, Wattam, Brooker & Kelly, 2000; Finkelhor, 1979; Smith & Israel, 1987), whereas other research among clinical samples of rape victims found sibling incest less prevalent (13%) than incest perpetrated by a father or stepfather (33% and 38%, respectively) (Darves-Bornoz, Berger, Degiovanni, Gaillard & Lepine, 1999). However, professionals working in this field believe that because a parent or victim must file assault charges against the perpetrating sibling, many incidents go unreported (Finkelhor & Araji, 1986). Embarrassment, shame, denial, and unwillingness to report a son or daughter coupled with entrenched attitudes unsupportive of disclosure such as "we don't air our dirty laundry," "we can't break up the family," and "what happens in our home is a private, family matter" may be the underlying reasons that sibling incest is less reported than extrafamilial or other forms of intrafamilial abuse (Caffaro & Conn-Caffaro, 1998; Cyr, Wright, McDuff & Perron, 2002; Haskins, 2003). Therefore, among clinical samples of victims, the lower percentage attributed to sibling incest in some instances may be due to underreporting. Nevertheless, this view of sibling incest being a pervasive form of abuse is supported by other studies with male adolescent sex offenders that have shown comparatively higher proportions (30–39%) being classified as sibling incest offenders as compared to other types of sex offenses (O'Brien, 1991; Ryan, Miyoshi, Metzner, Krugman & Fryer, 1996).

Apart from the studies described, there is still a relative dearth of epidemiological research that has examined sibling incest specifically among large, representative samples. Two surveys, one of college students cited previously (Finkelhor, 1980) and one of a community sample (Russell, 1986), estimated prevalence rates for sibling abuse among female respondents of 15% and 2%. Both authors indicated, however, that the obtained prevalence rates were most likely underestimated and should be viewed with caution. In particular, the Russell (1986) study did not eliminate respondents who were an "only-child" in their families. Thus, the overall 2% prevalence rate was certainly underestimated, as many of the respondents could not possibly be a victim of sibling incest.

Clearly, so few studies have been conducted to document adequately the scope of sibling incest that we cannot be sure how widespread it is. More research using diverse and representative samples is warranted so that we can determine the extent to which the sibling incest taboo is being violated, understand better who is violating whom, and assess the deleterious effects so that preventive interventions and treatment programs can be devised and implemented.

Individual Factors

A number of significant etiological theories for adolescent sex offenders have been described previously (see Chapter 22; Gilmartin, 1994; Luzes, 1990). These theories have included social learning theory, feminist theory, and psychodynamic theory, to name a few, and vary with respect to their level of analysis from psychological, to sociopsychological, to cultural. Unfortunately, no one singular model has emerged that has been validated empirically and explains the development of sibling incest in adolescents. Rather from these theories many factors have been examined in isolation such as psychopathy, poor social skills, inconsistent friendship patterns, poor social adjustment, prior sexual victimization, traditional sex roles, family dysfunction, and family abuse in an attempt to explain and understand sibling incest.

One psychological theoretical perspective in particular, which has been discussed and examined in the adolescent sex offender literature and in the incest literature, is *blockage theory*. Blockage theorists posit that people who because of poor social skills, inconsistent friendships, or poor social adjustment are "blocked" from having their emotional and physical needs met via normal social interactions (Finkelhor, 1984). To fulfill their needs, they instead force, persuade, or coerce inappropriate and traumatic interactions with younger siblings (in the case of sibling incest), or with either a son or daughter (in the case of parent–child incest); thus, sexually, emotionally, or physically victimizing their sibling or child. In the case of sibling incest offenders, a younger sibling in the household provides easy access to a person who can provide the emotional and sexual satisfaction the offender desires and needs. This perspective implies that adolescent sibling incest offenders who molest siblings may not have the necessary skills to cultivate meaningful peer relationships; therefore, it is easier to fulfill their needs with a sibling. They may have the desire to pursue outside peer relationships, but they may lack the skills to do so.

Empirical support for the blockage perspective is provided by studies with sibling incest offenders. As most cases of sibling incest involve older brothers molesting their younger sisters (Caffaro & Conn-Caffaro, 1998), most of these studies involve male perpetrators. O'Brien (1991) compared adolescent incest offenders with adolescent child molesters (extrafamilial) and with nonchild offenders on their social skills. Based on clinical interviews, he was able to characterize their degree of social functioning. He found that the group of adolescent incest offenders had a significantly higher proportion of adolescents who were evaluated as undersocialized (64%) compared to the group of nonchild offenders (37%); however, there was no difference between the percentage of undersocialized adolescents in the group of child molesters (57%) and the group of sibling incest offenders. Undersocialized was operationally defined as having few friends and poor social skills. These results support the view that adolescent sex offenders (both incest offenders and extrafamilial offenders) may be unable to achieve a normal degree of peer involvement and friendships due to their poor social skills. Consequently, many may turn to their siblings or younger children outside the family to fulfill their needs.

Other studies that have examined the psychological functioning of sex offenders may provide indirect evidence for blockage theory. For example, Adler & Schutz (1995) reported on 12 male sibling incest offenders referred to a hospital-based, outpatient psychiatric clinic for treatment. More than half (58%) had a history of conduct disordered behavior aside from the incest that included behavioral problems in school and learning disorders. Psychiatric diagnoses were quite prevalent among the sample of adolescents where 42% met criteria for conduct disorder; 17% were diagnosed with attention-deficit/hyperactivity disorder (ADHD), and 42% met criteria for depressive disorder. Similarly, Becker, Kaplan, Cunningham-Rathner, and Kavoussi (1986) interviewed 22 male adolescent incest sexual perpetrators from an outpatient clinic. A majority of these offenders (74%) had one or more psychiatric diagnoses, which included conduct disorder, attention-deficit disorder (ADD), drug abuse, adjustment disorder, social phobias, dysthymia, and post-traumatic stress disorder (PTSD). Together these results suggest that the adolescent offenders in these studies may have experienced a low degree of social functioning. In other words, although it was not evaluated directly in these studies, it may be plausible that because of their psychological deficits, the adolescent sex offenders were also socially deficient.

Family, Social, and Community Factors

An intuitive and popular theory of child abuse is the *intergenerational transmission of abuse,* one of the earliest theories of abuse, which has become the most widely accepted theory of abuse. This perspective suggests that there is a cycle of abuse that is transmitted across generations: Children who grow up in families where abuse is perpetrated on them by a parent will in turn become abusers who abuse their own children. This theory has been applied extensively to understand the causative factors for the physical abuse of children where many studies have provided support for the notion that "violence begets violence" (see Egeland, 1993; Kaufman & Zigler, 1993). Although these studies have documented transmission estimates ranging from 18% to 70%, some of the studies that obtained rates at the higher end of the spectrum were considered methodologically flawed. For example, most studies that documented high transmission rates were retrospective, and examined groups of abusers without using comparison groups. Without a comparison group, it is impossible to ascertain the percentage of abused children who grow up and do not become abusers. The results are therefore inconclusive. A more accurate estimate using methodologically strong designs has been derived and puts the rate more at 30% (Kaufman & Zigler, 1993).

Regarding the issue of sibling incest, the research is also mixed and inconclusive. O'Brien (1991) found in his study that adolescent sibling incest offenders were more likely to have been sexually victimized by a family member than extrafamilial child sex offenders and nonchild sex offenders: Of the adolescent offenders who were sexually molested as children, two thirds of the sibling incest offenders compared to one-half of the child molesters and less than twenty percent of the nonchild offenders had been abused by a family member. Nevertheless, overall, the majority of the sibling incest offenders had not been sexually abused by a family member. For the intergenerational transmission of abuse theory to be confirmed as a causative theory, most adolescents who are sibling incest offenders would have been victims of intrafamilial abuse. Only a minority of adolescent incest offenders in the O'Brien (1991) study was sexually abused by family members; thus, this finding constitutes evidence consistent with the theory, but does not necessarily confirm or disconfirm the theory. Interestingly, both parents of the sibling incest offenders had higher prevalence rates of childhood sexual abuse then either the parents of extrafamilial child molesters and the nonchild offenders, although the rates still constituted a minority (36% for mothers of offenders and 10% for fathers of offenders). Although it is unclear whether the mothers and fathers were sexually abused by a family member or by someone outside the family, this evidence suggests that sexual abuse may be passed down from one generation to the next, but perhaps indirectly. In this instance, how specifically the cycle of abuse is sustained is equivocal. A history of maternal sexual victimization and maternal physical victimization has been documented in other studies of adolescent sex offenders as well (Adler & Schutz, 1995; Becker et al., 1986; Kaplan, Becker & Martinez, 1990).

Another theory related to the intergenerational transmission of abuse has been called the *vampire syndrome* (O'Brien, 1991). It is similar to the intergenerational transmission theory in that the vampire syndrome also connotes the notion that abuse begets abuse. Yet, it differs in that the perpetrator does not necessarily have to be a family member. It simply suggests that offenders were first victims. Research has provided some evidence to suggest that prior sexual victimization may be a contributing factor, but not necessarily a causative factor (O'Brien, 1991; Pierce & Pierce, 1987; Smith & Israel, 1987; Smith, 1988). O'Brien (1991) found rates of prior sexual victimization to be much higher than found in the general population: 42% of sibling incest offenders, 40% of extrafamilial child molesters, and 29% of nonchild sex offenders. Other studies have found similar results. For example, Rayment-McHugh and Nisbet (2003) conducted a study that compared male adolescent sex offenders (extrafamilial) to male adolescent sibling incest offenders. They found that sibling incest offenders were more likely than nonsibling offenders to have had a child protection history and to have been victims of child sexual assault. Worling (1995) also compared adolescent male sex offenders to sibling incest offenders. He found groups did not differ significantly on measures of individual functioning, but there were significant more sibling incest offenders who reported a history of child sexual abuse (CSA) than nonsibling offenders. In another study, Pierce and Pierce (1987) investigated 37 cases of adolescent sex offenders and found that for the sizable portion that had committed sibling incest, many were victims of prior sexual victimization and abuse. Smith and Israel (1987) also explored family dynamics among 25 families referred to the Boulder County Colorado Sexual Abuse Team. They found that 52% of the sibling incest offenders were victims of either intrafamilial or extrafamilial sexual abuse. Yet, in one study of 12 sibling incest offenders, only one adolescent offender reported prior sexual victimization by an uncle and none reported prior extrafamilial sexual victimization; however, there was a preponderance of physical abuse. Eleven out of the 12 sibling incest offenders had been physically abused by one or both parents (Adler & Schutz, 1995). Collectively these studies suggest that the mechanism underlying the vampire syndrome could be unresolved early experiences of sexual or physical trauma, which in turn may lead to subsequent acts of sexual offending.

Many studies of incest sibling offenders have examined other factors related to family functioning to determine the etiological significance of these contextual variables. Parental rejection and abuse (Bank & Kahn, 1982; Breer, 1987; Canavan et al., 1992; Smith, 1988), marital conflict or discord (Adler & Schutz, 1995; Worling, 1995), authoritarian parenting styles characterized by high levels of physical punishment (Worling, 1995), negative family atmosphere (Worling, 1995), parental favoritism (Caffaro & Conn-Caffaro, 1998; Haskins, 2003), less overall satisfaction with family relationships (Worling, 1995), high levels of alcohol or substance abuse (O'Brien, 1991), poor parental sexual boundaries (Smith & Israel, 1987), and hypersexualized environments (Caffaro & Conn-Caffaro, 1998) have been found among the families of sibling incest offenders. Moreover, the presence of financial stress, disability, and/or illness has also been identified as a risk factor among many families of sibling incest offenders (Adler & Schutz, 1995).

Clearly, the literature indicates that the many dynamics of a dysfunctional family contribute significantly, to adolescents' becoming incest offenders, but there is no clear consensus as to the mechanism by which this phenomenon takes place. Some speculate that children in these families learn to behave in sexually inappropriate ways because of the collective feelings of distress, despair, and helplessness character-istic of dysfunctional families. It is also plausible that older siblings are merely seeking to fulfill basic human emotional needs of nurturance and comfort that have not been met by parents. The unavailability of parents—both emotionally and physically—can also contribute to a heightened emotional bonding between siblings where, unfortu-nately, in some instances, the act of seeking comfort becomes sexualized and turns to sibling incest.

A clinical case study conducted by Haskins (2003) of one family in which a 13-year-old adolescent boy sexually abused his younger 11-year-old sister was con-ducted and provides some insight into how these dynamics manifest into sibling incest. In this particular family, the mother had been a victim of father–daughter incest and had never received treatment to deal adequately with the emotional and psychological effects of her sexual abuse. Her own mother had been disabled and her father sought to fulfill his emotional and sexual needs through her for a period of eight years beginning at age 8. Consequently, the mother came to view men as "dis-gusting, sexual perverts" and projected her attitudes and beliefs onto her husband and son, even going so far as to discuss her own sexual abuse with her children. Her first husband, the father of her two children, was viewed with "anger and disgust" and was described as "lazy and sexually perverted" (Haskins, 2003, p. 342). Her sec-ond husband, the stepfather to her children, was obsequious and submissive to her wishes as he also was a victim of childhood physical abuse at the hands of an alco-holic mother. Both parents were emotionally unavailable to their children and failed to provide nurturance and security. Yet, the mother chronically favored her "good" daughter over her "bad" son. The stepfather was apathetic and allowed himself to be controlled and dominated and was withdrawn from the family. As far as the sib-ling incest was concerned, the son had molested his sister sexually for six months. The sister finally revealed to her mother that her brother had been coming into her bed at night, touching her genitals and penetrating her vagina and anus digitally. The mother took action immediately and called the police to have her son removed.

This case study and other similar studies of incest perpetrators, victims, and their families (Abrahams & Hoey, 1994; Laviola, 1992; Smith & Israel, 1987) show with a high degree of consistency that family dynamics play a key role in creating the context for sibling incest to occur. In this example, unresolved childhood abuse issues afflicting the parents contributed to an overarching dynamic of emotional neg-lect, verbal abuse, inappropriate response patterns, dysfunctional relational patterns, and maladaptive coping strategies (Haskins, 2003). Although many case studies have illuminated several contributing family factors with a degree of consistency, the literature has not revealed any one single factor that alone can explain the occurrence of sibling incest. Rather, sibling incest is the result of a complex interplay of intrapsychic, intergenerational, and intrafamilial dynamics (Ascherman & Safier, 1990). Children raised in households that exemplify some or many of these characteristics are not having their basic emotional needs met, are typically not being nurtured properly, are perhaps being both verbally and physically abused, and are learning impaired ways of behaving. As a consequence, to gain some mastery over their lives and situation, to have their needs fulfilled, or to "act out" their aggression and frustration, many of these children end up committing sibling incest with their younger sibling, or becoming the victims of incest (Laviola, 1992).

Evidence-Based Treatment Interventions in Community Settings

What Works

Empirical evidence regarding intervention effectiveness for sibling incest offenders in community settings is lacking in the literature, and therefore, cannot be described.

What Might Work

Interventions for sibling incest offenders in community-based settings are similar in approach and content to programs provided in residential treatment facilities. The best strategy that might work to treat sibling incest offenders is a *family systems approach*, where assessment and treatment of both the offender and family is critical to the healing process and to insure that the family dynamics underlying the sibling incest are rectified. Additionally, in the case of offenders placed in residential facilities, a family systems approach is essential for the reunification of the family. Two main differences between residential treatment interventions and community-based interventions are the setting in which treatment is provided (inpatient versus outpatient) and in the number of therapeutic sessions provided. Sibling incest offenders treated in the residential treatment center represent the more serious offenders; therefore, they receive typically more individual and group therapeutic sessions than offenders treated on an outpatient basis (Rich, 2003).

What Does Not Work

The literature on community-based interventions for sibling incest offenders does not describe any programs that have been evaluated empirically and were deemed as ineffective.

Evidence-Based Treatment Interventions in Residential Settings

Sibling incest is perhaps the most underreported (Carter, 1998) and the least studied type of adolescent sex offense (Smith & Israel, 1987), yet the research presented in this chapter suggests that sibling incest may be as common or more prevalent than other forms of incest and/or sexual abuse. In the past 20 years, treatment programs for adolescent sex offenders have proliferated, and many experts working in the field are moving towards adopting a public health approach to the issue

(Longo, 2003); however, interventions designed for the specific treatment of adolescent sibling incest offenders are scant, and for the most part have not been evaluated empirically. In general, treatment interventions for sibling incest offenders are similar to programs for general sex offenders, but because sibling incest involves the victimization of a resident family household member, the treatment approach must encompass special consideration for the victim. The literature on treatment for sibling incest offenders comprises mainly case studies that describe the various treatment modalities used to treat individual sibling incest offenders and their families. In this section, we present some of the common guidelines for assessment and treatment of the adolescent sibling incest offender that have been described among these case studies and highlight the unique aspects of treating sibling incest. A caveat must be issued though that these guidelines for assessment and treatment must be taken as illustrative rather than as proven models of best practice.

What Works

To date, treatment interventions for sibling incest offenders have mostly been single-case studies and have not been implemented on a wide scale. Empirically derived evaluation of treatment effects, therefore, is not available. Thus, we cannot say definitively what works for sibling incest.

What Might Work

Similar to the assessment of extrafamilial adolescent sex offenders, the first step with adolescent sibling incest offenders is for a multidisciplinary team of professionals (i.e., police officer, social worker, probation officer, therapist, victim advocate, and judiciary) to gather critical information regarding the nature and degree of the offense so that a determination can be made regarding the safety of the victim. Then, depending on the severity and chronicity of the abuse perpetrated, treatment would be implemented in either a residential facility or community-based mental health clinic. The former venue indicates that the abuse was serious enough (e.g., sexual penetration occurred) and chronic in nature that the perpetrator needed to be removed from the home and "placed" in a residential facility. The latter venue indicates that the abuse was less serious and perhaps of short duration, enabling the adolescent offender to remain in the family household given adherence to strict safety guidelines instituted by the team.

Although researchers are working on a typology of adolescents who sexually abuse, the lack of a typology that characterizes adolescent sibling incest offenders necessitates that each case be viewed as exceptional. In addition, according to Robert E. Longo, a renowned expert in the field, "not all sexual abusers are the same . . . a one-size-fits-all approach will not work with youth at risk" (Longo, 2003, p. 505). Consequently, the treatment plan should be tailored to meet the unique features of the case. This can be accomplished by conducting a thorough and careful family-based risk assessment (Caffaro & Conn-Caffaro, 1995). The risk-assessment is critical for the development of the treatment plan, for determining whether the offender should be removed from the household, and for developing a plan for reunification. Notwithstanding, removal of the perpetrator is the most often prescribed course of action (Hargett, 1998). In these instances the adolescent is placed in a residential treatment facility as a ward of the state. Critical information regarding the role of the parents in the incestuous activity determines whether the family can be reunified. If the parents were deemed nonoffending (i.e., were not implicated in the abuse), then the eventual reunification of the family becomes one goal of the treatment plan. If, however, it was determined that the parents intentionally participated in some way in the incestuous activity (i.e., covered up the activity; tolerated or allowed the activity to occur; encouraged the activity), then reunification of the family may not be possible (Hargett, 1998).

The *Sibling Abuse Interview* (SAI) (Caffaro & Conn-Caffaro, 1995) is a family-based risk assessment tool that can be used to glean information from six key areas: (1) the offender's motivation for the abuse and for treatment; (2) the family's ability to take responsibility for the incestuous activity; (3) the family's reaction to disclosure of the activity; (4) the family's ability to protect the victim; (5) sources of support for the victim; and (6) evidence of divided loyalties among children and parents (Caffaro & Conn-Caffaro, 1995). In-depth interviews must be conducted with the victim, the offender, parents, and other siblings. The therapist conducting the assessment must first consider the wishes of the victim before meeting with the entire family, and also consider the influence of the family's culture and religious background when performing the assessment interviews.

Treatment goals for the adolescent sibling incest offender are similar in scope to the treatment goals of the general sex offender outlined in the previous chapter (see Chapter 22), with the addition of one more vital goal: the offender must also acknowledge and disclose his incestuous sexual behaviors and those behaviors must match with the victim's account. This is an important step for the offender to take, as many times sibling incest offenders will minimize the degree and frequency of their activities and even try to implicate their victims as co-conspirators in the incest. The research supports the view that siblings seldom initiate incest simultaneously (Bank & Kahn, 1982) and that sibling incest is not benign (Cole, 1982). Thus, clear documentation that the offender has defined his abusive sexual behavior accurately and that they match the disclosures of the victim must be obtained. This step is a prerequisite to the reunification of the family and allowing the offender to be placed back in the home.

Because the victim is a family member involved directly with the therapeutic process, she is essentially integral to the process. Conducting an interview with the victim enables the garnering of specific details pertaining to her fear of the offending sibling, the nature of the sibling relationship, whether she assumes responsibility for the incest, and whether the sibling offender was psychologically abusive as well (Caffaro & Conn-Caffaro, 1995). This information is helpful not only for the development of her treatment plan and recovery, but also in devising treatment for the sibling offender.

Interviews with the parents must also be conducted where the therapist will assess the strengths, weaknesses, and character of the marital relationship and their parenting style. We reported previously that a dysfunctional parental subsystem characterizes many families in which sibling incest occurs. Assessing the myriad and overlapping intrapsychic and intrafamilial factors that have merged to create such a climate is imperative to treating sibling incest effectively (Ascherman & Safier, 1990). Ineffective communication patterns, lack of intimacy between the couple, poor parental structure and support, abusive parenting, displayed favoritism, and negative emotional interactions between couples and their children are etiologic factors contributing to the incest and represent the clinical issues to be addressed in family therapy. Parents must be taught how to communicate their needs to each other and to their children, encourage communication with their children, address preferential treatment of certain children, provide boundaries and structural guidelines for their children to avoid the potential for incest to reoccur, learn nonabusive and supportive methods of parenting, and model appropriate behavior. While this therapeutic process occurs, supervision of the children must be monitored by the therapist or other designated professionals to insure the safety of the victim.

Once assessment of the offender, victim, and family has been completed, treatment must be implemented accordingly. Treatment modalities can be multimodal, using a combination of individual therapy, group sessions, and family sessions and can incorporate forms of cognitive-behavioral and psychodynamic therapies (see Chapter 22 for details of these therapies). Standards of care for juvenile sex offenders have been developed and can be applied (see Bengis et al., 1999). The most important consideration is to address both the "individual and system factors that contributed to the incestuous behavior" (O'Brien, 1991, p. 90). Implementation of a family systems framework such as the one outlined in this section appears to be the best approach. Although this approach has not been well documented in the literature, several case studies of sibling incest that implemented a family systems approach have been described and suggest that this approach may be effective in resolving the underlying causes of the incest and its adverse effects (Caffaro & Conn-Caffaro, 1995; Carter, 1998; Hargett, 1998; Haskins, 2003). As devastating as sibling incest is for the victim, for the family, and for the offender, one positive aspect is that if treatment goals are met and reconciliation of the perpetrator and victim have been achieved (i.e., both have readjusted and overcome adversarial reactions), then with an adequate aftercare component instituted (i.e., weekly family counseling; providing formal roles for outsiders to act as monitors) reunification of the family can be attained.

What Does Not Work

The literature on sibling incest treatment approaches is scant and at this juncture does not reveal treatment approaches that have been tried and deemed ineffective.

Psychopharmacology

Using psychopharmacological treatment approaches specifically for sibling incest offenders has not been documented in the literature.

The Prevention of Sibling Incest Offenses

What Works

At this time, prevention programs specifically for sibling incest have not been derived or implemented. In today's world, where even the most inappropriate and personal topics are readily discussed publicly, sibling incest is still considered a taboo topic difficult to discuss, assess, and to research. Consequently, more theoretical and empirical research is needed before primary prevention strategies can be developed and implemented.

What Might Work

We cannot ignore the etiologic role of culture and society in sibling incest. Because it is young girls rather than boys who are overwhelming the victims of sibling incest, it becomes clear that "the family is not the only social institution which plays a role in causing and perpetuating the problem" (Gilmartin, 1994, p. 291). Most modern societies also embrace patriarchy, a system in which men hold the institutional power and control and women and children are devalued. In addition to treatment approaches, social change efforts should be undertaken that address the cultural issues of male power and sexual privilege. A public education media campaign is one avenue in which large-scale attitudinal change could be achieved and has been used as a means of social change for various social issues such as domestic violence (see Klein, Campbell, Soler & Ghez, 1997). Although constructing appropriate messages regarding pervasive societal attitudes requires the consideration of many factors, this approach when used in conjunction with other programs could be effective in combating the cultural aspects underlying sibling incest.

School-based prevention programs could also be used by incorporating activities that address male privilege and power in conjunction with activities that focus on prevention of all forms of sexual abuse including incest. Notwithstanding all of the complexities involved in designing age-appropriate sexual abuse prevention programs (see Reppucci & Haugaard, 1993, for a comprehensive discussion), special care must be taken for programs designed specifically to combat incest. It may be unethical to use strategies that hold young female victims responsible for protecting themselves from the sexual advances of more powerful perpetrators with whom there is a trusted relationship.

Another prevention approach that may be less invasive or controversial could be a community-based prevention program that targets families who have older brother–younger sister sibling dynamics. This approach could be couched as part of a comprehensive healthy families initiative where in addition to sibling incest other issues could be addressed. Prevention programs would target health-care providers, parents, and educators (i.e., anyone who comes into contact with families and children) and attempt to raise awareness of the individual and familial risk factors associated with sibling incest and which also underlie other negative health-related outcomes (e.g., adolescent sex offenses, delinquency, substance abuse, etc). Educating the community of the risk factors for sibling incest should be the first step in any type of prevention program.

What Does Not Work

The literature does not describe a primary prevention program for sibling incest; thus, there has not been evaluation research that would indicate what does not work.

Recommendations

For the most part, the existence of an incest taboo in most modern societies prevents the sexual abuse of young girls by family members. Violations do occur, however. Although we could not say with a high degree of certainty how often and how many girls are victimized, research has indicated that the sequelae of incest are serious. When the violation is brother–sister incest, offenses transcend mere child's sex play. The effects of sibling incest are not only deleterious, but also clinically significant and may last well into adulthood. Etiological factors involve an interaction of individual and family pathology. As demonstrated in this chapter, the implications for treatment are straightforward. Programs must be designed to address the dysfunction in both offenders and the family environment. A family systems approach was described and, although not rigorously evaluated, at this juncture constitutes the best practice in treating adolescents who commit sibling incest. We cannot emphasize enough the importance of instituting a family systems approach. This must be implemented whether the adolescent is treated in a residential treatment facility or in a community-based facility. The family is the social environment in which sibling incest offenders engage in their behavior. Consequently, without an emphasis on changing the family dynamics we cannot hope to change the individual sibling incest offender who is embedded within it.

Also duly noted in this chapter was the paucity of epidemiological and etiological research on sibling incest. A necessary next step calls for an expansion of research efforts. First, epidemiological studies with representative samples are warranted to document the scope. Second, subsequent research on etiology must include factors at the societal level. Developing a broader ecological perspective of this phenomenon will greatly enhance our understanding of the complex interactions between individuals and their many environments, and reveal how these interactions maintain or perpetuate sibling incest. Such a comprehensive level of scope and understanding can then lead to more effective multidimensional treatment and prevention programs.

References

Abrahams, J., & Hoey, H. (1994). Sibling incest in a clergy family: A case study. *Child Abuse & Neglect, 18*(12), 1029–1035.

Adler, N.A., & Schutz, J. (1995). Sibling incest offenders. *Child Abuse & Neglect, 19*(7), 811–819.

Ascherman, L.I., & Safier, E.J. (1990). Sibling incest: A consequence of individual and family dysfunction. *Bulletin of the Menninger Clinic, 54*(3), 311–322.

Bank, S.P., & Kahn, M.D. (1982). *The Sibling Bond.* New York: Basic Books.

Becker, J.V., Kaplan, M.S., Cunningham-Rathner, J., & Kavoussi, R. (1986). Characteristics of adolescent incest sexual perpetrators: Preliminary findings. *Journal of Family Violence, 1*(1), 85–97.

Bengis, S., Brown, A., Freeman-Longo, R.E., Matsuda, B., Ross, J., Singer, K., & Thomas, J. (1999). *Standards of Care for Youth in Sex Offense-Specific Residential Programs.* Holyoke, MA: NEARI Press.

Bevc, I., & Silverman, I. (1993). Early proximity and intimacy between siblings and incestuous behaviour: a test of the Westmarck hypothesis. *Ethology and Sociobiology, 14*, 171–181.

Breer, W. (1987). *The Adolescent Molester.* Springfield, IL: Charles C. Thomas.

Caffaro, J.V., & Conn-Caffaro, A. (1998). *Sibling Abuse Trauma: Assessment and Intervention Strategies for Children, Families, and Adults.* New York: The Haworth Press.

Canavan, M.M., Meyer, W.J., & Higgs, D.C. (1992). The female experience of sibling incest. *Journal of Marital & Family Therapy, 18*(2), 129–142.

Carter, G.S. (1998). Sibling incest: Time limited group as an assessment and treatment planning tool. *Journal of Child and Adolescent Group Therapy, 8*(2), 45–54.

Cawson, P., Wattam, C., Brooker, S., & Kelly, G. (2000). *Child Maltreatment in the United Kingdom: A Study of the Prevalence of Abuse and Neglect.* London: National Society for the Prevention of Cruelty to Children.

Cole, E. (1982). Sibling incest: The myth of benign sibling incest. *Women & Therapy, 1*(3), 79–89.

Cyr, M., Wright, J., McDuff, P., & Perron, A. (2002). Intrafamilial sexual abuse: brother-sister incest does not differ from father-daughter and stepfather-stepdaughter incest. *Child Abuse & Neglect, 26*(9), 957–973.

Darves-Bornoz, J.M., Berger, C., Degiovanni, A., Gaillard, P., & Lepine, J.P. (1999). Similarities and differences between incestuous and nonincestuous rape in a French follow-up study. *Journal of Traumatic Stress, 12*(4), 613–623.

de Jong, A.R. (1989). Sexual interactions among siblings and cousins: Experimentation or exploitation? *Child Abuse & Neglect, 13*(2), 217–279.

Egeland, B. (1993). A history of abuse is a major risk factor for abusing the next

generation. In R.J. Gelles & D.R. Loseke (Eds.), *Current Controversies on Family Violence*. Newbury Park: Sage.

Finkelhor, D.H. (1979). *Sexually Victimized Children*. New York: Free Press.

Finkelhor, D. (1980). Sex among siblings: A survey on prevalence, variety, and effects. *Archives of Sexual Behavior, 9*(3), 171–194.

Finkelhor, D. (1984). *Child Sexual Abuse: New Theory and Research*. New York: Free Press.

Finkelhor, D., & Araji, S.A. (1986). *Sourcebook on Child Sexual Abuse*. Newbury Park, CA: Sage.

Freud, S. (1955a). Beyond the pleasure principle. In J. Strachey (Ed.& Trans.), *The Standard Edition of the Complete Psychological Works of Sigmund Freud* (Vol. 18). London: Hogarth Press (original work published 1920).

Freud, S. (1955b). Totem and taboo: Some points of agreement between the mental lives of savages and neurotics. In J. Strachey (Ed.& Trans.), *The Standard Edition of the Complete Psychological Works of Sigmund Freud* (Vol. 13, pp. 1–162). London: Hogarth Press (original work published 1913).

Gilmartin, P. (1994). *Rape, Incest, and Child Sexual Abuse: Consequences and Recovery*. New York: Garland Publishing, Inc.

Gupta, G.R., & Cox, S.M. (1988). A typology of incest and possible intervention strategies. *Journal of Family Violence, 3*(4), 299–312.

Hargett, H. (1998). Reconciling the victim and perpetrator in sibling incest. *Sexual Addiction & Compulsivity, 5*(2), 93–106.

Haskins, C. (2003). Treating sibling incest using a family systems approach. *Journal of Mental Health Counseling, 25*(4), 337–350.

Henslin, J.M. (2001). *Down to Earth Sociology: Introductory Readings* (11th ed.). New York: Free Press.

Kaplan, M.S., Becker, J.V., & Martinez, D.F. (1990). A comparison of mothers of adolescent incest versus non-incest perpetrators. *Journal of Family Violence, 5*, 209–214.

Kaufman, J., & Zigler, E. (1993). The intergenerational transmission of abuse is overstated. In R.J. Gelles & D.R. Loseke (Eds.), *Current Controversies on Family Violence* (pp. 209–221). Newbury Park: Sage.

Klein, E., Campbell, J.C., Soler, E., & Ghez, M. (1997). *Ending Domestic Violence: Changing Public Perceptions/ Halting the Epidemic*. Thousand Oaks, CA: Sage.

Laviola, M. (1992). Effects of older brother-younger sister incest: A study of the dynamics of 17 cases. *Child Abuse & Neglect, 16*, 409–421.

Lodico, M.A., Gruber, E., & DiClemente, R.J. (1996). Childhood sexual abuse and coercive sex among school-based adolescents in a Midwestern State. *Journal of Adolescent Health, 18*, 211–217.

Longo, R.E. (2003). Emerging issues, policy changes, and the future of treating children with sexual behavior problems. *Annals of New York Academy of Sciences, 989*, 502–514.

Luzes, P. (1990). Fact and fantasy in brother^sister incest. *International Journal of Psycho-Analysis,17*(1), 97–113.

Malinowski, B. (1927). *Sex and Repression in Savage Society*. New York: Harcourt Brace.

O'Brien, M.J. (1991). Taking sibling incest seriously. In M.Q. Patton (Ed.), *Family Sexual Abuse. Frontline Research and Evaluation*. Newbury Park: Sage.

Pierce, L.H., & Pierce, R.L. (1987). Incestuous victimization by juvenile sex offenders. *Journal of Family Violence, 2*(4), 351–364.

Rayment-McHugh, S., & Nisbet, I. (2003, May 1-2). *Sibling incest offenders as a subset of adolescent sexual offenders*. Paper presented at the Child Sexual Abuse: Justice Response or Alternative Resolution Conference, Adelaide, South Australia.

Reppucci, N.D., & Haugaard, J.J. (1993). Problems with child sexual abuse prevention programs. In R.J. Gelles & D.R. Loseke (Eds.), *Current Controversies on Family Violence* (pp. 306–322). Newbury Park: Sage.

Rich, P. (2003). Juvenile Sexual Offenders: *Understanding, Assessing and Rehabilitating*. Hoboken, NJ: John Wiley and Sons.

Risin, L.I., & Koss, M.P. (1987). The sexual abuse of boys: Prevalence and descriptive characteristics of childhood victimizations. *Journal of Interpersonal Violence, 2,* 309–323.

Rudd, J.M., & Herzberger, S.D. (1999). Brother-sister incest/father-daughter incest: A comparison of characteristics and consequences. *Child Abuse & Neglect, 23,* 915–928.

Russell, D. (1986). *The Secret Trauma: Incest in the Lives of Girls and Women.* New York: Basic Books.

Ryan, G., Miyoshi, T.J., Metzner, J.L., Krugman, R.D., & Fryer, G.E. (1996). Trends in a national sample of sexually abusive youths. *Journal of the American Academy of Child & Adolescent Psychiatry, 35*(1), 17–25.

Shepher, J. (1983). *Incest: A Biosocial View.* New York: Academic Press.

Smith, H., & Israel, E. (1987). Sibling incest: A study of the dynamics of 25 cases. *Child Abuse & Neglect, 11,* 101–108.

Smith, W.R. (1988). Delinquency and abuse among juvenile sexual offenders. *Journal of Interpersonal Violence, 3,* 400–413.

Stark, E. (1984). The unspeakable family secret. *Psychology Today,* 38–46.

Tower, C. (1996). *Child Abuse and Neglect* (3rd ed.). Boston: Allyn and Bacon.

Tsun, O.K. (1999). Sibling incest: a Hong Kong experience. *Child Abuse & Neglect, 23*(1), 71–79.

Westermarck, E. (1889). *The History of Human Marriage.* New York: Allerton Press.

Wolf, A.P. (1995). *Sexual Attraction and Childhood Association: A Chinese Brief for Edward Westermarck.* Stanford: Stanford University Press.

Worling, J.R. (1995). Adolescent sibling-incest offenders: Differences in family and individual functioning when compared to adolescent nonsibling sex offenders. *Child Abuse & Neglect, 19*(5), 633–643.

Chapter 24

Treatment of Gangs/Gang Behavior in Adolescence[1]

Mark B. Borg, Jr. and Michael R. Dalla

Introduction

Youth gangs constitute the largest component of criminally active adolescent peer groups in the United States (Howell, 2003a). Applying primary prevention and health promotion models to this topic is a complex matter, especially in light of the guiding definition of primary prevention and health promotion used in this volume, which is "those planned actions that help participants prevent predictable problems, protect existing states of health and healthy functioning, and promote desired goals for a specified population" (paraphrased from Gullotta & Bloom, 2003, p. 9). Research is also hindered by the general lack of agreement among researchers on a common definition of an adolescent gang, the validity of current gang theories, associated risk and resiliency factors, and effective strategies for dealing with adolescent gang behavior (Howell, 2003b).

The latest findings show that no single technique effectively prevents, ameliorates, or suppresses gang activity (Curry & Decker, 2003; Howell, 2003a; Klein, Maxson & Miller, 1995; Knox, 1995; Thornberry, Krohn, Lizotte, Smith & Tobin, 2003). Instead, a range of specifically targeted programs and services have been shown to be much more effective in light of established patterns of delinquency, crime, and gang affiliation (Catalano & Hawkins, 1996; Greenwood, Model, Rydell & Chiesa, 1996; Hawkins, Herrenkohl, Farrington, Brewer, Catalano, Harachi & Cothern, 2000; Lipsey, Wilson & Cothern, 2000). Nevertheless, the majority of strategies (especially within the juvenile criminal justice system) have emphasized suppression techniques that tend to reinforce individual gang member commitment and to strengthen gang affiliation and identity (Howell, Egley & Gleason, 2002).

Historical evidence showing the ineffectiveness of suppression techniques can be traced to Thrasher's (1927) early research into gangs, in which he proposed that gangs themselves serve as a suppression technique against actual and perceived

[1] The authors would like to thank Jon Lindemann for his thoughtful comments and suggestions on this chapter.

519

threats—physical, racial, ethnic, or socioeconomic—in hostile environments. Cohen and Vila (1996) observed that "if it were not for gang rivalries, hostile police and [suppressing] neighbors, there would be little to hold these groups together save for the thrill-seeking derived from delinquent behavior" (p. 133).

Before describing a comprehensive and integrated "treatment approach" to gangs, we present an overview of (a) the demographics and primary organizational issues of adolescent gangs and (b) the characteristics, behaviors, and family and their community backgrounds of adolescent gang members. Based on our assertion that gangs—as "street organizations"—rarely respond favorably to the current array of prevention, intervention, and suppression "treatments" (Branch, 1997; Curry & Decker, 2003; Howell, 2003a), we instead focus our treatment approach on the individual, familial, and community characteristics and behaviors that previous researchers have identified.

Overview

A yearly survey published by the National Youth Gang Center (the only source of nationally compiled gang data) uses Spergel and Curry's (1995) gang prevention, intervention, and suppression classifications.[2] They have identified five general strategies that American agencies have historically used to address the gang problem: (a) community organizing (including mobilization and empowerment); (b) social intervention (e.g., outreach, counseling, crisis intervention); (c) service provision (e.g., job training, tutoring); (d) suppression (enforcement, arrest, and incarceration); and (e) organizational change and development (response programs, case management, advocacy).

Howell (2003a) believes that these five strategies can be boiled down to three: prevention, intervention, and suppression. According to his analysis,

> Prevention efforts reduce the number of youths who join gangs at the same time that intervention in gang careers with treatment/rehabilitation removes youths from gangs, while suppression strategies (especially graduated sanctions)—within this combination—can weaken gangs and help thwart their recruitment efforts, serving to help diminish the presence and influence of gangs in the community (pp. 88–89).

Howell (2003a) suggests that *windows of opportunity* for gang prevention, intervention, and suppression exist throughout childhood until the ages of 14–15—peak ages for gang involvement (Esbensen & Winfree, 1998; Huff, 1998). According to Lahey, Gordon, Loeber, Stouthamer-Loeber, and Farrington (1999), the intervention opportunity window overlaps with the prevention window that extends into later ages. Intervention efforts include programs and policies aimed at reducing conduct problems, failure in school, delinquency (juvenile and violent), and gang membership. Early interventions target children and young adolescents showing initial involvement in a number of problem behaviors (Hill, Howell, Hawkins & Battin-Pearson, 1999; Loeber & Farrington, 1999), while treatment or rehabilitation interventions (combined with graduated sanctions) are used with adolescents who are more advanced in terms of gang involvement and violent delinquency (Krohn, Thornberry, Rivera & Le Blanc, 2001).

---

[2]Spergel and Curry developed a classification system based on a comprehensive study of 254 criminal justice, community-based, and grass-roots organizations dealing with the youth gang problem in 45 counties in the United States.

Theoretical Perspectives

Racism-Oppression Theories

Racism and societal oppression have long been considered key reasons for the establishment of gangs (Vigil, 2002). It is generally assumed that when social forces and institutions fail to function effectively, street subcultures—gangs—are formed to fill the void (Vigil, 1988). According to racism-oppression theorists, the list of important causal determinants and reinforcing agents of gang activity in America include (a) patterns of ethnic conflict and competition; (b) our country's social structure and institutionalized patterns of race relations; (c) acts of accommodation to an affluent society by the poor and minorities; and (d) individual experiences, patterns of enduring racial conflict, and perceptions of racism and oppression (Knox, 1995; Vigil, 1988).

Vigil (1988) originated the concept of *multiple marginalities* to describe persons having more than one minority group status—for instance, a disabled African American female who lives in a ghetto—who regularly face complex mixes of prejudicial and discriminatory experiences. Multiple marginality involves clusters of interrelated socioeconomic, cultural, psychological, and ecological factors that may include inadequate living conditions, stressful personal and family changes, and a combination of racism and cultural repression in schools and communities. Along this line, Majors and Billson (1992) have posited that

> Joining a gang is a way to organize and make sense of the marginal world of the inner city neighborhood . . . For black males [and members of other ethnic minorities] who have been locked out of the social and economic mainstream, running with a gang can be a form of social achievement (p. 50).

These theories imply that gangs will exist as long as ethnic or racial oppression exists. For whites, gang membership is less a matter of racial or ethnic subjugation than competition with minorities in a context of mutually disagreeable economic conditions. In his broad overview of gang theories, Knox (1995) asserted that racism-oppression theory "is remarkably predictive" in determining the onset and persistence of American gangs in correctional, educational, and community settings" (p. 91). According to this theoretical approach, gangs—and other social problems— will remain a symptom of a society that ignores social justice issues and the needs of certain populations in favor of large-scale oppression and discrimination against marginalized citizens (Fromm, 1955; Rappaport & Seidman, 1986; Sloan, 1996; Vigil, 2002; Zizek, 2002).

Developmental Theories

The majority of contemporary researchers appears to favor development theories for understanding the individual, family, and community factors that contribute to the gang problem in America (Curry & Decker, 2003; Howell, 2003a; Loeber & Farrington, 1999; Thornberry et al., 2003). Current developmental theories have emerged from a sociological framework of examining human experience known as the *life-course perspective* (Baltes, 1987; Elder, 1985), which views human development across an entire lifespan, and focuses on individual progress according to age-graded and culturally defined roles and social transitions. In the United States, young people are expected to complete their education, begin their careers, then get married and start families—patterns of social development and social institutions that are described as *trajectories* and *pathways*. The word *transition* is used to describe short-term changes in social roles within long-term trajectories—for example, divorce, dropping out of school, or desistance from gang affiliation.

Elder (1985) has described life courses as being structured by webs of generally consistent, interlocking trajectories that are occasionally interrupted by transition life events that can include everything from marriage to being arrested. "Off-age" (i.e., not considered age-appropriate) transitions can produce disorder (Thornberry et al., 2003); individual adaptations to these changes are considered important because they lead to different trajectories (Sampson & Laub, 1993). From a life-course perspective, childhood, adolescence, and adult experiences are viewed as parts of a continuous process of change that are dependent on the consequences of earlier behavioral patterns and the influences of risk factors in family, school, and community domains.

In the 1980s, criminologists began using the life course perspective to formulate developmental theories of juvenile delinquency (Farrington, 2000; Thornberry et al., 2003).[3] Developmental theories are gaining greater acceptance due to the usefulness of viewing offending "careers" over time. They can be used to study causal or risk factors that in turn are used to explain the onset, escalation, de-escalation, and desistance components of individual gang members' careers (Loeber & Stouthamer-Loeber, 1986). Developmental theories assume that "delinquent careers are not predetermined but are malleable, changing as the person's life unfolds" (Thornberry et al, 2003, p. 2). Howell (2003a) adds that the developmental process that produces a gang member "is affected by numerous factors in childhood and adolescence" (p. 49). We therefore assume that transitions (including change-points or milestones) provide opportunities for alternative and healthier pathways that families and communities can use to steer at-risk adolescents away from lives of crime and gang membership.

Organizational Theories

Organizational theories are associated with the study of formal and complex organizations and bureaucracies (Thornberry et al., 2003). While many social scientists view gangs as social networks that embed their members in deviant routines and isolate them from prosocial arenas, the application of organizational theory is difficult because "Gangs are more than small groups and less than bureaucracies" (Knox, 1995, p. 233). Yet, if we accept Krohn's (1986) suggestion that all social networks constrain the behaviors of their members to be consistent with the group's dominant behavioral themes, it seems worthwhile to apply organizational theory to adolescent gangs. There are other methodological issues that make researching gangs as organizations particularly tricky—for instance, the use of crime statistics as "organizational data" removes most gang organizational functions from the purview of researchers. In other words, organizational theory suggests that we shift our analysis away from the individual and toward the group, yet access to gangs for purposes of data collection remains extremely limited if not impossible.

---

[3] Thornberry et al.'s (2003) developmental theory of gang involvement is considered the most powerfully illustrative theory of the life-course consequences of adolescent gang behavior (Howell, 2003a).

Still, there are at least two good arguments in support of applying organizational theories to adolescent gangs: first, they are considered well-formulated groups with both internal and external regulatory mechanisms; and second, there is considerable evidence showing that they are more than just loosely constructed collections of marginalized individuals—for example, many gangs are multigenerational and show signs of community stability, despite qualitative differences in cross-generational membership (Branch, 1997).

But despite the paucity of organizational gang theory research, analyses of gangs in terms of organizational characteristics have been effectively used for classifying their risk dimensions and for understanding the many ways that gangs, as organizations, strive for and develop greater sophistication.[4] At the same time, much of the information that is overlooked in traditional and contemporary gang theories seems very pertinent to assessing the gang problem in America. We agree with Branch's (1997, p. 4) assertion that "misconceptions about gangs and their [organizational] dynamics have been responsible for the failure to develop effective assessment and intervention strategies."

Gangs as Facilitating Environments for Delinquent Behavior

The perspective of gangs as facilitating environments for delinquent behavior is based on organizational theory. According to this view, "because gangs clearly connote groups that have a deviant or criminal orientation, a strong relationship between gang membership and high rates of involvement in delinquency and drug use is hardly surprising" (Thornberry et al., 2003, p. 96). Gangs manifest their facilitation component through their normative structures and group processes, resulting in high rates of delinquency, drug use, and other kinds of deviant and criminal behaviors (Deschenes & Esbensen, 1999; Hagedorn, 1998). Researchers who use this theoretical perspective have suggested that group norms and group processes that revolve around such dimensions as status, solidarity, cohesion, and exposure to risky and violent situations are likely to increase delinquent acts among gang members (Klein, Maxson & Miller, 1995; Miller & Brunson, 2000; Rosenfeld, Bray & Egley, 1999).

Clinical Theories

Clinical theories—defined by Branch (1997) as theories that are normally applied in clinical and family interventions—have been uniformly overlooked in association with adolescent gangs, perhaps because of the historical failures of the prevention, intervention, and suppression techniques that have been applied to gangs as organizations. Furthermore, this perspective challenges psychological theories regarding the characteristics of individual gang members—i.e., that they are hyperactive, conduct-disordered, cognitively impaired, impulsive, and sociopathic. There is considerable evidence suggesting that gang members have none of these traits, at least not wholly,

---

[4] Pertinent issues in any organizational analysis of gangs include level of organization; leadership structure; territoriality; internal organization; external organization; religious or political affiliations; written rules, constitutions, and literature; ethnic homogeneity; shifts in membership; role definitions; level of cohesion; level of morale, normative consensus; membership expectations; level of stability; leadership quality; recurrent crime patterns; age-graded participation; gender-graded participation; offensive patterns; initiation rites; subcultural diffusion; and strength (Knox, 1995).

since "street organizations" (as some gang members like to call them) have certain cognitive, behavioral, organizational, and leadership guidelines that discourage such behavior. These guidelines suggest that gang members must be able to interact with others in ways that are rewarding to the entire organization; at times, members must set aside their individual needs in order to achieve group goals. Other membership requirements include the capacity to function within a set of limits (either loosely or well-articulated), fidelity, understanding gang membership nuances, and delaying gratification—all evidence supporting the idea that extremely individualistic, sociopathic, impulsive, and narcissistic individuals may not function well as gang members (Branch, 1997). These qualities contradict more traditional gang theory and demand more detailed analysis regarding the application of organizational theory to prevention, intervention, and suppression strategies.

Definitional Issues

There are no universally accepted definitions of youth gang, gang membership, or gang behavior. Thrasher (1927, p. 5), considered the first gang researcher, noted that "no two gangs are just alike; [they take on] an endless variety of forms." We will suggest that all contemporary gang researchers still agree with Thrasher's observation, yet state and local jurisdictions continue to develop their own "universal" definitions of what constitutes a gang. For our purposes, we will use two definitions that we consistently encountered throughout the literature.[5] The first was established by Thrasher (1927), who characterized gangs in behavioral terms: face to face meetings, "milling," movement through space as a unit, and conflict and planning. Such collective behavior results in the development of tradition, an unreflective internal structure, an *esprit de corps*, solidarity, moral, group awareness, and territorial attachment.

Thrasher's definition has been disputed, modified, and completely reworked over more than seven decades. We will offer Jankowski's (1991) definition as being sufficiently comprehensive in terms of the major issues that we will address in this chapter:

> A gang is an organized social system that is both quasi-private and quasi-secretive and whose size and goals have necessitated that social interaction be governed by a leadership structure that has defined roles; where the authority associated with these roles has been legitimized to the extent that social codes are operational to regulate the behavior of both leadership and the rank and file; that plans and provides not only for the social and economic services of its members, but also for its maintenance as an organization; that pursues such goals irrespective of whether such action is legal or not; and that lacks a bureaucracy (pp. 28–29).

Collectively, these organizational definitions present a broad overview of what constitutes a gang,[6] yet defining adolescent gangs remains a slippery task for at least three reasons: (a) individual gangs tend to evolve and adapt over time to meet the

---

[5] Many frequently cited gang definitions are better considered as organizational assessments.
[6] Another issue concerning the definition of gangs has to do with graffiti, which is among the most significant ways that gangs have of defining themselves, delineating their territory, and communicating both within intra- and across inter-gang boundaries (Knox, 1995). In fact, crime specialists dealing with gangs often interpret graffiti in specific communities to assess the level of threat—as gangs often pass messages of threat and retaliation through graffiti (Jackson, 1998). To detail the issue of gang-related graffiti goes beyond the scope of this chapter, but detailed accounts of this issue can be found in Leet, Rush, and Smith (2000) and Phillips (1999).

demands of environments that often become increasingly hostile to their presence (Hagedorn, 1994; Horowitz, 1990; Taylor, 1990); (b) there has recently been a proliferation of "hybrid" gangs—that is, gangs whose membership is ethnically and racially diverse, and that include both male and female members (Miller & Brunson, 2000; Starbuck, Howell & Lindquist, 2001); and (c) ways in which youth gangs have been portrayed in the popular media (e.g., the films *Colors* and *Boyz in the Hood*), which are based on stereotypes rather than scientific knowledge (Howell, 2003a; Miethe & McCorkle, 1997).

The second definition that consistently shows up in the literature was developed by the U.S. Department of Justice's Office of Juvenile Justice and Delinquency Prevention (OJJDP); this definition has gained general acceptance within the criminal justice system. As restated by Howell (1997), a youth gang is a "self-formed association of peers having the following characteristics: a gang name and recognizable symbols, identifiable leadership, a geographic territory, a regular meeting pattern, and collective actions to carry out illegal activities" (p. 1).

Incidence Rates

At the time this chapter was being written, the 2001 *National Youth Gang Survey* edited by the OJJDP (Egley, 2002) was considered the most current and valid source of information on gang incidence rates (Howell, 2003b; Thornberry, 2003).[7] All cities with populations of 250,000 or more reported gang activity in 2001, as did 85% of cities with between 100,000 and 249,999 residents; 65% between 50,000 and 99,999; 44% between 25,000 and 49,999; and 20% between 2,500 and 24,999. Thirty-five percent of all suburban counties and 11% of all rural counties reported gang activity in 2001, and 95% of all jurisdictions reporting gang activity in 2001 also reported gang activity in previous surveys (conducted yearly since 1996). Approximately 3,000 jurisdictions across the country were believed to have experienced some form of gang activity in 2001 (Egley & Major, 2003).

Various surveys of urban adolescents indicate that between 14% and 30% join a gang for some period of time (Howell, 2003a). The data reveal an age range for gang members of between 12 and 24; membership is believed to be expanding at the very top and bottom of this range, but more so at the top, meaning that most youth gang members are actually young adults. (Howell, 1997; Thornberry et al., 2003). According to the National Youth Gang Survey, 94% of all gang members in the U.S. in 2001 were male, and 39% of all youth gangs had female members (Egley, 2002). Age, race, and ethnicity statistics are available from the 1996, 1998, and 1999 surveys. Respondents to the 1996 survey reported that 50% of all gang members were juveniles (17 years of age or younger). According to the 1999 and 2000 surveys, 47% of all gang members were Hispanic, 31% African American, 13% white, 7% Asian, and 2% "other" (Egley, 2002). Egley (2002) and Egley and Major (2003) have both reported that the racial/ethnic/gender distribution of gang members has varied little since these surveys began.

---

[7] The 2001 survey contains data from a) 1,216 police departments serving cities with populations of at least 25,000; b) 661 suburban and county police and sheriff's departments; c) a randomly selected sample of 398 police departments serving cities with populations ranging from 2,500 to 25,000; and d) a randomly selected sample of 743 rural county police departments. Of 3,018 departments that received a questionnaire, 2,560 (85%) returned a completed form (Egley & Major, 2003).

Available data for cities with populations of 25,000 or more residents show that 42% reported increases in gang membership and 45% reported increases in the number of active gangs from the two preceding survey years. In comparison, cities with populations of 100,000 or more that have gang-related problems consistently reported increasing numbers of gang members throughout all the years that the survey has been conducted (Egley & Major, 2003).

A significant number of cities that reported gang activity also reported gang-related homicides in 2001, including 69% of those cities with populations of 100,000 or more and 37% with populations between 50,000 and 99,999. More than half of all homicides in Los Angeles (59%) and Chicago (53%) were described as gang-related in 2001. The total number of gang-related homicides (698) in these two cities alone was greater than the total number of gang-related homicides (637) reported by 130 other cities with populations of 100,000 or more (Egley & Major, 2003).

Sixty-three percent of jurisdictions with gang-related problems also reported that gang members had returned to their jurisdictions in 2001 following periods of incarceration. More than two-thirds of these jurisdictions stated that the return of incarcerated gang members affected their existing gang problems—specifically, increases were noted in violent crime (63%) and drug trafficking (68%) by local gangs. Just over one-third (34%) of these jurisdictions reported that they did not have any community programs to assist gang members who were returning from prison, and another 35% did not mention whether or not they had such programs (Egley & Arjunan, 2002).

Risk and Resiliency Factors

The available evidence shows that resiliency factors are clearly outweighed by gang-related risk factors, not only in terms of the actual factors influencing risk and resilience, but also regarding the research efforts in both areas. In Howell's (2003a) words, "Research on protective factors has been slower to develop than risk factor studies, in part because of the absence of a standard for determining what constitutes [resilience]" (p. 90). Furthermore, individual, family, and community factors are highly intertwined and difficult to disentangle in the context of risk and resiliency research (Benard, 1991).

Several characteristics have been shown to predict gang membership and behavior. Tremblay and LeMarquand (2001) found that boys with chronic histories of physical aggression commonly exhibit cognitive-behavioral problems (i.e., inappropriate automatic reactions to situations). Such problems often lead to school failure, which is a strong predictor of gang membership (Hill, Howell, Hawkins & Battin-Pearson, 1999). Individual characteristics that are thought to have links with cognitive-behavioral problems include learning disabilities, hyperactivity, conduct problems, and lack of self-control (e.g., impulsivity, risk-seeking tendencies, and physical problem-solving tendencies); many of these same characteristics have been identified as key risk factors for gang membership (Esbensen, Huizinga & Weiher, 1993; Hill, Howell, Hawkins & Battin-Pearson, 1999; Howell, 2003b). The list of characteristics that predict gang membership also includes illegal gun ownership (Bjerregaard & Lizotte, 1995; Lizotte, Krohn, Howell, Tobin & Howard, 2000; Lizotte, Tesoriero, Thornberry & Krohn, 1994) and early involvement in delinquency, alcohol/drug use, early dating and precocious sexual activity, and mental health problems (Thornberry et al.,

2003). Thornberry et al. (2003) also found that youngsters (particularly boys) who experience numerous negative/stressful life events—failing a course at school, being suspended from school, breaking up with a boyfriend/girlfriend, having a major fight or problem with a friend, etc.—are also more likely to join gangs.

In short, children and adolescents with conduct disorders or who show worsening antisocial behavior as early as the first grade are at high risk of joining gangs (Esbensen, Huizinga & Weiher, 1993). These children are often identified as learning-disabled and show evidence of developing deviant life-styles at an early age (Hill, Howell, Hawkins & Battin–Pearson, 1999). The most dedicated gang members exhibit low self-control and tendencies toward risk-seeking behavior (Knox, 1995). Regardless of gender, future gang members are more likely to have conduct problems at a very young age, to develop delinquent beliefs, to cultivate delinquent friends, to begin dating early, and to become involved in drug use in late childhood and early adolescence (Thornberry et al., 2003). However, Howell (2003a) has also found evidence that a significant number of the youngest gang members "are good kids, from good families . . . are good students . . . [and] do not remain in gangs for long" (p. 90).

Some minor discrepancies in gang-related risk factors have been noted in terms of gender and race/ethnicity. However, at least one researcher has analyzed available data and concluded that risk factors for gang membership are very similar between adolescent girls and boys (Deschenes & Esbensen, 1999; Thornberry et al., 2003). In addition, Howell (2003b) has recently reported that for both genders, a strong association exists between having deficits in multiple developmental domains and the likelihood of joining a gang.

Evidence that risk and resiliency factors operate differently for members of different ethnic and racial groups has been presented by Spergel and Curry (1995) and Walker-Barnes and Mason (2001), among others. In terms of "multiple marginalities," ethnic minority and impoverished adolescents appear to be particularly at-risk for gang membership. Although it remains clear that socioeconomic status and the effects of discrimination are the most powerful factors affecting risk and resilience (Vigil, 2002), there is much less clarity regarding the association between socioeconomic status and discrimination on the one hand and race/ethnicity/gender on the other. Thus, it has been suggested that criminal statistics regarding race and ethnicity should not be used to confirm differences in rates of gang participation but to confirm differences in arrest rates for gang-related offenses. There is considerable evidence showing that adolescents of color, irrespective of gang membership, are more likely to be detained and arrested than their Caucasian counterparts (Howell, 2003b; Vigil, 2002). It has also been noted that in early developmental phases, ethnic identity is a factor in individual associations with collectives (including youth gangs) for the purpose of resolving one's sense of personal identity. Individuals who feel socially marginalized often try a variety of approaches to resolving such crises—for example, affiliating themselves with others they perceive as being most like themselves. On the other hand, such affiliations may be related to a specific developmental phase, and may later lead to full participation in healthy expressions of ethnic identity—a powerful factor in resisting the appeal of gangs (Branch, 1997).

Some resiliency factors may simply be the opposite of risk factors—for instance, low parental support is considered a risk factor, while high parental supervision is recognized as a resiliency/protective factor. Some evidence has been offered showing that resilience factors can interact with risk factors to reduce the likelihood of a child or adolescent joining a gang (Henderson, Benard & Sharp-Light, 1999). Researchers continue to work toward establishing which resiliency factors are most likely to buffer risk factors (Bjerregaard & Smith, 1993; Howell, 2003b; Maxson, Whitlock & Klein, 1998; Thornberry et al., 2003; Wyrick, 2000).

In the individual domain, support for personal skills, social skills, and self-efficacy is strongly correlated with resilience in young people who are at risk for gang involvement (Durlak, 1998; Howell, 2003a). Also, some of the membership characteristics we have described as being requirements for gang functioning—impulse control, fidelity, and delayed gratification—are also considered resiliency factors (Branch, 1997). Seeing that risk and resiliency factors are intertwined among individual, family, and social domains, developmental theories may be helpful in assessing the trajectories of individual life paths, especially for identifying key transition points for intervention. Assessing the impact of such transitions as entering high school or dating can be used to predict risk and emphasize resiliency by increasing support from such institutions as the family, school, or community agencies.

Family Factors

Key family risk factors for gang membership include structure (e.g., broken homes) and poverty (Hill, Howell, Hawkins & Battin-Pearson, 1999; Howell, 2003b). Poor family management—including low parental supervision, lack of control or child monitoring (Le Blanc & Lanctot, 1998), and abuse/neglect (Thornberry et al., 2003) are also strong predictors. Interestingly, a high level of psychological control in the form of manipulative and guilt-based actions on the part of parents is also considered a risk factor for gang membership (Walker-Barnes & Mason, 2001). While it may seem obvious that the involvement of other family members (especially siblings and cousins) in gang activity would be a strong predictor, there is very little in the way of research evidence supporting this assumption (Egley, 2002). What research has been conducted to date shows that this factor is particularly strong in Latino communities in East Los Angeles and the American Southwest, and to a lesser extent in African American communities in South Central Los Angeles (Vigil, 1983, 1988). There is also strong evidence that immigrants from countries that have recently suffered from the effects of war (examples include Vietnam and Nicaragua) are particularly vulnerable to gang affiliation (Vigil, 2002).

The primary resiliency factor associated with family context is good parent–child relationships, including the positive involvement of parents, consistent interaction between parents and children, and family bonding (Catalano & Hawkins, 1996; Durlak, 1998; Farrington, 1993). Benard (1991) has identified the most important family resilience factors as caring relationships, parents sending high expectation messages to their children, and parents giving their children meaningful opportunities to contribute to a family's well-being. Additional factors that have been identified as enhancing resiliency in a family context include income, cohesion, shared interests and activities, communication, flexibility, safe and adequate housing, and conflict resolution skills (Henderson et al., 1999).

Social and Community Factors

Most contemporary gang theorists list the three most important contexts affected by social and community risk and resiliency factors as school, peers, and community (Curry & Decker, 2003; Howell, 2003a; Thornberry et al., 2003; Vigil, 2002). All three are contexts in which gang members show high levels of alienation (Esbensen, Osgood, Taylor, Peterson & Freng, 2001; Howell, 2003b).

At least two sets of researchers believe that the strongest school-related risk factor for gang membership is low achievement in elementary school (Hill, Howell, Hawkins & Battin-Pearson, 1999; Le Blanc & Lanctot, 1998), which indicates low academic aspirations (Hill, Howell, Hawkins & Battin-Pearson, 1999; Howell, 2003b) and a low degree of commitment to education (Le Blanc & Lanctot, 1998; Thornberry et al., 2003). Two other factors that have been identified as contributing to gang affiliation are the negative labeling of youngsters by teachers (Esbensen, 2000) and feeling unsafe at school (Gottfredson & Gottfredson, 2001). Furthermore, Howell and Lynch (2000) found that increased security measures at schools do not necessarily reduce gang presence.

Regarding peer risk factors, Thornberry et al. (2003) describe associations with peers who engage in delinquent acts as one of the strongest risk factors for gang membership, particularly for boys. Another strong risk factor is associations with aggressive peers—whether or not they are involved in delinquency (Lahey, Gordon, Loeber, Stouthamer-Loeber & Farrington, 1999; Lyon, Henggeler & Hall, 1992). The lack of adult supervision of child or adolescent interactions with friends is integrally related to the influence of delinquent friends on a youngster's decision to join a gang (Le Blanc & Lanctot, 1998).

Longitudinal studies have shown that the strongest community or neighborhood risk factors for gang membership are the availability of drugs, the presence of troubled neighborhood youth, a youngster's sense of feeling unsafe in a neighborhood, low neighborhood attachment, low level of neighborhood integration, local poverty, and neighborhood disorganization (Howell, 2003a). Researchers have long acknowledged that gangs tend to cluster in high-crime and socially disorganized neighborhoods (Fagan, 1996; Short & Strodtbeck, 1965; Vigil, 1988). Virgil (2002) has suggested that during adolescence, many individual and family protective factors are strongly influenced by the level of disorganization in a neighborhood (Vigil, 2002); this includes the clustering of existing gangs in such communities.

Peer modeling, high-quality schools and teachers, clear and consistent social norms, and effective social policies in the community domain are all considered strong resiliency factors for potential gang members (Durlak, 1998; Howell, 2003a). Resiliency factors that can be supported by a community (especially when implemented within families and schools) are (a) strong social support, (b) setting clear and consistent boundaries, (c) filling free time with creative activities that emphasize prosocial values, (d) emphasizing commitment to a child's well-being and development, (e) stressing social competencies, and (f) supporting a child's sense of positive identity (including cultural identity) (Henderson et al., 1999). Furthermore, setting high but realistic expectations and opportunities for meaningful participation in schools and communities is strongly associated with resiliency (Benard, 1991).

In the same manner that increased family support during significant adolescent transitions can increase resiliency, there are many opportunities for social and community institutions to intervene and increase support at predictable points during an individual's life path. Such institutions as schools, churches, community organizations, and even the criminal justice system have the potential to provide support to adolescents as they make decisions that may or may not send them off on trajectories leading to gang affiliation.

However, despite the long list of social and community factors that influence risk and resiliency, the literature consistently states that adolescents who live in poor neighborhoods are demographically—if not psychologically—at greater risk of gang affiliation (Howell, 2003a; Thornberry et al., 2003). According to the evidence we have reviewed, it seems as though race and ethnicity are weaker determinants of risk margins or access to resiliency factors than such group association factors as residing in poor neighborhoods, acting according to stereotypical behavioral scripts, and being targeted by law enforcement agencies.

Evidence-Based Treatment Interventions in Community Settings

There is considerable disagreement about the potential to achieve social improvements through community organizations (Howell, 2003a), especially in light of Short's (1990) reminder that "communities, too, have careers in delinquency" (p. 224). In a subsequent analysis of critical features of the youth gang problem, Short (1996) identified individual characteristics and group processes that must be taken into account when developing prevention and intervention programs. Short claimed that community factors contributing to gang delinquency and violence consist of macro- and microlevel influences, with the macrolevel forces including the spread of gang culture, youth culture, and a growing underclass. Quantifying these forces is a difficult task, but it is important that they serve as a backdrop in the development of community-based "treatment" efforts (Howell, 1999, 2003a). There is some evidence indicating that intensive community-based sanctions are more effective than restrictive and expensive confinement policies in reducing adolescent gang incidents and recidivism (Howell, 2003b). This is an important concept, considering that long-term confinement is the equivalent of "residential treatment" for many gang members.

What Works

In their *National Assessment of Youth Gangs Survey*, Spergel and Curry (1995) suggested that community organization mobilization is the most effective strategy for dealing with adolescent gangs, but only when social opportunities are also provided. They recommended that communities create locally based youth agencies to provide a continuum of services to gang and non-gang youth (Howell, 2003b; Thornberry et al., 2003). This idea became the cornerstone for Howell's (2003a) *Comprehensive Strategy Framework* (CSF), which combines prevention, intervention, and suppression techniques with a strong emphasis on specific community contexts. The strategy encompasses all of the major treatment areas covered in this chapter and is currently the primary method used by the juvenile criminal justice system. It has been thoroughly evaluated by numerous researchers and is discussed in detail in a later section.

It is widely recognized that to be effective, community-based treatment must target the weaknesses and strengths of specific community structures beyond the gang problem—employment, schools, social services, health programs, and the like

(Howell, 1999; Klein, Maxson, & Miller, 1995). Of the handful of effective programs for reducing gang involvement that have been identified in resiliency studies, one that stands out is the *Health Realization/Community Empowerment program* (Mills, 1993; Mills & Spittle, 2001)—a program that combines prevention, intervention, and building relationships between communities and agency resources, including law enforcement. This program has been shown to be effective in reducing crime, delinquency, and gang involvement in some of the United States' most disturbed neighborhoods, including South Central Los Angeles, Oakland, and the Bronx (Benard, 1999; Borg, 2002; Henderson et al., 1999).

What Might Work

Gang interventions in community settings that serve to prevent, redirect, or reduce gang members and membership generally enlist the efforts of local citizens, youth agencies, community organizations, and the criminal justice system. The emphasis has been on indigenous leadership to combat delinquency and to provide the community with a sense of involvement (Knox, 1995). There has been little evidence, however, to support the effectiveness of these programs (Howell, 1998; Thornberry et al., 2003). One such large-scale program—*Mobilization for Youth* started in New York City in the 1960s—was seen to provide short-term success but failed to achieve lasting reform (Klein, 1995). In brief, community interventions, which are historically difficult to evaluate, have not shown significant evidence in reducing the number of gangs or the level delinquency—especially those that take on the gang problem directly (i.e., through criminal justice interventions).

However, there is evidence that community-based interventions that take a less direct approach might be effective in reducing adolescent gang membership (Howell, 1995; Goldstein & Huff, 1993). Such programs often focus on providing social opportunities and include a broad spectrum of educational and job-related opportunities. The most promising educational programs are those that use the school as the base for a multifaceted approach that addresses school performance, anti-gang education, and the building of self-esteem (Klein, Maxson & Miller, 1995; Moore, 1991). Community interventions that are school-based programs have shown to be effective in changing attitudes and increasing knowledge about gang issues, but their effect on behavioral change is unclear (Thornberry et al., 2003). Moreover, most of these programs are directed at marginal or peripheral youth rather than committed gang members (Hawkins, Catalano & Miller, 1992).

The successful strategies we identified combine prevention, intervention, and suppression efforts. When we consider programs that might work, we will speculate on whether or not strategies applied to larger inner-city populations could be applied in suburban and rural settings, where incidence rates have been increasing over the past decade (Egley, 2002). Testing these strategies in these settings will become increasingly important if this pattern continues, but very few efforts have been made to date.

What Does Not Work

The prevailing opinion among researchers is that the "get tough on crime" approach (e.g., three strikes law, zero tolerance, etc.) has failed to reduce the gang (or any other crime) problem (Howell, 2003a; Klein, Maxson & Miller, 1995). It is our opinion that suppression techniques without prevention and intervention do not work and very often backfire since they tend to increase the intensity of perceived threats to gangs, and cause them to become even more intractable. For this reason, we believe that suppression techniques—including the psychiatric hospitalization of gang-affiliated youth—have been generally counterproductive.

Evidence-Based Treatment Interventions in Residential Settings

Considerable contradictions mark the treatment of adolescent gang members in residential settings. The most common residential "treatment" has long been incarceration; however, up to 80% of incarcerated adolescents have disorders that meet criteria for *DSM-IV* mental disorders (Cocozza & Skowyra, 2000) and up to 50% of adolescents in psychiatric hospitals are admitted because of behavioral problems rather than mental disorders (Howell, 2003a; Weithorn, 1988).

What Works

In light of the failure of incarceration and other suppression techniques, residential treatment for adolescent gang members must incorporate prevention and intervention—the second and third components of Howell's (2003a) *Comprehensive Strategy Framework* (CSF). It seems most important to provide some form of aftercare whenever an adolescent has been placed in and released from residential treatment in order to prevent relapses into gang behaviors and to reduce recidivism (Greenwood et al., 1996). An important aspect of the CSF is its "graduated sanctions" approach to suppression and incarceration. Krisberg and Howell (1999) have suggested that "the appropriate mix of residential and home-based services for different types of offenders" (p. 364) might provide a useful initial framework for determining what works for different types of offending and gang-prone youth. When connected to prevention and intervention programs, graduated sanctions have proven effective for reducing adolescent gang behavior and gang affiliation (Egley & Major, 2003; Esbensen, 2000; Howell, 2003a). Currently, this is a strategy being employed by the juvenile criminal justice system to target adolescent gang behaviors.

To be effective, however, the components of any graduated sanctions system must match the developmental history of an adolescent's delinquent career as well as the risk of recidivism. When offenders persist in committing serious and violent acts of delinquency, their positions in the graduated sanctions system should be advanced, and rehabilitation systems must become more intensive and structured. In the CSF, the five levels of sanctions are (a) immediate intervention (e.g., counseling, probation) with first-time misdemeanors and nonviolent felony offenders and non-serious repeat offenders; (b) intermediate sanctions for first-time serious or violent offenders, including more intensive supervision and probation; (c) community confinement; (d) secure corrections for serious, violent, and chronic offenders; and (e) aftercare (Howell, 2003a). These gradations form a continuum of intervention options that require a matching continuum of treatment options that include referral and disposition resources. Intensive aftercare programs are critical to the success of such systems at all sanction levels (Howell, 2003a).

What Might Work

As we have emphasized throughout this chapter, residential treatment interventions that address adolescent gang behavior must be part of a broader strategy that includes prevention and suppression. Although the OJJDP continues to apply such strategies in large cities, the applicability of these strategies to suburban and rural adolescents is still being debated (Egley, 2002; Curry & Decker, 2003). Recent studies of migration patterns have shed new light on strategies that might work in those geographic locations (Thornberry et al., 2003). While the CSF and other combined strategy approaches appear applicable to these new patterns, empirical studies need to be conducted to support their validity. Other residential treatment programs for adolescent gang members that have shown various degrees of beneficial results include wilderness challenge programs (Lipsey, Wilson & Cothern, 2000), restitution programs (Roy, 1995), and specialized facilities for specific behavioral problems (Reich, Culross & Behrman, 2002). These approaches require more thorough evaluation.

What Does Not Work

Many prevention programs inadvertently create deviant peer groups (as often occurs in prisons) when they establish and run such activities as anger management classes (Lipsey, Wilson & Cothern, 2000). Being placed in one of these groups is often perceived as a form of punishment (Howell, 2003b), and such experiences can have iatrogenic effects—that is, the problem being addressed can be inadvertently made worse by the treatment procedure. Still, despite the large number of studies showing that punishment is ineffective for juvenile offenders (especially gang members), incarceration remains the most prevalent form of "residential treatment" for this population (Howell, 2003a; Klein, Maxson & Miller, 1995; Thornberry et al., 2003). Ever since the mid-19th century, advocates of incarceration alternatives have argued that prisons breed crime (Foucault, 1977; Krisberg & Austin, 1993; Krisberg & Howell, 1999), yet defenders of juvenile corrections continue to claim that confinement exerts a deterrent effect (DiIulio, 1995; Murray & Cox, 1979; Rhine, 1996).

Researchers have reported that the most ineffective forms of residential treatment are boot camps (MacKenzie, 2000), large custodial facilities (Krisberg & Howell, 1999), and long prison terms—especially for adolescents sent to adult facilities (Howell, 1997, 2000, 2003a). Psychiatric hospitalization for adolescent gang members has been described as the worst form of residential treatment (Howell, 2003a; U.S. Department of Health and Human Services [USDHHS], 2001) and one that does more harm than good (Burns, Hoagwood & Mrazek, 1999; Weithorn, 1988).

Psychopharmacology

The effects of medication on childhood and adolescent behavioral problems—especially violence and delinquency—are still very much in need of research and evaluation (Howell, 2003a; Wasserman, Miller & Cothern, 2000). The few studies that have been conducted on the long-term benefits of medication treatment for either chronic or acute violence and delinquency in adolescents have not specifically addressed gang-related issues (Burns et al., 1999; Howell, 2003a). When applied to aggression and delinquency, psychopharmacology typically focuses on physical acts of aggression (Rippon, 2000). Lynn and King (2002, p. 305[8]) have noted that "aggression and violence are often not precisely defined, and their [psychopharmacological] study is complicated as a result."

A primary issue in addressing adolescent delinquency and aggression is that both are viewed as symptoms in the constellation of psychiatric disorders that includes attention-deficit/hyperactivity disorders, conduct disorder, and oppositional defiant disorder. Aggression and delinquency can also occur in post-traumatic stress disorder, psychotic disorders, mood disorders, seizure disorders, pervasive developmental disorders, mental retardation, and traumatic brain injuries (Fava, 1997). Furthermore, in terms of psychopharmacological studies, aggression and associated delinquencies are poorly understood in terms of their neurobiological underpinnings (Lynn & King, 2002). There is some consistency in research results concerning interactions among multiple neurotransmitter, neuroendocrine, and hormonal systems and their mechanisms for regulating aggression, impulsivity, and other behaviors that are commonly associated with gang activities (De Felipe, Herrero & O'Brien, 1998).[9]

The Prevention of Adolescent Gang Formation and Gang Behavior

No one has yet discovered an effective strategy for preventing the formation of youth gangs (Howell, 2000, 2003a). As we have argued in preceding sections, we believe that in order to be effective, prevention must be considered as one part of a comprehensive strategy that also addresses intervention and suppression concerns. Here we describe several programs organized outside the juvenile criminal justice system that are considered exemplars of the prevention component of the CSF.

What Works

We believe that the only prevention techniques that work are those that combine prevention efforts with intervention and suppression strategies. Hawkins et al. (2000) have proposed the following set of principles to guide the programming of prevention efforts: (a) address known risk factors for delinquency, violence, and substance abuse; (b) make clear connections between program activities and risk reduction goals; (c) attempt to strengthen protective factors while reducing risk; (d) address risk reduction activities before they become predictive of later problems; (e) provide intervention strategies that target individuals and communities that are exposed to multiple risk factors; (f) take a multifaceted approach to addressing key risk factors affecting a community; and (g) include members of all racial, cultural, and socioeconomic groups that will be affected.

While a number of prevention strategies have been developed to augment the CSF, three programs stand out as examples of a prevention component that could be

---

[8]This statement could be considered ironic, since aggression, conduct problems, and antisocial behavior account for one-third to one-half of all child and adolescent referrals to psychiatric clinics (Lynn & King, 2002).

[9]It is important to note that the vast majority of the available studies used laboratory animals (Lopez, Vazqueuz, Chalmers, & Watson, 1997).

viewed as reducing the necessity of implementing intervention and suppression components. All three programs were analyzed in detail during the development of the CSF (Egley, 2002; Howell, 2003a).

1. The *Gang Resistance Education and Training* (G.R.E.A.T.) program. G.R.E.A.T. is a school-based gang prevention program that is currently delivered to 365,000 public middle school students in the United States (Howell, 2003a). The program places particular emphasis on cognitive-behavioral skills training, social skills development, refusal skills training, and conflict resolution. It has been found to have positive long-term effects on reducing gang membership and delinquency (Esbensen & Osgood, 1999; Esbensen et al., 2001; Howell, 2003a).

2. The *Montreal Preventive Treatment Program,* designed to address antisocial behavior in 7-, 8-, and 9-year-old boys from low-income families who display disruptive behavior problems in kindergarten. This program has successfully demonstrated that a combination of parent training and childhood skills development can steer children away from gangs. The training uses coaching, peer modeling, self-instruction, reinforcement contingencies, and role-playing to build skills. Evaluations have identified short- and long-term gains, including lower delinquency rates, less substance abuse, and less gang involvement at the age of 15 (Howell, 2000; Moore, 1998; Tremblay, Masse, Pagani & Vitaro, 1996).

3. The *Gang Prevention Through Targeted Outreach Program,* developed by the Boys and Girls Clubs of America. At-risk youth are identified and recruited into the program through direct outreach efforts and school referrals. Training is offered in character and leadership development, health and life skills, the arts, sports, fitness, and recreation. An evaluation of this program showed decreases in gang and delinquent behaviors, more positive adult and peer relationships, and positive changes in the participants' achievements in school (Arbreton & McClanahan, 2002; Esbensen, 2000; Howell, 2003a).

Two clinical approaches have been found to be effective in preventing child and adolescent antisocial behavior, delinquency, and associations with delinquent peers. The first is known as *multisystemic therapy* (MST) (Henggeler, Schoenwald, Bourduin, Rowland & Cunningham, 1998). Based on a family preservation model, MST focuses on improving parental control and involvement with their children, and emphasizes the formation of a care continuum between families and community cares systems.[10] The second is *Functional Family Therapy* (FFT) (Alexander, Barton, Schiavo & Parsons, 1976; Alexander & Parsons, 1973), which uses behavioral techniques such as clear specification of rules and consequences, contingency contracting, use of social reinforcement, and token economy, as well as more cognitively based interventions (e.g., examining attributions and expectations) to increase communication and mutual problem-solving within the family as a whole. In well-controlled studies, both MST and FFT have shown to be effective in improving family communication and in lowering recidivism of youth with histories of minor delinquency as well as those with more serious behavior problems (Mihalic, Irwin, Elliott, Fagan & Hansen, 2001; Wasserman, Miller & Cothern, 2000).

---

[10] Because of its emphasis on care continuums, MST is frequently used to augment the OJJDP Comprehensive Strategy (Howell, 2003a; Sutphen, Thyer & Kurtz, 1995).

What Might Work

In terms of prevention, what might work raises issues similar to those reviewed in previous sections, especially in regard to strategies that account for certain gang-related migration patterns. Potentially successful approaches include the use of peer leaders to serve as anti-gang and anti-delinquency role models, especially in partnership with teachers who are charged with applying the curriculum (Howell, 2003a).[11] Other prevention approaches believed to be effective but not yet evaluated include Midnight Basketball, community service, and community enrichment programs (Gottfredson and Gottfredson, 2001; USDHHS, 2001).

A strategy that has shown mixed results is community policing. Because there are so many different versions of this approach (Peak & Glensor, 1999), it is not possible to present a coherent overview in this chapter. However, it appears that the most successful community police interventions have been those that support community resiliency efforts, did the most to build relationships between individual police officers and community residents, and used suppression only as a last-ditch option (Howell, 2003a).

What Does Not Work

Scare tactics, perhaps the most common approach to preventing adolescent gang behavior, simply do not work (Howell, 2003a). Viewed as pre-suppression tactics, their failure lends further support to our assertion that prevention and intervention must be incorporated into any successful anti-gang strategy. The failure of some generously funded and widely implemented programs support this assertion, the most famous being the *Drug Abuse Resistance Education* (D.A.R.E.) program. Its success is widely acclaimed despite an ever-increasing number of reports attesting to its ineffectiveness as a substance abuse prevention program.[12]

Zero-tolerance policies are social control policies grounded in a philosophy of deterrence. They encourage punishment for any infraction of codes of conduct on the part of children and adolescents. In terms of gang-related behaviors, such policies have been implemented to address drug use, vandalism, threatening speech, and gun crimes in communities throughout the United States, but especially in low-income neighborhoods (Curry & Decker, 2003; Stimmel, 1996). The ineffectiveness of zero-tolerance policies may be due to a combination of their close relationship with suppression strategies and their demand for immediate and severe punishment for every single infraction of codes, rules, and laws, which taxes overburdened community resources.

---

[11]The use of peer leaders without adult/teacher supervision has proven to be uniformly ineffective (Gottfredson & Gottfredson, 2001; Howell, 2003a).

[12]D.A.R.E. has grown into a $227-million/year enterprise that hires 50,000 police officers to teach its curriculum (Gottfredson & Gottfredson, 2001). Mixed results have been reported from at least 20 rigorous evaluations of the D.A.R.E. program (Howell, 2003a). The three most rigorous studies, each of which used a random design, were conducted by Clayton, Cattarello, and Johnstone (1996); Rosenbaum, Flewelling, Bailey, Ringwalt, and Wilkinson (1994); and Rosenbaum and Hanson (1998). The results of these studies showed conclusively that D.A.R.E. is ineffective in achieving its stated goals.

Recommendations

Recent surveys have underscored the general lack of successful gang prevention, intervention, or suppression programs in the United States (Howell, 2003a; Thornberry et al., 2003). Klein, Maxson, and Miller (1995) concluded that "much of our local response and most of our state and federal responses to gang problems are way off base—conceptually misguided, poorly implemented, half-heartedly pursued" (p. 19). We believe his assertion remains true today.

An extraordinary amount of time, effort, and money has been expended since Thrasher's (1927) initial explorations of the gang problem in America, and most researchers who have reviewed the enormous amount of available information have concluded that the problem can only be successfully controlled through a combination of prevention, intervention, and suppression (Egley, 2002; Howell, 2003a; Thornberry et al, 2003). Based on that conclusion, Howell (2003a) has developed what he refers to as a *Comprehensive Strategy Framework* (CSF)—an integrated approach to the adolescent gang issue that has been described as the "best practice" for dealing with the adolescent gang problem by the U. S. Department of Justice's Office of Juvenile Justice and Delinquency Prevention (OJJDP) (Egley, 2002).

The CSF is a two-tiered system for responding proactively to juvenile delinquency, crime, and gang behavior. In the first tier, prevention and early intervention programs are used to prevent and mitigate initial acts of delinquency. If these efforts fail, then the juvenile justice system (the second tier) must respond to delinquency by addressing the recidivism risk factors and treatment needs of adolescent gang members.

The CSF is based on the following principles:

- Families must be strengthened in terms of their primary responsibilities to instill moral values and to provide guidance and support to children. Where no functional family unit exists, it is imperative to establish family surrogates and to provide them with adequate resources for guiding and nurturing their charges.
- "Core" social institutions, such as schools, churches, and community organizations require additional support for their efforts in developing capable, mature, and responsible youth. The collective goal of these institutions should be to ensure that children have opportunities and support for becoming productive, law-abiding adults.
- When delinquent/gang behaviors occur, timely intervention is required to prevent first-time or very young offenders from becoming chronic offenders or committing more serious and violent crimes. Under an authoritative umbrella that includes police, intake, and probation agencies, initial intervention efforts should be established around family and other core societal institutions. In addition to ensuring appropriate responses, juvenile justice system authorities should act quickly and firmly when formal adjudication procedures and sanctions are required.
- Serious, violent, and chronic juvenile offenders who have committed felony offenses or who have failed to respond to intervention and nonsecure community-based treatment and rehabilitation services must be identified. Offenders who are considered threats to community safety may require placement in more secure community-based facilities (Howell, 2003a).

Unlike many other gang prevention and control programs, the CSF is research-based, data-driven, and outcome-focused. It is a framework that is based on decades of research findings and a synthesis of program evaluations; its focus is on empowering communities to assess their own gang problems and needs, then provide guidance for using the data to design and implement their own comprehensive strategies. The CSF was established on the premise that local ownership of programs and strategies breeds success (Tolan, Perry & Jones, 1987).

The CSF is considered "comprehensive" in the following respects:

- It encompasses the entire juvenile justice enterprise—prevention, intervention, and suppression—in the form of graduated sanctions.
- While it specifically targets serious, violent, and chronic offenders, it provides a framework for dealing with all juvenile offenders as well as at-risk children and adolescents.
- It calls for an integrated, multi-agency response to childhood and adolescent problems that promotes a unified effort on the part of the juvenile justice, mental health, child welfare, education, and law enforcement systems and community organizations.
- It links all juvenile justice system resources in an interactive manner, reflecting the belief that comprehensive juvenile justice is not a zero-sum game.
- It guides jurisdictions in developing response continuums that parallel offender and gang member careers, beginning with early intervention and followed by a combination of prevention and graduated sanctions. Such a continuum allows a community to organize an array of programs that corresponds to how gang member careers develop over time.

A continuum of programs aimed at specific points in a gang member's career or an at-risk adolescent's life course has a much better chance of succeeding than any single intervention. Programs are needed that address family risk factors during the preschool years; school-focused interventions are required from preschool through elementary school; and programs that buffer the exposure of adolescents to delinquent and gang peer influences are required during the junior and senior high school years. Prevention, intervention, and suppression strategies that counter individual, family, and community risk factors for joining gangs are clearly needed at all points of a young person's life course.

References

Alexander, J.F., Barton, C., Schiavo, R.S., & Parsons, B.V. (1976). System-behavioral intervention with families of delinquents: Therapist characteristics, family behavior and outcome. *Journal of Consulting and Clinical Psychology, 44*, 656–664.

Alexander, J.F., & Parsons, B.V. (1973). Short-term behavioral intervention with delinquent families: Impact of family process and recidivism. *Journal of Abnormal Psychology, 81*, 219–225.

Arbreton, A.J.A., & McClanahan, W. (2002). *Targeted Outreach: Boys and Girls Clubs of America's Approach to Gang Prevention and Intervention*. Philadelphia: Public/Private Ventures.

Baltes, P.B. (1987). Theoretical propositions of life-span developmental psychology: On the dynamics between growth and decline. *Developmental Psychology, 23*, 611–626.

Benard, B. (1991). *Fostering Resiliency in Kids: Protective Factors in the Family, School, and Community*. Portland, OR: Western Center for Drug-Free Schools and Communities.

Benard, B. (1999). Fostering resiliency in communities: An inside out process. In N. Henderson, B. Benard & N. Sharp-Light (Eds.) *Resiliency in Action*. San Diego, CA: Resiliency In Action.

Bjerregaard, B., & Lizotte, A.J. (1995). Gun ownership and gang membership. *Journal of Criminal Law and Criminology, 86*, 37–58.

Bjerregaard, B., & Smith, C. (1993). Gender differences in gang participation, delinquency, and substance use. *Journal of Quantitative Criminology, 9*, 329–355.

Borg, Jr., M.B. (2002). The Avalon Gardens Men's Association: A Community Health Psychology Case Study. *Journal of Health Psychology, 7*, 345–357.

Branch, C.W. (1997). *Clinical Interventions with Gang Adolescent and Their Families*. Boulder, CO: Westview Press.

Burns, B.J., Hoagwood, K., & Mrazek, P.J. (1999). Effective treatment for mental disorders in children and adolescents. *Clinical Child and Family Psychology Review, 2*, 199–254.

Catalano, R.F., & Hawkins, J.D. (1996). The social development model: A theory of antisocial behavior. In J.D. Hawkins (Ed.) *Delinquency and Crime: Current Theories* (pp. 149–197). New York: Cambridge University Press.

Clayton, R.R., Cattarello, A.M., & Johnstone, B. (1996). The effectiveness of D.A.R.E: 5-year follow-up results. *Preventive Medicine, 25*, 307–318.

Cocozza, J.J., & Skowyra, K. (2000). Youth with mental health disorders: Issues and emerging response. *Juvenile Justice, 7* (1), 3–13.

Cohen, L.E., & Vila, B.J. (1996). Self-control and social control: An exposition of the Gottfredson-Hirschi/Sampson-Laub debate. *Studies on Crime and Crime Prevention, 5*, 125–150.

Curry, G.D., & Decker, S.H. (2003). *Confronting Gangs: Crime and Community*. Los Angeles, CA: Roxbury.

De Felipe, C., Herrero, J.F., & O'Brien, J.A. (1998). Altered nociception, analgesia and aggression in mice lacking the receptor for substance P. *Nature, 392*, 394–397.

Deschenes, E.P., & Esbensen, F. (1999). Violence and gangs: Gender differences in perceptions and behaviors. *Journal of Quantitative Criminology, 15*, 63–96.

DiIulio, J. (1995). Arresting ideas. *Policy Review* (pp. 1–15). Washington, DC: Heritage.

Durlak, J.A. (1998). Common risk and protective factors in successful prevention programs. *Journal of Orthopsychiatry, 68*, 512–520.

Egley, A., Jr. (2002). *National Youth Gang Survey Trends from 1996 to 2000*. Washington, DC: Office of Juvenile Justice and Delinquency Prevention (OJJDP).

Egley, Jr, & Arjunan, M. (2002). *Highlights of the 2000 National Youth Gang Survey*. Washington, DC: OJJDP.

Egley, A., Jr., & Major, A.K. (2003). *Highlights from the 2001 National Youth Gang Survey*. Washington, DC: OJJDP.

Elder, G.H. (1985). Perspectives on the life course. In G.H. Elder (Ed.), *Life Course Dynamics* (pp. 23–49). Ithaca, NY: Cornell University Press.

Esbensen, F. (2000). *Preventing Adolescent Gang Involvement: Risk Factors and Prevention Strategies*. Washington, DC: OJJDP.

Esbensen, F., Huizinga, D., & Weiher, A.W. (1993). Gang and non-gang youth: Differences in explanatory variables. *Journal of Contemporary Criminal Justice, 9*, 94–116.

Esbensen, F., & Osgood, D.W. (1999). Gang Resistance Education and Training: Results from the national evaluation. *Journal of Research in Crime and Delinquency, 36*, 194–225.

Esbensen, F., Osgood, D.W., Taylor, T.J., Peterson, D., & Freng, A. (2001). How great is G.R.E.A.T.? Results from a longitudinal quasi-experimental design. *Criminology and Public Policy, 1*, 87–117.

Esbensen, F., & Winfree, L.T. (1998). Race and gender differences between gang and nongang youths: Results from a multisite survey. *Justice Quarterly, 15*, 505–526.

Fagan, J. (1996). Gangs, drugs, and neighborhood change. In C.R. Huff (Ed.), *Gangs in America* (2nd edition, pp. 39–74). Thousand Oaks, CA: Sage.

Farrington, D.P. (1993). *Protective Factors in the Development of Juvenile Delinquency and Adult Crime*. New York: Cambridge University Press.

Farrington, D.P. (2000). Explaining and preventing crime: The globalization of knowledge. *Criminology, 38*, 1–24.

Fava, M. (1997). Psychopharmacologic treatment of pathologic aggression. *Psychiatry Clinical North America, 20*, 427–451.

Foucault, M. (1977). *Discipline and Punish: The Birth of the Prison*. New York: Vintage.

Fromm, E. (1955). *The Sane Society*. London: Routledge and Kegan Paul.

Goldstein, A.P., & Huff, R.C. (Eds.) (1993). *The Gang Intervention Handbook*. Champaign, IL: Research Press.

Gottfredson, G.D., & Gottfredson, D.C. (2001). *Gang Problems and Gang Programs in a National Sample of Schools*. Ellicott City, MD: Gottfredson Associates.

Greenwood, P.W., Model, K.E., Rydell, C.P., & Chiesa, J. (1996). *Diverting Children from a Life of Crime: Measuring Costs and Benefits*. Santa Monica, CA: RAND.

Gullotta, T.P., & Bloom, M. (2003). Evolving definitions of primary prevention. In T.P. Gullotta & M. Bloom (Eds.), *Encyclopedia of Primary Prevention and Health Promotion* (pp. 9–15). New York: Kluwer Academic/Plenum Publishers.

Hagedorn, J.M. (1988). *People and Folks: Gangs, Crime and the Underclass in a Rustbelt City*. Chicago: Lakeview.

Hagedorn, J.M. (1994). Homeboys, dope fiends, legits, and new jacks. *Criminology, 32*, 197–217.

Hawkins, J.D., Catalano, R.F., & Miller, J.Y. (1992). Risk and protective factors for alcohol and other drug problems in adolescence and early adulthood: Implications for substance abuse prevention. *Psychological Bulletin, 112*, 64–105.

Hawkins, J.D., Herrenkohl, T.I., Farrington, D.P., Brewer, D.D., Catalano, R.F., Harachi, T.W., & Cothern, L. (2000). *Predictors of Youth Violence*. Washington, DC: OJJDP.

Henderson, N., Benard, B., & Sharp-Light, N. (Eds.) (1999). *Resiliency in Action*. San Diego, CA: Resiliency In Action.

Henggeler, S.W., Schoenwald, S.K., Bourduin, C.M., Rowland, M.D., & Cunningham, P.B. (1998). *Multisystemic Treatment of Antisocial Behavior in Children and Adolescents*. New York: Guilford.

Hill, K.G., Howell, J.C., Hawkins, J.D., & Battin-Pearson, S.R. (1999). Childhood risk factors for adolescent gang membership: Results from the Seattle Social Development Project. *Journal of Research in Crime and Delinquency, 36*, 300–322.

Horowitz, R. (1990). Sociological perspectives on gangs: Conflicting definitions and concepts. In R. Huff (Ed.), *Gangs in America* (pp. 37–54). Newbury Park, CA: Sage.

Howell, J.C. (1995). *Guide for Implementing the Comprehensive Strategy for Serious, Violent, and Chronic Juvenile Offenders*. Washington, DC: OJJDP.

Howell, J.C. (1997). *Youth Gangs*. Washington, DC: OJJDP.

Howell, J.C. (1999). Promising programs for youth gang violence prevention and intervention. In R. Loeber & D.P. Farrington (Eds.) *Serious and Violent Juvenile Offenders: Risk Factors and Successful Interventions* (pp. 284–312). Thousand Oaks, CA: Sage.

Howell, J.C. (2000). *Youth Gang Programs and Strategies*. Washington, DC: OJJDP.

Howell, J.C. (2003a). *Preventing and Reducing Juvenile Delinquency: A Comprehensive Framework*. Thousand Oaks, CA: Sage.

Howell, J.C. (2003b). Youth gangs: Prevention and intervention. In P. Allen-Meares & M.W. Fraser (Eds.), *Intervention with Children and Adolescents: An Interdisciplinary Perspective* (pp. 493–404). Boston, MA: Allyn & Bacon.

Howell, J.C., Egley, A., Jr., & Gleason, D.K. (2002). *Modern-Day Youth Gangs*. Washington, DC: OJJDP.

Howell, J.C., & Lynch, J. (2000). *Youth gangs in school*. Washington, DC: OJJDP.

Huff, C.R. (1998). *Comparing Criminal Behavior of Youth Gangs and At-Risk Youth*. Washington, DC: National Institute of Justice.

Jackson, L. (1998). *Gangbusters: Strategies for Prevention and Intervention*. Lanham, MD: American Correctional Association.

Jankowski, M. (1991). *Islands in the street: Gangs and American urban society*. Berkeley, CA: University of California Press.

Klein, M.W., Maxson, C.L., & Miller, J. (Eds.) (1995). *The Modern Gang Reader*. Los Angeles, CA: Roxbury.

Knox, G.W. (1995). *An Introduction to Gangs*. Bristol, IN: Wyndham Hall Press.

Krisberg, B., & Austin, J. (1993). *Reinventing Juvenile Justice*. Newbury Park, CA: Sage.

Krisberg, B., & Howell, J.C. (1999). The impact of juvenile justice system and prospects for graduated sanctions in a comprehensive strategy. In R. Loeber & D.P. Farrington (Eds.), *Serious and Violent Juvenile Offenders: Risk Factors and Successful Interventions* (pp. 346–366). Thousand Oaks: Sage.

Krohn, M.D. (1986). The web of conformity: A network approach to the explanation of delinquent behavior. *Social Problems, 33*, 581–593.

Krohn, M.D., Thornberry, T.P., Rivera, C., & Le Blanc, M. (2001). Later careers of very young offenders. In R. Loeber & D.P. Farrington (Eds.), *Child Delinquents: Development, Intervention, and Service Needs* (pp. 67–94). Thousand Oaks, CA: Sage.

Lahey, B.B., Gordon, R.A., Loeber, R., Stouthamer-Loeber, M., & Farrington, D.P. (1999). Boys who join gangs: A prospective study of first gang entry. *Journal of Abnormal Child Psychology, 27*, 261–276.

Le Blanc, M., & Lanctot, N. (1998). Social and psychological characteristics of gang members according to gang structure and its subcultural and ethnic makeup. *Journal of Gang Research, 5* (3), 15–28.

Leet, D.A., Rush, G.E., & Smith, A.M. (2000). *Gangs, Graffiti, and Violence: A Realistic Guide to the Scope and Nature of Gangs in America*. Cincinnati, OH: Copperhouse.

Lipsey, M.W., Wilson, D.B., & Cothern, L. (2000). *Effective Interventions for Serious and Violent Juvenile Offenders*. Washington, DC: OJJDP.

Lizotte, A.J., Krohn, M.D., Howell, J.C., Tobin, K., & Howard, G.J. (2000). Factors influencing gun carrying among young urban males over the adolescent-young adult life course. *Criminology, 38*, 811–834.

Lizotte, A.J., Tesoriero, J.M., Thornberry, T.P., & Krohn, M.D. (1994). Patterns of adolescent firearms ownership. *Justice Quarterly, 11,* 51–73.

Loeber, R., & Farrington, D.P. (Eds.) (1999). *Serious and Violent Juvenile Offenders: Risk Factors and Successful Interventions.* Thousand Oaks, CA: Sage.

Loeber, R., & Stouthamer-Loeber, M. (1986). Family factors as correlates and predictors of juvenile conduct problems and delinquency. In M.H. Tonry & N. Morris (Eds.), *Crime and Justice: An Annual Review of Research.* Chicago: University of Chicago Press.

Lopez, J.F., Vazqueuz, D.M., Chalmers, D.T., & Watson, S.J. (1997). Regulation of 5-HT receptors and the hypothalamic-pituitary-adrenal axis. *Annual of the New York Academy of Science, 836,* 106–134.

Lynn, D., & King, B.H. (2002). Aggressive behavior. In S. Kutcher (Ed.), *Practical Child and Adolescent Psychopharmacology* (pp. 305–327). Cambridge, UK: Cambridge University Press.

Lyon, J.M., Henggeler, S.W., & Hall, J.A. (1992). The family relations, peer relations, and criminal activities of Caucasian and Hispanic-American gang members. *Journal of Abnormal Child Psychology, 20,* 439–449.

MacKenzie, D.L. (2000). Evidence-based corrections: Identifying what works. *Crime & Delinquency, 46,* 457–471.

Majors, R., & Billson, M. (1992). *Cool Pose: The Dilemmas of Black Manhood in America.* New York: Lexington.

Maxson, C.L., Whitlock, M.L., Klein, M.W. (1998). Vulnerability to street gang membership: Implications for prevention. *Social Service Review, 72* (1), 70–91.

Miethe, T.D., & McCorkle, R.C. (1997). *Evaluating Nevada's Anti-Gang Legislation and Gang Prosecution Units.* Washington, DC: National Institute of Justice.

Mihalic, S., Irwin, K., Elliott, D., Fagan, A., Hansen, D. (2001). *Blueprints for Violence Prevention.* Washington, DC: OJJDP.

Miller, J., & Brunson, R.K. (2000). Gender dynamics in youth gangs: A comparison of male and female accounts. *Justice Quarterly, 17,* 419–448.

Mills, R.C. (1993). *The Health Realization Model: A Community Empowerment Primer.* Alhambra, CA: California School of Professional Psychology.

Mills, R.C., & Spittle, E. (2001). *The Wisdom Within.* Renton, WA: Lone Pine.

Moore, J.W. (1991). *Going Down to the Barrio: Homeboys and Homegirls in Change.* Philadelphia: Temple University Press.

Moore, J.W. (1998). Understanding youth street gangs: Economic restructuring and the urban underclass. In M.W. Watts (Ed.) *Cross-Cultural Perspectives on Youth and Violence* (pp. 65–78). Stamford, CT: JAI.

Murray, C., & Cox, L. (1979). *Beyond Probation.* Beverly Hills, CA: Sage.

Peak, K.J., & Glensor, R.W. (1999). *Community Policing and Problem Solving: Strategies and Practices.* Upper Saddle River, NJ: Prentice Hall.

Phillips, S.A. (1999). *Wallbangin': Graffiti and Gangs in L.A..* Chicago: University of Chicago Press.

Rappaport, J., & Seidman, E. (Eds.) (1986). *Redefining Social Problems.* New York: Plenum Press.

Reich, K., Culross, P.L., & Behrman, R.E. (2002). Children, youth and gun violence: Analysis and recommendations. *Future of Children, 12* (2), 5–19

Rhine, E. (1996). Something works: Recent research on effective correctional programming. *The State of Corrections: 1995 Proceedings.* Lanham, MD: American Correctional Association.

Rippon, T.J. (2000). Aggression and violence in the health care profession. *Advanced Nursing, 31,* 452–460.

Rosenbaum, D.P., Flewelling, R.L., Bailey, S.L., Ringwalt, C.L., & Wilkinson, D.L. (1994). Cops in the classroom: A longitudinal evaluation of D.A.R.E. *Journal of Research in Crime and Delinquency, 31,* 3–31.

Rosenbaum, D.P., & Hanson, G.S. (1998). Assessing the effects of school-based drug education: A six-year multilevel analysis of Project D.A.R.E. *Journal of Research in Crime and Delinquency, 35,* 381–412.

Rosenfeld, R., Bray, T.M., & Egley, A., Jr. (1999). Facilitating violence: A comparison of gang-motivated, gang-affiliated, and non-gang youth homicides. *Journal of Quantitative Criminology, 15,* 495–516.

Roy, S. (1995). Juvenile restitution and recidivism in a midwestern county. *Federal Probation, 59* (1), 55–62.

Sampson, R.J., & Laub, J. (1993). *Crime in the Making: Pathways and Turning Points through Life.* Cambridge, MA: Harvard University Press.

Short, J.F., Jr. (1990). New wine in old bottles? Change ands continuity in American gangs. In C.R. Huff (Ed.), *Gangs in America* (pp. 223–239). Newbury Park, CA: Sage.

Short, J.F., Jr. (1996). *Gangs and Adolescent Violence.* Boulder, CO: Center for the Study and Prevention of Violence.

Short, J.F., Jr., & Strodtbeck, F.L. (1965). *Group Process and Gang Delinquency.* Chicago: University of Chicago Press.

Sloan, T. (1996). *Damaged Life: The Crisis of the Modern Psyche*. London: Routledge.

Spergel, I.A., & Curry, G.D. (1995). The National Youth Gang Survey: A research and development process. In M.W. Klein, C.L. Maxson, & J. Miller (Eds.), *The Modern Gang Reader* (pp. 254–265). Los Angeles, CA: Roxbury.

Stimmel, B. (1996). *Drug Abuse and Social Policy in America*. New York: Haworth.

Starbuck, D., Howell, J.C., & Lindquist, D.J. (2001). *Hybrid and Other Modern Gangs*. Washington, DC: OJJDP.

Sutphen, R.D., Thyer, B.A., & Kurtz, P.D. (1995). Multisystemic treatment of high-risk juvenile offenders. *International Journal of Offender Therapy and Comparative Criminology, 39*, 329–334.

Taylor, C. (1990). *Dangerous Society*. East Lansing, MI: Michigan State University Press.

Thornberry, T.P., Krohn, M.D., Lizotte, A.J., Smith, C.A., & Tobin, K. (2003). *Gangs and Delinquency in Developmental Perspective*. Cambridge, UK: Cambridge University Press.

Thrasher, F. (1927). *The Gang: A Study of 1,313 Gangs in Chicago*. Chicago: University of Chicago Press.

Tolan, P.H., Perry, M.S., & Jones, T. (1987). Delinquency prevention: An example of consultation in rural community mental health. *American Journal of Community Psychology, 15*, 43–50.

Tremblay, R.E., & LeMarquand, D. (2001). Individual risk and protective factors. In R. Loeber & D.P. Farrington (Eds.), *Child Delinquents: Development, Intervention, and Service Needs* (pp. 137–164). Thousand Oaks, CA: Sage.

Tremblay, R.E., Masse, L., Pagani, L., & Vitaro, F. (1996). From childhood physical aggression to adolescent maladjustment: The Montreal Prevention Experiment. In R.D. Peters & R.J. McMahon (Eds.), *Preventing Childhood Disorders, Substance Abuse, and Delinquency* (pp. 268–298). Thousand Oaks, CA: Sage.

United States Department of Health and Human Services (2001). *Youth Violence: A Report of the Surgeon General*. Rockville, MD: USDHHS.

Vigil, J.D. (1983). Chicano gangs: One response to Mexican urban adaptation in the Los Angeles area. *Urban Anthropology, 12*, 45–75.

Vigil, J.D. (1988). *Barrio Gangs: Street Life and Identity in Southern California*. Austin, TX: University of Texas Press.

Vigil, J.D. (2002). *A Rainbow of Gangs: Street Cultures in the Mega-City*. Austin, TX: University of Texas Press.

Walker-Barnes, C.J., & Mason, C.A. (2001). Ethnic differences in the effect of parenting on gang involvement and gang delinquency: A longitudinal, hierarchical linear modeling perspective. *Child Development, 72*, 1814–1831.

Wasserman, G.A., Miller, L.S., & Cothern, L. (2000). *Prevention of Serious and Violent Juvenile Offending*. Washington, DC: OJJDP.

Weithorn, L.A. (1988). Mental hospitalization of troublesome youth: An analysis of skyrocketing admission rates. *Stanford Law Review, 40*, 773–838.

Wyrick, P.A. (2000). *Vietnamese Youth Gang Involvement*. Washington, DC: OJJDP.

Zizek, S. (2002). *Welcome to the Desert of the Real*. London: Verso.

Chapter 25

Homicide

Michael J. Furlong, Vanessa M. Nyborg, and Jill D. Sharkey

Introduction

ALBANY, NY (Troy Record)—**Teen Pleads Guilty in Death of Infant.** A 16-year-old girl was arrested on felony charges of criminally negligent homicide in connection with the death of her newborn daughter. The arrest comes after a two-month joint investigation conducted by Colonie Police, the Albany County District Attorney's Office and the Albany County Coroner's Office and culminates with a pathology report that claims King unintentionally had played a part in her baby's death. According to the report, the baby suffered from a "severe infection," which already compromised her chances of survival at birth and the alleged failure on King's part to immediately call an ambulance further contributed to the infant's death. It wasn't until the teenager's mother came home and saw blood on her daughter that emergency medical services was called. In fact, the girl's parents didn't even know their daughter was pregnant until they saw the dead child in the girl's bedroom. McDermott also thinks the report shows that King unintentionally wrapped the child in towels in a way that caused the baby to struggle for air.

The incidence of adolescents committing homicide is alarming for any society because of the social, economic, and cultural damage it causes. Whenever these acts occur, societies pause to consider why a youth at a stage of life that should involve self-discovery and exploration felt the need to murder. Though a relatively rare event, adolescent homicide has significant implications for society in terms of the care and treatment of its children. This chapter examines historical trends in adolescent homicide, what is known about adolescents who commit homicide, and prevention programs designed to reduce homicide and behavior leading to its outcome.

Homicide is the act of unlawfully killing another human being, a definition that differentiates acts of homicide from legally sanctioned killing, such as capital punishment or deaths caused by war or death due to reckless or unintentional acts. In the United States, murder is the most heinous crime one can commit; however, not all people who kill are the most persistently dangerous or violent criminals, because about 20% of all homicides involve intimates (spouse, kin, or dating relationship) and are not part of a broader pattern of criminal behavior (U.S. Department of Justice, 2000). However, the penalties and lack of rehabilitation efforts for even the youngest perpetrator of homicide are far more significant than for any other crime. Because people and societies differ in their perceptions of violence and their acceptance of it, this chapter focuses primarily on homicide committed in the United States, which is ranked third behind sub-Saharan Africa and Latin America in world rankings in 1990 (Mercy & Hammond, 1999).

In the absence of significant social unrest, conflict, or war, adolescent homicides should be rare events—as they are in most industrialized countries. However, as with homicides in general, the adolescent homicide rate in the United States far exceeds that of any other modern industrial nation. For example, in 1993, the overall homicide rate per 100,000 for ages 15–24 in the USA was 15.3 compared to 3.1 in Canada and 0.4 in Japan (McGonigal, 2001). This pattern holds for adolescents aged 10–17—in 1993, for example, 7% of homicides in Canada were attributed to adolescents, compared to 14% in the United States (Heide, 2000). During the late 1980s and early 1990s, the adolescent homicide rate increased dramatically in the USA across all youth ages 14 to 17 (see Figure 1). African American youth during that time period were ten ten times more likely to be victims of homicide according to the Centers for Disease Control (Whitaker, 2000). Overall, these increases were associated with the use of firearms (the availability of which distinguished the United States from other nations) and homicides of known acquaintances and strangers (Snyder & Sickmund, 1999).

Between 1993 and 1999 adolescent homicide arrests in the United States decreased by 68% (Snyder, 2000). Putting these figures into perspective, in 1999, there were about 1,400 juveniles (aged 10–17) arrested for homicide in the USA, which compares to 3,800 in 1993. Arrests of juveniles for homicide were about 5 per 100,000, the lowest level since 1980 (Snyder, 2000). Much of this decline was due to substantial decreases among African American males.

Homicide is the second-leading cause of death for people aged 10–19. In 1999, a total of 1,797 youth under the age of 18 were murdered (Department of Justice, 2002).

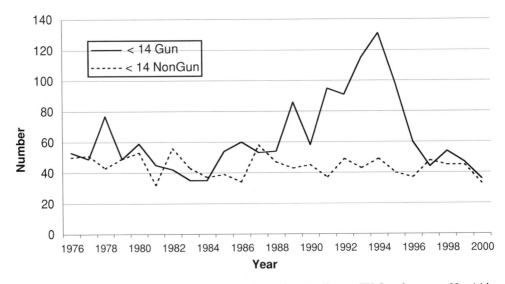

Figure 1. Annual number of homicides for youth aged 14 and under. (Source: FBI, Supplementary Homicide Reports, 1976–2000. Retrieved December 4, 2003, from http://www.ojp.usdoj.gov/bjs/homicide/homtrnd .htm.)

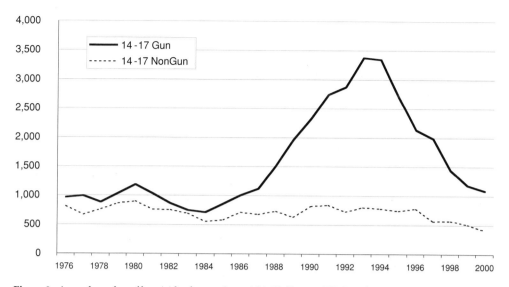

Figure 2. Annual number of homicides for youth aged 14–17. (Source: FBI, Supplementary Homicide Reports, 1976–2000. Retrieved December 4, 2003, from http://www.ojp.usdoj.gov/bjs/homicide/homtrnd.htm.)

In 2000, that number was 1,574. Nearly one in four murders of juveniles involved a juvenile offender. There is a large increase when moving to the 18–24-year-old category (DOJ, 2002). With regard to offenders, in 1999, 1,168 youth under the age of 18 were known murder offenders (DOJ, 2002). In 2000, that number was 1,006. Again, the largest increase is among the 18–24-year-old category.

It is important to consider the circumstances in which a homicide was committed when examining causes, correlates, and potential interventions for youth at-risk

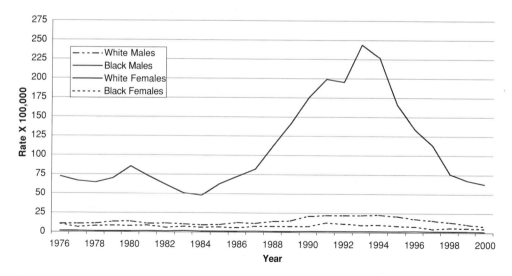

Figure 3. Annual homicide rate per 100,000 by gender and race for youth aged 14–17. (Source: FBI, Supplementary Homicide Reports, 1976–2000. Retrieved December 4, 2003, from http://www.ojp.usdoj.gov/bjs/homicide/homtrnd.htm.)

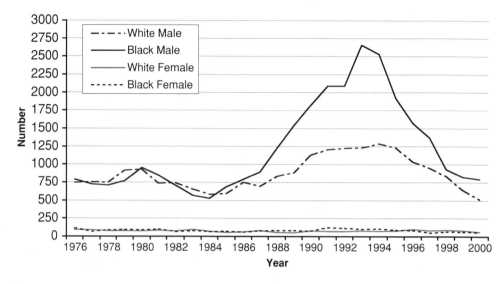

Figure 4. Annual number of homicides by gender and race for youth aged 14–17. (Source: FBI, Supplementary Homicide Reports, 1976–2000. Retrieved December 4, 2003, from http://www.ojp.usdoj.gov/bjs/homicide/homtrnd.htm.) http://www.fbi.gov/ucr/02cius.htm (2002 data); http://www.fbi.gov/ucr/01cius.htm (2001 data); other data from http://www.ojp.usdoj.gov/bjs/homicide/homtrnd.htm.)

to commit homicide. The number of homicides in which the circumstances were unknown has tripled since 1976 (DOJ, 2002). Homicides resulting from arguments have declined since 1976, but remain the most frequently cited, whereas murders involving gang violence has increased more than sixfold since 1976. Homicide circumstances of those under 18 include

- 32.8% gang related
- 15.6% felony murder
- 12.0% drug related
- 10.9% sex related
- 6.9% Argument
- 5.1% Workplace

Individual Factors

ALEXANDRIA, VA (AP)—**'Good,' White Teens Clash, too.** Alexandria police are investigating the beating death of a T.C. Williams High School junior. Investigators said several teenagers attacked Schuyler Jones, 16, but they think the attack was unplanned and unrelated to gang violence. Two Fairfax County teenagers will be tried as adults, but the case against the 17-year-old who police say orchestrated the attack will remain in juvenile court. The 17-year-old had a long-standing dispute with Jones, police said.

Developmental Pathways

Through longitudinal studies, researchers have described the development pathways of boys' delinquent behavior. Youth manifest antisocial behavior by engaging in less serious behaviors at early ages, persisting in these behaviors as they grow up, and later accelerate into more serious antisocial behaviors. In addition, only a small number of youth that begin along an antisocial pathway end up reaching its advanced stages (Kelley, Loeber, Keenan & DeLamatre, 1997). Older teens have the highest homicide victimization and offending rates (DOJ, 2002). The victimization rate for 14–17-year-olds has increased almost 150% from 1985 to 1993.

Though not focused specifically on youth who commit homicide, a number of theories provide information about how a child develops antisocial or violent behavior (youth may commit serious aggravated assaults that do not result in the death of the victim). Kelley and colleagues (1997) describe a developmental pathway model in which boys move along toward increasingly deviant behaviors in three distinct but related ways. The *overt* pathway includes those youth most likely to commit homicide. Youth enter the overt pathway at a young age through bullying peers and picking on others. These lower-level physical behaviors move into physical fighting, which in turn can lead to other violence such as rape, assault, and homicide. In this pathway, boys most likely to reoffend are those with multiple offenses, who begin at an early age, and whose severity of offenses increases over time. Patterson, Reid, and Dishion (1992) also offer a theory of delinquency centered on stages of development. In their model, poor parenting practices such as lack of management skills, ineffective discipline, and lack of monitoring promotes coercive and manipulative ways of responding to the world. When such a child reaches school age, his or her abrasive manner of interpersonal interaction leads to peer rejection. In addition, the child learns to use coercive techniques to avoid challenging tasks. As the child grows more alienated from peers and school, their natural tendency is to seek out similar peers with whom they continue antisocial behaviors, including truancy, substance abuse, and increasingly more delinquent behaviors. In this model, family factors, emotional functioning, academic performance, and substance abuse are all factors correlated with antisocial behaviors, including violence toward others.

Empirically Identified Factors Associated with Youth Who Kill

Lipsey and Derzon (1998) provide a review through synthesis of predictors of serious and violent offenses from longitudinal research studies. They found that variables differed depending on age at assessment. For offenders between the ages of 6 and 11, committing a general offense ($r = .38$) and substance use ($r = .30$) were the strongest predictors of future serious and violent offending. For offenders between the ages of 12 and 14, lack of social ties ($r = .39$), antisocial peers ($r = .37$), and committing a general offense ($r = .26$) were the strongest predictors of later serious and violent offending. Additional factors are positively correlated with subsequent offending. Within the realm of antisocial behavior, physical violence, aggression, person crimes, problem behavior, and substance use were identified as predictors. Personal characteristics included having a low IQ, poor school attitude and performance, and psychological conditions such as high activity level, impulsiveness, and psychopathology.

An analysis of 112 juveniles who committed murder revealed that around 43% had significant school problems and 9% were previously diagnosed with a learning disorder (Darby, Allan, Kashani, Hartke & Reid, 1998). Additionally, 30% had been evaluated prior to the crime by a mental health professional and 6% had been psychiatrically hospitalized prior to the offense. A history of aggressive behavior was common among the majority of the youth and 67.9% had previous contact with the authorities (Darby et al., 1998). Alcohol and illegal drug use were also common.

Homicides committed by adolescents are rare outside the United States and studies are often based on case examples. Nevertheless, it is important to examine factors associated with juveniles who commit homicide in other countries in order to have a broad understanding of this phenomenon. One study examined the characteristics of samples of adolescent murderers. Busch, Zagar, Hughes, Arbit, and Bussell (1990) compared a sample of 71 English adolescents convicted of homicide to 71 non-violent adjudicated adolescents. They found that the homicide-convicted group were more likely to (a) have a criminally violent family member (58% vs. 20%), (b) be involved in a youth gang (41% vs. 14%), (c) abuse alcohol (38% vs. 24%), and (d) have general cognitive ability test scores two standard deviations below the mean (21% vs. 10%). In a study of 72 adolescents from the United States, Cornell, Benedek, and Benedek (1987) compared homicide perpetrators to a separate group of non-violent delinquents. The juveniles arrested for homicide were a diverse group with no clear, single behavior pattern. Interestingly, the non-violent juvenile offenders had the most at-risk profile with the poorest mental health status. Other studies have examined adolescent violent offending as part of a developmental process and these studies offer additional insights about the etiological processes and accompanying prevention strategies for youthful homicide offenders.

Gender

Most victims and offenders are male (DOJ, 2002). Males were 3.2 times more likely than females to be murdered in 2000. Males were 10 times more likely to commit murder in 2000:

- Male offender/male victim   65%
- Male offender/female victim   25%
- Female offender/male victim   7.2%
- Female offender/female victim   2.6%

Although males most often commit violent offenses, recent studies show that female violence is increasing (Bilchik, 1999a). Research on female perpetrators indicates differences in the types of and motivations for homicide between boys and girls. Females are more likely to commit murder as a result of an argument or murder by poison (DOJ, 2002). Loper and Cornell (1996) analyzed data from homicide reports collected between 1984 and 1993 by the FBI in order to investigate this difference. Offense patterns indicate that girls mostly victimized family members, with 54% being infant offspring, and 24% being a parent. In contrast, only 8% of boys' victims were family members. When compared to boys, girls used a firearm significantly less frequently (32.2% vs. 82.3%). Girls were also involved more often in conflict-related homicides (79.3%) than crime-related homicides (20.7%). In contrast, boys were more often involved in crime-related homicides (57.3%) than conflict-related homicides (42.7%). Boys were also more likely to kill someone of the same gender (86%) than were girls (42%). These results point to extreme levels of emotional angst being experienced by girls who commit homicide and highlight the need for gender-specific prevention programs. Unfortunately, much of the research on preventing such violence has focused mainly on males. Programs teaching coping skills and the management of stressful life circumstances such as teen pregnancy may be warranted (Loper & Cornell, 1996).

Ethnicity

Homicide is the leading cause of death for African Americans aged 15–24 and the second-leading cause for Hispanics aged 15–24. Young black males continue to be disproportionately represented in both homicide victimization and offending numbers (CDC, 2002). Based on data from 1998, a 15-year-old urban African American male faces a probability of being murdered before reaching his 45th birthday that ranges from 8.5% in DC to 2.0% in Brooklyn, NY (Davis & Muhlhausen, 2000). By contrast, the death rate for U.S. soldiers in WWII was 2.5% and 1.2% during the Vietnam War.

Family Factors

PHOENIX, AZ (AP)—**Teen Arrested for Murder of Reds' Stenson** A 19-year-old man has been arrested on suspicion of homicide, robbery and kidnapping in the death of Cincinnati Reds outfielder Dernell Stenson, and police are seeking another suspect. Stenson's body was found in a street in the Phoenix suburb of Chandler early Wednesday after a night out with some teammates from the Arizona Fall League. He had been shot, then run over and apparently dragged some distance by his own SUV. Riddle's half brother Kevin Riddle, 43, was found driving Stenson's SUV about two hours after the body was discovered, and he was booked for investigation of possession of stolen property, police said.

Family characteristics include antisocial and abusive parents, poverty, and parent–child relationships characterized by low supervision, low warmth, and punitive discipline (Lipsey & Derzon, 1998). One review of the empirical research literature found that a family history of criminal behavior, substance abuse, family management problems, family conflict, and parental attitudes supporting criminal behavior and substance use were related to youth violence (Kashani et al., 1999). Other familial factors included modeling of aggressive behavior by parents, overly harsh parental discipline, insufficient monitoring, and low warmth. Furthermore, adolescents who were abused as children commit more violence than those who were not and those youth growing up in homes with multiple forms of violence (i.e., spousal abuse and child abuse) commit higher rates of violent offenses than youth coming from homes with less violence (Kashani et al., 1999).

An analysis of 112 juveniles who committed homicide revealed that few had parents who were married, many of their family members (e.g., father, mother, sibling) had been previously convicted of a crime, and drug use was fairly common among their family members (Darby et al., 1998). Moreover, youth who were abused by a family member tended to be white, younger, and were more likely to experience suicidal ideation or attempt suicide prior to the commission of the homicide (Darby et al., 1998). Females who committed homicide were more likely to report abuse than males (Darby et al., 1998).

Parricides

Parricide, which is the murder of a parent or close relative, accounts for about 2% of all homicides (Hillbrand et al., 1999). Offenders are usually white, middle-class males without a history of prior criminal offense. Parricides usually involve a single-victim: fathers outnumber mothers as the target 2:1. Precipitating risk factors leading to parricide include severe abuse, family, and community ignorance or denial of the abuse, and presence of guns (Hillbrand et al., 1999).

In a review of 10 studies that examined adolescents who had killed their parents, Heide (1993) discusses three types of parricide offenders: the severely abused child, the severely mentally ill child, and the dangerously antisocial child. Adolescent parricide offenders do include those who are severely mentally ill or dangerously antisocial, but in smaller frequencies compared to severely abused children. Components of child maltreatment pervasive in some families that also may lead to parricide are physical, sexual, emotional, and verbal abuse, and physical, medical, and emotional neglect. She asserts that ascertaining the driving force behind a parricide is complex, but factors in the family that often contribute to the homicides include a pattern of violence, easy access to guns, and alcoholism or heavy drinking. Adolescent offenders expressed helplessness in coping with stress in the home and feelings of isolation and suicidal ideation. They had failed in their attempts to get help with little (if any) adult intervention, and had failed in their efforts to escape, with a history of running away (Heide, 1993).

Infanticide

Rates of infanticide, which is the killing of an infant, have increased in the United States over the past 25 years. Parents or close family members commit the majority of child homicides (Pritchard & Butler, 2003). In the United States, between 1974 and 1999, there was a 78% increase in male baby, and a 44% increase in female baby, homicides. Changes in the infant homicide rates are indicative of increased family pathology such as family discord, teen pregnancy, poverty, and drug abuse. Hypotheses about why rates of child homicide have increased in the United States, but not in other countries, focus on increased poverty among vulnerable families and that child protective services are less able to prevent such problems (Pritchard & Butler, 2003).

Neonaticide, which is murder of an infant in the first 24 hours of life, is a rare crime that is not well understood, but often has a specific related circumstance such as unplanned pregnancy, shame, rejection, economic hardship, or age of the parent(s) (Schwartz & Isser, 2001). Neonaticide is more likely when a woman neither expects, nor understands her pregnancy. Consequences for such a crime are varied, often depending on evidence available to press charges. It is most likely that a parent who kills a newborn child will be sentenced to jail. As with other types of homicide, psychotherapeutic programs and psychiatric therapy are rarely provided. In the case of neonaticide, long-term imprisonment does not act as a deterrent and is in most cases unnecessary for preventing future acts of homicide (Schwartz & Isser, 2001). Rather, it is argued that a therapeutic intervention would most efficiently and successfully prevents the future incidence of such a crime. Two primary preventions for neonaticide are pregnancy education and prevention and that every pregnant mother receives adequate medical and psychological prenatal care (Schwartz & Isser, 2001).

Social and Community Factors

MIDDLETON, WI (AP)—**Teen Accused Of Killing Middleton Jogger 'Ordinary Kid'.**
Authorities said the Middleton High School graduate ate hallucinogenic mushrooms
and smoked pot with friends Saturday while celebrating his birthday and then "freaked
out," and tried to drive home. On the way, he allegedly hit and killed a jogger. The student faces more than 90 years in prison after being charged with multiple counts, including first degree-reckless homicide.

Gangs

Gang-related activities markedly contribute to the incidence of adolescent homicide. Nationally, one-quarter of the victims of gang-related killings are under age 18
(DOJ, 2002). In Los Angeles County in 1998, gangs played a role in almost 80% of
adolescent homicides (Bilchik, 1999a). In addition, only five communities in the United
States (Los Angeles, Chicago, Houston, Detroit, and New York), all with a significant
gang presence, accounted for 25% of all known juvenile homicide offenders in 1997
(Loeber, Farrington & Waschbusch, 1998). Moreover, the incidence of gang violence
involving guns has increased after 1980 (DOJ, 2002). Programs aimed at decreasing
rates of homicide must consider gang influences and develop unique treatments to
intervene with this population.

School-Associated Homicides

Although school-associated violent deaths represent less than 1% of all homicides
and suicides that occur among school-aged children (CDC, 2002), the 2003–2004
school year for the nation's public schools had seen 18 violent deaths by the end of
October. This shows an increase from the previous two school years. Although more
violence prevention funds were initially given following the 9–11 incident, this
funding has dropped by 41%. David Osher notes, "an increased emphasis on academic skills is putting children at risk because schools often ignore their social and
emotional needs" (Toppo, 2003). Most school-associated violent deaths occur at the
start of the school day, during lunch period, or at the end of the school day (CDC,
2002). More than 6% of high school students surveyed had carried a weapon during
the preceding 30 days (CDC, 2002). Of the 28 school shootings that took place
between 1982 and 2001, twenty took place in states that voted Republican in the last
presidential election, states which are more "gun friendly" (Kimmel & Mahler, 2003).
Kimmel and Mahler (2003) note that all but two two of the shootings were perpetrated by white males with a history of being constantly bullied, beat up, teased, and
threatened by their peers.

Firearms

Homicides are most often committed with guns, especially handguns (DOJ,
2002). In 1999, a total of 82% of homicide victims 15–19 years old were killed with
a handgun. A majority of United States juvenile homicide victims are killed with
a firearm, with percentages ranging from 79% to 83% in various communities

(Bilchik, 1999a). In a Los Angeles survey of adolescent males living in high-risk neighborhoods, 25% of youth surveyed indicated that they knew several places to get a gun in their neighborhood, and 7% indicated that they could secure one in less than an hour (Bilchik, 1999a).

A review of the literature on firearm availability and homicide found that individuals in households with guns are at a markedly higher risk for homicide victimization, especially from family, intimates, and acquaintances (Hepburn & Hemenway, 2004). The review notes that individuals who carry guns are more prone to binge drink and act aggressively and inappropriately. Of particular relevance, the association of handgun sales with homicides was stronger for younger males than older males. Compared to other high-income countries, the United States firearm rate was 11 times higher than that of all other countries and its female homicide rate was five times higher (Hepburn & Hemenway, 2004). Within the United States, even after controlling for poverty, unemployment, alcohol consumption, urbanization and crime levels, for both genders, and for age, states with more guns experience significantly higher homicide rates (Hepburn & Hemenway, 2004). The combination of easy access to firearms and their pivotal role in homicides makes gun accessibility an important issue in considering how to reduce homicide rates.

Alcohol and Substances

Alcohol availability and advertising are disproportionately concentrated in ethnic minority communities (Alaniz, 1998; Scribner et al., 1995). In one study, alcohol availability was examined by city block groupings (one block grouping = four city blocks; these were considered to be a "neighborhoods"). Alcohol availability was measured by counting the number of bars and liquor stores in each neighborhood. Whites accounted for 53% of the population and only two of their "neighborhoods" had a concentration of alcohol outlets. By contrast, Latinos accounted for 29% of the population and 29 of their "neighborhoods" were found to have high concentrations of alcohol availability. African Americans accounted for only 4% of the population but 13 of their neighborhoods had a high concentration of alcohol availability. Vietnamese accounted for 13% of the population and a high concentration of alcohol availability was found in nine of their "neighborhoods" (Alaniz, Cartmill & Parker, 1998).

Research has shown a relationship between alcohol availability, consumption, and violence in these communities. In neighborhoods with no alcohol outlets the arrest rate for Latino youth was 1.19 per 1,000 compared to 2.67 arrests per 1,000 for neighborhoods with at least one, and there were 18.67 arrests per 1,000 for neighborhoods with the highest concentration of alcohol outlets (Alaniz et al., 1998). Among African Americans the homicide rate was 24% higher in a neighborhood with two liquor stores compared to a neighborhood with one (Scribner et al., 1995). Moreover, the alcohol marketed in these communities comes in the form of high-alcohol content, large products (e.g., 40- or 64-oz. malt liquor), and have cheaper prices (Wallace, 1999).

An examination of the Pittsburgh Youth Study found that a substantial number of youth report being under the influence when committing illegal acts (White et al., 2002). Around 42% percent of adolescents reported being under the influence when engaged in gang fighting, 37% when they've attacked another person, and 49% when strong-arming another person. Aggressive offenses were more often related to alcohol than marijuana use. Heavy alcohol and drug users were more serious offenders, were more impulsive, and had more deviant peers (White et al., 2002).

Exposure to Violence

Bell and Jenkins (1993) assert that community violence occurs in a public way. They cite that in Chicago over half of the city's homicides occurred in a public area (i.e., street, park). Consistent with this, studies of children living in central cities have found increasing levels of exposure to violence. In one study, African American students between the ages of 10 to 19 from Chicago's south side reported on their encounters with violence (Uehara, Chalmers, Jenkins, & Shakoor, 1996). Seventy-four percent of the respondents reported having witnessed a robbery, shooting, stabbing, and/or killing. Forty-seven percent of victim types represented people known to the respondents (i.e., friends, family, classmates, or neighbors). Of those victims that were known to the respondent, 77.5% were subject to extreme forms of violence (i.e., robbed, shot, stabbed, or raped). Almost half of the respondents reported that they have been victims of at least one form of violent crime, such as robbery, having a knife or gun pulled on them, being shot, or being raped. Furthermore, 32.6% reported that they currently carry a weapon. This study found overlap between participants in violence and witnessing violence (86%). There was also overlap in the number of victims who have witnessed violence (84%). Carrying a weapon was also significantly associated with witnessing violence.

Guerra, Huesmann, and Spindler (2003) found that exposure to community violence increases children's aggressive behavior and normative beliefs supporting aggression. A related study found that recent exposure to community violence along with a history of receiving traumatic news, direct victimization in the community, and associations with deviant peers increase the risk for criminal offending among young adults (Eitle & Turner, 2002). Moreover, male respondents were more likely than females to report violent victimizations and the prevalence was substantially greater for African Americans.

In his work, Garbarino (1995) has found many similarities between children growing up in war zones around the world and the experiences of American children growing up amid chronic community violence. Some of the similarities between the two groups of children are as follows:

- In both, gangs offer some sense of belonging, security, and solidarity in a hostile world.
- Women, particularly mothers, are in a desperate situation. They are under enormous amounts of stress and have few economic resources.
- Children and youth have diminished prospects for the future. This lack of a positive future orientation produces depression, rage, and disregard for human life.

Evidence-Based Treatment Interventions

SAN ANTONIO, TX (San Antonio Express)—**Teen to be tried as adult in deaths.** A judge Friday ordered a 16-year-old boy facing capital murder charges to be tried as an adult for shooting and killing a mother and her teenage son during a car robbery in February at a South Side apartment. Ramos has a limited mental capacity and was designated as a special education student, Ugarte argued. Ramos was on probation for a previous crime when he allegedly committed double homicide.

What Works

Evidence-based treatment interventions for juveniles who commit homicide do not currently exist. As will be discussed further below, most often youth are sentenced to a correctional facility.

What Might Work

In terms of what might work, Bilchik (1999b) emphasized the importance of transitioning from individual programs to more broadly focused programs. He also recommended a revitalized system that not only holds youth accountable for crime, but helps change their path towards a positive direction (Bilchik, 1998). This occurs through his three stated goals for the juvenile justice system (a), accountability; (b) enabling capability, productivity, and responsibility; and (c) protecting the community. Clearly, this must be a community-wide effort supported by legislators. Bilchik (1998) suggests that interventions be consistent, efficient, and appropriate by including (a) assessment, (b) a range of treatment services, and (c) increasingly severe sanctions and intensive treatment. Unique programs should be tailored to different clusters of crime (e.g., sex offenders, gang members, drugs, racial, females, disabilities). Finally, intensive aftercare services are necessary to monitor and treat juveniles, and to integrate offenders successfully into the community where they can become productive citizens.

What Does Not Work

Most often juveniles who murder are sentenced to severe penalties such as life in jail or the death penalty (Whitaker, 2000). These youth generally do not receive the mental health services they require given the prevalence of psychiatric disability among the population (Crespi, & Rigazio-DiGillo, 1996). Related to society's reaction to such a heinous crime, there is often no differentiation in sentence based on type of crime committed, even when circumstances differ drastically from retaliation against an abusive parent to open fire upon a group of school children.

Prison costs more than $20,000 per year per individual, where inmates experience and commit a variety of hateful violent crimes (Whitaker, 2000). Arguments for life imprisonment include protecting society from harm and deterring others from committing a similar crime. Though the increase in numbers of individuals incarcerated has been dramatic, the crime rate has not gone down. According to Whitaker, the death penalty costs approximately $20 million per case and does not act as a deterrent to perpetrators. Furthermore, race of the victim appears to affect the decision to apply the death penalty. Though African Americans account for half of all murder victims, only 11% of executed murderers from 1977 to 2000 had victimized an African American, whereas 85% murdered a European American. Finally, between 1980 and 1995, the prison population of California rose from 23,5111 to 126,140, and more funds were allocated to prisons than to the University of California system.

Psychopharmacology

SHEBOYGAN, WI (Sheboygan Press)—**Teen talked of prophesy, aliens.** A 19-year-old accused of murdering his father and shooting a police officer told police he was embarking on a personal war against the world related to a prophesy placed on the Internet by aliens. Jason B. Larson, charged with murdering his father and with five counts of attempted homicide, told police he suffers from schizophrenia. He was placed in The Crisis Center—a group home for people with mental-health issues—a month ago after attempting to castrate himself, police said. He told police about a Catholic prophesy he read on the Internet years ago in which the Virgin Mary is supposed to resurrect herself and expose Satan, the report said. He said he didn't believe the prophesy, because it was written by aliens, and that the Virgin Mary actually would become the anti-Christ. Because of his belief, someone would try to kill him unless he waged war in the world, the report said. Larson told police he killed his father to get possession of his father's guns, so he could use the weapons in his war. He said his personal war against the world would continue until God told him what to do, according to authorities.

Given that those who commit homicide may have comorbid mental health disorders, medication is important in the managing of symptoms. In looking at the intersection of violence and metal illness, researchers note that co-occurring substance abuse is perhaps the most important mechanism linking the two (Swartz et al., 1998). They note that the combination of medication noncompliance and substance abuse was the strongest predictor of serious violent behavior in an adult psychiatric population. Individuals who abused alcohol and substances were at the highest risk for violence (Swartz et al., 1998).

In their examination of Prozac in the reduction of aggressive behavior, Barratt and Slaughter (1998) found that it significantly reduced verbal and indirect impulsive aggression against objects, but it did not reduce aggression toward others.

Yarvis (1990) argues that the psychiatric health of an individual is the foundation of functioning that mediates all other factors affecting the risk of committing an act of homicide. Studies have found varying rates of psychopathy among samples of killers, including schizophrenia, substance abuse, antisocial personality disorders, and dissociative reaction. In his own study, Yarvis found a far higher degree of axis I and axis II conditions among 100 California murders that in a community sample. Of the total sample of murders, 86% had an axis I disorder, including substance abuse conditions (35%), schizophrenia (21%), conduct disorder (4%), sexual sadism (3%), and mental retardation (2%). In addition, 74% had axis II disorders, including antisocial disorder (38%), borderline disorder (18%), and paranoia (5%). Though there were not many different axis I and axis II diagnoses found among all the participants, the distribution of diagnoses appeared to differ based on several factors, including circumstances of the crime, gender, prior criminal history, and relationship to the victim. Results indicated that treating psychosis would potentially prevent some types of homicide, such as female murderers, and men who know their victims, but not other types, such as those who commit robberies and rapes involving strangers. Results indicate that pharmacological interventions for psychiatric diagnoses are warranted in many cases, and the particular intervention would depend on the particular psychiatric diagnosis.

The Prevention of Homicide

ST. PAUL, MN (Pioneer Press)—**Girl, 14, Kills Infant** A 14-year-old St. Paul, MN, girl secretly gave birth at home, strangled her newborn baby and hid the body in a shoebox, authorities said Friday. Police said the teen became pregnant during a relationship with a 22-year-old man. She apparently delivered the baby girl at home Thursday, then used a sock to strangle the infant. The girl's family reportedly told investigators they were unaware of the pregnancy. The case marks the third time in the past three months that a young child has died at the hands of a parent in St. Paul. Minnesota is one of 44 states with a program that allows mothers to legally drop off unwanted infants at any hospital with no questions asked.

What Works

In a time of continuing concern about serious and chronic youth violence, it is crucial to identify general treatment approaches as well as prevention programs that show evidence of success and promise. Research in this area has attempted to pinpoint common elements within successful programs that can reduce serious and chronic youth violence (e.g., Catalano, Loeber & McKinney, 1999; Centers for Disease Control and Prevention, 2000; Tolan & Guerra, 1998). Although research has identified various characteristics found in effective intervention programs, only four of the most common are discussed in addition to examples of programs that address these common characteristics. It is important to note that these programs focus on reducing identified risk factors that contribute to aggressive and violent behavior and serious delinquency in their efforts to prevent homicide.

Successful prevention programs target multiple risk factors that affect violent youth and become obstacles toward decreasing their maladaptive behavior (e.g., poverty, serious illness, poor parenting, poor academic achievement, and gang affiliation). Effective delinquency prevention programs typically range from two to five years in length. Longer intervention programs affect multiple predictors of delinquency, whereas brief interventions might only have time to affect single risk factors (Yoshikawa, 1994). Another aspect of successful programs is that they maintain a level of cultural sensitivity in the support services they provide to delinquent youth and their families. By maintaining this cultural competence, the needs of all youth and families considered "at risk" are addressed. A third aspect of exemplary programs is that they include program evaluation. Studies to evaluate program effectiveness must examine how the interventions were implemented and adequately examine their effectiveness in addressing the needs of high-risk populations (Foote, 1997; Tate, Reppucci & Mulvey, 1995; Tolan & Guerra, 1998). Finally, successful interventions target risk factors that individual youth encounter in a variety of settings (e.g., within the individual youth, within the youth's close interpersonal relationships, within proximal social contexts, or within greater societal macrosystems; Fraser, 1996; Tolan & Guerra, 1998).

MULTISYSTEMIC THERAPY.   One well-researched example of a cross-context intervention is *multisystemic therapy* (MST) developed by Henggeler and colleagues (1999). MST focuses on familial problems, including difficulties experienced with parenting techniques and family cohesion and organization. It can be considered a prevention program when it is used to intervene with youth who show signs of chronic, violent antisocial behavior in order to prevent future homicide. MST draws upon validated treatment strategies such as strategic family therapy and cognitive behavioral therapy. The program targets interpersonal, familial and extrafamilial factors, which can contribute to serious violent and delinquent behavior. MST's success in decreasing serious antisocial behavior comes from its highly individualized and flexible interventions. The program uses an individualized treatment-planning strategy to address the unique needs and circumstances of each adolescent and his or her family. When compared to individual therapy, MST has been found to be more effective in decreasing antisocial behaviors and adjustment problems and has established both short- and long-term success with chronic, serious and violent youth (Borduin, 1999).

COGNITIVE-BEHAVIORAL PROGRAMS. Programs that focus on particular risk factors that impact youth (e.g., difficulty with self-control and problem-solving skills) are often based on a cognitive-behavioral approach. This approach seeks to decrease antisocial and violent behavior by changing the social cognitive mechanisms linked with such behavior. An example of such an approach is the *Viewpoints Training Program*, which focuses on improving social problem-solving skills, increasing self-control, changing beliefs and attitudes about violence, and enhancing perspective taking (Tate et al., 1995; Tolan & Guerra, 1998). This 12-session, small-group training program attempts to teach youth appropriate responses to conflict. Guerra and Slaby (1990) examined the effectiveness of this program with 120 juvenile offenders randomly assigned to the Viewpoints program, an attention-control group, or a no-treatment group. Their results showed decreases in aggressive as well as impulsive behavior, with increases in problem solving skills for the participants of the Viewpoints program.

BEHAVIOR CONTINGENCY PROGRAMS. Promising programs in this area implement strategies that include behavior modification techniques. These approaches focus on changing behavior through such techniques as direct reinforcement, contingency contracting, and modeling. The volunteer *Buddy System program* is an example of an individualized behavior modification program that partners youth with volunteers to address a range of academic and behavioral problems (Catalano et al., 1999). With the assistance of a volunteer, the youth participates in a variety of weekly behavioral support activities. In addition to 12 hours of initial training, the mentors later attend biweekly training sessions on behavior management throughout the duration of the program. These volunteers work with their assigned youth, submit reports on their youth's behavior, complete weekly logs, and collaboratively complete weekly assignments (Catalano et al., 1999). An evaluation of the program demonstrated a decrease in truancy when mentors implemented various methods of reinforcement for appropriate behaviors (Fo & O'Donnell, 1975).

SOCIAL NETWORK-FOCUSED PREVENTION PROGRAMS. Influencing a youth's close interpersonal relations (e.g., family and peers) is a strategy to reduce adolescent violence. Family interventions have repeatedly reduced antisocial behavior by focusing on behavior management and family relations. *Multisystemic therapy*, previously described in this chapter, is a very successful example of a family focused and comprehensive prevention program (Henggeler et al., 1999). Another successful program attentive to the needs of families is the *Prenatal and Infancy Nurse Home-Visitation program*. Each family is assigned an individual nurse, who stays with the family during pregnancy. The nurse visits the home once a week after registration into the program for the first month and then every other week through delivery. Once the baby is born, home visits are made once a week for the first six weeks, then every other week for the first two years of the infant's life. The nurses monitor the health and well-being of the mother while providing parenting instruction and other activities in order to promote the physical, cognitive, and emotional development of the children in the home (Muller & Mihalic, 1999). This intervention is designed to help mothers manage their children and their own lives more effectively, reducing the stress typically experienced after the birth of their children. This program has been shown to reduce verified reports of child abuse and neglect by 79%, reduce maternal behavior problems due to alcohol and drug abuse by 44%, and reduce future arrests of the children involved in the program by 56% (Olds, Hill, Mihalic & O'Brien, 1998). Evidence of child abuse, neglect, and parental alcohol and drug abuse are risk factors that have been known to contribute to juvenile violence and chronic delinquency. A third family program is *functional family therapy* (FFT). This is a complete family program that assists families in changing their communication, interaction and problem solving patterns (Muller & Mihalic, 1999). Functional Family Therapy is a short-term intervention that targets at-risk adolescents, 11–18 years old, and their families. The program has worked successfully with youth who have a variety of problems from conduct disorders to serious criminal offenses. Depending on the severity of the case, 8–30 hours of direct service are provided by a wide range of interventionists (e.g., degreed mental health professionals, mental health technicians, trained probation officers). Functional Family Therapy has been reported to be a cost-effective program, with significant treatment effects including a reduction in recidivism rates from 40% to 75% (Alexander et al., 1998).

SOCIAL CONTEXT INTERVENTIONS.   Other general strategies to prevent adolescent violence and homicides include those interventions that focus on the adolescent's immediate social setting. These programs seek to transform aspects of the youth's social context that encourage or reinforce serious violent or antisocial behavior. An equally important emphasis is on identifying those social influences that interfere with the development of more positive behaviors (Tolan & Guerra, 1998). These programs are community-based and involve schools, neighborhoods, and communities. One such program, which has been recognized as exemplary by the United States Office of Education, Safe and Drug-Free Schools Expert Panel, is *Positive Action Through Holistic Education* (PATHE; Gottfredson, 1986). The program's main objective is to improve the school environment so as to enhance students' attitudes toward school, improve academic achievement, and consequently reduce juvenile delinquency and violence. Teams of teachers, school staff, students as well as community members implement school-improvement programs. These teams participate in ongoing training in and collaborative review of school curriculum and discipline policies. The program promotes various academic, school climate, and career-oriented innovations, and provides counseling and academic services for students demonstrating particular academic or behavioral needs. High school students involved in the PATHE program have demonstrated decreases in delinquency, drug use, school suspensions, and punishment (Catalano et al., 1999). Another exemplary program is *Project Care*. This program uses classroom management and cooperative learning techniques to reduce the incidence of delinquent behavior within a middle school setting (Catalano et al., 1999). Teams of teachers, administrators, school staff, and parent volunteers are involved in the program. After two years of implementation, students reported a significant decrease in delinquency, while teachers found improvements in classroom discipline (Gottfredson, 1987).

Other community and neighborhood programs with promising results have sought to increase the motivation of high-risk students to attend school and participate in prosocial community activities (Tolan & Guerra, 1998). The *Big Brothers, Big Sisters of America* (BBBSA) mentoring program serves at-risk youth from 6 to 18 years old who are from single-parent homes. The goal of the program is to provide the youth with a consistent and stable relationship (Muller & Mihalic, 1999). An adult volunteer and child meet weekly for three to five hours over the course of a year or more. A professional case manager outlines goals identified in an initial interview with the child or adolescent that will guide the activities of the relationship. Goals can include developing stable relationships with adults, siblings, parents, and peers as well as improving school attendance, academic performance, and personal hygiene. These goals are developed into an individualized case plan. An 18-month study comparing 500 youth participants of BBBSA with 500 youth randomly assigned to a control group (youth not matched with a BBBSA mentor) found that youth participants were less likely to use drugs or assault another child or adult. BBBSA youth improved their school attendance, grades, and their relationships with family members and peers (McGill, Mihalic & Grotpeter, 1998). A similar mentoring program in Hawaii, *The Buddy System*, previously addressed in this chapter, also uses mentoring relationships with at-risk youth to promote appropriate behavior and reduce truancy (Catalano et al., 1999). Mentoring programs, which expose at-risk youth to positive adult role models, serve as a key protection against future violence and antisocial behavior (Centers for Disease Control and Prevention, 2000).

Several community-based programs focus on adolescent drug, tobacco, and alcohol use, which are risk factors for delinquency and antisocial behavior in at-risk youth. An example of such a program is the *Midwestern Prevention Project* (MPP) in Kansas City, which is designed to prevent substance abuse in at-risk middle and junior high school students. Over a five-year period, the program included a media campaign, school curriculum, parent education, community organization, and changes in local health policy supporting the goals of the intervention (Muller & Mihalic, 1999). The program was first introduced in the schools and provided students with direct skills training on resistance to drug use. Teachers and other adults provided indirect skills training on prevention practices, while community efforts supported non-drug use. The implementation of MPP resulted in decreases of daily tobacco, marijuana, and alcohol use with students through the 12th grade (Pentz, Mihalic & Grotpeter, 1998), all behaviors positively associated with aggression. *Project Northland* in Minnesota similarly combines an educational curriculum and community-based interventions, in addition to parent education, in order to prevent alcohol use among at-risk adolescents (Catalano et al., 1999). This three-year program integrates individual, parent, peer, and community training and targets sixth- through eighth-grade students. In the sixth grade, students collaborate with their parents on assignments regarding adolescent alcohol use. In seventh grade, the curriculum emphasizes resistance skills and normative expectations concerning adolescent alcohol use. During eighth grade, students become community activists by making recommendations to the community regarding strategies for the prevention of teen alcohol use. A program evaluation found that youth who participated in the program versus those students who had not participated demonstrated lower scores on their tendency to use alcohol, and on peer influence to use alcohol. An increase was noted in scores relating to students' communication with their parents about the consequences of drinking (Catalano et al., 1999).

What Might Work

GUN CONTROL.   Gun control is a hotly debated topic in the United States, the only industrialized nation to allow the private possession of handguns (Sherman, 2000). In reviewing the issue of reducing gun violence, Sherman (2000) notes that research into the effects of various gun policies is limited. Epidemiological studies show that using conviction history to control gun sales is not useful because individuals with no criminal history commit a majority of gun-related crimes. In addition, it is important to note that most gun violence occurs in areas where gun possession is prevalent (Sherman, 2000). Such information about the nature of gun crimes allows for the informed analysis of what types of innovative policies may help reduce gun violence. Sherman (2000) argues that what works to reduce gun violence is having police patrol high-density gun crime areas and mandating background checks in order to restrict gun sales in stores. What "does not work" includes gun-buyback programs. What is promising includes virtual bans on private handgun ownership and bans on the sale of new assault weapons. Additional ideas for effective programs include bans on high-caliber guns, ammunition controls, waiting periods for ammunition, and national one-gun-a-month laws.

LAW ENFORCEMENT.   With regard to the police's role in preventing homicide, one study found that when police adopted a problem-oriented philosophy that sought involvement, support, and approval from the residents of the community, there was a decrease in both the nature and frequency of homicides (White, Fyfe, Campbell & Goldkamp, 2003). These decreases were especially noted in those homicides that were directly targeted by the intervention (i.e., homicides that occur outdoors, gun homicides). Moreover, reductions were also noted in other types of violence (i.e., robbery, aggravated assault, and rape; White et al., 2003). Likewise, the *Hollenbeck initiative* in Los Angeles sought to bring together law enforcement and community-based and faith-based organizations (RAND, 2003). Following the initiative, decreases were noted in violent crimes, gang crimes, and gun crimes. A few areas of improvement were noted including that the intervention never developed dynamically or in response to changing needs, and that the project did not succeed in getting the working group participants to view the intervention as its own (as opposed to RAND's project) and seek to continue it (RAND, 2003).

What Does Not Work

As discussed in the previous section, programs with proven effectiveness to reduce adolescent aggressive behavior universally have taken a "contextual" approach. By this, we mean that they have multiple components and they consider most instances of violence, including homicide, to be the result of a long-term developmental process that is influenced by multiple social contexts and circumstances. As such, effective interventions have focused not only on the social competence of the youth, but on family, school, and community contexts as well. Given this status of violence prevention, it is perhaps not surprising that ineffective programs do not take such a holistic and contextual approach.

For example, traditional psychotherapy, psychiatric hospitalization, institutional placement, and psychopharmacological management have not shown consistently to prevent adolescent violence or homicide. In addition, group therapy, although considered to be a more cost-effective approach in comparison to individual therapy, has no evidence regarding its effectiveness in reducing antisocial or violent behavior in at-risk youth (Tate et al., 1995; Tolan & Guerra, 1998). Social casework, which combines individual counseling with close supervision and coordination of social services, has not proven to be effective in preventing serious antisocial and violent behavior (Tolan & Guerra, 1998).

State curfew ordinances, designed to reduce juvenile crime, have also been found to be ineffective in lowering homicide victimization rates (Fried, 2001). Although juvenile crime rates dropped during curfew hours, they were accompanied by increases in crime rates during the afternoon hours. Moreover, juvenile crime usually peaks around 3:00 PM on school days (Fried, 2001).

Ward (1995) asserted that although social science researchers point to the importance of cultural factors that can either augment or attenuate the likelihood of violent behavior, for the most part violence prevention programs tend either to ignore or oversimplify the influence of cultural factors. Ward advocates creating violence prevention programs that encourage African American teens to develop and act in accord with their developing ethical principles against the injustice and inequality for African Americans and other disenfranchised groups. These programs should encourage prosocial conduct towards other African Americans and towards all whom they encounter (Ward, 1995). In a similar argument, Dodge (2001) asserts that many interventions have been developed by white middle-class interventionists for a white middle-class target population who have presumed that these programs are appropriate for other groups. Dodge (2001) advocates the development of comprehensive, culturally sensitive violence prevention programs.

Recommendations

JEFFERSON CITY, MO (AP)—**Boy, 6, Suspected in Grandfather's Death** A 6-year-old boy suspected of shooting his grandfather to death with a .22-caliber rifle has a history of mental illness and attacking family members, authorities said. James Zbinden, 59, was found dead at his home Friday after his grandson ran into the street and flagged down a neighbor, Cole County Sheriff John Hemeyer said. The boy, who has not been identified, is being evaluated at a mental-health facility. An autopsy Saturday showed Zbinden bled to death from a single gunshot wound near his armpit. Hemeyer said Zbinden and the boy were alone together Friday when the boy apparently found a gun that family members thought was no longer in the house. Hemeyer said it was unclear what led up to the attack. "This is a kid who has attacked family members before with no provocation," Hemeyer said. The boy had been released last Monday from a central

Missouri mental-health facility where he was admitted after attacking another family member, Hemeyer said. Past assaults have involved the boy's younger siblings and his parents, Hemeyer said. He also said the boy has used knives during previous attacks. Before his legal counsel halted the interview, the boy indicated to authorities that he was responsible for Zbinden's death, Hemeyer said.

Adolescent aggression and homicide is disturbing because when it occurs in any culture, it suggests that some aspects of the youth development and socialization processes have gone awry. Juvenile homicide is a particular problem in the United States, although rates of violence have decreased by more than two-thirds between 1994 and 1999 as a result of multilevel prevention programs aimed at high-risk youth. Despite these recent successes, there continues to be recurring incidents of adolescent homicide, most of which are unknown to the public. Given continued pubic concern about youth violence, there has been a growing interest in profiling the "typical" homicide offender. Such a practice is dubious due to the comparatively low incidence of homicide and the many variations in the types of adolescent homicide (Furlong, Bates & Smith, 2001). What continues to be needed is an in-depth analysis of homicide in order to learn more about the different types of adolescent homicide (e.g., relationship-based, gang-associated, drug-involved, and revenge-driven killings). Intensive case studies (e.g., Gabarino, 2000) are necessary in order to determine what contexts and conditions are associated with homicide. It is crucial to examine contextual and environmental elements in order to understand how to provide preventive support to those at risk for such violent acts.

Several neglected areas in understanding youth antisocial behavior need to be addressed through research. First, the ecology that supports violent behaviors must be examined. Homicide is promoted, in part, by basic beliefs and societal values surrounding violence and used as a means to solve problems. Owning guns is seen as a right, revenge is seen as being appropriate for "evening the score." Perpetrators of extreme acts of violence are highly visible in the media and justified homicide is often glorified (e.g., movie action heroes). These values are prevalent not only in the media, but in our communities, schools, and homes, fostering conditions where violence can occur. Even school shooters receive an abundance of attention for their crimes. Second, it is necessary better to understand the relationship between delinquency, antisocial behaviors, aggression, and homicide for diverse youth. Homicide may be viewed as one possible outcome of a developmental trajectory that begins in early childhood (Moffitt, Caspi, Dickson, Silva & Stanton, 1996). Factors that maintain this trajectory should be examined for diverse populations of youth, such as females and various cultural groups. Finally, a balanced research focus necessitates the consideration of youth assets as they affect outcomes. The influence of protective factors in decreasing the likelihood of a homicidal act should be investigated in order to increase the sensitivity of screening procedures to determine which components would enhance prevention and treatment programs.

From what is currently known about homicidal behavior, it is clear that multiagency, multisystematic and school-community options must be available for those youth showing multiple risk signs. Efforts to prevent homicide should be invested in providing a comprehensive, coordinated continuum of services necessary to respond to youth needs at every level. Successful programming will involve a four-tiered system. At the first level, the targets are community-wide beliefs and values. Expectations of appropriate behavior must be made explicit and demonstrated by adult role models. Second, comprehensive community services must be made available for all youth in need of support where early intervention is key. Third, those youth most at risk for homicide must be provided with more intensive services. These youth are likely to experience extraordinary life challenges from which few children should be expected to thrive without support. Finally, it must be recognized that there are some adolescents who will not respond to preventive efforts throughout childhood and may require more intensive services later in adolescence. These youth may need to be removed from their current environments (community contexts) and provided opportunities to learn new social and life skills in a different social setting. Public resources should be made available to support local community programs that provide a full continuum of services to youth who are beginning to manifest or already are showing warning signs of chronic and violent behaviors.

Programs that have proven the most effective in reducing adolescent violence and homicide are those that include social competence and problem-solving skills training combined with efforts to improve social support across family, community, and school contexts. The successes of these programs support efforts to continue their refinement and their expansion in order to kindle hope for the elimination of adolescent homicide.

References

Alaniz, M.L. (1998). Alcohol availability and targeted advertising in racial/ethnic minority communities. *Alcohol Health and Research World, 22,* 286–290.

Alaniz, M.L., Cartmill, R.S., & Parker, R.N. (1998). Immigrants and violence: The importance of neighborhood context. *Hispanic Journal of Behavioral Sciences, 20,* 155–174.

Alexander, J., Barton, C., Gordon, D., Grotpeter, J., Hansson, K., Harrison, R., Mears, S., Mihalic, S., Parsons, B., Pugh, C., Schulman, S., Waldron, H., & Sexton, T. (1998). *Blueprints for Violence Prevention, Book Three: Functional Family Therapy.* Boulder, CO: Center for the Study and Prevention of Violence.

Barratt, E.S., & Slaughter, L. (1998). Defining, measuring, and predicting impulsive aggression: A heuristic model. *Behavioral Sciences and the Law, 16,* 285–302.

Bell, C., & Jenkins, E. (1993). Community violence and children on Chicago's Southside. *Psychiatry, 56,* 46–54.

Bilchik, S. (1998). A juvenile justice system for the 21st century. *Crime and Delinquency, 44*(1), 89–91.

Bilchik, S. (1999a). *Juvenile violence research. Report to congress.* Washington DC: Office of Juvenile Justice and Delinquency Prevention. NCJ176976.

Bilchik, S. (1999b). *Promising strategies to reduce gun violence.* Washington, DC: Office of Juvenile Justice and Delinquency Prevention. NCJ173950.

Borduin, C.M. (1999). Multisystemic treatment of criminality and violence in adolescents. *Journal of the American Academy of Child and Adolescent Psychiatry, 38,* 242–249.

Busch, K.G., Zagar, R., Hughes, J.R., Arbit, J., & Bussell, R.E. (1990). Adolescents who kill. *Journal of Clinical Psychology, 46,* 472–485.

Catalano, R.F., Loeber, R., & McKinney, K.C. (1999). *School and community interventions to prevent serious and violent offending.* Washington, DC: Office of Juvenile Justice and Delinquency Prevention, U.S. Department of Justice.

Centers for Disease Control and Prevention. (2000). *Best Practices of Youth Violence Prevention: A Sourcebook for Community Action.* Atlanta, GA: U.S. Department of Health and Human Services.

Centers for Disease Control and Prevention. (2002). *Youth violence.* Retrieved January 26, 2004, from http://www.cdc.gov/ncipc/factsheets/yvfacts.htm

Cornell, D.G., Benedek, E.P., & Benedek. D.M. (1987). Characteristics of adolescents charged with homicide: Review of 72 cases. *Behavioral Sciences & the Law, 5,* 11–23.

Crespi, T.D., & Rigazio-DiGillo, S.A. (1996). Adolescent homicide and family pathology: Implications for research and treatment with adolescents. *Adolescence, 31*(122), 353–367.

Cunningham, P.B., & Henggeler, S.W. (2001). Implementation of an empirically based drug and violence prevention and intervention program in a public school setting. *Journal of Clinical Child Psychology, 30,* 221–232.

Darby, P.J., Allan, W.D., Kashani, J.H., Hartke, K.L., & Reid, J.C. (1998). Analysis of 112 juveniles who committed homicide: Characteristics and a closer look at family abuse. *Journal of Family Violence, 13,* 365–375.

Davis, G.G., & Muhlhausen, D.B. (2000). Young African American males: Continuing victims of high homicide rates in urban communities. *The Heritage Foundation,* CDA00-05.

Department of Justice. (2002). *Homicide trends in the United States.* Retrieved October 29, 2003, from http://www.ojp.usdoj.gov/bjs/homicide/homtrnd.htm

Dodge, K. (2001). The science of youth violence prevention: Progressing from developmental epidemiology to efficacy to effectiveness to public policy. *American Journal of Preventative Medicine, 20,* 63–70.

Eitle, D., & Turner, R.J. (2002). Exposure to community violence and young adult crime: The effects of witnessing violence, traumatic victimization, and other stressful life events. *Journal of Research in Crime and Delinquency, 39,* 214–237.

Fo, W.S., & O'Donnell, C.R. (1975). The Buddy System: Effect of community intervention on delinquent offenses. *Behavior Therapy, 6,* 522–524.

Foote, J. (1997). *Expert panel issues report on serious and violent juvenile offenders.* Washington, DC: Office of Juvenile Justice and Delinquency Prevention, U.S. Department of Justice.

Fraser, M.W. (1996). Aggressive behavior in childhood and early adolescence: An ecological-developmental perspective on youth violence. *Social Work, 41,* 347–357.

Fried, C.S. (2001). Juvenile curfews: Are they an effective and constitutional means of combating juvenile violence? *Behavioral Sciences and the Law, 19,* 127–141.

Furlong, M.J., Bates, M.P., & Smith, D.C. (2001). Predicting school weapon possession: A secondary analysis of the Youth Risk Behavior Surveillance Survey. *Psychology in the Schools, 38,* 127–140.

Garbarino, J. (1995). The American war zone: What children can tell us about living with violence. *Developmental and Behavioral Pediatrics, 16,* 431–435.

Gabarino, J. (2000). *Lost Boys: Why Our Sons Turn to Violence and How We Can Save Them.* New York: Vantage.

Gottfredson, D.C. (1986). An empirical test of school based environmental and individual interventions to reduce the risk of delinquent behavior. *Criminology, 24,* 705–731.

Gottfredson, D.C. (1987). An evaluation of an organization development approach to reducing school disorder. *Evaluation Review, 11,* 739–763.

Guerra, N.G., Huesmann, L.R., & Spindler, A. (2003). Community violence, social cognition, and aggression among urban elementary school children. *Child Development, 74,* 1561–1576.

Guerra, N.G., & Slaby, R.G. (1990). Cognitive mediators of aggression in adolescent offenders: 2. Intervention. *Developmental Psychology, 26,* 269–277.

Heide, K.M. (1993). Weapons used by juveniles and adults to kill parents. *Behavioral Sciences and the Law, 11,* 397–405.

Heide, K.M. (2000). *Young Killers: The Challenge of Juvenile Homicide.* Thousand Oaks, CA: Sage.

Henggeler, S.W., Rowland, M.D., Randall, J. Ward, D.M., Pickrel, S.G., Cunningham, P.B., Miller, S.L., Edwards, J., Zealberg, J.J., Hand, L.D., & Santos, A.B. (1999). Home-based Multisystemic Therapy as an alternative to the hospitalization of youth in psychiatric crisis: Clinical outcomes. *Journal of the American Academy of Child and Adolescent Psychiatry, 38,* 1331–1339.

Hepburn, L.M., & Hemenway, D. (2004). Firearm availability and homicide: A review of the literature. *Aggression and Violent Behavior. 9,* 417–440.

Hillbrand, M., Alexandre, J.W., Young, J.L., & Spitz, R.T. (1999). Parricides: Characteristics of offenders and victims, legal factors, and treatment issues. *Aggression and Violent Behavior, 4,* 179–190.

Kashani, J.H., Jones, M.R., Bumby, K.M., & Thomas, L.A. (1999). Youth violence: Psychosocial risk factors, treatment, prevention, and recommendations. *Journal of Emotional and Behavioral Disorders, 7,* 200–211.

Kelley, B.T., Loeber, R., Keenan, K., & DeLamatre, M. (1997). *Developmental pathways in boys' disruptive and delinquent behavior.* OJJDP Juvenile Justice Bulletin, Office of Juvenile Justice and Delinquency Prevention. (NCJ165692)

Kimmel, M.S., & Mahler, M. (2003). Adolescent masculinity, homophobia, and violence: Random school shootings 1982–2001. *American Behavioral Scientist, 46,* 1439–1458.

Lipsey, M.W., & Derzon, J.H. (1998). Predictors of violent or serious delinquency in adolescence and early adulthood: A synthesis of longitudinal research. In R. Loeber & D.P. Farrington (Eds.), *Serious and Violent Juvenile Offenders: Risk Factors and Successful Interventions* (pp. 86–105). Thousand Oaks, CA: Sage.

Loeber, R., Farrington, D.P., & Waschbusch, D.A. (1998). Serious and violent offenders. In R. Loeber & D.P. Farrington (Eds.), *Serious and Violent Juvenile Offenders: Risk Factors and Successful Interventions* (pp. 13–29). Thousand Oaks, CA: Sage.

Loper, A.B., & Cornell, D.G. (1996). Homicide by juvenile girls. *Journal of Child and Family Studies, 5,* 323–336.

McGill, D.E., Mihalic, S.F., & Grotpeter, J.K. (1998). *Blueprints for Violence Prevention, Book Two: Big Brothers and Big Sisters of America.* Boulder, CO: Center for the Study and Prevention of Violence.

McGonigal, M.D. (2001). *Violence prevention programs.* Retrieved January, 26, 2004, from [http://www.courses.ahc.umn.edu/medical-school/InMd/Gun%20Violence%20and%20You/ sld001.htm]

Mercy, J.A., & Hammond, R.W. (1999). Combining action and analysis to prevent homicide: A public health perspective. In M.D. Smith & M.A. Zahn (Eds.), *Homicide: A Sourcebook of Social Research.* Thousand Oaks, CA: Sage.

Moffitt, T.E., Caspi, A., Dickson, N., Silva, P., & Stanton, W. (1996). Childhood-onset versus adolescent-onset antisocial conduct in males: Natural history from ages 3–18 years. *Development and Psychopathology, 9,* 399–424.

Muller, J., & Mihalic, S. (1999). *Blueprints: A violence prevention initiative.* Washington, DC: Office of Juvenile Justice and Delinquency Prevention, U.S. Department of Justice.

Olds, D., Hill, P., Mihalic, S., & O'Brien, R. (1998). *Blueprints for Violence Prevention, Book Seven: Prenatal and Infancy Home Visitation by Nurses.* Boulder, CO: Center for the Study and Prevention of Violence.

Patterson, G.R., Reid, J.B., & Dishion, T.J. (1992). *Antisocial Boys.* Eugene, OR: Castalia.

Pentz, M.A., Mihalic, S.G., & Grotpeter, J.K. (1998). *Blueprints for Violence Prevention, Book One: The Midwestern Prevention Project.* Boulder, CO: Center for the Study and Prevention of Violence.

Pritchard, C., & Butler, A. (2003). A comparative study of children and adult homicide rates in the USA and the major western countries 1974–1999: Grounds for concern? *Journal of Family Violence, 18,* 341–350.

RAND. (2003). *Reducing Gun Violence: Results from an Intervention in East Los Angeles.* Santa Monica, CA: RAND.

Schwartz, L.L., & Isser, N.K. (2001). Neonaticide: An appropriate application for therapeutic jurisprudence? *Behavioral Sciences & the Law, 19,* 703–718.

Scribner, R.A., MacKinnon, D.P., & Dwyer, J.H. (1995). The risk of assaultive violence and alcohol availability in Los Angeles County. *American Journal of Public Health, 85,* 335–340.

Sherman, L.W. (2000). *Reducing Gun Violence: What Works, What Doesn't, What's Promising. Presentation at Perspectives on Crime and Justice: 1999–2000 Lecture Series, National Institute of Justice, IV.* Washington, DC: U.S. Department of Justice.

Snyder, H.N. (2000, December). *Juvenile arrests 1999.* Washington, DC: OJJDP Juvenile Justice Bulletin, Office of Juvenile Justice and Delinquency Prevention. (NCJ 185236)

Snyder, H.N., & Sickmund, M. (1999). *Juvenile Offenders and Victims: 1999 National Report.* Washington, DC: Office of Juvenile Justice and Delinquency Prevention.

Swartz, M.S., Swanson, J.W., Hiday, V.A., Borum, R., Wagner, R., & Burns, B.J. (1998). Taking the wrong drugs: The role of substance abuse and medication noncompliance in violence among severely mentally ill individuals. *Social Psychiatry and Psychiatric Epidemiology, 33,* S75–S80.

Tate, D.C., Reppucci, N.D., & Mulvey, E.P. (1995). Violent juvenile delinquents: Treatment effectiveness and implications for future action. *American Psychologist, 50,* 777–781.

Tolan, P., & Guerra, N. (1998). *What Works in Reducing Adolescent Violence: An Empirical Review of the Field.* Boulder, CO: University of Colorado, Center for the Study and Prevention of Violence.

Toppo, G. (2003, October 21). Violent deaths surge in schools across US. *USA Today.* Retrieved October 28, 2003, from *http://www.azcentral.com*

Uehara, E., Chalmers, D., Jenkins, E., & Shakoor, B. (1996). African American youth encounters with violence: Results from the community mental health council violence screening project. *Journal of Black Studies, 26,* 768–781.

United States Department of Justice. (2000). *Intimate Partner Violence.* Washington, DC: Bureau of Justice Statistics (NCJ178247). Retrieved February 22, 2004, from *http://www.ojp.usdoj.gov/bjs/abstract/ ipv.htm*

Wallace, J.M. (1999). The social ecology of addiction: Race, risk, and resilience. *Pediatrics, 103,* 1122–1127.

Ward, J. (1995). Cultivating a morality of care in African American adolescents: A culture-based model of violence prevention. *Harvard Educational Review, 65,* 175–188.

Whitaker, L.C. (2000). Social inducements to paralethal and lethal violence. In *Understanding and Preventing Violence: The Psychology of Human Destructiveness* (pp. 27–72). Boca Raton, FL: CRC Press.

White, M.D., Fyfe, J.J., Campbell, S.P., & Goldkamp, J.S. (2003). The police role in preventing homicide: Considering the impact of problem-oriented policing on the prevalence of murder. *Journal of Research in Crime and Delinquency, 40,* 194–225.

White, H.R., Tice, P.C., Loeber, R., & Stouthamer-Loeber, M. (2002). Illegal acts committed by adolescents under the influence of alcohol and drugs. *Journal of Research in Crime and Delinquency, 39,* 131–152.

Yarvis, R.M. (1990). Axis I and Axis II diagnostic parameters of homicide. *Bulletin of the American Academy of Psychiatry and the Law, 18,* 249–269.

Yoshikawa, H. (1994). Prevention as cumulative protection: Effects of early family support and education on chronic delinquency and its risks. *Psychological Bulletin, 115,* 28–54.

Chapter 26

Adolescent Pregnancy

Brent C. Miller, Rayna Sage, and Bryan Winward

Introduction

Adolescent pregnancy and childbearing remain at high levels and are problems in the United States even though rates have declined substantially since the early 1990s (Manlove et al., 2002). Teen pregnancy and birth rates in the United States still are about one-third higher than those in England and Wales, and are more than twice the rates in Canada (Singh & Darroch, 2000). Rates of teen pregnancy and births in any of these countries are 5 to 10 times higher than in countries such as Denmark, Korea, and Japan (Singh & Darroch, 2000).

Adolescent *pregnancy* is a problem in advanced societies mostly because it leads to premature childbearing and parenthood. Early *childbearing* is problematic because it poses increased risks to the health and well-being of infants born to young mothers, and to young mothers themselves. Teen *parenthood* is problematic because of its early timing: coming before the extended education and training that is expected in advanced societies, early parenthood interrupts the social and economic preparations of young parents, constrains their life chances and productivity, and imposes costs on society to support families formed before they are likely to be self sufficient (Maynard, 1996).

Teen pregnancy, childbirth, and parenthood are sequential events that begin with sexual and contraceptive behaviors. Figure 1 portrays this chain of behaviors and events. Several points of prevention and intervention are possible, beginning with prevention of pregnancy through lowering pregnancy risk behaviors (reducing sexual intercourse and/or increasing effective contraceptive use). Prevention of adolescent pregnancy is generally preferable to intervention after pregnancy occurs, because the later interventions are more strongly value-laden (e.g., abortion) or life-altering in their potential consequences (e.g., adoption and teen parenthood interventions). So, the focus of major efforts in this area are on preventing teen pregnancy (see the National Campaign to Prevent Teen Pregnancy at *www.teenpregnancy.org*).

If pregnancy prevention fails and teens become pregnant, abortion can be thought of as an intervention to prevent teen childbearing. Similarly, adolescent

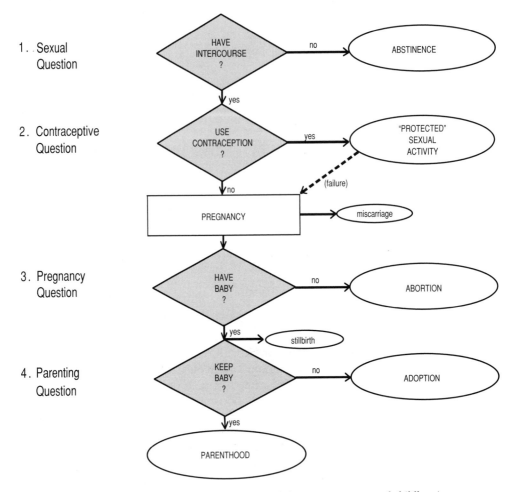

Figure 1. Major issues and turning points in adolescent pregnancy and childbearing.

parenthood can be avoided by making an adoption plan, although infant adoption has become very rare (Miller and Coyl, 2000). The ways in which adolescent pregnancies are resolved in the United States are approximately 55% live births, 30% abortions, and 14% miscarriages (Henshaw, 2003).

The following sections include a review of individual, family, and community factors that increase or decrease the risk of adolescent pregnancy. It is important to recognize that the major proximal determinants of adolescent pregnancy are having sexual intercourse without using effective contraception. Consequently, the risk and protective factors for adolescent pregnancy work through these major determinants, and closely related factors such as the frequency of intercourse and consistency of contraceptive use. The following sections are condensed because there are literally hundreds of factors that influence risk of adolescent pregnancy; interested readers are referred to Kirby and Ryan (2004) for a comprehensive summary of adolescent pregnancy risk and protective factors.

Individual Factors

Many individual factors can be linked to an increased risk of adolescent pregnancy. These individual factors can be conceptualized under three broad categories dealing with (a) the inherent characteristics, (b) values and choices, and (c) experiences in adolescents' lives that influence lifelong outcomes.

Inherent Characteristics

Some researchers have explored genetic and biological contributions to adolescent sexual behavior and pregnancy. Three primary areas of investigation have emerged: (1) genetics and heredity; (2) hormone levels in relation to sexual motivation and behaviors; and (3) the role of early pubertal development.

Researchers have reported correlations between mother, daughter, and sister ages of menarche (Garn, 1980; Mott, Fondell, Hu, Kowaleski-Jones & Menaghan, 1996; Newcomer & Udry, 1984) and noted that mothers' young age at first intercourse predicts sons' and daughters' having intercourse before age 14 (Mott et al., 1996). Behavior-genetic models of age at first intercourse indicate that genetic influences account for some of the variance in both early and late onset of first sexual intercourse (Rodgers, Rowe & Buster, 1999). A relationship between dopamine receptor genes and age at first intercourse also has been reported (Miller, Pasta, MacMurray, Chiu, Wu & Comings, 1999). Research by Udry and colleagues (Udry, Talbert & Morris, 1986; Udry, 1988) showed that free testosterone hormone levels are related to sexual motivation and behavior among teens. There is little evidence, however, that changes in boys' testosterone levels directly affected their sexual behavior over three years; pubertal development was a much stronger predictor of sexual ideation and behavior than changes in testosterone levels (Halpern, Udry, Campbell & Suchindran, 1993).

As teens become older they are more likely to engage in sex. Some of this age effect is biological, including physical maturity and higher hormone levels. There are also social causes of the age effect such as more pressure from others to have sex, changes in perceived norms about sex, and increased opportunity to have sex, which comes from greater independence of older ages (Kirby & Ryan, 2004). Several investigators have noted a relationship between early pubertal development, age of first intercourse, and subsequent adolescent sexual behavior and pregnancy (Flannery, Rowe & Gulley, 1993; Zabin, Smith, Hirsch & Hardy, 1986). Halpern et al. (1993) reported that early pubertal development was a significant predictor of adolescent males' transition to intercourse, and the risk ratio was about twice as great for earlier-versus later-maturing boys. Miller, Norton, Fan, and Christopherson (1998) also reported that early development relative to peers was related to a higher level of sexual behavior two years later. Both theory and research findings suggest that early pubertal development is associated with early involvement in intimate relationships, including sexual involvement with larger numbers of sexual partners, and an increased likelihood of teen pregnancy (Alan Guttmacher Institute, 1994).

African American and Hispanic youth have sex at younger ages than whites and are thus more likely to become pregnant and have children in adolescence (Kirby, 2001). This difference is largely due to differences in socioeconomic level, community, and opportunity, but these contextual characteristics don't entirely explain the increased risk. Kirby (2001) noted that cultural values such as the Hispanic's culture

placing a greater emphasis on families can also have an impact. Adolescents identifying themselves with Hispanic culture might feel more inclined to have unprotected
sex or give birth if pregnancy occurs due to influences that are part of that culture.

Values and Choices

Teens who feel that education is important, attend school regularly, have plans
for education after high school, and who get good grades postpone having sex to
later ages, use contraception more frequently, and are thus less likely to become pregnant during adolescence. Similar protective effects are found for female teens who
are involved in extracurricular activities such as sports, drama, or music outside of
the classroom after school (Kirby, 2001).

Teens who participate in religious activities, describe themselves to be religious,
and who have strong religious affiliations are much less likely to participate in sexual
activity at any given age. This may be due to the impact that religion has on a teen's
behavior or that teens who engage in sexual behavior are less likely to participate in
religious activities (Whitehead, 2001).

Teen drug or alcohol use is a risk factor for participating in unprotected sex
and becoming pregnant. Teen drug and alcohol use puts teens at risk in two ways:
first, by exposing them to individuals and environments where risky behavior is
observed; and second, because the substances impair their ability to make rational
decisions about sex and contraception (Kirby, 2001). When teens choose to date at an
early age, date often, have a larger number of romantic partners, and go steady at an
early age, they place themselves at an increased risk of having sex because they have
both greater opportunities and greater pressures to have sex (Kirby & Ryan, 2004).

Adolescents' sexual attitudes, beliefs, and skills also affect their sexual behavior
and risk for teen pregnancy. Teens who have permissive attitudes toward sex,
believe there are social and personal benefits if they engage in sex, don't care if their
friends and families know they have had sex, or lack the confidence necessary
to avoid having sex, are more likely to engage in risky sexual behaviors and less
likely to use contraception than their counterparts who lack these permissive attitudes (Kirby, 2001).

Peers also influence whether or not teens engage in risky sexual behavior. When
peers do poorly in school, participate in delinquent behavior, and are unattached to
positive community structure, teens within that peer group are more likely to engage
in sex. The effect of peers goes beyond their actions. If teens simply believe that their
peers are engaging in sex, and not using contraception, those teens are more likely to
engage in sex and not use contraception themselves (Kirby, 2001).

Traumatic Experiences in the Lives of Adolescents

Recent studies have found that traumatic child or adolescent experiences, especially sexual abuse, are related to higher adolescent pregnancy risk (Miller, Benson &
Galbraith, 2001), both through earlier onset of voluntary sexual intercourse (Browning
& Laumann, 1997; Miller, Monson & Norton, 1995; Small & Luster, 1994) and through
less consistent use of contraception (Roosa, Tein, Reinholtz & Angelini, 1997).

Childhood sexual abuse may prematurely initiate sexual developmental processes
for girls, altering subsequent life course transitions (Browning & Laumann, 1997).

Many girls who experience childhood sexual abuse initiate early voluntary sexual intercourse (Boyer & Fine, 1992), choose older male partners, and lack refusal skills necessary for avoiding unwanted sexual relationships (Friedrich, 2002; Russell, 1986). Some researchers have hypothesized that the relation between early sexual abuse and poor outcomes is cyclical, in that girls who are victimized as children lack necessary cognitive, psychological, and emotional resources for making responsible or protective choices about dating and sex in their teen years (Browning & Laumann, 1997; Miller et al., 1995). This can lead to further victimization in the form of date rape, violence, and unwanted pregnancy.

Family Factors

A broad range of family variables affect adolescent pregnancy risk through sexual and contraceptive behavior. Family influences include (a) the contextual and structural features of families (e.g., parent's education, marital status, sibling composition) and (b) family processes, relationships, or practices of parenting (e.g., parental support, control, or supervision of teenagers).

Family Structural Influences

Families provide structural contexts in which children grow up usually having primary relationships with one or two biological parents, and with or without older and younger siblings. With respect to parents' marital status, many studies consistently show that living with a single parent is related to adolescents' being more likely to have had sexual intercourse (Miller et al., 2001). Relatedly, many studies show earlier onset of intercourse, and a few studies show less contraceptive use, among teens in single parent families. Several investigators have gone beyond the bivariate relationship to show that single or divorced parents' more permissive sexual attitudes (Thornton & Camburn, 1987), lesser parental supervision, and parents' own dating activity (Whitbeck, Simons & Kao, 1994) help explain why adolescents in some single parent families are at increased risk of pregnancy. Other investigators have reported that the number of parents' relationship transitions or number of changes in parents' marital status, and time lived with single parents, are related to teens' risk of pregnancy (Capaldi, Crosby & Stoolmiller, 1996; Miller et al., 1997; Wu & Martinson, 1993).

Having older siblings also is related to higher risk of adolescent pregnancy (see Miller et al., 2001), apparently through younger siblings' earlier onset of sexual intercourse (Rodgers & Rowe, 1988; Rodgers, Rowe & Harris, 1992; Widmer, 1997). This effect is not due to having older siblings older per se, because the influence on younger sibs' pregnancy risk behaviors is strongest if older siblings have had sexual intercourse, and especially if older sisters have experienced an adolescent pregnancy or birth (East, 1996a,b; East, Felice & Morgan, 1993; East & Shi, 1997; Widmer, 1997).

There is abundant evidence that parents' social and economic status (SES) is related to adolescent pregnancy (Miller et al., 2001); adolescents whose parents have higher education and income are more likely both to postpone sexual intercourse and to use contraception.

Parent–Child Relationships

Many researchers have investigated the association between adolescents' sexual behavior and family process variables such as parental warmth, support, parent–child closeness, or connectedness (Miller et al., 2001). There is marked consistency in this body of about two dozen studies; all but a few indicate that parent–child closeness is associated with reduced adolescent pregnancy risk through teens' remaining sexually abstinent, postponing intercourse, having fewer sexual partners, or using contraception more consistently. For example, parent–child connectedness or closeness is related to both daughters' and sons' postponement of sexual intercourse (Jaccard, Dittus & Gordon, 1996; Resnick et al., 1997; Weinstein & Thornton, 1989), and to more consistent contraceptive use by sexually active teens (Jaccard et al., 1996).

Most of the evidence shows that parental supervision and monitoring of children is another important relationship dimension related to adolescents' sexual behaviors in ways that would lower their risk of pregnancy (see Miller et al., 2001). More specifically, family rules and household routines (Danziger, 1995; Ku, Sonenstein & Pleck, 1993), parental supervision of dating activities (Hogan & Kitagawa, 1985), and parental monitoring of teens (Luster & Small, 1994, 1997; Small & Luster, 1994; Upchurch, Aneshensel, Sucoff & Levy-Storms, 1999) all have been associated with teens not having intercourse, having a later sexual debut, or having fewer sexual partners. Parental supervision and control might also reduce teen pregnancy indirectly by decreasing teens' association with high-risk peers, and by lowering teen alcohol and drug use, thereby decreasing teenagers' unprotected sexual intercourse.

A possible explanation for the few contrary findings in this area is that parental control is multidimensional; and it is associated with negative teen outcomes if it is excessive or coercive (Barber, 1996; Gray & Steinberg, 1999). In fact, it has been reported that intrusive maternal control is related to early age of first sexual intercourse (Miller et al., 2001) and parents' psychological control is related to high-risk behavior among sexually active daughters (Rodgers, 1999).

Parent–child communication is another dimension or process in family relationships, and its association with adolescent pregnancy risk has been investigated in more than 30 studies (see Miller et al., 2001). Results across these studies are so variable and discrepant that no simple, direct effect is discernible. There is little or no agreement between what parents and teens perceive to have been communicated between them (Newcomer & Udry, 1985), and there is no consistency in findings about whether parents' or teens' reports of their communication are related to adolescent pregnancy risk. In most studies that have tested these relationships by parent and child gender, mothers' communication is more likely to be associated with adolescent pregnancy risk variables than father's communication, and there is a stronger effect for daughters than for sons.

Several important conceptual and methodological issues complicate our understanding of the association between parent–child communication and adolescent pregnancy risk (Jaccard, Dittus, & Litardo, 1999). One is the temporal ordering of variables; there is a theoretical basis for prior parent–child sexual communication to predict more responsible adolescent sexual behavior, especially if parents disapprove of their child's having sex and there is a close parent–child relationship. On the other hand, if teen sexual behaviors are known to, or suspected by parents, they might begin or intensify their communication with teens about sex and contraception.

Further, associations between parent/teen communication and adolescent sexual behavior are moderated by parents' values. Researchers (Jaccard et al., 1996; Luster & Small, 1997; Miller et al., 1998) have demonstrated that parents' sexual values, in combination with parent–child communication, have an important effect on adolescents' intercourse experience.

Mediating mechanisms have been identified that could help explain how parent/child relationships (especially closeness and supervision) influence adolescents' sexual behavior. For example, in one study (Scaramella, Conger, Simons & Whitbeck, 1998) the effects of parental warmth and involvement in the seventh grade were shown to affect teen pregnancy status in 12th grade through intervening mechanisms such as deviant peer affiliations, substance use, delinquency, and academic competence. Results of other studies indicate that parent–child closeness is related to mediating mechanisms such as teens' attitudes about having intercourse, teens' depression, impulse control, academic and prosocial activities, and teens' use of substances and association with sexually active peers, all of which are related to adolescent sexual behavior and pregnancy. In particular, several investigators (Benda & DiBlasio, 1991; Feldman & Brown, 1993; Whitbeck, Conger & Kao, 1993; Whitbeck, Hoyt, Miller & Kao, 1992) have suggested that a lack of closeness in the parent–teen relationship increases the negative influence of peers on adolescent sexual activity. On the positive side, parent–child closeness and involvement can reduce teen sexual behavior by enhancing educational achievement, providing youth with opportunities to develop prosocial skills, and helping teens acquire a sense of competence and worth (Ramirez-Valles, Zimmerman & Newcomb, 1998).

Social and Community Factors

In addition to more proximal individual and family influences on adolescent pregnancy risk, community factors have been shown to play a role in adolescent decision-making (Corcoran, Franklin & Bennett, 2000; Denner, Kirby, Coyle & Brindis, 2001; Moore & Chase-Lansdale, 2001; Upchurch et al., 1999). Researchers have suggested that racial differences in teen pregnancy rates can better be understood in the context of the impoverished environments where many minorities reside (Moore & Chase-Lansdale, 2001), suggesting that concentrated community poverty and increased social isolation creates an environment with norms and values that deviate from the mainstream. According to this framework, community members create and maintain a structural system that dictates social norms, including those related to adolescent sexual behavior and childbearing.

Youth in low-income and working-class neighborhoods have higher rates of adolescent sexual intercourse (Upchurch et al., 1999) and teen pregnancy (Moore & Chase-Lansdale, 2001) than teens in middle and upper-class neighborhoods. Additionally, more adolescents are at risk for STIs and pregnancy in neighborhoods with high ethnic heterogeneity than neighborhoods with ethnic homogeneity (Denner et al., 2001; Upchurch et al., 1999). A final important component is the perceived danger or ambient hazards present in the community (Moore & Chase-Lansdale, 2001; Upchurch et al., 1999). Adolescents who perceive more crime, drug and alcohol use, and overall dangers in their neighborhood are more likely to engage in sexual intercourse; even when neighborhood socioeconomic status, racial diversity, family structure, parent–child relationship quality, and gender are considered (Upchurch et al., 1999).

Some research suggests that the community can also provide protection for minority, low-income youth (Denner et al., 2001; Moore & Chase-Lansdale, 2001; Upchurch et al., 1999). Latino girls growing up in Latino neighborhoods with strong homeland ties and social networks were the least likely to engage in sexual intercourse when compared to several other groups of adolescents (Denner et al., 2001). Upchurch and colleagues (1999) also found that minority girls experience protection from their community resources, especially when perceived ambient hazards are low.

Evidence-Based Treatment Interventions in Community Settings

Findings regarding the effectiveness of community intervention programs in lowering teen pregnancy have been modest (Weatherley, 1991). To provide an overview of what works, what might work, and what does not work, one must first ask, "What is the desired outcome?" There have been three main approaches to programming for teen parents and their children.

The first, and most common, approach is to assist adolescent parents in achieving economic self-sufficiency through continued education and employment training (Bos & Fellerath, 1997a; Granger & Cytron, 1999). The 1996 welfare reform act included special provisions regarding teen parents and economic self-sufficiency (Grisham & Levin-Epstein, 2003; Granger & Cytron, 1999; Klaw, Rhodes & Fitzgerald, 2003; Zaslow & Eldred, 1998). The second approach to enhancing parent and child well being is to increase parenting knowledge and skills through home-based programs or early childhood centers (Crean, Hightower & Allan, 2001; Klerman, Baker & Howard, 2003; Wagner & Clayton, 1999). These programs focus on increasing positive child outcomes through improving parent–child interactions. The final approach to teen–parent programming has been to target parent and child health through wellness clinics and contraceptive use (Akinbam, Cheng & Kornfeld, 2001; Klerman et al., 2003). In addition to these three primary goals, most programming for adolescent parents includes secondary components for enhancing other areas of development, but resources dedicated to secondary goals often are very limited.

What Works

Comprehensive approaches that include continued education, employment services, access to and education about contraceptives, and parenting training have demonstrated the most positive outcomes for maternal and child well-being (Akinbam et al., 2001; Bos, Polit & Quint, 1997b; Crean et al., 2001; Klerman et al., 2003; Love et al., 2002; Wagner & Clayton, 1999). Although comprehensive community approaches are very expensive to deliver, large investments in early interventions may actually save money over the long term (Maynard, 1996). The following discussion is of programs that have been shown to encourage economic sufficiency, to enhance teens' ability to parent, or have improved maternal and child health.

ENHANCING ECONOMIC SELF-SUFFICIENCY: TEENAGE DEMONSTRATION PROJECT. The Teenage Demonstration Project, designed for mothers younger than 20 who had experienced only one pregnancy and who were accessing welfare services for the first time, has been described as the most cost efficient and economically promising program for teen mothers and their families (Granger & Cytron, 1999). This was a mandatory program in which teen welfare recipients were subject to financial sanctions if they did not comply with education or job training requirements (Granger & Cytron, 1999). Intense case management was coupled with intermittent parenting workshops to meet program goals of decreasing welfare dependency through increased employment and self-sufficiency. A secondary goal of this program was to increase positive parenting behaviors.

Rigorous evaluation of this program showed long-term increases in employment for participating mothers, with earnings averaging $79 more per month (Kisker, Rangarajan & Boller, 1998). Welfare dependency also decreased for mothers who had dropped out of high school prior to enrolling in the program. While these economic findings are promising, the Teenage Demonstration Project did not have a measurable impact on literacy, education attainment, subsequent pregnancies, or parenting skills (Granger & Cytron, 1999; Klerman et al., 2003).

BUILDING CAPACITY FOR PARENTING: EARLY CHILDHOOD CENTERS. A strong parenting program and having easy access to quality early-childhood centers with a parenting component have been shown to be moderately successful in achieving the dual goals of improving parenting skills and completing high school, especially for certain subgroups (Crean et al., 2001; Love et al., 2002; Stephens, Wolf & Batten, 1999; Webster-Stratton, 1998). Based on the social learning model, these programs are designed to provide parents with much needed childcare, formal guidance about child development and parenting, and positive role modeling of constructive adult–child interaction. Early childhood centers appear to be most successful in improving parent and child outcomes when they are school-based (Stephens et al., 1999).

One of the most established programs of this type is Early Head Start, which currently serves 55,000 children in 664 communities (Love et al., 2002). Early Head Start is designed to serve all low-income families with children up to 3 years old, regardless of parental age, but it has shown specific success in serving adolescent parents and their children. A large-scale evaluation indicated that participating parents provided their children with more emotional support, home environments that were more conducive to language and learning, and were more likely to read to their children than parents who did not participate in Early Head Start (Love et al., 2002). Participating parents were also less likely to engage in negative parenting and had knowledge of a wider range of discipline options than non-participating parents. Researchers found that the positive parenting differences measured when the children were 2 years old were related to positive child outcomes a year later (i.e., better cognitive and language scores).

Evaluations of similar programs serving teen parents showed that participating parents were much more likely to graduate from high school (Crean et al., 2001), engaged in less negative parenting behaviors and more positive parenting, and were more involved in their children's schools (Webster-Stratton, 1998) than those who did not participate.

MATERNAL AND CHILD HEALTH: THE SPECIAL SUPPLEMENTAL NUTRITION PROGRAM FOR WOMEN, INFANTS, AND CHILDREN (WIC). Although the WIC program is not age-specific, teen parents and their children accounted for about 15% of the 8 million participants served in 2002 (Williams et at., 2002). About half of the 15% were mothers under the age of 18, or children born to those mothers (Kresge, 2003). Some suggest young parents and their children are at more risk for problems related to nutritional deficiencies than older parents and their children (Gupta, Venkateswaran, Gorenflo & Eyler, 1999). Research has indicated that WIC families, compared to eligible non-WIC families, show several benefits, including decreased premature births, increased infant birth weight (Kowaleski-Jones & Duncan, 2002), higher infant intake of iron and vitamin C, regular medical care, and on-time immunizations (Besharov & Germanis, 2000). Although some studies indicate that low-income mothers are less likely to breast-feed, about 35% of WIC mothers breastfeed, approximately the same portion as non-eligible mothers (Besharov & Germanis, 2000). In addition, participating adolescent mothers reported improved eating habits, especially young Hispanic mothers (Williams et al., 2002). The most significant gains were among the poorest WIC families (Besharov & Germanis, 2000).

What Might Work

ENHANCING ECONOMIC SELF-SUFFICIENCY: NEW CHANCE. New Chance was developed to meet various needs of adolescent parents through a "one-stop shop" approach; it costs about $9,000 per participating family (Bos et al., 1997b). Although the main focus is on creating economic self-sufficiency through academic success, New Chance also offers career and employment preparation, job placement, work experience, family planning, and childcare referrals (Bos et al., 1997b). Workshops on parenting, communication, and decision-making are additional components of New Chance (Zaslow & Eldred, 1998). This program was initially designed to serve teen mothers and their children for up to 18 months; however, the average length of stay in the program was about six months (Granger & Cytron, 1999).

Rigorous evaluation has shown that participating mothers take part in activities that increase self-sufficiency more often than mothers who did not participate. Specifically, New Chance mothers were more likely to obtain a GED than non-participating mothers (Granger & Cytron, 1999). However, long-term follow-up indicated there was no impact on adult literacy skills, employment, welfare dependency, parenting, subsequent pregnancies, or children's cognitive development (Bos et al., 1997b). This program raised important issues about unintended consequences, when researchers found that mothers who participated in this program were more likely to report negative child behaviors (Granger & Cytron, 1999). However, Zaslow and Eldred (1998) observed improved parenting behaviors among mothers participating in New Chance.

BUILDING CAPACITY FOR PARENTING: PARENTS AS TEACHERS. *Parents as Teachers* is a program developed to serve parents of all ages, but some programs have been tailored to serve adolescent parents (Wagner & Clayton, 1999). This program is delivered primarily through weekly home visits where parents are taught about normal child development and how best to foster positive child growth. This program is designed to increase parenting knowledge, skills, positive parenting attitudes, child wellness, and normal child development (Wagner & Clayton, 1999). For the demonstration project serving adolescent parents, evaluations showed a minimal increase in acceptance of normal child behavior, immunizations, and child cognitive development and a decrease in child abuse and neglect cases at the two-year follow-up (Wagner & Clayton, 1999). However, these differences were most apparent for teens who were receiving intensive case management, in addition to the parenting education.

MATERNAL AND CHILD HEALTH: TEEN–TOT PROGRAMS.   Another way to reach teen mothers and their children is through public health clinics. These types of programs have been called "teen–tot" programs because of their emphasis on mother and child well-being. Akinbam et al.'s (2001) review of four clinic-based programs designed to encourage high school completion, self-sufficiency, positive parenting, wellness, and to decrease subsequent pregnancy, found that most of the programs showed increased short-term education attainment, better health-care behavior, and improved contraceptive use among teen mothers who participated in the program. Additionally, there were fewer subsequent pregnancies reported among participants 18 months later. Teen–tot programs were the only interventions that were able to reduce the likelihood of subsequent pregnancies and that enhanced the health of both mothers and their children (Akinbam et al., 2001).

What Does Not Work

It is not possible to state definitively that a program approach "does not work," when most programmatic efforts to improve the lives of young parents and their children show at least some positive results depending on the target population and the context. Some approaches have demonstrated fewer benefits than other approaches, especially among those most at risk for poor outcomes such as families headed by mothers who had dropped out of high school (Bos & Fellerath, 1997b).

Evidence-Based Treatment Interventions in Residential Settings

What Works

There has been a renewed interest in residential interventions that once were common in the United States. Because there has been very little research done to evaluate residential treatment interventions for teen pregnancy, it is not possible to identify what works.

What Might Work

In 1863 Abraham Lincoln signed a charter to protect wayward females and orphans by establishing privately funded rescue homes (Sylvester, 1995). Because such homes were intended to be a temporary solution to the problems of teen parenthood, it was expected that young women would stay no longer than six months. The common practice, however, seemed to be that young women stayed for one to two years (Nathanson, 1991). Initially these homes placed an emphasis on marriage to the fathers of the children, trying to establish a more permanent solution to the difficulties of single parenthood. The marriage emphasis was gradually abandoned in favor of training young mothers for employment in the work force (Sylvester, 1995). Professional social workers placed heavy emphasis on licensing requirements for maternity homes mandated by state law and insisted they serve a purpose beyond concealing unmarried mothers (Nathanson, 1991). Group homes during this era provided young mothers with a place of residence, stable income, and allowed women to keep their children with them (Sylvester, 1995).

The New Deal of the 1930s transferred welfare responsibilities away from the private sector to the public, adopting a new school of thought that blamed social inequities for causing poverty and unwed motherhood. The New Deal instituted mother pensions which initially were intended for widows and orphans, but which were quickly extended to unwed mothers (Sylvester, 1995). During the 1940s, welfare services began to focus their attention away from maternity homes and more upon prenatal services. By the 1970s, government sponsored maternity homes gradually were eliminated (Sylvester, 1995).

Today the difficulties of teen mothers' not becoming self-sufficient, not delaying subsequent pregnancies, and not assisting their children in early development has sparked a renewed interest in reestablishing maternity group homes. These new group homes for young mothers have been labeled *Second Chance Homes,* defined as apartments or group homes which combine housing and assistance for both teen mothers and children (DHHS, 2000). Second Chance Homes allow minor teens, who have been displaced out of their parent's homes, to meet the TANF requirement that the teen live with a responsible adult in order to qualify for welfare benefits. These homes offer access to child care, education, job training, counseling, and advice on parenting and life skills (SPAN, 2001). Second Chance homes can potentially address a wide variety of needs for teenage mothers in areas such as pregnancy, health of newborns, maternal well-being, economic self-sufficiency, parenting style, and child development (DHHS, 2000). Funding of $33 million dollars requested by President Bush in his 2002 budget was approved by the House and Senate for the years 2003–2007 in the form of competitive state block grants. This program offers grants to faith and community-based programs to provide Second Chance Homes and programs for teens and their children (SPAN, 2001).

Several challenges are faced by Second Chance Homes. The first challenge is that teen mothers come into the homes with a wide variety of needs. Some only need a place to stay, a chance to further their education, or employment training. Others have needs relating to physical or sexual abuse, violence, and poverty. Consequently, Second Chance Homes need to be equipped to offer a flexible and comprehensive program, and not just a core set of standardized services (DHHS, 2000). Secondly, program staff feel that teen mothers need socialization, nurturing, structure, and discipline in order to make positive changes. This is sometimes achieved by having young mothers sign contracts to obey house rules (Sylvester, 1995), and participation in many forms of activity is mandated throughout the day. This strictness is reportedly related to some young mothers' dropping out of the program, causing them to go back to a poor family structure, boyfriends, or negative habits. Thirdly, these homes need to coordinate their services with other community, state, and federal programs. Working together can provide a more comprehensive umbrella so that all of the needs of teen mothers are better met. Because the entire program hinges on having well trained and efficient staff, the final challenge is to develop staff so that they can address the varied issues facing teen mothers (DHHS, 2000).

Psychopharmacology

The use of psychopharmacological agents for the prevention or treatment of adolescent pregnancy is not appropriate.

The Prevention of Teen Pregnancy

What Works

Hundreds of teen pregnancy prevention programs designed to reduce unintended pregnancy among adolescents have been implemented, resulting in many evaluation studies of varying quality. However, the discrepant research designs and results of these studies have left the effectiveness of the interventions in doubt. There is a growing consensus about which programs work, but it is not cleat that any programs meet the most stringent criteria of having shown effectiveness three or more times in a rigorous experimental evaluation design.

What Might Work

Fortunately, there have been several major recent efforts to summarize the results of primary prevention program evaluations. Substantial efforts have been made to identify effective teen pregnancy prevention programs by four groups: National Campaign to Prevent Teen Pregnancy; Child Trends; Program Archive on Sexuality, Health, and Adolescence; and Advocates for Youth. Some of their efforts have been coordinated, and certainly the lists of effective programs they identified are overlapping. However, the lists of effective programs range widely, from only 8 (Kirby, 2001) to 19 (Advocates for Youth, 2003) to 20 (Manlove et al., 2001, 2002) to 41 (Solomon & Card, 2004).

Reasons for discrepancies in the lists of effective programs are detailed in Solomon and Card (2004); somewhat simplified, those compiling lists of effective programs used somewhat different criteria for what was considered to be a program (which varies by targeted outcome, approach, and participant age range) and somewhat different criteria for what evaluation criteria (research design and methods) would be accepted as showing evidence for effectiveness. In this section several different views of what might be effective teen pregnancy prevention programs are discussed, concluding with a consolidated picture of program effectiveness.

In 1997 the National Campaign to Prevent Teen Pregnancy published a review and assessment of teen pregnancy prevention programs entitled *No Easy Answers* (Kirby, 1997), which concluded that evaluation studies had almost all failed to find sustained effects on teen pregnancy and the behaviors that lead to teen pregnancy. The situation had improved markedly a few years later when the National Campaign to Prevent Teen Pregnancy published *Emerging Answers* (Kirby, 2001). Larger and more rigorous studies of selected sex and HIV education programs reported sustained positive effects on pregnancy risk behaviors for as long as three years; one program (Children's Aid—Carrera) that combined sexuality education and youth development showed pregnancy reduction for three years; other service learning (Teen Outreach) and sex and HIV education programs (Reducing the Risk) also reduced sexual risk-taking and teen pregnancy in several settings; and some short educational and clinical interventions that included one-on-one counseling showed evidence for increasing contraceptive use (Kirby, 2001).

Child Trends issued two reports (Manlove et al., 2001, 2002) in which prevention programs were graded "what works," "what does not work," and "mixed reviews," based on a systematic analysis of prevention programs targeted at initiation of sexual intercourse, use of condoms, use of contraceptives, and prevention of pregnancy and birth. Manlove and colleagues concluded that one program (*Reach for Health* or *Teen Outreach*) which included voluntary community service and related activities postponed the initiation of sexual intercourse. Several programs also showed strong evidence for preventing teen pregnancies and births. These were Teen Outreach (described above)(Allen & Philliber, 2001); an intensive early-childhood program for low-income families (Abcedarian), (Campbell & Ramey, 1994) that reduced teen pregnancies and births as well as out-of- wedlock births by age 27 (High/Scope, Perry Preschool) (Luster & McAdoo, 1996); and a home visiting program (Cole, Kitzman, Olds & Sidora, 1998) where nurses visited expectant teens before and after their babies were born, and which showed better child and maternal outcomes and reduced subsequent pregnancies.

Advocates for Youth (2003) published *Science and Success: Sex Education and Other Programs that Work to Prevent Teen Pregnancy*, using a methodology very similar to Kirby (2001). However, primarily because Advocates used less stringent criteria for length of followup to show duration of effects, 19 programs were included in their assessment of effective programs (vs. 8 programs identified by Kirby, 2001).

The list of effective programs developed by the Program Archive on Sexuality, Health, and Adolescence (PASHA) was derived by submitting candidate programs to a five-member scientific expert panel for review and scoring (Card, Niego, Mallari & Farrell, 1996). Most of the PASHA selected programs include replication kits consisting of the materials actually needed to set up and evaluate the programs. The PASHA group of effective programs is much larger (n = 41) than the others primarily for two reasons; it included programs targeted for STD/HIV prevention as well as teen pregnancy, and it accepted change in attitudes, values, and intentions (as opposed to behavior) as preliminary evidence of effectiveness for younger teens (ages 15 and under).

Another rigorous and methodologically demanding analysis of primary prevention studies was based on a systematic review of 26 evaluations conducted as randomized controlled trials between 1970 and 2000 (DiCenso, Guyatt & Griffith, 2002). To be included, studies had to be based on randomly assigned treatment and control groups and include outcome measures of sexual intercourse, contraceptive use, or pregnancy status. To tighten the design further, studies were excluded if they were based on older (college student) populations, second pregnancies, or measured only knowledge or attitudes rather than behavior. This systematic review methodology also gave a quality rating to each study based on four criteria, and statistically combined study findings using odds ratios and confidence intervals. The results of this very carefully controlled systematic review were quite consistent, but disappointing. "Primary prevention strategies evaluated to date do not delay the initiation of sexual intercourse, improve use of birth control among young men and women, or reduce the number of pregnancies in young women" (DiCenso et al., 2002).

What Does Not Work

Programs that don't work suffer from one or more of the following problems: (1) the short length of time the program has been implemented, (2) a poor evaluation design not addressing key issues (e.g., no control group, a lack of replication, inadequate sample size), or a (3) lack of a clear definition of what it means to be effective.

Recommendations

Community Interventions for Adolescent Parents and Their Children

Unfortunately, there is no magic recipe for intervention that will eradicate poor outcomes for adolescent parents and their children. However, following some general principles, and offering selected services will improve the lives of adolescent parents and their children. Comprehensive Quality Programming (CQP) provides practical guidance for prevention and intervention programming whether the intended outcomes are increased self-sufficiency, improved parenting, or enhanced maternal and child health (Nation et al., 2003). Table 1 provides a brief explanation of the eight essential components of CQP.

In addition to generally effective programming practices, the programs that were previously identified as those "that work" (i.e., Teen Parent Demonstration Project, early-childhood centers, and WIC) included three "bare-minimum" components that appear to be critical in assisting adolescent parents and their children. First, programs should be easily accessible and publicized. Some suggest the best place for adolescent parent programming to take place is on campus at high schools (See Stephens et al., 1999). Next, all programs for teen parents should include intensive case management. Finally, programs should either directly offer tangible resources (e.g., money, childcare, food vouchers) or make successful referrals to community partners which can provide these valuable resources.

The remaining program components depend on the specific needs in the community of adolescent parents. Contextual factors should drive program design and emphasis, given limited available resources. Additional support offered to teen parents with some success has often included education and job training, formal parenting or child development training, and quality, low-cost childcare. Successful programs offered more comprehensive support and intervention for adolescent parents and their children.

Residential Interventions for Adolescent Mothers and Their Children

Residential intervention options for teen mothers are extremely limited at this time. Renewed interest in *Second Chance Homes* provides an option aimed specifically at teen mothers. Second Chance Homes seem to be a program that might work for teen mothers displaced from their homes, but data are still preliminary. Displaced teen mothers are a vital group to target not only for the teen and child, but also preventing teens from having subsequent pregnancies, which multiply their difficulties.

Table 1. The Comprehensive Quality Programming approach

Accountability Questions	Strategic Planning	Explanation
1. Why is an intervention needed?	NEEDS ASSESSMENT	Application of validated assessment tools to gauge specific needs of youth or families in a defined community
How does the program use scientific knowledge and "best practice" of what works?	CONSULT SCIENCE LITERATURE AND PROMISING PRACTICE PROGRAMS	Synthesizing a body of significant literature that provides guidance of antecedents, correlates, and supportive intervention or prevention strategies
How will this new program fit with other programs you already offer?	FEEDBACK ON COMPREHENSIVENESS AND FIT OF PROGRAM	Becoming familiar with other services in the community that would compliment the target prevention or intervention efforts
How will the program be carried out?	PLANNING	Creating a written contract of how the program is expected to proceed, defining benchmarks of program implementation, and how the attainment of benchmarks will be assessed
How well was the program carried out?	PROCESS EVALUATION	Continuous tracking of program indicators related to the previously defined benchmarks; a bi-annual synthesis of this information is helpful until the program is well established
How well did the program work?	OUTCOME AND IMPACT EVALUATION	Upon full implementation, rigorously designed outcome evaluations that include a control comparison group should be conducted
What can be done to improve the program in the future?	LESSONS LEARNED	Retrospective consideration of possible changes that are needed to improve the impact of the program that is based on both process and outcome evaluations
What can be done to institutionalize the program?	PROGRAM DURATION, SUSTAINABILITY, AND ADAPTATION	Once a program is shown to be effective, implementers can pursue additional local, state, and national level support for wider implementation and adaptation for additional contexts

Table 2. Elements of Effective Adolescent Pregnancy Prevention Programs

Core Elements	Potential Additions
Targets a specific age range from junior high through high school*****	Family involvement**
Curriculum-based program time intensity ranged from 5 to 40 hours per year****	Intense youth development focus (including community service, 3–5 after-school hours per day, self-reflection activities, referral to social services, summer program)*
Sex education, HIV prevention, and/or health promotion curriculum****	Values clarification*
School-based****	Family, school, and community partnerships*
Experiential activities for enhancing refusal and avoidance skills***	Gender-specific classrooms*
Educator training***	Community-based*

*Number of stars indicates how many of the five programs had this element
Adapted from Nation et al., (2003).

The economic costs of these residential programs are reasonable and promise benefits that could reduce society costs in the long run.

There are more than 100 Second Chance Homes nationwide. Early research shows that less than 1% of Second Chance Home residents become pregnant while living in the home, and later subsequent pregnancies remain low where they have been evaluated. Two-thirds of residents continued with education or job training after leaving the home, nearly half had found work, and almost one-third of residents were off welfare rolls (SPAN, 2001). Studies also report that participants in these homes have higher rates of school completion, lower child abuse and neglect, and improved health of both the mother and the child when compared to state averages (DHHS, 2000).

Preventing Adolescent Pregnancy

Five programs have been identified by multiple groups as having the strongest evidence of effectiveness in preventing adolescent pregnancy. These are (1) *Be Proud! Be Responsible! A Safer Sex Curriculum; (2) Becoming a Responsible Teen; (3) Children's Aid Society—Carrera Program; (4) Reach for Health Community Youth Service;* and *(5) Safer Choices: A School-Based HIV Prevention Program.* An important caveat about these five programs are that they have been most rigorously tested with urban, mostly African American youth (Alford, 2003).

Core elements of the five most effective programs (Table 2) included targeting a specific age range; delivering 5–40 hours of HIV prevention, sex education, and/or health promotion curricula per year; being school-based; having trained educators deliver the curricula; and engaging students in experiential activities (See Alford, 2003). Additional complementary components utilized by some of the successful programs included family involvement, intense youth development, clarification of youth sexual values, community partnership building and/or community-based programming, and gender-specific classrooms (Alford, 2003).

References

Advocates for Youth. (2003). *Science and Success: Sex Education and Other Programs that Work To Prevent Teen Pregnancy.* Washington DC: Advocates for Youth.

Akinbam, L.J., Cheng, T.L., & Kornfeld, D. (2001). A review of teen-tot programs: Comprehensive clinical care for young parents and their children. *Adolescence, 36*(142), 381–393.

Alan Guttmacher Institute. (1994). *Sex and America's Teenagers.* New York: Author.

Allen, J.P. & Philliber, S. (2001). Who benefits most from a broadly targeted prevention program? Differential efficacy across populations in the Teen Outreach program. *Journal of Community Psychology, 29*(6), 637–656.

Alford, S. (2003). *Science and Success: Sex Education and Other Programs that Work To Prevent Teen Pregnancy.* Washington, DC: Advocates for Youth.

Barber, B.K. (1996). Parental psychological control: Revisiting a neglected construct. *Child Development, 67,* 3296–3319.

Benda, B.B., & DiBlasio, F.A. (1991). Comparison of four theories of adolescent sexual exploration. *Deviant Behavior, 12*(3), 235–257.

Besharov, D.J., & Germanis, P. (2000). Evaluating WIC. *Evaluation Review, 24*(2), 123–190.

Bos, J.M., & Fellerath, V. (1997a). *LEAP: Final Report on Ohio's Welfare Initiative To Improve School Attendance Among Teenage Parents.* New York: Manpower Demonstration Research Corporation.

Bos, J., Polit, D., & Quint, J. (1997b). *New Chance: Final Report on a Comprehensive Program for Young Mothers in Poverty and Their Children.* New York, NY: Manpower Demonstration Research Corporation.

Boyer, D., & Fine, D. (1992). Sexual abuse as a factor in adolescent pregnancy and child maltreatment. *Family Planning Perspectives, 24*(4), 4–19.

Browning, C., & Laumann, E. (1997). Sexual contact between children and adults: A life course perspective. *American Sociological Review, 62,* 540–560.

Campbell, F.A., & Ramey, C.T. (1994). Effects of early intervention on intellectual and academic achievement: A follow-up study of children from low-income families. *Child Development, 65,* 684–699.

Capaldi, D.M., Crosby, L., & Stoolmiller, M. (1996). Predicting the timing of first sexual intercourse for at-risk adolescent males. *Child Development, 67,* 344–359.

Card, J.J., Niego, S., Mallari, A., & Farrell, W.S. (1996). The program archive on sexuality, health & adolescence: Promising "prevention programs in a box." *Family Planning Perspective, 28*(5), 210–220.

Cole, R., Kitzman, H., Olds, D., & Sidora, K. (1998). Family context as a moderator of program effects in prenatal and early childhood home visits. *Journal of Community Psychology, 26,* 37–48.

Corcoran, J., Franklin, C., & Bennett, P. (2000). Ecological factors associated with adolescent pregnancy and parenting. *Social Work Research, 24*(1), 29–39.

Crean, H.F., Hightower, A.D., & Allan, M.J. (2001). School-based child care for children of teen parents: Evaluation of an urban program designed to keep young mothers in school. *Evaluation and Program Planning, 24,* 267–275.

Danziger, S.K. (1995). Family life and teenage pregnancy in the inner-city: Experiences of African-American youth. *Children and Youth Services Review, 17,* 183–202.

Denner, J., Kirby, D., Coyle, K., & Brindis, C. (2001). The protective role of social capital and cultural norms in Latino communities: A study of adolescent births. *Hispanic Journal of Behavioral Sciences, 23*(1), 3–21.

DHHS. (2000). *Second Chance Homes: Providing services for teenage parents and their children.* Retrieved November 3, 2003, from *www.aspe.os.dhhs.gov/hsp/2ndchancehomesoo/*

DiCenso, A., Guyatt, G., & Griffith, W.L. (2002). Intervention to reduce unintended pregnancies among adolescents: Systematic review of randomised controlled studies. *British Medical Journal, 324,* 1426–1435.

East, P.L. (1996a). Do adolescent pregnancy and childbearing affect younger siblings? *Family Planning Perspectives, 28*(4), 148–153.

East, P.L. (1996b). The younger sisters of childbearing adolescents: Their attitudes, expectations, and behaviors. *Child Development, 67,* 267–282.

East, P.L., Felice, M.E., & Morgan, M.C. (1993). Sisters' and girlfriends' sexual and childbearing behavior: Effects on early adolescent girls' sexual outcomes. *Journal of Marriage and the Family, 55,* 953–963.

East, P.L., & Shi, C.R. (1997). Pregnant and parenting adolescents and their younger sisters: The influence of relationship qualities for younger sister outcomes. *Journal of Developmental and Behavioral Pediatrics, 18,* 84–90.

Feldman, S.S., & Brown, N.L. (1993). Family influences on adolescent male sexuality: The mediational role of self restraint. *Social Development, 2*(1), 15–35.

Flannery, D.J., Rowe, D.C., & Gulley, B.L. (1993). Impact of pubertal status, timing, and age on adolescent sexual experience and delinquency. *Journal of Adolescent Research, 8*(1), 21–40.

Friedrich, W.N. (2002). *Psychological Assessment of Sexually Abused Children and Their Families.* Thousand Oaks, CA: Sage.

Garn, S.M. (1980). Continuities and change in maturational timing. In O.G. Brim & J. Kagan (Eds.), *Constancy and Change in Human Development* (pp. 113–162). Cambridge: Harvard University Press.

Granger, R.C., & Cytron, R. (1999). Teenage parent programs: A synthesis of the long-term effects of the New Chance Demonstration, Ohio's Learning, Earning, and Parenting Program, and the Teenage Parent Demonstration. *Evaluation Review, 23*(2), 107–145.

Gray, M.R., & Steinberg, L. (1999). Unpacking authoritative parenting: Reassessing a multidimensional construct. *Journal of Marriage and the Family, 61,* 574–587.

Grisham, C., & Levin-Epstein, J. (2003). *Teen Parents and Temporary Assistance for Needy Families: A Summary of Recent Congressional Action.* Washington, DC: Center for Law and Social Policy.

Gupta, S., Venkateswaran, R., Gorenflo, D.W., & Eyler, A.E. (1999). Childhood iron deficiency anemia, maternal nutritional knowledge, and maternal feeding practices in a high-risk population. *Preventative Medicine, 29,* 152–159.

Halpern, C.T., Udry, J.R., Campbell, B., & Suchindran, C. (1993). Testosterone and pubertal development as predictors of sexual activity: A panel analysis of adolescent males. *Psychosomatic Medicine, 55,* 436–447.

Henshaw, S.K. (2003). *U.S. Teenage Pregnancy Statistics with Comparative Statistics for Women Aged 20–24.* New York: The Alan Guttmacher Institute.

Hogan, D.P., & Kitagawa, E.M. (1985). The impact of social status, family structure, and neighborhood on the fertility of Black adolescents. *American Journal of Sociology, 90*(4), 825–855.

Jaccard, J., Dittus, P.J., & Gordon, V.V. (1996). Maternal correlates of adolescent sexual and contraceptive behavior. *Perspectives on Sexual and Reproductive Health, 28*(4), 159–185.

Jaccard, J., Dittus, P.J., & Litardo, H.A. (1999). Parent-adolescent communication about sex and birth control: Implications for parent-based interventions to reduce unintended adolescent pregnancy. In L.J. Sever, W.B. Miller & L. Sever (Eds.), *Advances in Population: Psychological Perspectives* (Vol. 3). London: Jessica Kingsley Publishers.

Kirby, D. (1997). *No Easy Answers: Research Findings on Programs to Reduce Teen Pregnancy.* Washington DC: National Campaign to Prevent Teen Pregnancy.

Kirby, D. (2001). *Emerging Answers.* Washington, DC: National Campaign to Prevent Teen Pregnancy.

Kirby, D., & Ryan, J. (2004). *Risk and Protective Factors Affecting Teen Sexual Behavior, Pregnancy, Childbearing, and Sexually Transmitted Diseases: Which Are Important? Which Can You Change?* Washington, DC: National Campaign to Prevent Teen Pregnancy.

Kisker, E.E., Rangarajan, A., & Boller, K. (1998). *Moving Into Adulthood: Were the Impacts of Mandatory Programs for Welfare-Dependent Teenage Parents Sustained After the Programs Ended?* Princeton, NJ: Mathematica Policy Research.

Klaw, E.L., Rhodes, J.E., & Fitzgerald, L.F. (2003). Natural mentors in the lives of African American adolescent mothers: Tracking relationships over time. *Journal of Youth and Adolescence, 32,* 223–232.

Klerman, L.V., Baker, B.A., & Howard, G. (2003). Second births among teenage mothers: Program results and statistical methods. *Journal of Adolescent Health, 32,* 452–455.

Kowaleski-Jones, L., & Duncan, G.J. (2002). Effects of participation in the WIC program on birthweight: Evidence from the National Longitudinal Survey of Youth. *American Journal of Public Health, 92*(5), 799–804.

Kresge, J. (2003). *WIC Participants and Program Characteristics: Executive Summary.* Alexandria, VA: United States Department of Agriculture.

Ku, L., Sonenstein, F.L., & Pleck, J.H. (1993). Neighborhood, family and work: Influences on the premarital behaviors of adolescent males. *Social Forces, 72,* 479–503.

Love, J.M., Kisker, E.E., Ross, C.M., Schochet, P.Z., & Brooks-Gunn, J. (2002). *Making a Difference in the Lives of Infants and Toddlers and Their Families: The Impacts of Early Head Start.* Washington, DC: U.S. Department of Health and Human Services.

Luster, T., & McAdoo, H. (1996). Family and child influences on educational attainment: A secondary analysis of the high/scope. *Developmental Psychology, 32,* 26–40.

Luster, T., & Small, S.A. (1994). Factors associated with sexual risk-taking behaviors among adolescents. *Journal of Marriage and the Family, 56,* 622–632.

Luster, T., & Small, S.A. (1997). Sexual abuse history and number of sex partners among female adolescents. *Family Planning Perspectives, 29*(5), 204–211.

Manlove, J., Terry-Humen, E., Papillo, A.R., Franzetta, K., Williams, S., & Ryan, S. (2001). *Background for Community-Level Work on Positive Reproductive Health in Adolescence: Reviewing the Literature on Contributing Factors*. Washington, DC: Child Trends.

Manlove, J., Terry-Humen, E., Papillo, A.R., Franzetta, K., Williams, S., & Ryan, S. (2002). *Preventing Teenage Pregnancy, childbearing, and Sexually Transmitted Diseases: What the Research Shows*. Washington, DC: Child Trends.

Maynard, R.A. (1996). *Kids Having Kids: A Robin Hood Foundation Special Report on the Costs of Adolescent Childbearing*. New York: Robin Hood Foundation.

Miller, B.C., Benson, B., & Galbraith, K.A. (2001). Family relationships and adolescent pregnancy risk: A research synthesis. *Developmental Review, 21*, 1–38.

Miller, B.C., & Coyl, D.D. (2000). Adolescent pregnancy and childbearing in relation to infant adoption in the United States. *Adoption Quarterly, 4*, 3–25.

Miller, B.C., Monson, B.H., & Norton, M.C. (1995). The effects of forced sexual intercourse on white female adolescents. *Child Abuse and Neglect, 19*, 1289–1301.

Miller, B.C., Norton, M.C., Curtis, T., Hill, E.J., Schvaneveldt, P., & Young, M.H. (1997). The timing of sexual intercourse among adolescents: Family, peer, and other antecedents. *Youth and Society, 29*, 54–83.

Miller, B.C., Norton, M.C., Fan, X., & Christopherson, C.R. (1998). Pubertal development, parental communication, and sexual values in relation to adolescent sexual behaviors. *Journal of Early Adolescence, 18*, 27–52.

Miller, W.B., Pasta, D.J., MacMurray, J., Chiu, C., Wu, H., & Comings, D.E. (1999). Dopamine receptor genes are associated with age at first sexual intercourse. *Journal of Biosocial Science, 31*, 43–54.

Moore, M.R., & Chase-Lansdale, P.L. (2001). Sexual intercourse and pregnancy among African American girls in high-poverty neighborhoods: The role of family and perceived community environment. *Journal of Marriage and the Family, 63*, 1146–1157.

Mott, F.L., Fondell, M.M., Hu, P.N., Kowaleski-Jones, L., & Menaghan, E.G. (1996). The determinants of first sex by age 14 in a high-risk adolescent population. *Family Planning Perspectives, 28*(1), 13–18.

Nathanson, C.A. (1991). *Dangerous Passage: The Social Control of Sexuality in Women's Adolescence*. Philadelphia: Temple University Press.

Nation, M., Crusto, C., Wandersman, A., Kumpfer, K.L., Seybolt, D., Morrissey-Kane, E., & Davino, K. (2003). What works in prevention: Principles of effective prevention programs. *American Psychologist, 58*, 45–64.

Newcomer, S.F., & Udry, J.R. (1984). Mothers' influence on sexual behavior of their teenage children. *Journal of Marriage and the Family, 46*, 477–485.

Newcomer, S.F., & Udry, J.R. (1985). Parental marital status effects on adolescent sexual behavior. *Journal of Marriage and the Family, 49*, 235–240.

Ramirez-Valles, J., Zimmerman, M.A., & Newcomb, M.D. (1998). Sexual risk behavior among youth: Modeling the influence of prosocial activities and socioeconomic factors. *Journal of Health and Social Behavior, 39*, 237–253.

Resnick, M.D., Bearman, P.S., Blum, R.W., Bauman, K.E., Harris, K.M., Jones, J., et al. (1997). Protecting adolescents from harm: Findings from the National Longitudinal Study on Adolescent Health. *Journal of American Medical Association, 278*, 823–832.

Rodgers, J.L., & Rowe, D.C. (1988). Influence of siblings on adolescent sexual behavior. *Developmental Psychology, 24*, 722–728.

Rodgers, J.L., Rowe, D.C., & Buster, M. (1999). Social contagion, adolescent sexual behavior, and pregnancy: A nonlinear dynamic EMOSA model. *Developmental Psychology, 34*(5), 1096–1113.

Rodgers, J.L., Rowe, D.C., & Harris, D.F. (1992). Sibling differences in adolescent sexual behavior: Inferring process models from family composition patterns. *Journal of Marriage and the Family, 54*, 142–152.

Rodgers, K.B. (1999). Parenting processes related to sexual risk-taking behaviors of adolescent males and females. *Journal of Marriage and the Family, 61*, 99–109.

Roosa, M.W., Tein, J., Reinholtz, C., & Angelini, P.J. (1997). The relationship between childhood sexual abuse and teenage pregnancy. *Journal of Marriage and the Family, 59*, 119–130.

Russell, D.E.H. (1986). *The Secret Trauma: Incest in the Lives of Girls and Women*. New York: Basic Books.

Scaramella, L.V., Conger, R.D., Simons, R.L., & Whitbeck, L.B. (1998). Predicting risk for pregnancy by late adolescence: A social contextual perspective. *Developmental Psychology, 34*, 1233–1245.

Singh, S.A., & Darroch, J.E. (2000). Adolescent pregnancy and childbearing: Levels and trends in developed countries. *Family Planning Perspective, 32*, 14–23.

Small, S.A., & Luster, T. (1994). Adolescent sexual activity: An ecological, risk-factor approach. *Journal of Marriage and the Family, 56*, 181–192.

Solomon, J., & Card, J.J. (2004). *Making the List: Understanding, Selecting, and Replicationg Effective Teen Pregnancy Prevention Programs*. Washington, DC: National Campaign to Prevent Teen Pregnancy.

SPAN. (2001). *Second Chance Homes in the Federal Budget*. Retrieved October 10, 2003, from *www.span-online.org*

Stephens, S.A., Wolf, W.C., & Batten, S.T. (1999). *Improving Outcomes for Teen Parents and Their Young Children by Strengthening School-Based Programs: Challenges, Solutions, and Policy Implications*. Washington, DC: Center for Assessment and Policy Development.

Sylvester, K. (1995). *Second-chance homes: Breaking the cycle of teen pregnancy*. Retrieved November 3, 2003, from *www.ppionline.org/documents/2ndchance.pdf*

Thornton, A., & Camburn, D. (1987). The influence of the family on premarital sexual attitudes and behavior. *Demography, 24*, 323–340.

Udry, J.R. (1988). Biological predispositions and social control in adolescent sexual behavior. *American Sociological Review, 53*, 709–722.

Udry, J.R., Talbert, L.B., & Morris, N.M. (1986). Biosocial foundations for adolescent female sexuality. *Demography, 23*(2), 217–230.

Upchurch, D.M., Aneshensel, C.S., Sucoff, C.A., & Levy-Storms, L. (1999). Neighborhood and family contexts of adolescent sexual activity. *Journal of Marriage and the Family, 61*, 920–933.

Wagner, M.M., & Clayton, S.L. (1999). The Parents as Teachers Program: Results from two demonstrations. *The Future of Children, 9*(1), 91–115.

Weatherley, R.A. (1991). Comprehensive services for pregnant and parenting adolescents: Historical and political considerations. *Evaluation and Program Planning, 14*(1–2), 17–25.

Webster-Stratton, C. (1998). Preventing conduct problems in Head Start children: Strengthening parenting competencies. *Journal of Consulting and Clinical Psychology, 66*(5), 715–730.

Weinstein, M., & Thornton, A. (1989). Mother-child relations and adolescent sexual attitudes and behaviors. *Demography, 26*, 563–577.

Whitbeck, L., Conger, R., & Kao, M. (1993). The influence of parental support, depressed affect, and peers on the sexual behaviors of adolescent girls. *Journal of Family Issues, 14*, 261–278.

Whitbeck, L., Hoyt, D., Miller, M., & Kao, M. (1992). Parental support, depressed affect, and sexual experiences among adolescents. *Youth and Society, 24*(2), 166–177.

Whitbeck, L.B., Simons, R.L., & Kao, M. (1994). The effects of divorced mothers' dating behaviors and sexual attitudes on the sexual attitudes and behaviors of their adolescent children. *Journal of Marriage and the Family, 56*, 615–621.

Whitehead, B.D. (2001). *What's God Got To Do with Teen Pregnancy Prevention?* Washington, D.C.; National Campaign to Prevent Teen Pregnancy.

Widmer, E.D. (1997). Influence of older siblings on initiation of sexual intercourse. *Journal of Marriage and the Family, 59*, 928–938.

Williams, R.L., Hersey, J., Kavee, J., Smith, D., Bell, L., Bellamy, H., et al. (2002). *Adolescent WIC participants study: Volume 1, final report* (No. WIC-02-ADOL). Alexandria, VA: United States Department of Agriculture.

Wu, L.L., & Martinson, B.B. (1993). Family structure and the risk of a premarital birth. *American Sociological Review, 58*, 210–232.

Zabin, L.S., Smith, E.A., Hirsch, M.B., & Hardy, J.B. (1986). Ages of physical maturation and first intercourse in black teenage males and females. *Demography, 23*(4), 595–605.

Zaslow, M.J., & Eldred, C.A. (1998). *Parenting Behaviors in a Sample of Young Mothers in Poverty: Results of the New Chance Observation Study*. New York: Manpower Demonstration Research Corporation.

Chapter 27

School Failure

Peter W. Dowrick and Natalie Crespo

Introduction

School failure is an important worldwide issue, leading to underemployment (unemployment or job dissatisfaction) and a lower quality of life. The overall drop-out rate in the United States is 10–25%, depending on how it is reckoned. But it is common for the most struggling high schools to lose 25–50% of their students between 9th and 12th grade, and on any given day, 10–20% of the student body will be absent from school. Overkall, rates of drop-out and truancy have remained steady for a decade but have increased in some areas, especially in low-income families and among other subpopulations. Drop-out and truancy are the topics covered in this chapter. Many methods of keeping adolescents in regular attendance at school are widely reported but not thoroughly evaluated.

Definitions

The term *to drop out* is widely used in reference to youth who do not finish high school, or it can be used to refer to the phenomenon itself (usually one word, *drop-out*). That raises the question, What does it mean to finish? In the United States, students are expected to complete 12 grades. Students in 12th grade (usually aged 17 or 18 years) who meet standards set by their school or district receive a graduation diploma or a certificate of completion. Other parts of the world are different. In many countries, the last three years of high school are optional. There are often national examinations, at different levels, in these years, enabling youth aged 15 or 16 to leave school with viable credentials. Thus internationally, the term *dropping-out* may refer either to leaving school before passing any recognized exams, or to leaving unqualified to pursue employment opportunities of personal fulfillment (Dowrick, 2003).

Even within a single country, how and when drop-out is measured greatly influences the reports of incidence and the perceived magnitude of the problem. Moreover, drop-out should not be seen as a single event. Although there is a moment in time when circumstances meet some criterion for drop-out, it is usually the cumulation of a long-term process of increasing alienation from the school system (Srebnik & Elias, 1993).

Most high schools in the US set goals of 90–95% average daily attendance; struggling schools typically reach about 88%. Within the broad spectrum of *absenteeism*, the term *truancy* simply means being absent from school without permission—also referred to as *absenteeism*. It is the interpretation of "permission," and its vagaries across schools and age groups, that creates confusion. For example, one school district may expect a parental letter of explanation for an absence of up to three days, and a physician's note beyond that. Another may set different time limits or require different levels of explanation. (In my last year at high school, I [first author] would write "please excuse Peter's absence" [without saying why] and sign it myself, as I was privately boarding away from my parents and all the teacher wanted was a letter on file.) Thus thousands of days may not be counted that might otherwise be included under strict definitions and monitoring of truancy. While nearly all schools diligently document absences, most will pursue issues of truancy only when it is a significant and obvious problem for individual students. Up to *one-third* of all absences may be classified as truant, depending on the local definition.

As noted, this chapter focuses on drop-out and truancy. More generally *school failure* may be defined as drop-out in any form, truancy, being suspended or expelled, failing, or repeating classes, or not "graduating" by age 19 (or 22 with certain disabilities) in the US public school system, or the equivalent outcomes elsewhere.

Incidence of Drop-Out

The US Department of Education reported a "completion" rate of 86% in 18–24-year-olds in the year 2000 (National Center for Education Statistics; NCES, 2002a). The implied converse figure, a 14% drop-out rate, is socially important—because it indicates how many young adults for whom school has been unsuccessful. Even if some of these individuals enroll in night school in their 40s and complete a General Education Development (GED) award, as some do, the publicly mandated school system has failed to provide work- and life-relevant fundamental education in a timely way. Other ways to measure this phenomenon include the "event" drop-out rate, referring to the percentage of students aged 15–24 in 10th–12th grade who left school in the past year, without a certificate (5%). The "status" drop-out (12%), is the percentage of 16–24-year-olds who left school incomplete, regardless of when they left. All these rates fell by about one-third in the 1960s but reverted by a few percentage point in the 1970s and have changed little since (NCES, 2002a).

Another socially important way to measure drop-out is to track those entering ninth grade who quit school within the subsequent four years ("cohort" rate). This method of measurement is favored by some (e.g., Fitzpatrick & Yoels, 1992), because it indicates a failure by the school system even though at least one-third of such drop-outs are temporary. On the other hand, this measure overlooks those who drop out before ninth grade, an incidence that can be significant for some populations (e.g., migrant farm workers; Martinez & Cranston-Gingras, 1996). Interstate differences are large; recent completion rates varied from 74% (Arizona) to 95% (Maine). Drop-out is significantly greater in the southern United States (NCES,

2002a). It would seem investigations of state differences would tell us much about risk and protective factors in school failure, but little causal analysis is available except that the drop-out rate is 44% among foreign-born Latino youth. The NCES methods of reporting drop-out, especially for African Americans, have been seriously challenged by the Manhattan Institute for Policy Research (Greene, 2002), who put the graduation rates much lower based on differences in definitions and sampling.

An appreciation of the incidence of drop-out is further complicated by the practice of school districts' typically identifying a student as dropped out by such definitions as "absent for 30 consecutive school days without a request for transcripts from another school." While such criteria are functional for schools, they are simply different from those used by NCES in national reports.

Rates vary considerably across schools and social conditions (Dowrick, 2003). In small high schools in stable communities, over 90% of students finish; in large high schools in less stable, low-income communities, fewer than 50% complete in four years. Youth living in families with incomes in the lowest 20% are six times as likely as their peers from the top 20% in the income distribution to drop out of high school (NCES, 2002a). Youth with disabilities are more than five times as likely to drop out of school. Drop-out rates also vary across the major ethnic and linguistic groups. Asian Americans have significantly lower rates than European Americans. The rate for African Americans is 50% higher; for Latinos and Native Americans, three or four times higher (Meece & Kurtz-Costes, 2001). Boys are less likely to graduate than girls, and this difference increases within the settings and groups most at risk.

Internationally, success in school is highly dependent on what the country can afford and on government priorities. Industrialized countries tend to have rates comparable to those in the United States. Many other countries do not have free and widely accessible schooling. In these places, high school *attendance* may be as low as 5% of any age group, favoring the (wealthy) boys, especially where the girl's job in life is to procreate and support family. In the two most populated countries in the world, China and India, high school attendance for girls in rural areas is less than 5%, although educational prospects are far better in the cities (Bhakta, Hackett & Hackett, 2002; Zhou, Zhang, Liu, Ma & Peng, 2001).

Implications

For individuals who do not finish or regularly attend school, there is an expected lower quality of life; nationally, there is lost productivity. Those who finish high school are more likely to get well-paid jobs, to gain higher education of their choice, and to participate in the democratic process (Dowrick, 2003). Whereas the drop-out rate has decreased from the levels of 40 years ago, the consequences have increased in that the earning power of educationally unqualified youth has been *halved* in that time. Youth who drop out spend more time in jail and less time in shopping malls (personal spending is a major factor in economic growth). If a program that costs $700,000 prevents one drop-out, it breaks even with the costs to the individual and society (lost wages, public and private benefits). If that would-be drop-out were also diverted from becoming a heavy drug user and career criminal, $1.700,000 would be a fair price (based on Cohen, 1998; 2004 dollar equivalents).

Theories to Guide Prevention and Practice

Adolescents become truant or likely to drop out when they *dislike school*, combined with either (a) weak incentives to stay or (b) strong incentives to leave (Dowrick, 2003). Many risk and resilience factors contribute to liking or disliking school, and to the incentives to stay or leave (Vallerand, Fortier & Guay, 1997). Most published research indicates that *combinations* of factors, never single factors, are needed for dropping out of school to occur.

Why might youth dislike school? The most important reasons are being academically unsuccessful and/or experiencing negative social outcomes. The two can overlap because poor grades and repeating classes are damaging when the failure is emotionally *felt* through shame or separation from a peer group. Contributors to academic failure include learning disabilities (one of the most cited risk factors; Tobler, 2000), especially when literacy skills are well below par. Other contributors are negative attitudes towards education by peers or family. For youth in trouble at school, there emerges a vicious cycle, in which the institutional response to an aberrant behavior sets up a negative emotional reaction to create more trouble.

When are there weak incentives to attend school? The value of school seems less important when one's parents and family members have little education, unless the family is outspoken in promoting more education. Incentives to stay in school are weakened when pupils' anticipations of the future are bleak or empty (Dowrick, Tallman & Connor, 2004). Failing and expecting failure are interrelated, as the theory of self-efficacy makes clear (Bandura, 1993). As a consequence, teachers can encourage or discourage school participation on the basis that *they* can succeed with students who are struggling. Many youth who believe in the value of education find their school incompatible and hostile towards their goals (Dowrick, 2003).

What are the incentives to be somewhere other than school? Peers are a significant influence, as truancy is seldom a solitary activity (Corville-Smith, Ryan, Adams & Dalicandro, 1998). Sometimes immediate needs or short-term opportunities will tip the balance for students who are discontent (Jordan, Lara & McPartland, 1996). These opportunities can range from openings to earn just minimum wage in a local retail franchise, to life-changing enticements to sell illicit drugs. Girls may skip school or leave because of pregnancy. Youth in low-income families may feel a responsibility to contribute a regular paycheck to the household. Such is frequently true in low income communities and among migrant farm workers.

Individual Factors

There has been considerable research on the factors contributing to drop-out. From the individual's viewpoint, the most general risks posed to succeeding in school are academic performance (poor grades, repeating a grade, low literacy; Vallerand et al., 1997) incompatibility with school (ethnic, linguistic, social; Vitaro, Larocque, Janosz & Tremblay, 2001), and misconduct and drug use (Rosenthal, 1998). See Table 1 for a list of risk and resilience factors believed to have the greatest influence on school success or failure.

Table 1. Factors of Risk and Resiliency in School Failure (Dropout and Truancy). (Items represent a short list of the most important factors identified in studies and reviews).

Risk	Resiliency
Individual factors influencing risk and resiliency	
Incompatible with school	
Feeling ignored	Feeling valued by teachers, etc.
Poor school performance	Belief in the future, value of education
Low literacy	High literacy
Low self-efficacy	High self-efficacy
Misconduct, delinquency, drug use	Sports/extracurricular activity
Family factors influencing risk and resiliency	
	Parent is involved in child's education
Low family socioeconomic status (SES)	High family SES
Receives public assistance	
Unstable employment	Stable employment
Being (or having) a teen parent	Family support for a teen parent
Social and community factors influencing risk and resiliency	
Neighborhood factors	
Low neighborhood SES	High neighborhood SES
Few employment opportunities	Visible employment opportunities
Adults and peers with low achievement	Adults and peers with high achievement
School factors	
Culturally mismatch	Culturally relevant instruction
Tracking with low achieving peers	Supportive mentor or teacher

Special populations have additional risk factors. Although disabilities are predictive of dropping out, low intelligence, measured by IQ, is not as predictive as the risks listed above. In the United States, the term "learning disabilities" refers, not to overall cognitive deficits as it does in other countries, but to an uneven development in which there is a discrepancy between core academics and other areas of performance. This learning disorder is frustrating and contributes to a dislike of school (Tobler, 2000). There is little evidence that learning disability, on its own, leads to drop-out. Other risk factors—from the individual, family, school, or community—are necessary to act in combination with learning difficulties to produce negative outcomes. Many studies have examined the large representation of youth with emotional and behavioral disorders (EBD) in the drop-out statistics. Youth with EBD experience school failure in more ways and more often than students in any other category (Rylance, 1997). These youth also experience the worst post-school outcomes, such as unemployment, criminal involvement, or family dysfunction.

Research on high school failure in mainstream families also indicates how many factors contribute. In a study of hundreds of "middle class drop-outs," there were high rates of mental health disorders, substance abuse, family problems, learning disorders, and difficult relationships at school (Franklin & Streeter, 1995). Involvement with drugs or other delinquency often occurs among truant youth and increases the risk of dropping out of school (see Chapter 27). However, drug use on its own poses a small risk; youth dealers are five times more likely to quit school than nondealers involved with drugs (Dembo et al., cited by Centers & Weist, 1998). Drug abuse is an important marker, but part of a pattern that includes family stress.

A frequently cited reason for disliking school is being unsuccessful in school organized activities (Battistich & Hom, 1997).

But many students experiencing some failure do stay in school and "complete." Results of research in this area are typified by Finn and Rock (1997), who studied 1,800 high school students from ethnic minority families in low-income neighborhoods, systematically sampled from a large number of schools. They measured 'school engagement' (i.e., liking school) for students identified as succeeding in school (vs. failing), while eliminating other personal and family differences. They found large, significant differences in the levels of engagement, with evidence for disliking school being a strong predictor of skipping school and/or dropping out.

In many countries, immigrants who speak another language are much more likely to drop out of school. Studies in Canada have found drop-out rates up to 75% for second-language learners, rates correlating inversely with proficiency in the language of instruction (Worrell, 1997).

There is considerable research related to the importance of self-efficacy—belief that one can succeed—and perseverance in the face of adversity. Having a specific positive image of the future may be crucial to remaining engaged in a challenging situation (Dowrick, 1999). For example, Dowrick et al. (2004) found superior outcomes for special needs students when they made videos explicitly of the youths' "futures plans" to show what their lives could look like in five years' time. In an extensive review of positive youth development programs, Catalano, Berglund, Ryan, Lonczak, and Hawkins (2002) expressed disappointment that few well-documented interventions addressed the resilience factor of positive futures (although nearly all addressed self-efficacy). The multiple ways in which a belief in a positive future may be developed and the role it plays in success at school are topics for further research.

Family Factors

The family environment has a considerable influence on academic success. Of the many family factors contributing to risk and resiliency, most are related to the child's developmental progress and socioeconomic environment. Factors such as social and economic status (SES) and employment status of parents are key to a student's risk of failure. Also important is the type of family environment in which a child is raised. For example, children who are in foster homes or who have unstable family lives are at increased risk of school failure. Being a teenage mother increases the risk that she will drop out of school. This risk is carried over to the next generation, as children of teenage mothers also perform poorly in school. The influence of the family is both developmental and social—how and where the child grew up.

Parents' involvement in their children's education can have a positive effect. Large data studies have indicated a positive influence of parental involvement on youth staying in school, even when the youth have low academic achievement or are from low income families (e.g., Jimerson, Egeland, Sroufe & Carlson, 2000). Parents tend to be less involved in the educational support of their sons than with that of their daughters (Carter & Wojtkiewicz, 2000). Parent involvement and child outcomes are affected by parenting style and by the family's socioeconomic status. Often parents from foreign or low-SES backgrounds will defer to the teacher's authority in making decisions regarding their child's education and avoid advocating for change in the school setting (Fischer & Dowrick, 2003).

Instability in the family environment is a significant risk factor. High school (9th–12th grade) students whose families receive public assistance have a 25% greater risk of dropping out of school (Orthner & Randolph, 1999). Family stability is important—more important than status. Children of parents who remain unemployed and on welfare are more likely to succeed than children of parents who fluctuate between employment and joblessness. Research on teenagers in foster care indicates a higher than usual rate of personal problems and difficulty in school such as suspension, expulsion, and repeating a grade. A study by Zima, Bussing, Freeman, Yang, Belin, and Forness (2000) found that 25% of the students in foster care experienced these difficulties. Pong and Ju (2000) found that instability in family structure also increased dropout risk beyond the financial instability that often comes with family changes such as divorce and break-up. They report the risk to be higher if the change results in households headed by a single mother.

The risk generated by having a child while in high school depends on the available support system and the mother's values and academic goals (Stevenson, Maton & Teti, 1998). If there is family support available to the mother, including some childcare, the mother is more likely to return to school. Success then depends largely on the mother's previous academic success and educational goals. Overall, a mother's individual risk factors (as discussed in the previous section) modify her likelihood of success or failure. Children whose mothers gave birth to them as teenagers are more likely to perform poorly on academic tests and to be held back a grade in school. Teenage parenthood is related to factors such as lower SES and larger family size, which affect the academic success of children. However, the impact of the risk is only half as great for the child as it is for his or her teenage mother (Levine, Pollack, & Comfort, 2001).

Children often achieve education equal to that of their parents and siblings. A study by McCaul, Donaldson, Coladarci, and Davis (1992) with a large number of public school drop-outs indicated significant economic factors: rural students left school most often to get a job or to get married; urban students most frequently reported leaving school to support families or because friends were dropping out. Here we see an overlap in family and social factors.

Social and Community Factors

Where a family lives has an influence on risk and resiliency. Neighborhoods with low socioeconomic status are associated with an increase in school drop-out and truancy. Low-SES areas have limited employment opportunities, high family mobility, and many adults with low educational attainment. Communities in which educational attainment is not valued and consequently not achieved are communities in which children are more likely to drop out of school (South, Baumer & Lutz, 2003). The reverse of these factors also promotes resiliency. Community examples of high educational participation and attainment serve as protective factors for youth. Schools that serve these neighborhoods are often fraught with poor teaching and high teacher attrition, leading to students' feeling detached from school and more attracted to deviant behaviors.

An important influence on students' academic success is peer educational behavior. A student whose peers are frequently truant or have already dropped out of school is more likely to participate in the same activities. That is, affiliation with deviant or dropped-out peers has a strong effect, presumably through modeling and engagement in activities incompatible with school-based education (Vitaro et al., 2001). Low social acceptance by peers has been identified as a risk factor in some studies and not in others—it may be a marker of behavior and academic problems or it may be a summary of them.

In their relationships with students, teachers also have the potential to influence resiliency. Teaching can improve achievement when it is culturally relevant and conducted in a way in which students are supported and challenged. Youth whose peers attend school regularly and graduate are likely to do the same. Social and environmental surroundings have a great deal of influence in the risk and resiliency of adolescent school failure. Collective school efficacy (administrators and teachers' beliefs that they can get good academic outcomes) is just as important as the self-beliefs of students (Bandura, 1993). For example, a comparison across 79 elementary schools showed that students from "disadvantaged" backgrounds, based on family income, education, and ethnicity, performed significantly better in schools in which staff reported high levels of belief that they could produce excellent academic standards of student achievement. On the other hand, students are less likely to attend school and more likely to drop out where teachers have low expectations of themselves or their students.

Many neighborhood and community factors are related to risk and resiliency. Neighborhoods with few employment or career opportunities and many community members who have had little academic success create risk factors. Such characteristics can be offset by the presence of adult, and older peer, role models. These factors are especially relevant for minorities. Family incomes that place in the top third among African Americans place in the poorest third of white families (Vartanian & Gleason, 1999). Individuals from such families experience less exposure to and fewer benefits from resiliency factors in their communities and local schools.

School size can affect the achievement of students. "Optimal" high school size has been found to be dependent on community factors such as SES. Schools in poorer communities benefit from being even smaller than those in more affluent communities. High school size in high-SES communities is best limited to 1,000 pupils. In low-SES areas, schools should be much smaller, around 600 students, to achieve equity in student success (Howley, Strange, & Bickel, 2000). Note that many high schools with significant school failure problems have 2,000 to 5,000 students.

Students benefit from having positive relationships with adults in the community, although mentoring alone has not been shown to have valuable effects. In peer and adult mentoring relationships, it is important to consider who is mentoring. Peers have a great influence on student performance. Mentoring can be detrimental to failing students when they are introduced to new peers who are also doing poorly (O'Donnell, Tharp & Wilson, 1993). But mentoring is helpful when it includes positive role modeling, genuine caring, and skill building. Naturally occurring mentoring relationships, for example, with relatives or teachers, are often mentioned by at-risk students as a reason that they succeeded in school.

Teachers have the opportunity to influence students to re-engage in academics by challenging them and providing opportunities for them to succeed. Teachers and schools also have a responsibility to provide culturally relevant instruction and environment for students. This task can be difficult in schools with diversity—that is, multiple cultures to which to respond. However, culturally relevant education can make a great difference in students' achievement.

Teaching in a culturally relevant way results in a higher level of student engagement in school activities (Nation et al., 2003). Education requires working with, rather than against, cultural norms. For example, Hawaiian school children have been noted to test their teacher's authority rambunctiously, behavior known locally as "to act" (at home, parents will admonish: "No act!"). Teachers have found that everyone wins if they use the students' natural energies and tendency to learn collaboratively (versus competitively), and their interpersonal structures and hierarchies (D'Amato, 1988). Minority students begin school with enthusiasm, but these feelings are often lost early on, and by high school it can be too late.

Involvement with drugs, as noted above, is an individual risk factor. Communities with drug gangs pose additional risks by offering financial incentives to leave school. At least one in six teenagers in the big cities of United States had some involvement in drug dealing in the 1990s (Centers & Weist, 1998). Accurate evidence for youth income from these activities is difficult to determine—but the monthly earnings are reliably at least four times those of other income opportunities in the same neighborhoods.

Community members, culture, and schools are all intertwined in adolescents' educational experience. Communities that provide encouragement and models for school success can influence children to complete high school and contribute to their plans for postsecondary education or employment. Overall the findings remind us of the need for multiple characteristics and events to be present for truancy and dropout to occur, or to be prevented (Battin-Pearson, Newcomb, Abbott, Hill, Catalano & Hawkins, 2000).

Evidence-Based Treatment Interventions in Community Settings

Individualized assistance of some intensity may be necessary to make a difference in educational outcomes for youth who have dropped out—or have been been "dropped," e.g., expelled or placed in a restrictive institution (VanDenBerg & Grealish, 1996). In the early 1990s, MacFarquhar, Dowrick, and Risley (1993) collected data from 15 programs in 12 states through structured interviews with experts in the field. These programs were for the most seriously emotionally disturbed youth, who required multiple agency support and were frequently sent to out-of-state institutions. The average youth had four prior psychiatric hospitalizations and up to 100% had quit school at least once after extensive truancy, although most were attending an institutionally provided school program. The objectives of these individualized assistance programs are to return the child to his or her home community and a regular public school by providing suitable "wrap-around services."

The programs whose staff and administrators were interviewed reported up to 100% success in these objectives, although not always permanently. For example, the Alaska Youth Initiative reported all 35 youth placed out of state were returned to community-based living in Alaska in 1991–1992, at one-third the cost of institutional placement. (Within four years, over 30 of these youth were maintained in the community until they aged out of the child mental health system.) Nationwide, 75% of administrators identified the top factor in success as using either an interagency team or the talent and commitment of staff.

Program leaders concurred in identifying the following 13 key features:

1. Program services are tailored to fit the youth, not the youth fit into the existing services.
2. Services are youth and family centered.
3. Flexible funding to permit flexibility in programming.
4. Programs work under a policy of unconditional care.
5. Collaborative planning and management.
6. Normalization is emphasized throughout all treatment.
7. Use a community-based care approach.
8. Intensive case management.
9. Funding must be extensive enough to provide whatever services are needed for significant effect with an individual.
10. Treatment planning and implementation strive toward less restrictive alternatives.
11. Accountability.
12. Services based on appropriate outcome data.
13. Specifically trained and supported staff.

Evidence-Based Treatment Interventions in Residential Settings

A completely different approach is the use of alternative schools (which may or may not be residential) provided in about 40% of school districts, often presented as a last chance before being expelled (NCES, 2002b). Some students become less "at risk," but many do not even return to their home schools (US General Accounting Office, 2002). Positive behavior change and academic improvement are frequently achieved in these schools, but then lost when the youth returns to the neighborhood school, unless attendance was voluntary *and* the students had already shown high levels of persistence in their studies (Lange & Lehr, 1999). Losing the gains on returning to the home school is readily explained by two factors: a lack of effort to transfer the new skills to the home environment, and the likelihood of negative peer influence.

By contrast, some minority groups do well in alternative settings (Nyberg, McMillin, O'Neill-Rood & Florence, 1997). For children of migrant farm workers (Latinos), the US Department of Education has a residential program that appears quite popular and effective (Martinez & Cranston-Gingras, 1996). This program is essentially a boarding school offering strong support in bilingual education. Given that it is government sponsored and the population has unique features (extreme transience, in particular), it seems difficult to generalize its success to other settings.

Findings in European countries are similar, although the interpretation and institutional responses to some specific issues can be quite varied. For example, Britain and Sweden have proactive programs for absenteeism, which is not seen as a problem in Germany (Carroll, 1995).

Psychopharmacology

Some medications are widely used for mental health disorders that interfere with succeeding in school. For example, amphetamines (such as methylphenidate/Ritalin) are widely used for attention-deficit/hyperactivity disorder; fluoxetine/Prozac is used for teenage depression; risperidone /Risperdol for conduct disorder. Adolescent disorders amenable to psychopharmacology are not listed among the main predictors of school failure, with the exception of conduct disorder. In our widespread review of the literature, we could find no systematic attempts to incorporate medications into treatment programs for drop-out or truancy.

The Prevention of School Failure

What Works

There are a number of recent reviews of prevention programs that bear on this topic. For example, Catalano et al. (2002), with support from a National Institute of Child Health and Human Development grant and a number of notable consultants, reviewed 77 "positive youth development" programs with published field research. They identified 25 programs that met standards for high-quality evaluation research, with statistically effective outcomes in comparison conditions and adequate size and design. Other recent reviews related to the prevention of school failure include those by Prevatt and Kelly (2003), South et al. (2003), Baker et al. (2001), Hatch (2000), Goldschmidt and Wang (1999), Orthner and Randolph (1999), and reviews of reviews by Greenberg et al. (2003) and Nation et al. (2003). In taking a close look at the original prevention studies, only a handful report findings in terms of drop-out data (and only one, for Big Brothers Big Sisters, with truancy data; Tierney, Grossman & Resch, 1995).

It is notable that no prevention program with drop-out data has been thoroughly evaluated three times in experimental designs with published replications. However, some interventions such the *Valued Youth* project have one solid evaluation reported, with additional claims of many replications and "comparable evaluations" that are not published. Other interventions, such as the *Seattle Social Development Project* (O'Donnell, Hawkins, Catalano, Abbott & Day, 1995), have been replicated with promising data related to school success—but not specifically drop-out. Our analysis is that effective programs to improve attendance and staying in school, as supported by data, include at least five of the design features listed below. That is, if programs are defined by their characteristics, not by their labels, then we can identify replications of effective programs.

CHARACTERISTICS THAT WORK.
1. Instruction in academic and other learning with high-quality mentoring.
2. Activities valued by youth, with implied positive futures.
3. Additional resources with dollars and community connections.
4. Family involvement, plus cultural respect and adaptations.
5. School-wide policies and emphasis on subsets of local risk and resilience factors.

6. Strategies based on theory and best practices, in which implementation is sustained and data driven, with fidelity.
7. Youth choices and self-determination.

The effective programs, with above characteristics, are comprehensive in two ways. First, they systematically include most if not all the possible constituents. That is, programs in some way include (1) the school (policy, structure, administrators); (2) the classroom (teachers, aides, curriculum); (3) the family; (4) the community (agencies, businesses); and (5) students and their peers. Secondly, effective programs are customized to the individuals and the setting. That is achieved by another list of five *must* considerations: (1) cultural differences and cultural enhancements; (2) social, emotional, and physical climate, and 'personal value'; (3) creating futures and self-efficacy; (4) finances, resources, and opportunities; and (5) standards, performance, and accountability. See Table 2 in the Conclusion section of this chapter for the application of these findings as a means to develop local best practices.

Published reviews and specific studies contribute to these findings. Gottfredson (2001) indicates that multilevel studies show student outcomes are up to 35% better on the basis of a *school effect*; that is, school effects often swamp intervention effects, with implications for improving school organization and management, perhaps even before considering special programs for youth. Jordan and Nettles (2000) studied *out-of-school* effects. They found a positive effect (in 10th through 12th grade) from structured time with adults, and a negative effect from "hanging out" with peers. Effectiveness requires intensive or sustained programming. Interventions to address even highly specific risk factors are ineffective if they are 10 hours or less (Tobler, 2000). We have found 40 hours, with the willingness to provide twice that, is necessary to take many students out of the at-risk category in literacy (Dowrick & Yuen, 2005).

Srebnik and Elias, in 1993, concluded the strongest predictors of school failure were poor achievement and alienation from school, with family and community influences a distant third. They claimed that promoting school success was better than preventing failure, through such means as contributing to others by cross-age tutoring (cf. the Valued Youth Program, described below). They indicated the importance of timing in the application of interventions, considering the transition to middle school as most vulnerable. Others claim that family factors are among the strongest predictors (Kumpfer & Alvarado, 2003). In a review of the reviews, Nation et al. (2003) identified five characteristics for effective programming in the prevention of school failure: (1) comprehensive settings and methods (including skill training); (2) intensive "dose" and duration; (3) fostering positive relationships among peers and adults; (4) appropriate (developmental) timing; and (5) well-trained staff. Skill building and environmental/organizational change are also emphasized in a review by Greenberg et al. (2003). A somewhat different, but compatible emphasis is given by South et al. (2003), who claim that raising the educational aspirations and achievement of youth could have vast impact on drop-out, etc., by reversing what they call the epidemic effect in economically disadvantaged communities.

In a specific intervention evaluation of the *Quantum Opportunities Program (QOP)*, Hahn, Leavitt, and Aaron (1994) tracked randomly selected youth going into ninth grade from (primarily) single-parent, minority families on welfare. The program included peer tutoring, computer-assisted instruction, service/job opportunities, mentoring and family skills, and futures planning. Four years later, 63% of the QOP youth graduated versus 42% of the control group; the QOP youth earned five times as many awards, and the following year two and a half times as many went to college. Other programs with similar elements have had comparable results. For example, Graber, Amuge, Rush, and Crichlow (1995) reduced drop-out from 33% to 15%. While these programs do not have replications to qualify as 'proven,' collectively they contribute by their overlapping findings to the general model of *what works* presented here.

Numerous reports on programs for students with disabilities, with some consistency, identify the most effective strategies to be curriculum options (vocational training, internships), other school organization (e.g., class size), and family participation (e.g., Stodden, Dowrick, Gilmore & Galloway, 2003). Many of the better high school programs for students with emotional and learning disabilities attribute their success to an emphasis on vocational learning (Kohler, 1996). Parent involvement is effective when there are specific roles such as paid aide positions, voting membership of committees, or bringing cultural expertise to the classroom. These responsibilities require support and training to be effective (Martin, 1994). Youth at risk can develop educational roles that eventually serve themselves and others. For example, students who lack literacy development can develop their own skills in reading whilet becoming peer coaches for other students (Topping & Ehly, 1998).

Hundreds of programs related to the prevention of school failure have been developed, demonstrated, and either shelved or replicated without data or comparison conditions. Very few have been adequately documented to meet the "what works" criterion of this book. However, the following four programs have many of the key elements noted at the beginning of this section and in Table 2.

The *Teen Outreach* (TO) program, implemented multiple times in the past decade, has been consistently found to reduce school failure (and pregnancies) in high school (e.g., Allen & Philliber, 2001). It is designed with an emphasis on reducing (unwanted) pregnancies while keeping at risk youth at school, so it is interesting that pregnancy and academic failure are not directly addressed in the content of the program. Activities include volunteering (at least 20 hours), from peer tutoring to working as hospital aides; classroom small group discussion on topics selected to be of interest to teenagers. Trained facilitators select from the curriculum provided by Teen Outreach.

In a recent study (Allen & Philliber, 2001), there were about 3,200 participants, half of them "no treatment" controls. Teen Outreach participants were self-selected, and the control group was partly matched through nominations. Teen Outreach discussion groups were held in health or social studies classes, or after school. In this study, there were strong program effects on pregnancy, course failure, and suspensions. As noted, these outcomes are highly predictive of reducing school failure; unfortunately, drop-out and attendance were not directly reported.

The *Valued Youth Program* has been implemented extensively with indications of considerable effects on drop-out, especially among Latino youth with English as a second language. While the designers of the program identified 12–15 "critical elements" from the literature (Montecel, Supik & Montemayor, 1993), the main feature is to train middle school youth with high risk factors (including *poor* reading levels) to become reading tutors for elementary school students. The program also fosters

Peter W. Dowrick and Natalie Crespo

school-business relationships to provide financial support. Note that the evaluations appear to be self-published and that the early implementations (1984–88) and evaluations were sponsored by Coca Cola. Montecel et al. describe a study from the late 1980s that included approximately 200 youth, half of whom were assigned to a no-treatment control condition. (It is not clear if they were truly randomly selected, or just from two different school districts.) The youth assigned to be tutors were active for two years, sustaining 1% drop-out, compared with 12% in the control group. Tutors received pay (minimum wage), training, field trips, and public recognition for their "valued" contribution. The authors claim to have carried out comparable evaluations in numerous replications in multiple states.

A program to improve school climate by affecting adult–student relationships is *Check and Connect* (Sinclair, Christenson, Evelo & Hurley, 1998). It features drop-out prevention through mentoring, monitoring, and building effective transitions from middle to high school. It is "proven" in the sense that it and a number of other programs with similar features have been evaluated, producing good outcomes of lowered drop-out rates. It also addresses associated risk factors for students with learning disabilities and emotional and behavioral disorders. Overall, the procedures were shaped by the collaboration of school personnel, family and other community members, including university researchers and the pupils.

There are five features of note. First, adults with good cooperative skills are assigned as mentors or monitors for 25 students each. Secondly, the mentors check on the status of risk factors (attendance, conduct, academics) known to affect engagement with school. Thirdly, the mentors provide regular support for all students by means of feedback on progress and encouragement to stay in school. They also provide structured training in problem-solving for risky situations (e.g., tardiness). Fourthly, in situations where the monitoring indicates elevated risk, the students are provided with additional intensive problem-solving, including parent participation— on the basis of which they can receive specific academic support, or recreational or community opportunities. For example, tutoring could be arranged, if classes were being avoided because of difficult content. Finally, the system is initiated in seventh grade and continued in eighth grade and on to high school (ninth grade).

The results typical of this type of program indicate significantly positive outcomes for attendance and assignment completion, with modest effects on grades, conduct, and self-reported attitude toward school. Thus, such programs are helpful but by no means the entire answer.

One program to improve school outcomes with an academic overhaul, and also address some specific risk factors, is the *Seattle Social Development Project*. It has been well evaluated, beginning with young children and extended to all ages. It is a multiyear program addressing schools and families in low income communities. Compared with controls, children in a six-year evaluation showed greater school commitment and class participation; girls experimented less with drugs; boys improved their school work and social skills (O'Donnell et al., 1995).

The program is designed to decrease risk factors of academic failure, low commitment to school, early conduct disorders, family management problems, and involvement with antisocial peers. It is also designed to improve resilience factors: positive social bonds to school and family, through active involvement; belief in family and school values, through consistent reinforcement.

The program has recently been extended into the high schools. Teachers are trained in proactive classroom management, interactive teaching, cooperative learning, and problem-solving. This approach improves predictability of teacher–student interactions and increases the amount of praise, modeling, and appropriate student involvement. Youth are provided individual social skills interventions. Parents are offered skills training related to behavior, drugs, and homework. Overall results have been positive, if moderate, with respect to drop-out per se. Teachers improved their skills. Some of the children at risk benefitted academically, and some reduced their risky behavior (e.g., drug involvement).

Smaller learning communities in schools. High school size of 600 to 1,000 pupils correlates with the lowest rates of dropout (Howley et al., 2000). Given that many high schools now have enrollments of 1,500 to 5,000, the US Department of Education has called for initiatives to restructure these large schools with freshman academies, career tracks, block scheduling, etc., to reduce the negative effects of size. While this type of intervention is not a program per se, it incorporates most of the seven characteristics that work at a practical level. Evaluations have not been done with experimental designs, but through grant reporting and site reviews. It is salient that the strongest predictor of success identified by the Department of Education is described as the extent of "buy in" from all constituents; that is, the objectives and the spirit of the school reform must be understood and endorsed by the school administrators, teachers, students, families, and local community agencies (personal communication, competition manager, Office of Elementary and Secondary Education, January 2002).

What Might Work

This book provides testimony to the number of prevention programs for youth at risk for drug abuse, unwanted pregnancy, and other concerns. Many such programs appear to have an impact on school attendance and performance, but without reporting drop-out and truancy outcomes in detail. Thus they can provide information on promising but unproven interventions for school failure or success. As might be expected, a review such as the special issue of *Journal of Primary Prevention* (2000) reports many general strategies in common with the proven practices identified above in this chapter. Promising practices may also be provided by programs in elementary schools, given that school failure is a cumulative process almost always with its roots in the early grades. Such programs include *First Step to Success* (Walker, Stiller, Severson, Feil & Golly, 1998) and *Effective Behavior Supports* (Lewis, Sugai & Colvin, 1998), which are aimed at early intervention with childhood aggression in schools, thus improving the school climate and academic success of all students. Additional clues for improving interventions to prevent or treat school failure include—

1. *Small programs* may be twice as effective as large ones (Tobler, 2000).
2. *Intervening early* is frequently advocated (e.g., Reynolds, 1998). For example, teaching literacy should be implemented before a child starts to fail at other subjects (Dowrick, Power, Manz, Ginsburg-Block, Leff & Kim-Rupnow, 2001). For teenagers at risk, many of whom read below fifth-grade level, it is never too early and never too late to help.
3. *Peers may be better teachers* than teachers, for social and emotional learning programs (Richman, Rosenfeld & Bowen, 1998).
4. *Expand the use of school locations.* Schools have the potential to become community learning centers, at which students and local adults have opportunities to support each other educationally. Outside organizations can provide on-campus recreational and special expertise in prevention programs (Mahoney & Cairns, 1997). A well-evaluated

British project for school-based family social services has demonstrated a 50% reduction in truancy (Pritchard & Williams, 2001).

5. *Social skills training* is widely used, with much justification but modest outcomes. Generalization is notoriously poor for socials skills learned by role play in school settings; applications in daily life, as with cross-age mentoring, and digital technology to provide feedforward[1] of these skills give promising results (e.g., Embry, Flannery, Vazsonyi, Powell & Atha, 1996).

6. *Special populations* (e.g., ethnic minorities) may benefit more than others from an interactive approach that sets high expectations (Nyberg et al., 1997).

There are a number of straightforward approaches that should not be overlooked in the prevention of truancy. Examples include simple incentives (contingency management) and group counseling (Brooks, 2001), teachers' showing interest and empathy in students' lives, asking families to take an interest and rapidly reporting absences directly to parents (Epstein & Sheldon, 2002).

Promising strategies are similar internationally, except where the issues are strikingly different. For example, in one part of Namibia the goal is ensure that children stay in school at least three years and learn basic reading skills. Here they use a community-responsive approach to reduce discrimination by teachers and to accommodate the local language and culture (Pfaffe, 1995).

What Does Not Work

In the United States, and other countries where 85% of the population spends approximately 12 productive years in school, there is little evidence that small-scale or unitary approaches have much promise. For example, providing additional academic support for failing students will have little effect on dropout if other risk factors are not addressed. This situation is amply illustrated in a report by Hamovitch (1999). He describes a failed "afterschool compensatory" program for low-income African American students, attributing the failure to the emphasis on tutorials after school (more of the school day), without reflecting local culture and needs.

Attempts to address drugs and violence also have weak possibilities of preventing dropping out of school, although many of the positive youth development programs reviewed by Catalano et al. (2002) included reductions in alcohol, tobacco, and marijuana as part of their goals. These issues are tough to address, and programs have struggled to show an impact when linked to school difficulties (Dowrick, Leukefeld & Stodden, 2005).

Currently fashionable approaches of "zero tolerance" and adjudication do not work, whether for the youth or their parents. In a study of nearly 800 youth, three years after their release from correctional facilities, Haberman and Quinn (1986) found that about 1% were attending high school and less than 2% had 'completed' high school—thus 97% *had dropped out*. However, there are some long-established strategies for successful transition of juvenile offenders to the public school system and the home community. One example is the Juvenile Corrections Interagency Transition Model (Edgar, Webb & Maddox, 1987). The procedures focused on interagency awareness of the educational needs of youthful offenders, systematic steps for the

---

[1]Feedforward refers to personal images of success that have not yet occurred.

transfer of educational records between agencies, placement planning before the offender leaves the institution, and placement maintenance and communication when the youth returns to his or her home community.

Recommendations

Prevention and intervention strategies to reduce school failure must improve pupils' appreciation of school (how much they like school), and concurrently increase the incentives to stay and/or decrease the incentives to leave. That can be achieved by a comprehensive approach that includes consideration of—

1. culture,
2. school climate,
3. self-efficacy,
4. adding resources, and
5. performance.

At the same time, consideration is given to all constituents: students, the school, teachers, family, and the community. Table 2 provides the highlights of our recommendations for practice. It provides a school community with a simple tool to develop as comprehensive or as focused an approach to preventing and intervening

Table 2. A Matrix for the Development of Best Practices in the Prevention of School Failure and the Promotion of Success

	Cultural differences, enhancements	Social, emotional, & physical climate; personal value	Creating futures, self-efficacy	$$, resources, opportunity	Standards, performance, accountability
School (admin, policy)					
Classroom (tchrs, curric)	*				
Family		*b			
Community (agencies, businesses)				*	
Students		*a			

1. Set goals for each of the intersections above.
   Include considerations of transitions, art, spirituality, ethics, marginalization, teamwork, conduct, romance, employment, drugs, violence, as well as math, science, society, and sports.
2. Determine activities/programs to address the goals. Not all 1:1, but combined is better.
   Include consideration of self-determination, feedforward, leadership, and fun.
3. Get complete buy-in from all settings/constituents.
4. First, do just a one-year plan. Next year evaluate, do five-year goals, one-year goals, and programs.
5. Design primary prevention, school-wide programs. Or tailor to at-risk groups. Or both.
* It is not necessary to address all the boxes in the matrix (although several may be addressed with a single program). The ones marked * are the most essential.

with school failure (drop-out and truancy) as desired. As indicated, a school-based team would use the matrix annually to revise its goals and to plan what programs would meet those goals. The row and column headings, and the other considerations, are intended to ensure that the main elements from proven and promising practices are included in the plan. Although the matrix has 25 elements, in practice only, say, about half would need objectives/activities; just five, marked with an asterisk, are essential.

We recommend putting local effort into the following:

* Adequate assessment of where individual schools are in terms of criteria 1–5 above, and where the priorities and current resources are, to take appropriate action. If school climate is good, but the outcomes (e.g, grades, competitions) are poor, then that suggests refocusing on new objectives of performance. If the school is succeeding, then there may be individual life problems to be addressed.
* More data on what works and what does not. A number of programs are widely implemented but lack adequate data. There has been too little research that really addresses the causal relationships between efforts for improvement and the outcomes.
* Redistribute money and resources into at-risk communities. In a study of policy and school structure, Fitzpatrick and Yoels (1992) found spending per pupil to have the greatest effect of all factors on staying in school.
* Recognition that different programs for at-risk children and youth have considerable overlap. The chapters of this book provide the basis for a synthesis of programs, addressing such issues as drug abuse, delinquency, violence, and teen pregnancy, with those for school dropout and truancy. Eighty percent of prevention programs for personal or community issues in adolescence (drugs, etc.) have a major school-based component (Catalano et al., 2002).
* A huge effort in the United States in the last 15 years has gone into addressing dropout and related issues for students with disabilities, and the analysis of findings has remarkably little overlap with the recommendations from general education. The field would benefit from a synthesis here, too.
* Recognition that much of creating a good school is basic: a healthy environment and effective teaching. There have been big strides in knowledge of what makes an effective curriculum (design and expectations), how it is taught, and school-wide reform, that could be more consistently and conscientiously applied.

Some major changes could be made with the stroke of a legislator's pen or an executive action by a school district. These changes include:

* Building smaller high schools. If it is more expensive to build three campuses for 900 students than to maintain one campus for 2,700, it would be money well spent. There is growing advocacy to replace the separate levels of schools, which breed transition and school size problems, with K–12 schools (Howley et al., 2000).
* Change the hours of the school day to begin at 9:00 and end at 3:30, with universally available after-school sports practice and other activities. Most juvenile crime, pregnancies, and other risky behavior occur between 2:30 and dinner time.
* Make "Prevention of School Failure and the Promotion of Success" an ongoing effort with emphasis on applying currently proven or promising strategies with integrity. Prevention programs will not be successful as magic bullets, but must become a way of doing business.

There are considerable international differences in how "drop-out" is perceived and valued. There are also differences in approach. Broadly speaking, in the Americas most effort has gone into academics, vocational preparation, and cooperative behavior of students. In Europe there has been more emphasis on attitudes and friendships. In Asia and Africa the effort has been in creating opportunities socially and institutionally to attend school. These differences may be characterized as succeeding in schoolwork, enjoying school, and school availability (Dowrick, 2003). In any school system, all three considerations are essential, with emphasis depending on the local or national situation.

ACKNOWLEDGMENTS. Preparation of this article was partially supported by US Department of Education (Office of Elementary and Secondary Education), although no endorsement is implied of the views expressed herein. Please address correspondence to Peter W. Dowrick, Ph.D, Professor of Disability Studies, University of Hawaii at Manoa, 1776 University Av. UA4-6, Manoa, HI 96822, USA; <dowrick@hawaii.edu>.

References

Allen, J.P., & Philliber, S. (2001). Who benefits most from a broadly targeted prevention program? Differential efficacy across populations in the Teen Outreach Program. *Journal of Community Psychology, 29,* 637–655.

Bandura, A. (1993). Perceived self-efficacy in cognitive development and functioning. *Educational Psychology, 28,* 117–148.

Baker, J.A., Derrer, R.D., Davis, S.M., Dinklage-Travis, H.E., Linder, D.S., & Nicholson, M.D. (2001). The flip side of the coin: Understanding the school's contribution to dropout and completion. *School Psychology Quarterly, 16,* 406–426.

Battin-Pearson, S., Newcomb, M., Abbott, R., Hill, K., Catalano, R., & Hawkins, J.D. (2000). Predictors of early high school dropout: A test of five theories. *Journal of Educational Psychology, 92,* 568–582.

Battistich, V., & Hom, A. (1997). The relationship between students' sense of their school as a community and their involvement in problem behaviors. *American Journal of Public Health, 87,* 1997–2001.

Bhakta, P., Hackett, R.J., & Hackett, L. (2002). The prevalence and associations of reading difficulties in a population of South Indian children. *Journal of Research in Reading, 25,* 191–202.

Brooks, B.D. (2001). Contingency management as a means of reducing school truancy. *Education, 95,* 206–211.

Carroll, H.C.M. (1995). Pupil absenteeism: A northern European perspective. *School Psychology International, 16,* 227–247.

Carter, R.S., & Wojtkiewicz, R.A. (2000). Parental involvement with adolescents' education: Do daughters or sons get more help? *Adolescence, 35,* 29–44.

Catalano, R.F., Berglund, L., Ryan, J., Lonczak, H.S., & Hawkins, D. (2002). Positive youth development in the United States: Research findings on evaluations of positive youth development programs. *Prevention & Treatment, 5*(15). Retrieved January 2002, from http://journals.aps.org/prevention/volume5/pre0050015a.html.

Centers, N.L., & Weist, M.D. (1998). Inner city youth and drug dealing: A review of the problem. *Journal of Youth and Adolescence, 27,* 395–411.

Cohen, M.A., (1998). The monetary value of saving a high-risk youth. *Journal of Quantitative Criminology, 14,* 5–33.

Corville-Smith, J., Ryan, B.A., Adams, G.R., & Dalicandro, T. (1998). Distinguishing absentee students from regular attenders: The combined influence of personal, family, and school factors. *Journal of Youth and Adolescence, 27,* 629–649.

D'Amato, J. (1988). "Acting": Hawaiian children's resistance to teachers. *Elementary School Journal, 88,* 529–544.

Dowrick, P.W. (1999). A review of self modeling and related applications. *Applied and Preventive Psychology, 8,* 23–29.

Dowrick. P.W. (2003). School drop-outs; Adolescence. In T. Gullotta & M. Bloom (Eds.), *Encyclopedia of Primary Prevention and Health Promotion* (pp. 924–929). New York: Plenum.

Dowrick, P.W., Leukefeld, C., & Stodden, R.A. (2005). Early prevention of substance abuse by young children with school difficulties. *Journal of Primary Prevention, 25*, 309–328.

Dowrick, P.W., Power, T.J., Manz, P.H., Ginsburg-Block, M., Leff, S.S., & Kim-Rupnow, S. (2001). Community responsiveness: Examples from under-resourced urban schools. *Journal of Prevention and Intervention in the Community, 21*(2), 71–90.

Dowrick, P.W., Tallman, B.I., & Connor, M.E. (2004). Constructing better futures via video. *Journal of Prevention and Intervention in the Community, 24*, in press.

Dowrick, P.W., & Yuen, J.W.L. (2005). Literacy for the community, by the community. *Journal of Prevention and Intervention in the Community, 25*, in press.

Edgar, E.B., Webb, S.L., & Maddox, M. (1987). Issues in transition: Transfer of youth from correctional facilities to public schools. In C.M. Nelson, R.B. Rutherford, & B.I. Wolford (Eds.), *Special Education in the Criminal Justice System* (pp. 251–272). Columbus, OH: Merrill.

Embry, D.D., Flannery, D.J., Vazsonyi, A., Powell, K., & Atha, H. (1996). PeaceBuilders: A theoretically driven, school-based model for early violence prevention. *American Journal of Preventive Medicine, 12*, 91–100.

Epstein, J.L., & Sheldon, S.B. (2002). Present and accounted for: Improving student attendance through family and community involvement. *Journal of Educational Research, 95*, 308–318.

Finn, J., & Rock, D. (1997). Academic success among students at risk for school failure. *Journal of Applied Psychology, 82*, 221–234.

Fischer, M.J., & Dowrick, P.W. (2003). The interrelationship between schools and families: A Hawaiian middle school example. *The Community Psychologist, 36*(3), 45–49.

Fitzpatrick, K.M., & Yoels, W.C. (1992). Policy, school structure, and sociodemographic effects on statewide high school dropout rates. *Sociology of Education, 65*, 76–93.

Franklin, C., & Streeter, C.L. (1995). Assessment of middle class youth at-risk to dropout: School, psychological and family correlates. *Children & Youth Services Review, 17*, 433–448.

Goldschmidt, P., & Wang, J. (1999). When can schools affect dropout behavior? A longitudinal multilevel analysis. *American Educational Research Journal, 36*, 715–738.

Gottfredson, D.C. (2001). *Schools and Delinquency*. New York: Cambridge University Press.

Graber, C.F., Amuge, I.M., Rush, A., & Crichlow, W. (1995). New York State's Stay-in-School Partnership Program: Overview and evaluation. In I.M. Evans, T. Cicchelli, M. Cohen & N.P. Shapiro (Eds.). *Staying in school: Partnerships for Educational Change*. Baltimore: Paul H. Brookes.

Greenberg, M.T., Weissberg, R.P., O'Brien, M.U., Zins, J.E., Fredericks, L, Resnik, H., & Elias, M.J. (2003). Enhancing school-based prevention and youth development through coordinated social, emotional and academic learning. *American Psychologist, 58*, 466–474.

Greene, J.P. (2002). *High School Graduation Rates in the United States (Revised)*. New York: Manhattan Research Institute for Policy Research. Retrieved June 2004, from http://www. manhattan-institute. org/html/cr_baeo.htm#04.

Hahn, A., Leavitt, T., & Aaron, P. (1994). *Evaluation of the Quantum Opportunities Program. Did the Program Work?* Waltham, MA: Brandeis University Heller Graduate School Center for Human Resources.

Hatch, T. (2000). What does it take to break the mold? Rhetoric and reality in new American schools. *Teachers College Record, 102*, 561–589.

Haberman, M., & Quinn, L.M. (1986). The juvenile justice interagency transition model: Moving students from institutions to community schools. *Remedial and Special Education, 7*, 56–61.

Hamovitch, B. (1999). More failure for the disadvantaged: Contradictory African-American student reactions to compensatory education and urban schooling. *Urban Review, 31*(1), 55–77.

Howley, C., Strange, M., & Bickel, R. (2000). *Research About School Size and School Performance in Impoverished Communities*. Charleston, WV: ERIC Clearinghouse on Rural Education and Improvement (ERIC Report No. EDO-RC-00-10).

Jimerson, S.R., Egeland, B., Sroufe, L.A., & Carlson, B. (2000). A prospective longitudinal study of high school dropouts: Examining multiple predictors across development. *Journal of School Psychology, 38*, 525–549.

Jordan, W.J., Lara, J., & McPartland, J.M. (1996). Exploring the causes of early dropout among race-ethnic and gender groups. *Youth & Society, 28*(1), 62–94.

Jordan, W.J., & Nettles, S.M.. (2000). How students invest their time outside of school: Effects on school-related outcomes. *Social Psychology of Education, 3*, 217–243.

Kohler, P.D. (1996). *A Taxonomy for Transition Programming: Linking Research and Practice*. Champaign: University of Illinois, Transition Research Institute.

Kumpfer, K.L., & Alvarado, R. (2003). Family-strengthening approaches for the prevention of youth problem behaviors. *American Psychologist, 58,* 457–465.

Lange, C.M., & Lehr, C.A. (1999). At-risk students attending second chance programs: Measuring performance in desired outcome domains. *Journal of Education for Students Placed at Risk, 4,* 173–192.

Levine, J.A., Pollack, H., & Comfort, M.E. (2001). Academic and behavioral outcomes among the children of young mothers. *Journal of Marriage and the Family, 63,* 355–369.

Lewis, T.J., Sugai, G., & Colvin, G. (1998). Reducing problem behavior through a school-wide system of effective behavioral support: Investigation of a school-wide social skills training program and contextual interventions. *School Psychology Review, 27,* 446–459.

MacFarquhar, K.W., Dowrick, P.W., & Risley, T.R. (1993). Individualizing services for seriously emotionally disturbed youth: A nationwide review. *Administration and Policy in Mental Health, 20,* 165–174.

Mahoney, J.L., & Cairns, R.B. (1997). Do extracurricular activities protect against early school dropout? *Developmental Psychology, 33,* 241–253.

Martin, C.J. (1994). *Schooling in Mexico: Staying in or Dropping out*. Brookfield, VT: Ashgate.

Martinez, Y.G., & Cranston-Gingras, A. (1996). Migrant farmworker students and the educational process: Barriers to high school completion. *High School Journal, 80,* 28–38.

McCaul, E.J., Donaldson, G.A., Coladarci, T., & Davis, W.E. (1992). Consequences of dropping out of school: Findings from high school and beyond. *Journal of Educational Research, 85,* 198–207.

Meece, J.L., & Kurtz-Costes, B. (2001). Introduction: Schooling of ethnic minority children and youth. *Educational Psychologist, 36*(1), 1–7.

Montecel, M.R., Supik, J.D., & Montemayor, A. (1993). Valued youth program: Dropout prevention strategies for at-risk youth. *National Association for Bilingual Education (NABE). Annual Conference Journal, 1992–1993,* 65–80. Retrieved October 2003, from EDRS: http://www.edrs.com/Webstore/Download.cfm?ID=388062.

National Center for Education Statistics (NCES). (2002a). *Dropout Rates in the United States: 2000*. Washington, DC: US Department of Education.

National Center for Education Statistics (NCES). (2002b). *Public Alternative Schools and Programs for Students at Risk of Education Failure: 2000–01*. Washington, DC: US Department of Education.

Nation, M., Crusto, C., Wandersman, A., Kumpfer, K.L., Syebolt, D., Morrissey-Kane, E., & Davino, K. (2003). What works in prevention: Principles of effective prevention programs. *American Psychologist, 58,* 449–456.

Nyberg, K.L., McMillin, J.D., O'Neill-Rood, N., & Florence, J.M. (1997). Ethnic differences in academic retracking: A four-year longitudinal study. *Journal of Educational Research, 91,* 33–41.

O'Donnell, C.R., Tharp, R.G., & Wilson, K. (1993). Activity settings as the unity of analysis: A theoretical basis for community intervention and development. *American Journal of Community Psychology, 21,* 501–520.

O'Donnell, J., Hawkins, J.D., Catalano, R.F., Abbott, R.D., & Day, L.E. (1995). Preventing school failure, drug use, and delinquency among low-income children: Long-term intervention in elementary schools. *American Journal of Orthopsychiatry, 65,* 87–100.

Orthner, D.K., & Randolph, K.A. (1999). Welfare reform and high school dropout patterns for children. *Children and Youth Services Review, 21,* 881–900.

Pfaffe, J.F. (1995). The Village Schools Project: Ju/'hoan Literacy Programme and community-based education in Nyae Nyae, Namibia. *School Psychology International, 16,* 43–58.

Pong, S.L., & Ju, D.B. (2000). The effects of change in family structure and income on dropping out of middle and high school. *Journal of Family Issues, 21,* 147–169.

Prevatt, F., & Kelly, F.D. (2003). Dropping out of school: A review of intervention programs. *Journal of School Psychology, 41,* 377–395.

Pritchard, C., & Williams, R. (2001). A three-year comparative longitudinal study of a school-based social work family service to reduce truancy, delinquency and school exclusion. *Journal of Social Welfare and Family Law, 23*(1), 23–43.

Reynolds, A.J. (1998). Developing early childhood programs for children and families at risk: Research-based principles to promote long-term effectiveness. *Children and Youth Services Review, 20,* 503–523.

Richman, J.M., Rosenfeld, L.B., & Bowen, G.L. (1998). Social support for adolescents at risk of school failure. *Social Work, 43,* 309–323.

Rosenthal, B.S. (1998). Non-school correlates of dropout: An integrative review of the literature. *Children & Youth Services Review, 20,* 413–433.

Rylance, B.J. (1997). Predictors of high school graduation or dropping out for youths with severe emotional disturbances. *Behavioral Disorders, 23*(1), 5–17.

Sinclair, M.F., Christenson, S.L., Evelo, D.L., & Hurley, C.M. (1998). Dropout prevention for youth with disabilities: Efficacy of a sustained school engagement procedure. *Exceptional Children, 65*, 7–21.

South, S.J., Baumer, E.P., & Lutz, A. (2003). Interpreting community effects on youth educational attainment. *Youth and Society, 35*, 3–36.

Srebnik, D.S., & Elias, M. (1993). An ecological, interpersonal skills approach to dropout prevention. *American Journal of Orthopsychiatry, 63*, 526–535.

Stevenson, W., Maton, K.J., & Teti, D.M. (1998). School importance and dropout among pregnant adolescents. *Journal of Adolescent Health, 22*, 376–382.

Stodden, R.A., Dowrick, P., Gilmore, S., & Galloway, L.M. (2003). *A Review of Secondary School Factors Influencing Postschool Outcomes for Youth with Disabilities.* National Center for the Study of Postsecondary Educational Supports. Retrieved January 29, 2004, from http://www.rrtc. hawaii.edu/documents/products/phase1/043-H01.pdf

Tierney, J.P., Grossman, J.B., & Resch, N.L. (1995). *Making a Difference: An Impact Study of Big Brothers/Big Sisters.* Philadelphia, PA: Public/Private Ventures.

Tobler, N.S. (2000). Lessons learned. *Journal of Primary Prevention, 20*, 261–273.

Topping, K., & Ehly, S. (1998). *Peer-Assisted Learning.* Mahwah, NJ: Erlbaum.

US General Accounting Office. (2002). *School Dropouts: Education Could Play a Stronger Role in Identifying and Disseminating Promising Prevention Strategies (GAO-02-240).* Washington, DC: Author.

Vallerand, R.J., Fortier, M.S., & Guay, F. (1997). Self-determination and persistence in a real-life setting: Toward a motivational model of high school dropout. *Journal of Personality & Social Psychology, 72*, 1161–1176.

VanDenBerg, J.E., & Grealish, E.M. (1996). Individualized services and supports through the wraparound process: Philosophy and procedures. *Journal of Child and Family Studies, 5*, 7–21.

Vartanian, T.P., & Gleason, P.M. (1999). Do neighborhood conditions affect high school dropout and college graduation rates? *Journal of Socio-Economics, 28*, 21–42.

Vitaro, F., Larocque, D., Janosz, M., & Tremblay, R.E. (2001). Negative social experiences and dropping out of school. *Educational Psychology, 21*, 401–415.

Walker, H., Stiller, B., Severson, H., Feil, E., & Golly, A. (1998). First Step to Success: Intervening at the point of school entry to prevent antisocial behavior patterns. *Psychology in the Schools, 35*, 259–269.

Worrell, F.C. (1997). Predicting successful or non-successful at-risk status using demographic risk factors. *High School Journal, 81*(1), 46–53.

Zhou, W., Zhang, T., Liu, W., Ma, Y., & Peng, J. (2001). Research into girls' education in four western provinces of China. *Chinese Education and Society, 33*, 4–28.

Zima, B.T., Bussing, R., Freeman, S., Yang, X., Belin, T.R., & Forness, S.R. (2000). Behavior problems, academic skill delays and school failure among school-aged children in foster care: Their relationship to placement characteristics. *Journal of Child and Family Studies, 9*, 87–103

Chapter 28

Religious Cults

Joseph L. Calles, Jr., Maritza Lagos, Tatyana Kharit,
Ahsan Nazeer, Jody Reed, and Suhail Sheikh

Introduction

Cult—the word conjures up images of people who are not in the mainstream of society, who are strange, possibly even dangerous. Either through the media—or through direct experience—we have seen cult members, such as the Hare Krishnas, who wear saffron-colored robes, shave their heads, and try to collect money in public places. We have also seen the images of dead bodies—adults and children alike—who have been the victims of fringe ideology and charismatic, but misguided leaders, e.g., David Koresh and his Branch Davidians (Small, 1998). This chapter defines what a cult is, what leads young people to join them, and what can be done to keep that from happening. We also discuss what can be done to help those who have been adversely affected by their involvement in a cult.

There is no consensus on the definition of the word *cult*; the term is traditionally used to refer to any new religious movement [NRM] (Wieder, 1998). Even within established religions, there can be differences among members as to how dogma is established, interpreted, and expressed. There are, for example, numerous Christian *denominations*, and within any one denomination there can exist *sects*, which distinguish themselves from the parent group by adhering to different teachings. One way of a cult forms, therefore, is when novel beliefs conflict with the group's majority beliefs, making their continued stay within the group untenable.

The debate over how to define a *cult* is not solved by calling it a new religious movement (NRM). It has been elegantly argued (Robbins, 2000) that there are even problems in how one would define the terms *new, religious,* and *movement*. The Hare Krishna cult was "new" to Americans, but was actually a reworking of ancient Hindu beliefs. Therapy cults (e.g., est [Erhard Seminar Training]) are sometimes listed as NRMs, yet there is nothing religious about their beliefs or practices. "Movements" can refer to nonspecific phenomena (e.g., New Age) or to more discrete organizations, such as the Church of Scientology.

A more technical, research-based resource (Stark & Bainbridge, 1987) has distinguished a *cult movement* ("a deviant religious organization with novel beliefs and practices") from *cults*, which "are social enterprises whose primary purpose is to create, maintain, and exchange supernaturally based general compensators." These "compensators" are spiritual rewards that the cult member is promised to receive in the afterlife, and is willing to work towards and wait for.

Although religiously based cults are the most common type, there are many other kinds of cults, most of which can be subsumed under categories such as Christian variants, Eastern philosophical, satanic, racial, political, psychotherapeutic, and lifestyle (Singer, 1995).

Perhaps the most common way that society defines a cult is by the methods it uses to attract, retain, and influence its members. Many people equate cults with the use of "brainwashing" and intimidation. Due to scrutiny by the media and by law enforcement agencies, these methods have tended to change over time in order to avoid "bad press" and litigation. These changes are also made to address specific needs that the cult(s) may have, such as trying to increase income in the face of dwindling membership (Schwartz & Kaslow, 2001).

As more adults—especially elder adults—are recruited for their financial resources, younger people are still attractive for their naïveté, energy, and income-generating potential. It is this possibility of manipulation and misuse of younger people that concerns parents, governments, and members of mainstream religious groups. There are those in the law enforcement community, however, who caution against using societal perception as an important factor in defining a cult (Szubin, Jensen & Gregg, 2000).

Despite the need for calm and reason in approaching this subject, some European governments have initiated programs to investigate and outlaw "religious minorities," which are seen as a threat to traditional religious thought, thus causing a "moral panic" and subsequent legislation to prohibit certain religious organizations (Richardson & Introvigne, 2001). There is a certain unfortunate irony in this situation, since much of the impetus for it derives from the American concepts of "brainwashing" and "mind control," which have mostly been discounted in the United States.

These technicalities may make it difficult to distinguish what is potentially dangerous from that which is merely unusual. However defined, society's awareness of cults has become more prominent in recent decades. Although it has existed for centuries, cult activity has reemerged in contemporary society, sometimes with tragic results. An important question to ask therefore is, What places adolescents at risk for cult involvement?

Adolescence is the developmental period during which the dependency of youth diminishes and the responsibilities of adulthood increase (Hunter, 1998). It is a time of self-reflection, when young people try to understand who they are, what they are capable of doing—even why they exist at all. Even as their freedoms increase, certain privileges of adulthood remain unavailable to them. Their lives, therefore, can be a confusing mix of reality, possibility, and ambiguity. It is unknown what the actual incidence of cults trying to recruit adolescents is (nor is it known how many adolescents are born into cults and raised by its members). It has been noted, however, that "cults have traditionally drawn their members from adolescents or young adults, people who may be in that stage of life when confusion and uncertainty seems to accompany any action or belief" (Goodnough, 2000).

For any given adolescent, a combination of risk factors, extraordinary stressors, limited coping mechanisms, and/or insufficient support systems could place him/her at risk for coming under the influence of a cult. Some adolescents have felt most susceptible to the recruiting efforts by cults when they have (1) wanted quick answers for life's complicated questions; (2) had their self-confidence shaken by crisis; (3) not known quite how to act (i.e., found themselves in confusing situations); and/or (4) not known what to believe or value in their own lives (Porterfield, 1995).

The sections that follow will look at the interplay between risk factors and protective factors, as well as interventions to counter the effects of cult beliefs on individual adolescents.

Individual Factors

There are a number of risk factors which seem to influence individual susceptibility and vulnerability to cults:

Age

There are no consistent data regarding the specific ages at which people are at greater risk for cult recruitment. Commenting on a study that he and his colleagues did in 1980, Zimbardo (1997) noted that in their random survey of 1,000 high school students in the San Francisco area, 54% had been approached at least once to join cults.

Another author (Wright & Piper, 1986) has indicated that cults are most successful in recruiting individuals in late adolescence and young adulthood. In other words, being more "mature" does not necessarily reduce the vulnerability that we see in younger people. In fact, many developmental issues can persist in this "older" group, including lack of social experience, need for social acceptance, idealism vs. pessimism, and existential and identity struggles (Schwartz & Kaslow, 2001).

On a more optimistic note, due to scrutiny by the media and by various watchdog groups, contemporary cults have become more cautious in their recruiting efforts, making sure to focus on those of legal age (Schwartz & Kaslow, 2001).

Gender

There are no data on the male-to-female ratios of active cult memberships. One author (Levine, 1978) interviewed members of various religious cults, all of whom volunteered for the study. Of the 106 people interviewed, fifty-one (51) were females and fifty-five (55) were males, essentially an even distribution. Of potential relevance to this chapter, however, is that there was "a preponderance of girls in the younger age groups," where the ages of those interviewed ranged from 17 to 30 years (median age 21.5 years). One could interpret this, albeit cautiously, to mean that younger females may be more likely to join religious cults than are younger males. In the case of satanic cults, however, young males from abusive families seem to be especially vulnerable to their recruiting efforts (Belitz & Schacht, 1992).

Race

There is no good way to determine the racial/ethnic makeup of contemporary cults, as these groups tend not to let "outsiders" know of their inner workings. One can speculate, however, which racial/ethnic group(s) is/are most likely to be targeted for recruitment, based on known demographics. To begin with, "cults and new religious movements are looking increasingly to university students as a potential pool of devotees" (The Nationalist, 2003). Who are these students? In the United States for the years 1999–2000, it was shown that 68.5% of college undergraduates, aged 19–23, identified themselves as "white, non-Hispanic" (U.S. Commission on Civil Rights, 2002). It is reasonable to assume, therefore, that for those attending college, the majority of people who will be approached to join a cult will be white.

Situational Stress and Crisis

All people have to deal with a certain amount of life stressors. How well one does in handling a stressful situation has to do, in part, with whether this is a new occurrence, or whether this is another in a series of negative events. The experiencing of repeated stressors, and the accumulation of stress effects, can overwhelm a person's ability to adjust to them. Adolescents, by virtue of their incomplete emotional development, would be vulnerable at this point, making them more likely to see the promises of a cult as an answer to their problems, an escape from their suffering (Curtis & Curtis, 1993).

Personality Profile

Personality characteristics of an adolescent which may make him/her more susceptible to the lure of a cult might include identity confusion, ambivalence, avoidance, dependency, defiance, or a feeling of powerlessness (Hunter, 1998). Those with narcissistic personality styles may be especially vulnerable (Feldmann & Johnson, 1995). Even during normal adolescence there may be sudden changes in personality or behavior, such as withdrawal from home and social activities, the development of defiant attitudes, a decline in academic achievement, the assumption of an unusual style of dress, or interest in music with negativistic themes. If not recognized and addressed appropriately, this can lead to—or exacerbate—the adolescent's poor sense of self and need for peer approval, greatly increasing his/her vulnerability to negative, inappropriate, or potentially dangerous outside influence (Wieder, 1998).

Childhood Abuse or Neglect

A childhood marked by physical or sexual abuse and/or substandard care or neglect can play a decisive role in influencing an adolescent's development (Curtis & Curtis, 1993). An individual's subjective experiences or perceptions of past abuse (which may include incest, other types of sexual molestation, neglect, physical harm, and exposure to bizarre or ritualistic behavior) can cause emotional damage and produce psychological symptoms. Abuse and neglect can not only destroy self-esteem, but also lead to identity confusion, a feeling of disorientation, tenuous interpersonal boundaries, and intense neediness. Since some adolescent cult members will experience psychological and physical neglect and/or abuse (Schwartz & Kaslow, 2001), they may have considerable difficulty extricating themselves from that situation, as they were unable to escape from earlier traumas.

Substance Abuse

Severe childhood abuse and neglect may predispose adolescents to use alcohol and other drugs, increasing the risk of susceptibility to cults (Curtis & Curtis, 1993). Individuals who would usually not be easily influenced might be made more open to the negative messages of the cult while affected by drugs and alcohol (Ahmed, 1991). The use of drugs and alcohol tends to diminish internal controls, i.e., to cause disinhibition, to impair judgment, to affect decision-making adversely, and to encourage passive conformity. As the excessive use of drugs and alcohol seems to promote poor judgment and inappropriate behavior, vulnerable individuals who are involved with cults may demonstrate a self-defeating and potentially self-destructive pattern.

Psychological Disorder

It is tempting to characterize those who become involved with cults as having been psychologically disturbed, in some manner, prior to their joining the cult. However, most (two-thirds) of them seem not to have been seriously impaired before their cult experiences, and only about 5–6% of the remaining third demonstrated serious psychopathology beforehand (Singer, 1995).

The aforementioned use of substances by adolescents is a factor that does greatly increase the risk of developing psychological problems, especially behavioral problems, which may make the radical vision of the cult more appealing (Ahmed, 1991).

A history of abuse and/or neglect may predispose an adolescent to dissociation, a psychological "tuning out," which helped them to survive their past traumas. Unfortunately, the tendency to dissociate also renders an individual susceptible to psychological manipulation and indoctrination, the *modus operandi* of many fringe groups (Curtis & Curtis, 1993).

Depression, with or without self-harming behavior or suicidal preoccupation, has been seen in adolescents who are exploring participation in deviant subcultural groups (Clark, 1992). Of those adolescents and adults who joined cults, one-third showed some psychological disturbance before joining, the vast majority (94–96%) suffering from clinical depressions due to personal losses or developmental crises (Singer, 1995).

The presence of psychosis may not be a direct precursor for cult involvement. However, in one study (Bhugra, 2002) psychosis was related to a tendency to increase involvement in religious activities, especially by non-whites. The reasons for this were hypothesized to be an attempt to maintain self-esteem and acceptance by others in those experiencing psychic disintegration. This could indirectly increase an individual's vulnerability to recruitment into a NRM.

The issue of treatments for psychological disturbances that develop as a result of involvement in a cult will be addressed in later sections.

Family Factors

Family systems theory proposes that the family is a dynamic system, and that the behavior of any individual family member can be understood only in relation to the behavior of other family members and the interactions between subsystems (Walsh, 2003). Studies suggest that vulnerability to *external* influences and their effects on child adjustment may differ in different types of families, with the lowest risk for developing adjustment problems seen in those families with high rates of acceptance and consistency in discipline (Wolchik et al., 2000).

Exposure to stressors *within* the family increases the chances that its children will develop dysfunctional behaviors (Jackson et al., 2003). Adolescent externalizing behaviors (e.g., aggression, substance abuse) are associated with conflicted relationships with parents, siblings, and peers (Kim, Hetherington & Reiss, 1999). Research data has demonstrated that externalizing behaviors are higher both in children with divorced and remarried parents than in those with nondivorced parents (Dekovic, Janssens & Van Es, 2003). Joining a cult could be interpreted as defiance, which is a common externalizing behavior.

Parental divorce can be a significant stressor for the adolescent, and can have long-lasting effects (Allison & Furstenberg, 1989). The sequelae can be especially negative if divorce leads to non-involvement with the father. The time that the father is absent from the family is directly correlated to the amount of antisocial characteristics seen in the family's children (Pfiffner, McBurnett & Rathouz, 2001). Interestingly, involvement with a stepfather did not ameliorate the behavioral problems reported in the children. Conversely, overpermissiveness tends to produce a demanding and defiant adolescent (Ahmed, 1991).

Negative and conflicted relationships among siblings are also related to adolescent externalizing responses. It has been proposed that aggressive behavior in children may be initiated by inept parenting, but sustained and exacerbated by relations with siblings and peers (Kim, Hetherington & Reiss, 1999).

Detachment from family relationships precedes cult membership (Wright & Piper, 1986). Thus, parenting that provides clear and consistent expectations, structure, and limits that promote the development of healthy self-esteem and a sense of competency (Ahmed, 1991). Stable, mutually understanding and supportive interactions of family subsystems might diminish the susceptibility to cult involvement.

Eccentric Family Patterns

The family remains the primary influence in the development of a child's personality (Ahmed, 1991). The more aberrant, bizarre, and out of the mainstream family patterns become, the more likely they are to lead to susceptibility to cults. In what seems to be a counterintuitive correlation, studies have indicated that a significant number of cult members come from homes that are in the upper socioeconomic levels, rather than those from lower socioeconomic groups. These homes also tend toward an equitable balance between rights and responsibilities, and do not tend to be overly permissive or indulgent, nor otherwise dysfunctional (Hunter, 1998).

The ethnic or cultural isolation of some families, whose customs and practices are discordant with those of the greater community, and whose exposure to the outside world remains limited, will condition its members to its own philosophical, political, and religious views. To the extent that individuals are exposed in childhood to unusual and even bizarre family patterns, this may also increase susceptibility to cults.

There may be cases in which an adolescent is from a multigenerational cult family, where other family members are involved in cult activities, and who reinforce the adolescent's continued participation in the cult (Clark, 1992). Children who have been born and raised in families affiliated with a cult are isolated, have limited knowledge about the external world, and are unable to function autonomously (Langone & Eisenberg, 1993). Compared with adult or young adult cult members who have a more or less mature personality before entering the cult, people born and raised in cult-related families do not have a mature pre-cult personality (Langone & Eisenberg, 1993). The cult environment may also foster dependency in their members, such that they may rely on other people to make their decisions for them (Hassan, 1988). These people have trouble thinking and performing independently, and are unable to distinguish between healthy and unhealthy values.

Social and Community Factors

To understand the effects of society and culture on the person's vulnerability to join a cult, it is important to review some social theories. *Social influence theories* propose that the environment has a significant effect on human beings. According to the theory of *reasoned action* (Ajzen & Fishbein, 1980), behaviors are generated via the interactions of beliefs, attitudes, and intentions. *Cognitive dissonance theory* (Festinger, 1957) proposes that any situation that conflicts with a person's worldview causes a state of uncomfortable tension, which must be relieved. It is a well-known fact that under different kinds of stress people behave differently. In some circumstances, in order to reduce tension, people can be induced to adopt certain beliefs and behaviors that are quite different from those that were characteristic of them before the stress. *Social judgment theory* (Sherif, Sherif & Nebergall, 1965) proposes that these changes occur in small to moderate steps, using ego distortions to fit persuasive information into our categories of judgment. This is why even "stable" individuals, when exposed to overwhelming stressors, can become susceptible to the lure of cults.

Cult members come from all parts of society and there is no specific identifiable "type." Some investigators make the assumption that those who enter cults do so as an escape from a bad family situation, or to find a venue of peace and spiritual healing in the middle of a stressful, violent and unpredictable society. Some authorities also report that those who enter cults are "maladjusted, troubled or even psychiatrically ill beforehand" (West, 1993, p. 11). Other researchers argue against this, saying that people may become more susceptible to join a cult during periods of life change, e.g., after a move to a new city or starting college. One study (Deutsch & Miller, 1983) characterized some of these factors after examining four female members of a cult. Among them they mentioned idealism, the wish to unify others, a spiritual world view, and a tendency to "wish away" perceived threats.

Exactly why it is that some choose to join cults, while others do not, remains unsolved. However, some believe that the disintegration of the family and society plays a significant role in this. The emergence of cults has been viewed as the result of some crises within the culture, making people disillusioned with the current system of values and beliefs. New beliefs are embraced in order to replace the previous ideologies and to provide some stability for those who feel alienated by and from their culture.

Adolescence is a phase of personality development which is a relatively fragile construct, dependent heavily on fairly consistent feedback from others, especially in terms of peer approval. Although there are strong biological factors that govern the expression of violence, hatred, compassion, and responsibility, it is also through socially learned behaviors that these are modified.

Social and cultural context has great power to shape individual identity. Adolescents will consolidate their appreciation of "right and wrong" in their early adulthood, and this process is dependent on role models that have traditionally been provided by the family and society. However, with the slow disintegration of the family and society, studies indicate that it is the "non-shared environment" involving peer groups that provide moral and social cues to the child and not the "shared environment" of family, school and church. In the absence of well-defined cultural and moral standards, adolescents can become vulnerable to risk taking behaviors. They may oscillate between different moods and relationships. They may also attempt to test limits and express defiant and rebellious behavior (Ahmed, 1991).

Conversely, parents and teachers may put excessive burdens on the adolescent, creating an atmosphere that is extremely demanding and competitive, which in turn can lead to undesirable outcomes such as substance abuse, violence, and gang or cult membership (Hunter, 1998). In one study (Ahmed, 1991) adolescents were found to have feelings of alienation and powerlessness, leading to involvement in heavy drug use and heavy metal music, which glorifies violence and encourages sexual activities.

Adolescents who feel alienated, isolated, or that they do not belong to society, and also who lack a sense of personal positive identity are especially attracted to non-mainstream organizations. Resentment and anger toward authority figures is also a contributing factor (Ahmed, 1991). Cults satisfy certain needs of an individual which he or she cannot satisfy elsewhere. The knowledge adolescents seek in cults is almost invariably something that they cannot find in their society's schools or religion. They traditionally feel frustrated with the current state of society, show dissatisfaction with their state of living, desire change, and feel frustrated when this does not occur. They have weak cultural, religious, and community ties and feel powerless in this seemingly out-of-control world (Hunter, 1998).

Many cult groups play upon the naive idealism of young people and promise to improve their lives. Clinical experience and informal surveys indicate that a very large majority of cult joiners were experiencing significant stress (frequently related to normal crises of adolescence and young adulthood, such as romantic breakup, school failure, vocational confusion) prior to their cult conversion. Because their normal ways of coping were not working well for them, these stressed individuals were more vulnerable than usual during these periods.

The increasing use of the internet poses as a potential factor for cult involvement, albeit an indirect one (Knapp, 1997). As has been noted in one parent information handout (American Academy of Child and Adolescent Psychiatry, 1997a), "hours spent online is time lost from developing real social skills." The ensuing social incompetence in turn can cause an increase in loneliness, priming the adolescent to be prey for the cult recruiters. There is recent data, however, that contradicts this fear, coming to the conclusion that "home internet use has no adverse effects on children's social or psychological outcomes," at least in the low-income children that were studied (Jackson, von Eye & Biocca, 2003).

Evidence-Based Treatment Interventions in Community Settings

What Works

A review of the literature did not reveal a program that met the standard for what works.

What Might Work

When evaluating cults it is very important to obtain a comprehensive and clear knowledge of the concepts and activities of specific groups before making a priori judgments and absolute generalizations. Fringe religious and ideological cults are not necessarily damaging. Considering cults that can be potentially harmful, there are no systematic studies available to evaluate the effectiveness of existent interventions for cultists. It appears that contemporary interventions are empirical, practical techniques that are essentially based on reasoning and experience.

As there are currently no evidence-based models in this area, the points of view expressed here rest on various information resources, such as anecdotal clinical reports presented by psychotherapists and pastoral counselors, the clinical expertise of professionals, and the personal experiences of those formerly involved with mind control groups. They are also based on the personal accounts of people who purposely allowed themselves to be recruited into cults (e.g., investigative journalists) in order to see how they operated.

Interventions can be delivered at different stages of cult involvement:

- Prior to the conversion
- While the member is committed to the cult
- Facilitating the exit of cult members from cults
- Support recovery from cultic involvement of cult members who have defected voluntarily or involuntarily.

INTERVENTIONS PRIOR TO THE CONVERSION. This can be seen as primary prevention (see the later section on this topic) when the person might be starting to become attracted to the group but is not yet committed. Parents may be the ones looking for help at this stage. If the family or clinician is convinced about the potential damage the cult can exert upon the individual, this might be the critical time to intervene. All possible resources, including friends or authority figures close to the potential convert, might need to be mobilized (Levine, 1979). For the clinician, a thorough evaluation is indicated to assess whether there is a mental disturbance that may warrant treatment or appropriate referral. The process also can help to establish the person's baseline, to learn about the family dynamics and determine how best one can help.

INTERVENTIONS WITH CURRENT CULT MEMBERS. It appears that the elitist and suspicious tendencies of cults make it difficult for its members to seek medical or mental health assistance (Langone, 1996). The role of the concerned physician could be essentially the same for current members and former cultists and will be described below. For the mental health clinician, such as counselors, psychologists and psychiatrists, assistance to the cultist may have ethical implications. Some patients might not be ready or willing to consider that their involvement in the group may in any way influence his or her emotional state. In such cases, the clinician has to decide whether to confront the issue, avoid the issue, or work within the limits dictated by the patient's level of comfort. In cases where these dilemmas cannot be resolved, the person may need to be referred to another clinician. The decision will likely depend on the patient's presentation in terms of acuity, severity, and the clinician's critical and ethical analysis of the situation at hand. In his article "Clinical updates on Cults," Langone (1996) suggests that the clinician may find it helpful to get a chronological history that will allow the patient to see whether his or her current psychological state could be a consequence of the group's practices.

INTERVENTIONS TO FACILITATE DISAFFILIATION FROM THE CULT. In the book *Cults in our Midst* (Singer, 1995), the author states that most cult members will eventually leave their cults in one of three ways: (1) on their own, when they become disappointed because the cult is not what it said it was, and when the inconsistencies can no longer be disregarded. These members are called *walkaways*. (2) Members can be expelled by the cult and are called *castaways*. The reasons vary—some members are expelled because they break down mentally or physically or they are removed for economic or other reasons. This process can infuse fear in the remaining members. (3) *Exit counseling*. This is an intervention coordinated by nonmembers of the cult, usually family or friends and a team made up of exit counselors and former members. This team gives the cult member objective information and/or support that will allow reevaluation of her or his membership and commitment to the cult.

One more way to leave a cult is through a process called *deprogramming*. As opposed to exit counseling, this is an involuntary departure from a cult.

EXIT COUNSELING. This is a contractual, voluntary process carried out by an exit counselor. The intervention is intensive and entails a time-limited sharing of concrete information about the cult with the cultist. Ideally, the informational material will be presented in a way that is unbiased and understandable to the cultist. This would facilitate an informed reevaluation about their cult involvement in order to make informed decisions regarding their relationship and commitment to a cult. The counselor approaches the case as a family matter and invites the cultist to participate in reviewing the information provided to allow him or her and family to better comprehend and cope with their problem. The educational process also involves the family, concerned spouse, and/or relatives, who are usually the ones initiating the process of exit counseling. The families are furnished with significant information pertinent to their deliberations. This includes references, such as books, articles, audio and videotapes, people, and organizations with appropriate expertise (Clark et al., 1993). Although there are no data regarding the effectiveness of these resources, it makes intuitive sense that information presented in several modalities would enhance the learning process.

DEPROGRAMMING. The term *programming* was selected to describe the rapid changes the families were noticing in their family member's personality. The acquired *pseudo* (false) *personality* was not typical of the person they knew before they joined a cult. Deprogramming is a process of involuntary disaffiliation from the cult and can be divided into two phases. The first one is the preparatory phase. It consists of physical procurement of the person forcefully or through designed plans to draw the cultist away from their cult residency. The second one is the deprogramming phase. During this phase, the cultist is subjected to unidirectional confrontation, constant input, exhortation, and physical control of the environment until a substitution of the belief system about the cult is attained (Ungerleider & Wellisch, 1979, 1989). Proponents of these techniques say that they are effective, but claims are based on anecdotes, not on controlled scientific studies.

INTERVENTIONS TO SUPPORT RECOVERY. Whether the individual has walked away, been expelled, or been helped to leave the cult, invariably there are realistic concerns. In addition to the individual's own needs, conflicts, and sense of personal failure, he or she may experience relationship difficulties with their families and friends. The person may also struggle with adjustment to the new world, insecurities about his/her future, and the need to resume previous activities, e.g. school, work, etc. It is important that the counselors ensure that the former cultists receive a full medical examination before addressing the client's emotional needs (Robinson, 1997).

MEDICAL EVALUATION. The physician needs to perform a precautionary medical exam that includes a thorough history and complete physical examination. Signs of abuse and neglect should be considered and sought out. It is important to understand that events that we easily categorize as abusive, e.g. rape, may be perceived as normal experiences by the cultist or former cultist. This is especially true for the child raised in a cult, who had little exposure to the outside world (Langone & Eisenberg, 1993).

PSYCHIATRIC/PSYCHOLOGICAL EVALUATION. As mentioned previously, some adolescents who come from unhealthy families and have underlying psychiatric problems are predisposed to embrace the cults more readily. Activities in cults may reflect underlying psychopathology; therefore, a complete psychiatric evaluation is necessary for appropriate treatment (Ahmed, 1991).

In general, since a cult connection may not be readily noticeable, the physician or therapist can play a crucial role just by being alert to, and by asking about, possible involvement in cults (Lottick, 1995). This is especially true when the experienced traumas have not left obvious physical signs, but are being expressed as anxiety, depression, and/or psychosomatic complaints (Kliger, 1994).

Adolescents influenced by cult activities also may use drugs. Therefore, they need to be evaluated and referred to a substance abuse program if needed (Ahmed, 1991).

Post-cult recovery assistance may include individual therapy, support groups, residential rehabilitation centers, and psychiatric hospitalization. There are also support resources available on-line, such as The American Family Foundation, (www.aff.org), "a nonprofit, tax-exempt research center and educational organization. . . . to assist those who have been adversely affected by a cult-related experience" (Langone, 2000).

INDIVIDUAL PSYCHOTHERAPY.   Working with individuals who are recovering from cult involvement will likely require a departure from the traditional psychodynamic approach. A psychoeducational approach plays a crucial role in helping ex-cultists to understand how cults could have influenced their belief system, emotions, and behavior (Goldberg, 1993). The counselor should assist the client to direct attention to the unmet needs that made the cult attractive (Robinson, 1997). The therapist should provide a tolerant and safe environment for expression of memories, spontaneous reactions, and autonomous behavior. This would allow former cultists to regain their sense of independence and begin making independent life decisions that will facilitate their reintegration into society.

GROUP WORK WITH FORMER CULTISTS.   This intervention can be offered during the "post–mind control" phase, when the former cultist is striving to put his or her cult experiences into perspective (Goldberg & Goldberg, 1982). Some groups meet regularly; less formal groups meet as the need emerges and attendance at groups is not enforced. Members are free to attend to as many meetings as they wish. This would ideally encourage a sense of autonomy in contrast to the repression and dependency reinforced in the cult.

Support groups can be a favorable milieu where members have the opportunity to discuss their cultic involvement. Healthy self-assertion and interpersonal relationships are always encouraged and reinforced to promote emotional growth. The groups are thought to be a safe environment that will help former cultists to transition and adjust to society. They also provide its members support in their effort to overcome the sequelae of cultic involvement. The groups can be a source of networking with people who can offer experiential advice and support to former cultists experiencing difficulties.

Former cultists with good social support may return home and seek short-term or long-term individual therapy and/or attend support groups. They may also choose residential programs. The latter choice appears to be a better alternative if the home environment seems to be dysfunctional or inconsistent (Ahmed, 1991).

What Does Not Work

A review of the literature did not disclose any resource that specifically addressed what does not work. There is, however, some debate regarding whether or not the groups that monitor cults for violent activity inadvertently contribute to that violence (Barker, 2002).

Evidence-Based Treatment Interventions in Residential Settings

What Works

A review of the literature did not reveal a program that met the standard for what works.

What Might Work

Residential rehabilitation centers are places where clients can be self-referred, or referred by pastors, ministers, friends, or former cult members. Regardless of the disaffiliation method, the ex-cultist can have multiple unresolved issues generating distress (Martin, 1993). Some of these issues include grief over loss of friends, a sense of insecurity, and dependency issues, among others. The interventions at these centers involve a thorough assessment of the patients' stage of recovery and needs, followed by a individualized rehabilitation program designed to help the members to attain emotional, social, and spiritual stability (Martin, 1993). Occasionally, a member or ex-member becomes so disturbed—psychotic, violent, etc.—that hospitalization may be warranted (Clark, 1992).

In an attempt to allow the individual to express his or her feelings and thoughts, the milieu can be permissive of peculiar clothing and makeup. However, destructive behavior should not be tolerated.

As with other patients with aggressive behavior, the use of the quiet room and seclusion might be necessary, in order to ensure a safe environment where the individual can experience strong emotions without concerns of harmful behavior toward the self or others. Youth with satanic involvement may attempt to express and exhibit satanic material. The milieu should not permit this practice based on the principle that this material can be associated with violence, abuse, and alienation (Belitz & Schacht, 1992).

In addition to therapeutic, educational, and socialization experiences, young children may need case management to ensure coordination of all services received. The parents may be able to exercise this role, but sometimes the therapist or other helper may need to function as the child advocate when parents are not available or when they are struggling with their own post-cult issues (Langone & Eisenberg, 1993).

Evidence-based treatment interventions are not widely available. Systematic and scientific research that surveys and examines ex-cultist adults, and children born into cults, is needed in order to deal more efficiently with this problem. Research is also essential to test the efficacy of current interventions and ways that we could improve them (Robinson, 1997).

What Does Not Work

A review of the literature did not disclose any resource that specifically addressed what does not work.

Psychopharmacology

As stated previously, there is no one "type" of person who may become involved with a cult. Likewise, there are no distinct psychiatric conditions that place an individual at higher risk for joining a cult. Thus, there are also no specific medications that are indicated in the treatment of cult survivors. There are, however, some conditions that can develop as a result of being in a cult, and it is the pharmacological treatment of these particular disorders that will be addressed here.

Depression is quite common in this population, "particularly those from religious groups" (Goldberg, 1993), as opposed to survivors of other types of cults. The decision to use antidepressant medication will be determined by several factors. If the depression is mild to moderate in severity, using psychotherapy as the first treatment seems reasonable (American Academy of Child and Adolescent Psychiatry,

1998a). Medications would be considered in more severe cases of depression, especially if they are associated with suicidality, bipolar disorder, and/or psychosis, or if they interfere with participation in, or response to, psychotherapy. Antidepressant agents from the class known as selective serotonin reuptake inhibitors (SSRIs) are the medications of choice, mostly based on tolerability and safety.

Another common psychological reaction to cult involvement is post-traumatic stress disorder (PTSD) (Singer & Ofshe, 1990). There seems to be clinical consensus that treatment interventions should include exploration of the traumatic events, stress management, correction of cognitive distortions, and parental involvement (American Academy of Child and Adolescent Psychiatry, 1998b). Regarding the use of psychotropic medications for PTSD in younger people, there are no good empirical studies to guide the use of any particular agents. As with depression, psychotherapy is the recommended first step in the treatment of PTSD. Should there be prominent symptoms (e.g., profound sleep disturbances or autonomic hyperarousal) that are not amenable to psychotherapy, it would be up to the psychiatrist to make an informed, clinical judgment as to which medications to use, and to monitor carefully for adverse effects.

The use of mind-altering substances can be a precursor to cult involvement, a direct effect of cult involvement, or a risk factor for continued stay in a cult and/or the unsuccessful exit from a cult (Martin, 1993). Although there are no specific psychopharmacologic interventions for drug and alcohol addictions, it is important for the clinician to identify common co-morbid conditions, e.g., depression, which might benefit from treatment with medications (American Academy of Child and Adolescent Psychiatry, 1997b).

The Prevention of Cults

What Works

A review of the literature did not reveal a program that met the standard for what works.

What Might Work

Cults are difficult to study in an objective manner. As a result, it is even more difficult to develop preventive strategies to counter their development. Operating within ethical boundaries prevents us from studying them within the framework of clinical trials. The literature, thus far, consists of observational studies with an emphasis on identification and characterization of cults and fringe groups. Within this literature, there remain unanswered questions concerning prevalence. There are also questions as to whether conversion to a cult is a symptom of the declining family, or is the cause (Wright & Piper, 1986). Society's awareness of the presence of cults is primarily through the recognition of fringe behaviors, or as a result of forensic involvement by cult members. Because of this, and because of the ambiguity of what constitutes a cult, it is exceedingly difficult to make an accurate assessment of the prevalence of cult involvement, and it therefore complicates our ability to assess the effectiveness of preventive strategies.

Table 1. Cult Susceptibility Risk Factors

Risk Factors	Biological	Psychological	Social
Generalized ego weakness and emotional vulnerability	×	×	
Propensity towards dissociative states	×	×	
Tenuous, deteriorated, or nonexistent family relations and support systems		×	×
Inadequate means of dealing with exigencies of survival		×	×
History of severe child abuse or neglect	×	×	×
Exposure to idiosyncratic or eccentric family patterns		×	×
Proclivity toward abuse of controlled substances	×	×	×
Unmanageable and debilitating situational stress and crisis		×	×
Intolerable socioeconomic conditions		×	×

For the purpose of proposing preventive strategies, we have found the most useful observational studies to be those which established risk factors increasing the vulnerability of adolescents to indoctrination. As listed in Table 1 (Curtis & Curtis, 1993), there are nine risk factors which make adolescents more susceptible to joining cults.

If one is to use these risk factors as a model to establish strategic preventive interventions, then it must be acknowledged that the inability to study these phenomena realistically forces the development of intervention strategies based on speculation. We are aware that our suggestions are not based on an exact science, but rather a "logical" attempt to develop strategies that would counteract the specific risk factors. As described above, these risk factors do not neatly fit into a specific category. They are multifaceted issues that operate at various levels, within individuals, families, and communities. Even with the development and possible implementation of preventive strategies, there are limitations in terms of one's ability to assess the effectiveness of the interventions, i.e., if after these preventive strategies are implemented and assumed to have been effective, there is still no objective way to measure outcomes.

On the surface, these risks seemingly identify several relatively unconnected factors. However, closer examination would suggest that these factors can be grouped under specific, identifiable categories (refer to Table 1). Tracing each back to an etiology allows us to classify each as deriving from a biological, psychological, and/or social (biopsychosocial) origin. Within the specific risk factor categories, several share a combined origin. When analyzing these risk factors within the framework of the biopsychosocial model, one can note striking similarities to- and parallels with those of the multi-faceted, multilevel risk factors that span the lives of all individuals, families, and communities. Our proposal is that each risk factor—either direct or indirect—must be investigated thoroughly. More specific implications for the individual would be to apply the model and estimate the relative influence of each component of the model on that person's risk for cult involvement.

The individual factors, within each domain, contribute to the overall functional level of the individual and can, to a certain extent, determine the character, intensity, and duration of negative feelings and suffering. Viewing these issues within this framework can help us to understand how cults fit within this model of distress. This understanding can then be used to develop more effective preventative strategies.

Within the biopsychosocial framework, cults can be seen as providing needed support and services for its members. In terms of the social aspect, cults provide structure with rituals and guidelines for those who lack them at home. They also provide support through shelter and positive reinforcement for those participating.

Within the biological domain, cults provide acceptance and sometimes encouragement of certain biologically influenced behaviors, e.g., substance abuse. Several studies which have focused on the relationship between cults and psychopathology have yielded mixed results. One study (Ungerleider & Wellisch, 1979) did not find an association between cult membership and psychopathology. However, other studies (e.g., Kiev & Francis, 1964) have shown an association. Cults can provide acceptance of certain psychopathological conditions, particularly certain mood, thought, and personality disorders. For example, antisocial behavior or paranoid beliefs may not only be accepted, but encouraged.

As stated previously, developing interventions for prevention within the model is difficult. It would be financially impossible to address each risk factor individually; therefore, implementing strategies which would address each biological, psychological, and social domain would be more efficient. The overall strategy would be to provide a safety net for at risk individuals, families, and communities. Access to the necessary structure and support would ideally be available to individuals before their situation has deteriorated to the point where cults are looked upon as the only viable source of providing those services. Community organizations could be established to provide support for individuals and families in areas where families are no longer able to do so. Support in terms of addressing family violence, psychiatric disorders, and early diagnosis and treatment of medical illnesses and substance abuse would also reduce the risks for cult involvement.

What Does Not Work

A review of the literature did not disclose any resource that specifically addressed what does not work.

Recommendations

As can be seen from the information presented in this chapter, the factors that contribute to an individual's being attracted to, joining, staying with, and/or leaving a cult are diverse and complex in their interplay.

From a prevention point of view, resources in the greater social environment would ideally include programs and facilities to offer support—emotional, social, legal, financial, etc.—to adolescents and their families who are at risk, e.g., those experiencing a divorce. In the case of an absent parent, organizations such as Big Brothers Big Sisters of America (http://www.bbbsa.org) might offer the mentoring and role modeling needed to guide the adolescent toward healthy academic and occupational goals. Another essential component of prevention would be early recognition and treatment of high-risk behaviors, such as substance abuse, which if left untreated could contribute to adolescent involvement in a cult. Early intervention for depression also would likely reduce vulnerability to cult recruitment.

Treatment for those who are suffering the emotional sequelae of cult involvement begins with a comprehensive assessment of the individual and his/her immediate environment. Interventions should be multimodal and multispecialty, attending to whatever medical, psychological, and spiritual needs are identified. The treating clinician should keep an open mind regarding the use of any and all relevant resources in the community. Only with a coordination of care and services will the affected adolescents—and their families—have the best chance of making a full recovery.

References

Ahmed, M.B. (1991). High-risk adolescents and satanic cults. *Texas Medicine, 87,* 74–76.

Ajzen, I. & Fishbein, M. (1980). *Understanding Attitudes and Predicting Social Behavior.* Englewood Cliffs, NJ: Prentice-Hall, Inc.

Allison, PD. and FF. Furstenberg, Jr. (1989). How marital dissolution affects children: Variations by age and sex. *Developmental Psychology, 25,* 540–549.

American Academy of Child and Adolescent Psychiatry. (1997a). Children online. *Facts for Families* 59. Washington, D.C.

American Academy of Child and Adolescent Psychiatry. (1997b). Practice parameters for the assessment and treatment of children and adolescents with substance use disorders. *Journal of the American Academy of Child and Adolescent Psychiatry, 36,* 140S–156S.

American Academy of Child and Adolescent Psychiatry. (1998a). Practice parameters for the assessment and treatment of children and adolescents with depressive disorders. *Journal of the American Academy of Child and Adolescent Psychiatry, 37,* 63S–83S.

American Academy of Child and Adolescent Psychiatry. (1998b). Practice parameters for the assessment and treatment of children and adolescents with posttraumatic stress disorder. *Journal of the American Academy of Child and Adolescent Psychiatry, 37,* 4S–26S.

Barker, E. (2002). Watching for violence: A comparative analysis of the roles of five types of cult-watching groups. In D.G. Bromley, & J.G. Melton, (Eds.), *Cults, Religion & Violence.* NY: Cambridge University Press.

Belitz, G., & Schacht, A. (1992). Satanism as a response to abuse: The dynamics and treatment of satanic involvement in male youths. *Adolescence, 27,* 855–872.

Bhugra, D. (2002). Self-concept: psychosis and attraction of new religious movements. *Mental Health, Religion & Culture, 5,* 239–252.

Clark, C.M. (1992). Deviant adolescent subcultures: Assessment strategies and clinical interventions. *Adolescence, 27,* 283–293.

Clark, D., Giambalvo, C., Giambalvo, N., Garvey, K., & Langone, M.D. (1993). Exit counseling: A practical overview. In M.D. Langone (Ed.), *Recovery from Cults: Help for Victims of Psychological and Spiritual Abuse.* New York: W.W. Norton.

Curtis, J.M., & Curtis, M.J. (1993). Factors related to susceptibility and recruitment by cults. *Psychological Reports, 73,* 451–460.

Dekovic, M., Janssens, J.M.A.M., & Van Es, N.M.C. (2003). Family predictors of antisocial behavior in adolescence. *Family Process, 42,* 223–235.

Deutsch, A., & Miller, M.J. (1983). A clinical study of four Unification Church members. *American Journal of Psychiatry, 140,* 767–770.

Feldmann, T.B., & Johnson, P.W. (1995). Cult membership as a source of self-cohesion: Forensic implications. *Bulletin of the American Academy of Psychiatry and Law, 23,* 239–248.

Festinger, L. (1957). *A Theory of Cognitive Dissonance.* Stanford, CA: Stanford University Press.

Goldberg, L. (1993). Guidelines for therapists. In M.D. Langone (Ed.), *Recovery from Cults: Help for Victims of Psychological and Spiritual Abuse.* New York: W.W. Norton.

Goldberg, L., & Goldberg, W. (1982). Group work with former cultists. *Social Work, 27,* 165–170.

Goodnough, D. (2000). *Cult Awareness.* Berkeley Heights, NJ: Enslow Publishers, Inc.

Hassan, S. (1988). *Combating Cult Mind Control.* Rochester, VT: Park Street Press.

Hunter, E. (1998). Adolescent attraction to cults. *Adolescence, 33,* 709–714.

Jackson, L.A., von Eye, A., & Biocca, F. (2003). Children and internet use: Social, psychological, and academic consequences for low-income children. Retrieved January 10, 2004, from http://www.apa.org/science/psa/sbjacksonprt.html

Jackson, Y., Sifers, S.K., Warren, J.S., & Velasquez, D. (2003). Family protective factors and behavioral outcome: the role of appraisal in family life events. *Journal of Emotional and Behavioral Disorders, 11,* 103–111.

Kiev, A., & Francis, J.L. (1964). Subud and mental illness: psychiatric illness in a religious sect. *American Journal of Psychotherapy, 18,* 66–78.

Kim, J.E., Hetherington, E.M., & Reiss, D. (1999). Associations among family relationships, antisocial peers, and adolescents' externalizing behaviors: Gender and family type differences. *Child Development, 70,* 1209–1230.

Kliger, R. (1994). Somatization: Social control and illness production in a religious cult. *Culture, Medicine, and Psychiatry, 18,* 215–245.

Knapp, D. (1997). The internet as a God and propaganda tool for cults. Retrieved October 31, 2003, from http//: www.cnn.com/TECH/9703/27/techno.pagans/

Langone, M.D. (1996). Clinical update on cults. *Psychiatric Times.*

Langone, M.D. (2000). What should be done about the cults? *Paradigm,* Spring, 16–18. Retrieved December 26, 2003, from http//:www.onlineparadigm.com/archives/120_SP00_AD.GI.pdf

Langone, M.D., & Eisenberg, G. (1993) Children and cults. In M.D. Langone (Ed.), *Recovery from Cults: Help for Victims of Psychological and Spiritual Abuse.* New York: W.W. Norton.

Levine, S.V. (1978). Youth and religious cults: a societal and clinical dilemma. *Adolescent Psychiatry, 6,* 75–89.

Levine, S.V. (1979). Role of psychiatry in the phenomenon of cults. *Canadian Journal of Psychiatry, 24,* 593–603.

Lottick, E.A. (1995). Cult-proofing your patients: A guide to diagnosis, treatment, and referral of cult victims and survivors. *Pennsylvania Medicine,* 22–23.

Martin, P.R. (1993). Post-cult recovery: Assessment and rehabilitation. In M.D. Langone (Ed.), *Recovery from Cults: Help for Victims of Psychological and Spiritual Abuse.* New York: W.W. Norton.

Pfiffner, L.J., McBurnett, K., & Rathouz, P.J. (2001). Father absence and familial antisocial characteristics. *Journal of Abnormal Child Psychology, 29,* 357–367.

Porterfield, K.M. (1995). *Straight Talk About Cults.* New York: Facts on File, Inc.

Richardson, J.T., & Introvigne, M. (2001). "Brainwashing" theories in European parliamentary and administrative reports on "cults" and "sects." *Journal for the Scientific Study of Religion, 40,* 143–168.

Robbins, T. (2000). "Quo vadis" the scientific study of new religious movements? *Journal for the Scientific Study of Religion, 39,* 515–523.

Robinson, B. (1997). Cult affiliation and disaffiliation: Implications for counseling. *Counseling and Values, 41,* 166–173.

Schwartz, L.L., & Kaslow, F.W. (2001). The cult phenomenon: A turn of the century update. *The American Journal of Family Therapy, 29,* 13–22.

Sherif, C., Sherif, M., & Nebergall, R. (1965). *Attitude and Attitude Change: the social judgment-involvement approach.* Philadelphia: Saunders.

Singer, M.T., (1995). *Cults in our Midst.* San Francisco: Jossey-Bass Publishers.

Singer, M.T., & Ofshe, R. (1990). Thought reform programs and the production of psychiatric casualties. *Psychiatric Annals, 20,* 188–193.

Small, A. (1998). Our doomsday messiahs: Too much freedom for destructive cults. *Fresh Review, 12,* 1–12. Retrieved August 20, 2003, from http://maven.english.hawaii.edu/comp/small.pdf

Stark, R., & Bainbridge, W.S. (1987). *A Theory of Religion.* New York: Peter Lang.

Szubin, A., Jensen, C.J., & Gregg, R. (2000). Interacting with "cults": A policing model. *The FBI Law Enforcement Bulletin, 69,* 16–24.

The Nationalist. (2003). How to spot a cult at college. Retrieved January 3, 2004, from http://archives.tcm.ie/carlownationalist/2003/10/08/story18820.asp

Ungerleider, J.T., & Wellisch, D.K. (1979). Coercive persuasion (brainwashing), religious cults, and deprogramming. *American Journal of Psychiatry, 136,* 279–82.

Ungerleider, J.T., & Wellisch, D.K. (1989). Deprogramming (involuntary departure), coercion, and Cults. In M. Galanter (Ed.), *Cults and New Religious Movements,* Washington, D.C.: American Psychiatric Association.

U.S. Commission on Civil Rights (2002). Beyond percentage plans: The challenge of equal opportunity in higher education. Chapter 4: National trends in college enrollment. Retrieved January 3, 2004, from http://www.usccr.gov/pubs/percent2/ch4.htm

Walsh, F. (2003). Family resilience: a framework for clinical practice. *Family Process, 42,* 1–18.

West, L.J. (1993). A psychiatric overview of cult-related phenomena. *Journal of the American Academy of Psychoanalysis, 21,* 1–19.

Wieder, R. (1998). Cults. *Gale Encyclopedia of Childhood and Adolescence.* Retrieved December 31, 2003, from http://www.findarticles.com/cf_0/g2602/0001/2602000171/print.jhtml

Wolchik, S.A., Wilcox, K.L., Tein, J.Y., & Sandler, I.N. (2000). Maternal acceptance and consistency of discipline as buffers of divorce stressors on children's psychological adjustment problems. *Journal of Abnormal Child Psychology, 28,* 87–102.

Wright S.A. & Piper, E.S. (1986). Families and cults: Familial factors related to youth leaving or remaining in deviant religious groups. *Journal of Marriage and The Family, 48,* 15–25.

Zimbardo, P. (1997). What messages are behind today's cults? *APA Monitor, 5,* 14.

Epilogue

Thomas P. Gullotta and Gerald R. Adams

Every book has a voice. This handbook, written by scholars across the world, has several. In this last reflection, Gerald and I share with you the messages we heard as we read and reread this volume, and we offer our thoughts for the direction the behavioral health field should take over the next 20 years.

The first message that emerges is that this evidence-based handbook would not have been possible a decade ago. In one sense this volume stands as a tribute to the exhaustive work that has been undertaken in the last ten years. In another sense it documents the enormous gaps that exist in our knowledge of what works and what doesn't.

The reader cannot escape the realization that our knowledge is greatest where government and foundations have invested research dollars. Thus, we discover more evidenced-based practices in areas such as drug abuse and conduct disorder than in eating disorders or pervasive developmental delays. Next, successful treatment interventions are overwhelmingly behavioral in approach. This is not because humanistic or transpersonal approaches have been demonstrated to be ineffective but rather they have not been tested for effectiveness. There is a paucity of outcome research related to residential treatment. Further, little attention has been given to bridging the experience of young people from the residential to the community setting. Next, it is evident that the advent of new classes of medications have revolutionized the delivery of treatment services. Amazingly, trials are underway using psychotropic medications to prevent the onset of schizophrenia. It is truly a remarkable time. This said, most clinical drug trials are with adult populations, and our knowledge of their effectiveness with youth is sorely lacking. One needs only look at the controversy swirling around the use of antidepressants to see that lack of knowledge.

Given these messages, where should the field be heading over the next 20 years? First, foundations and governmental support should be extended to the development and testing of treatment and prevention approaches for more than the acting-out behaviors. Further, this volume was sorely lacking in discussing co-occurring disorders. The reality is the field lacks the theoretical framework to bridge the substance abuse world with depression, schizophrenia, conduct disorder, and scores of other dysfunctional behaviors. Thus, examples of integrated programming (not co-existing but integrated programming) are not to be found in the published literature. This fault must be corrected if progress is to occur.

Next, the vast majority of therapeutic interventions remain untested and possibly non-therapeutic. Yet, given the infancy of identifying effective practices, it is ill-advised to dismiss other therapeutic techniques just yet. Rather, we need to determine what interventions work, in what situations, and with whom. Further, there is little, if any, evidence to suggest that a pill a day will keep the disorder away. Rather, human contact found in the therapeutic relationship is a necessary ingredient to increasing the likelihood of improved health.

Anecdotal reports suggest that a quality residential setting can work but that the skills learned in those settings are soon forgotten when the youth returns to an unaltered living situation. We see value in the residential experience for some youth. Indeed, for a small subset of youth, the quality residential experience holds the greatest promise for a successful later life. This said, it remains to be demonstrated how the quality residential experience can be transferred to the community setting.

Who would have ever thought that a strep infection could cause a specific form of OCD known as PANDAS? We know that the syphilis bacteria causes dementia, that lead poisoning lowers intelligence, and that the AIDS retrovirus causes dementia. We do not know the effect that mercury from coal-burning generating plants or in childhood vaccines have on vulnerable children. We do know that pregnant women, nursing mothers, and infants are urged not to consume tuna fish because of exposure to mercury. We do not understand the adverse impact some antidepressants have on some youth by increasing their suicidal ideation. Clearly, we need to be much more aggressive in examining and policing the toxic elements in our environment and in understanding the effects of prescribed medication on the health of young people.

This handbook is a cautionary warning to those who would believe that a pill can solve the problems in living that individuals experience. We are a long way from that point (if, indeed, we ever reach it) and attention must be given to developing prevention and intervention practices that work. As our knowledge grows of the factors that contribute to health, the opportunity to develop universal interventions to encourage that health should be seized. As our knowledge of those at specific risk for disorders grows, we should (respecting ethical issues) make available interventions that ideally will prevent the onset of that disorder or lessen the impact of that disorder to permit that individual to maximize their life potential.

This brings us to two final observations—fidelity and dosage. Fidelity refers to the truthfulness with which an intervention is applied. In short, did you faithfully follow the directions? Dosage refers to the amount of the intervention received. In short, did you take all your prescribed medicine? There are scores of programs that work effectively in tightly controlled laboratory settings only to fail in community settings. A primary challenge to the field over the next 20 years will be designing prevention and intervention programs that are resilient to field tinkering and which are powerful enough to be applied with varying degrees of dosage.

Clearly, there are multiple challenges to advancing the effectiveness of our clinical and prevention practice. Still, this handbook documents the progress made to date and offers hope that over the next 20 years dramatic advances may be realized.

Index